BSAVA Manual of Rabbit Medicine

Editors:

Anna Meredith
MA VetMB PhD CertLAS DZooMed MRCVS
Exotic Animal and Wildlife Service,
Royal (Dick) School of Veterinary Studies
University of Edinburgh, Hospital for Small Animals,
Easter Bush Veterinary Centre
Roslin, Midlothian EH25 9RG

and

Brigitte Lord
BVetMed(Hons) CertZooMed MRCVS
Exotic Animal and Wildlife Service,
Royal (Dick) School of Veterinary Studies
University of Edinburgh, Hospital for Small Animals,
Easter Bush Veterinary Centre
Roslin, Midlothian EH25 9RG

Published by:

British Small Animal Veterinary Association
Woodrow House, 1 Telford Way,
Waterwells Business Park, Quedgeley,
Gloucester GL2 2AB

A Company Limited by Guarantee in England
Registered Company No. 2837793
Registered as a Charity

First published 2014
Reprinted 2016, 2018, 2019, 2021, 2023, 2024
Copyright © 2024 BSAVA

Illustrations on pages 6, 8, 10, 36 and 94 were drawn by S.J. Elmhurst BA Hons (www.livingart.org.uk) and are printed with her permission.

A catalogue record for this book is available from the British Library.

ISBN 978-1-905319-49-7

The publishers, editors and contributors cannot take responsibility for information provided on dosages and methods of application of drugs mentioned or referred to in this publication. Details of this kind must be verified in each case by individual users from up to date literature published by the manufacturers or suppliers of those drugs. Veterinary surgeons are reminded that in each case they must follow all appropriate national legislation and regulations (for example, in the United Kingdom, the prescribing cascade) from time to time in force.

Printed in the UK by Halstan & Co Ltd., Amersham HP6 6HJ
Printed on ECF paper made from sustainable forests

19598PUBS24

Other titles in the BSAVA Manuals series:

Manual of Avian Practice: A Foundation Manual
Manual of Backyard Poultry Medicine and Surgery
Manual of Canine & Feline Abdominal Imaging
Manual of Canine & Feline Abdominal Surgery
Manual of Canine & Feline Advanced Veterinary Nursing
Manual of Canine & Feline Anaesthesia and Analgesia
Manual of Canine & Feline Behavioural Medicine
Manual of Canine & Feline Cardiorespiratory Medicine
Manual of Canine & Feline Clinical Pathology
Manual of Canine & Feline Dentistry and Oral Surgery
Manual of Canine & Feline Dermatology
Manual of Canine & Feline Emergency and Critical Care
Manual of Canine & Feline Endocrinology
Manual of Canine & Feline Endoscopy and Endosurgery
Manual of Canine & Feline Fracture Repair and Management
Manual of Canine & Feline Gastroenterology
Manual of Canine & Feline Haematology and Transfusion Medicine
Manual of Canine & Feline Head, Neck and Thoracic Surgery
Manual of Canine & Feline Musculoskeletal Disorders
Manual of Canine & Feline Musculoskeletal Imaging
Manual of Canine & Feline Nephrology and Urology
Manual of Canine & Feline Neurology
Manual of Canine & Feline Oncology
Manual of Canine & Feline Ophthalmology
Manual of Canine & Feline Radiography and Radiology:
*   A Foundation Manual*
Manual of Canine & Feline Rehabilitation, Supportive and Palliative
*   Care: Case Studies in Patient Management*
Manual of Canine & Feline Reproduction and Neonatology
Manual of Canine & Feline Shelter Medicine: Principles of Health
*   and Welfare in a Multi-animal Environment*
Manual of Canine & Feline Surgical Principles: A Foundation Manual
Manual of Canine & Feline Thoracic Imaging
Manual of Canine & Feline Ultrasonography
Manual of Canine & Feline Wound Management and Reconstruction
Manual of Canine Practice: A Foundation Manual
Manual of Exotic Pet and Wildlife Nursing
Manual of Exotic Pets: A Foundation Manual
Manual of Feline Practice: A Foundation Manual
Manual of Practical Animal Care
Manual of Practical Veterinary Nursing
Manual of Practical Veterinary Welfare
Manual of Psittacine Birds
Manual of Rabbit Medicine
Manual of Rabbit Surgery, Dentistry and Imaging
Manual of Raptors, Pigeons and Passerine Birds
Manual of Reptiles
Manual of Rodents and Ferrets
Manual of Small Animal Practice Management and Development
Manual of Wildlife Casualties

RELATED TITLES

BSAVA Manual of Rabbit Surgery, Dentistry and Imaging

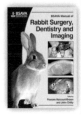

Edited by Frances Harcourt-Brown and John Chitty

- Anaesthesia and analgesia
- Radiography, ultrasonography, CT, MRI
- Surgical conditions and treatment
- Dental examination, problems and procedures
- Step-by-step Operative Techniques

BSAVA Manual of Exotic Pet and Wildlife Nursing

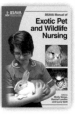

Edited by Molly Varga, Rachel Lumbis and Lucy Gott

- Husbandry and biology
- Ward design and management
- Inpatient care
- Nursing clinics
- Useful forms and questionnaires
- Client handouts

For further information on these and all BSAVA publications, please visit our website: **www.bsava.com**

Contents

Contributors

Wendy Bament BSc MSc RVN
Exotic Animal and Wildlife Service,
Royal (Dick) School of Veterinary Studies,
University of Edinburgh, Hospital for Small Animals,
Easter Bush Veterinary Centre, Roslin,
Midlothian EH25 9RG

John Chitty BVetMed CertZooMed MRCVS
Anton Vets, Unit 11, Anton Mill Road,
Andover, Hampshire SP10 2NJ

Kevin Eatwell BVSc(Hons) DZooMed(Reptilian)
DipECZM(Herp) DipECZM(Small Mammal) MRCVS
Exotic Animal and Wildlife Service,
Royal (Dick) School of Veterinary Studies,
University of Edinburgh, Hospital for Small Animals,
Easter Bush Veterinary Centre, Roslin,
Midlothian EH25 9RG

Sarah Elliott
Small Animal Practice, Langford Veterinary Services
and School of Veterinary Science, University of
Bristol, Langford, Bristol, BS40 5DU

Sally Everitt BVSc MSc(VetGP) PhD
Head of Scientific Policy, BSAVA

Kellie A. Fecteau MS PhD
Department of Biomedical and Diagnostic Sciences,
College of Veterinary Medicine,
University of Tennessee, 2407 River Drive,
Knoxville, TN 37996, USA

Gidona Goodman DVM MSc MRCVS
Exotic Animal and Wildlife Service,
Royal (Dick) School of Veterinary Studies,
University of Edinburgh, Hospital for Small Animals,
Easter Bush Veterinary Centre, Roslin,
Midlothian EH25 9RG

Frances Harcourt-Brown BVSc DipECZM
(Small Mammal) FRCVS RCVS
*Recognized Specialist in Rabbit Medicine
and Surgery*
30 Crab Lane, Harrogate,
North Yorkshire HG1 3BE

Joanna Hedley BVM&S DZooMed(Reptilian)
MRCVS
Exotic Animal and Wildlife Service,
Royal (Dick) School of Veterinary Studies,
University of Edinburgh, Hospital for Small Animals,
Easter Bush Veterinary Centre, Roslin,
Midlothian EH25 9RG

Emma Keeble BVSc DipZooMed(Mammalian)
MRCVS
*RCVS Recognized Specialist in Zoo and Wildlife
Medicine*
Exotic Animal and Wildlife Service,
Royal (Dick) School of Veterinary Studies,
University of Edinburgh, Hospital for Small Animals,
Easter Bush Veterinary Centre, Roslin,
Midlothian EH25 9RG

Tim Knott BVSc BSc CertVOphthal MRCVS
Bradley House, Rowe Veterinary Hospital,
Ferndene, Bristol BS30 9DT

Angela M. Lennox DVM DipABVP-Avian DipABVP-
Exotic Companion Mammal
Avian and Exotic Animal Clinic of Indianapolis,
9330 Waldemar Road, Indianapolis, IN 4626, USA

Brigitte Lord BVetMed(Hons) CertZooMed MRCVS
Exotic Animal and Wildlife Service,
Royal (Dick) School of Veterinary Studies,
University of Edinburgh, Hospital for Small Animals,
Easter Bush Veterinary Centre, Roslin,
Midlothian EH25 9RG

Elisabetta Mancinelli DVM CertZooMed MRCVS
Edinburgh

E. Anne McBride BSc PhD FRSA
Applied Animal Behaviour Unit,
School of Psychology,
University of Southampton,
Southampton SO17 1BJ

Anna Meredith MA VetMB PhD CertLAS DZooMed
MRCVS
Exotic Animal and Wildlife Service,
Royal (Dick) School of Veterinary Studies,
University of Edinburgh, Hospital for Small Animals,
Easter Bush Veterinary Centre, Roslin,
Midlothian EH25 9RG

Connie Orcutt DVM DipABVP
Medical Writer/Editor, 70 Centre Street,
Brookline, MA 02446, USA

Jenny Prebble BVSc MRCVS
South Yorkshire

Jenna Richardson BVM&S MRCVS
Exotic Animal and Wildlife Service,
Royal (Dick) School of Veterinary Studies,
University of Edinburgh, Hospital for Small Animals,
Easter Bush Veterinary Centre, Roslin,
Midlothian EH25 9RG

**Richard Saunders BSc BVSc MRCVS CBiol MSB
DZooMed(Mammalian)**
Veterinary Department, Bristol Zoo Gardens,
Clifton, Bristol BS8 3HA

Molly Varga BVetMed DZooMed MRCVS
*RCVS Recognized Specialist in Zoo and Wildlife
Medicine*
Cheshire Pet Medical Centre,
Holmes Chapel, Cheshire CW4 8AB

Petra Wesche DVM MSc (WAH)
Center for Veterinary Medicine,
Mississippi State University,
Starkville, MS 39759, USA

Foreword

It is only a few years since the diseases affecting pet rabbits were accorded only a small section in the Exotic Pets Manual when they were regarded as a minor species. In addition, student tuition about these animals was almost totally neglected at the majority of veterinary schools.

The increasing popularity of rabbits as household pets has seen them elevated to the position of a mainstream patient. This has increased the demands made upon practising veterinary surgeons to provide rabbits with the first class care that previously was only expected by the owners of dogs and cats.

Nobody could have predicted the enormous increase in knowledge, nor the demand for that information to be disseminated, that has taken place since the original *BSAVA Manual of Rabbit Medicine and Surgery* was published in 2002. The knowledge base is now so great that two BSAVA Manuals are necessary in order that all aspects of rabbit medicine and surgery might be covered – namely, the *BSAVA Manual of Rabbit Surgery, Dentistry and Imaging* and the *BSAVA Manual of Rabbit Medicine*.

The Editors, who are themselves recognized as pre-eminent clinicians and authorities on veterinary aspects of rabbits, have assembled up-to-date contributions from a truly international collection of distinguished authors. I am sure that the *BSAVA Manual of Rabbit Medicine* will come to be regarded not only as a well loved manual but also as an indispensable text on rabbit diseases and therapeutics.

The original intention of the BSAVA has not been lost, however, in that this book is definitely a Manual that the busy practitioner or student can refer to for succinct and readily available information and advice when needed. The addition of flow charts for the 'top 10' common conditions will be greatly appreciated and will often be referred to by both experienced clinicians and recent graduates alike. In addition, there are new chapters on subjects that have never been covered in previous BSAVA publications.

The Editors and the BSAVA Publications Committee are to be congratulated for all their expertise and commitment which has resulted in the production of this superb Manual. It is an absolute honour and privilege to be asked to write the foreword for this edition of the *BSAVA Manual of Rabbit Medicine*.

Alistair M Lawrie BVMS MRCVS

Preface

Rabbits make up a considerable and growing proportion of the caseload in small animal practice, and both interest and knowledge in rabbit medicine and surgery has grown rapidly in the last six years. In recognition of this increasing interest and available literature and expertise, the second edition of the *BSAVA Manual of Rabbit Medicine and Surgery*, published in 2006, has now been superseded by two separate volumes – the *BSAVA Manual of Rabbit Surgery, Dentistry and Imaging* and the *BSAVA Manual of Rabbit Medicine*.

The *Manual of Rabbit Medicine*, which is complementary to the new surgical manual, greatly expands and builds on the medical information given in the previous combined edition. The authors have provided a greater depth and breadth of coverage for practitioners seeking definitive and authoritative information to improve and refine the quality of veterinary care that they can provide for rabbits. We are confident that the two manuals now provide the most comprehensive and up-to-date coverage of all aspects of rabbit veterinary care currently available, in an easy-to-use, well illustrated format following the tried and tested BSAVA Manual template that is so popular.

Rabbit medicine has advanced dramatically in the last few years as we gain an increased understanding of the pathology of common diseases and a greater awareness of new conditions affecting this species and of the rabbit's response to both disease and treatment regimes. In particular, we now have a much better understanding of the differences in conditions seen in pet rabbits compared to research or commercial rabbits, on which a lot of the original literature was based. Pet rabbits are fed differently, have highly variable living conditions in a home environment, and are living far longer than ever before. There are seven new chapters, and many of the other chapters and sections have been updated and expanded. The introduction of new authors has brought fresh insights and opinions to several topics.

Rabbit medicine is still a challenging and exciting field to work in. We are optimistic that we can and should provide higher levels of care and best practice to approach those offered to our cat and dog patients, and that we can meet the expectations of rabbit owners for their much-valued pets.

This new rabbit medicine manual has two editors, so two families to thank for tolerating the seemingly endless task of proofreading and editing. These tasks were made easier by our enthusiastic and highly professional chapter authors, and we have greatly enjoyed working with them throughout the whole process of creating the Manual. Finally, we would like to thank the excellent editorial, illustration and production team at BSAVA for all their help and support.

Anna Meredith and Brigitte Lord
November 2013

Biology, anatomy and physiology

Anna Meredith

Biology

The domestic rabbit *Oryctolagus cuniculus* originated from the European wild rabbit. There are many other species of rabbit, belonging to 10 genera including *Oryctolagus*, and these, along with hares (genus *Lepus*) make up the family Leporidae, of the Order Lagomorpha, which also contains the pikas (family Ochotonidae). Rabbits are social, burrowing herbivores that are natural prey for a large number of carnivores. As a prey species they have evolved to be constantly vigilant, lightweight and fast-moving, with a highly efficient digestive system that enables them to spend the minimum time possible above ground, in danger of capture from aerial or terrestrial predators. However, even underground, a rabbit is still in danger of predation from mustelid carnivores such as weasels and stoats, and foxes will also dig up young rabbits from their nursery burrows. For the same reason, in order to avoid attracting predator attention, rabbit behaviour is not florid and overt and relies heavily on scent (see Chapter 5).

Over the centuries, humans have made use of the rabbit for food, sport and clothing, as a scientific model and as a hobby (the rabbit 'fancy'). The relationship between people and the European rabbit was first recorded by the Phoenicians over 3000 years ago. They termed the Iberian Peninsula '*i-she-phan-im*' (literally, 'the land of the rabbit'); the Romans converted this to the Latin form, *Hispania*, hence the modern word Spain. The wild rabbit has long been hunted as an important food item. It is unclear exactly when domestication first took place but this is believed to have occurred between the 5th and 10th centuries in southern Europe, probably by monks who kept them for food. In the 5th and 6th centuries newborn rabbits were classified as 'fish' by the Pope, so they could be eaten during Lent and other fasting periods. The Romans kept rabbits in walled enclosures (*leporaria*) and there is evidence that they brought them to Britain, but the species did not survive at this time. In Europe, and especially France, the process of domestication was well under way by the 5th century; and in the 12th century the Normans brought rabbits to Britain, where they became established and remain as both domestic and wild animals. People have also transported the rabbit throughout the world, to all continents except Antarctica, often with devastating effect; the absence of predators in Australia and New Zealand has led to rabbits becoming a pest species. The European rabbit has not become established in the wild in North America, however, where its ecological niche is filled by the cottontail (*Sylvilagus* spp.).

The keeping of rabbits as pets developed in Victorian times, and their popularity has grown enormously, leading to the current situation where rabbits are the third most popular mammalian pet in the UK and many other countries. Although traditionally kept mainly as a children's pet, increasing numbers are kept by adults and as house pets, and they have become well established as a true companion animal.

Originally, rabbits were referred to in English as coneys and only the young were termed rabbits. The origin of the term 'bunny' is not entirely clear but it is believed to be derived from the Gaelic word '*bun*' that means a stump or root, and which also refers to the tail of a rabbit or hare. Female rabbits are referred to as does, males as bucks and young rabbits as kits or kittens.

Breeds and varieties

All domestic rabbits are of the same species as the wild European rabbit (*Oryctolagus cuniculus*). With domestication came the development of different breeds and varieties.

- A breed is a group of related animals that are genotypically and phenotypically sufficiently similar to produce physically similar offspring when they are mated to each other (see Chapter 4). Most breeds of rabbit have breed standards, which are detailed descriptions of the characteristics of the ideal specimen. Breeds are not static and may evolve significantly over time.
- The 'variety' refers to a colour within a breed.

Breeds are created either through mutation, combining existing characters of two or more breeds, or by selective breeding for particular characteristics to such a degree that the resulting offspring are significantly different from the original stock. For example, the Rex breed emerged as the result of a mutation that caused an abnormality in the length of guard hairs in the coat. The guard hairs and undercoat of this breed are the same length, giving a velvety feel to the coat. Another example of a mutation is the Satin, where the hair scales are smooth and the hollow central portion of the hair fibre is absent, giving the coat a distinctive sheen. Lop breeds have soft ears that hang down and cannot be held erect. Giant breeds are becoming increasingly popular as pets and weigh approximately 5 kg or more.

In 2012, the British Rabbit Council (www.thebrc.org) recognized 81 breeds and over 500 varieties of rabbit in the UK (Figure 1.1), and more are being derived from selective breeding and mutation, although many pet rabbits are crossbreeds. In the UK, breeds are currently divided into Fancy (e.g. Himalayan, Dutch, Lop, English, Netherland Dwarf), Lop (e.g. Dwarf, English, French, Miniature), Normal Fur (e.g. Chinchilla, Beveren, New Zealand) and Rex (mainly different coat colours and patterns with basic Rex fur type). In the USA, the classification of breeds differs; links to a useful series of websites illustrating US breeds can be found on the website of the American Rabbit Breeders Association (www.arba.net).

Longevity and ageing

The life expectancy of the pet rabbit is commonly quoted as 5–10 years, but some individuals can live for up to 18 years, or more (Figure 1.2). The author has received confirmation of a 21-year-old pet rabbit. Wild rabbits do not generally survive beyond their first year, but there is a longevity record of 7.6 years for a wild rabbit from Australia.

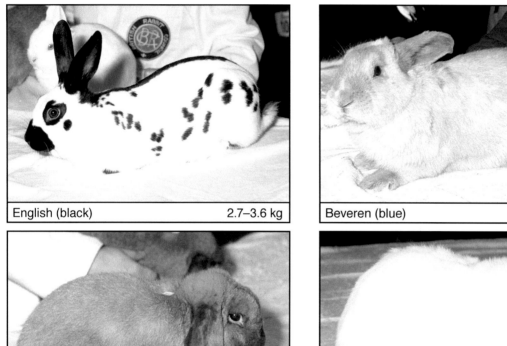

| English (black) | 2.7–3.6 kg |

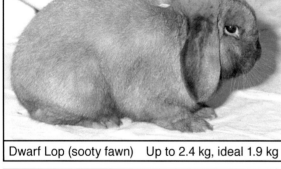

| Dwarf Lop (sooty fawn) | Up to 2.4 kg, ideal 1.9 kg |

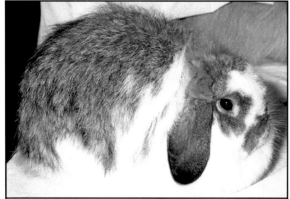

| Cashmere Lop (agouti broken) | Up to 2.4 kg |

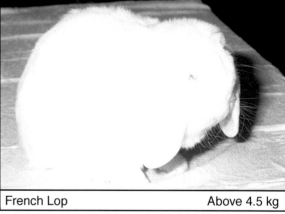

| Beveren (blue) | Above 3.6 kg |

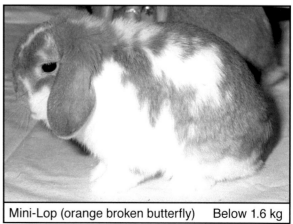

| French Lop | Above 4.5 kg |

| Mini-Lop (orange broken butterfly) | Below 1.6 kg |

1.1 Examples of breeds of domestic rabbit, showing typical adult bodyweight. (© CBC, University of Newcastle) (continues) ▶

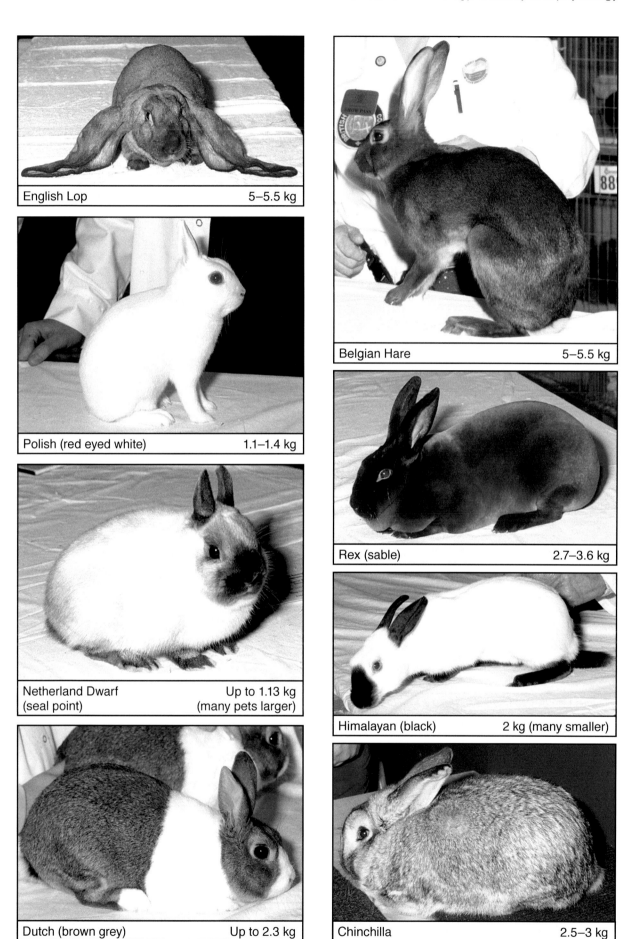

English Lop · 5–5.5 kg

Polish (red eyed white) · 1.1–1.4 kg

Netherland Dwarf (seal point) · Up to 1.13 kg (many pets larger)

Dutch (brown grey) · Up to 2.3 kg

Belgian Hare · 5–5.5 kg

Rex (sable) · 2.7–3.6 kg

Himalayan (black) · 2 kg (many smaller)

Chinchilla · 2.5–3 kg

1.1 (continued) Examples of breeds of domestic rabbit, showing typical adult bodyweight. (© CBC, University of Newcastle) (continues) ▶

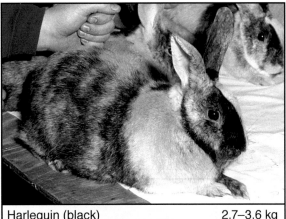

Harlequin (black)   2.7–3.6 kg

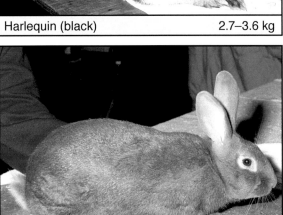

New Zealand Red   3.6 kg

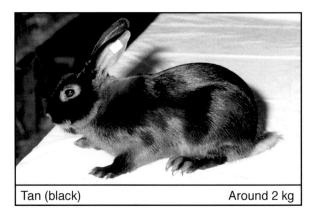

Tan (black)   Around 2 kg

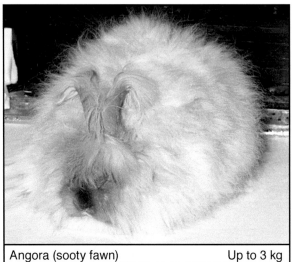

Angora (sooty fawn)   Up to 3 kg

1.1 (continued) Examples of breeds of domestic rabbit, showing typical adult bodyweight. (© CBC, University of Newcastle)

Parameter	Usual value
Heart rate	150–300 beats/minute
Respiratory rate	30–60 breaths/minute
Body temperature	38.5–40.0°C
Daily water consumption	50–150 ml/kg [a]
Daily urine production	20–350 ml/kg [a]
Bodyweight adult (breed dependent)	1–6 kg
Bodyweight newborn kit	30–80 g
Life expectancy	5–10 years

1.2 Physiological data for the rabbit. [a] Water intake and urine production are highly variable and dependent on diet.

In general it is not possible to age a rabbit once adulthood is reached (6–8 months in most breeds). However, experienced owners and breeders may use various criteria. The claws do not generally project beyond the fur until maturity, and the ears feel 'tougher' in animals over 2–3 years than in younger animals, in which the ears are much softer. These factors are highly variable, however, and no feature can be relied upon. Deciduous dentition is shed at birth, and permanent dentition is fully erupted from 3–5 weeks of age, so by the first presentation to a veterinary surgeon all teeth are generally permanent. Radiographic closure of the growth plates in rabbits occurs at between 20 and 30 weeks (in the New Zealand White).

Anatomy and physiology

Musculoskeletal system

The rabbit skeleton is light, making up only 7–8% of the bodyweight, compared with 12–14% in most other domestic mammals, although the calcium content is relatively higher in rabbits than in cats (Abdalla *et al.*, 1992). The bones are relatively brittle compared with those of the dog and cat, which can complicate orthopaedic surgery. Rabbit muscle is light pink in colour and overall muscle mass makes up over 50% of bodyweight.

The forelimbs are short and fine, and the radius and ulna are fused and clearly bowed. In contrast the hindlimbs are long and powerful. The pelvic limb muscles are concentrated in the proximal portion of the leg and make up 13% of the overall muscle mass, reflecting the need and ability for rapid acceleration and high-speed running to evade capture. The fibula extends over only half the length of the tibia and is fused with it. The forelimb has five digits and the hindlimb four. The plantar surface of the hindlimb from the tarsus distally is in contact with the ground at rest, but when running the rabbit is digitigrade. The pelvis is elongated, with a length-to-breadth ratio >2:1 and an oval obturator foramen and the acetabulum lying halfway between the front and back edge.

The spine is naturally curved and the ribs are flattened. The vertebral formula of the rabbit is C7 T12 L7 S4 C16, but 13 thoracic vertebrae and six lumbar vertebrae are seen in some animals. One study of 64 rabbits reported T12 L7 in 44%, T13 6L in 33% and T13 7L in 23% of rabbits (Greenaway *et al.*, 2001).

The body conformation of domesticated rabbits varies greatly depending on the breed, and can deviate widely from the wild type in both size and shape, from the squat or 'cobby' shape of the dwarf breeds to the lithe and lean ('racy') Belgian Hare (a breed of rabbit, not a hare). Skull morphology also varies widely, and this can lead to disease, especially dental problems, particularly in some dwarf breeds that have mandibular prognathism, causing incisor malocclusion (see Oral cavity and dentition, below). Breeds with a foreshortened skull (maxillary brachygnathism) also seem predisposed to nasolacrimal duct and dental problems. The temporomandibular joint (TMJ) of the rabbit is elongated longitudinally, allowing forward and backward as well as vertical and lateral movement.

Great care must be taken when handling rabbits. In addition to the pelvic limb muscles, the lumbar muscles are also powerful (9% of body mass), and osteoporosis may be present as a result of lack of exercise and/or low calcium intake. If rabbits are not handled securely, a kick with the powerful hindlegs can result in lumbar vertebral fractures (usually L6/L7), even in rabbits with normal bone density.

Nervous system

The nervous system of the rabbit is similar to that of other mammals, except that the spinal cord extends more caudally, for almost the entire length of the vertebral canal, and the cauda equina is much less pronounced. The spinal cord terminates at the level of S1–S3, but usually within the second sacral vertebra. In rabbits with a higher number of vertebrae (e.g. 13 thoracic and 7 lumbar) it will terminate more cranially than in those with fewer vertebrae.

Oral cavity and dentition

The upper lip of the rabbit is naturally cleft. The oral commissure is small and the oral cavity long and curved (Figure 1.3). The maximum gape is only 20–25 degrees and this, together with the presence of cheek folds across the diastema, makes visualization of the cheek teeth difficult in the conscious animal. The tongue is large and has a mobile rostral portion and a relatively fixed thicker caudal portion (torus). There are four pairs of salivary glands: parotid, submaxillary, sublingual and zygomatic.

The dental formula is I2/1 C0/0 P3/2 M3/3. Rabbits have six unpigmented incisor teeth, one in each mandible and two each side of the premaxilla. The second upper incisor is much smaller than the

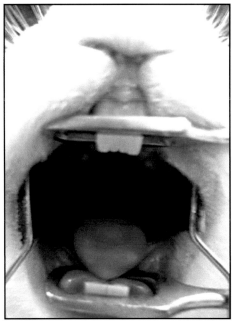

1.3 The rabbit's upper lip is cleft and the oral commissure is small, with a gape of only 25–30 degrees.

rest, commonly being referred to as a 'peg tooth', and is directly behind the first incisor. There is a diastema between the incisor and premolar teeth. The premolar teeth are similar in form to the molar teeth, and these are usually described together as the 'cheek teeth'. All the teeth are classified as elodont (continuously growing with no anatomical 'root') and hypsodont (high or long crowned). The clinical crown refers to the portion of the tooth above the gingival margin, and so-called roots are more correctly described as 'reserve crowns', with the active growing tip referred to as the apex (Figure 1.4). The periodontal ligament has fine collagen fibres that allow for continuous eruption of the tooth. Tooth anatomy is described in more detail in the *BSAVA Manual of Rabbit Surgery, Dentistry and Imaging*.

The incisor teeth are used with a largely vertical scissor-like slicing action. Enamel is present only on the labial surface of the tightly curved maxillary incisors, creating a chisel-like occlusal surface, but is present on both labial and lingual surfaces of the less curved mandibular incisors. The tips of the mandibular incisors lie just caudal to the maxillary incisors and touch the peg teeth. In addition to the normal biting action, rabbits will periodically grind the incisors together to help keep the occlusal surfaces correctly shaped. One study of two groups of 20 normal male pet rabbits has shown that there are only minor differences in the average clinical crown length between maxillary (6.1 ± 0.9 mm) and mandibular (6.4 ± 0.6 mm) incisors (Schumacher, 2011). Incisor wear, growth and eruption are balanced in a normal rabbit at a rate of 2 mm/week for the maxillary incisors and 2.4 mm/week for the mandibular incisors (Shadle, 1936).

The cheek teeth abut closely without any significant interproximal space to form a single functional

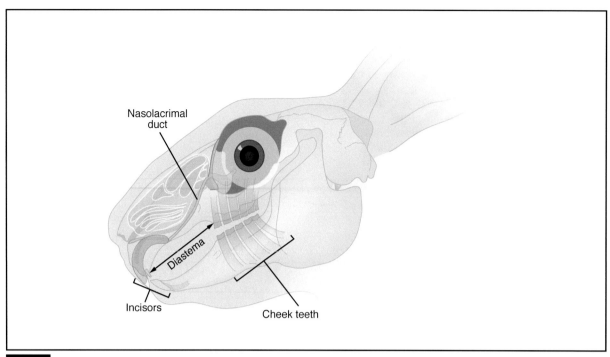

1.4 Diagram of the skull of a rabbit indicating the position of the teeth and the nasolacrimal duct.

occlusal grinding surface. On the buccal surface the enamel is deeply folded. As there are six maxillary and five mandibular cheek teeth on each side, each mandibular tooth occludes with two maxillary teeth, except for the smaller first and sixth maxillary cheek teeth. The mandible is narrower than the maxilla (anisognathism) and the occlusal surfaces are tilted laterally at an angle of approximately 10 degrees. The TMJ is located caudal and dorsal to the molar arcade and is oriented in a paramedian plane with an elongated condyle and a short, deep fossa, similar to that of the horse. Ingesta is ground by the cheek teeth with a wide lateral chewing action, concentrating on one side at a time. Chewing occurs at a rate of approximately 200 cycles per minute. The natural diet of grass is highly abrasive because it has a high content of silicate phytoliths, so there is rapid wear of the cheek teeth (approximately 3 mm per month), with equally rapid tooth growth and eruption. The food type affects the chewing action: natural vegetation is chewed with a wide lateral movement and a horizontal power stroke whereas pellets and grains are chewed with a more vertical power stroke (Weijs *et al.*, 1989; Figure 1.5). Mandibular teeth grow and erupt faster than maxillary teeth.

Skin and haircoat
Rabbit skin is delicate and easily torn. In most breeds, female rabbits possess a large fold of skin under the chin, known as the dewlap, from which they pull hair to line the nest before kindling (Figure 1.6). The toes and metatarsal areas are completely covered with hair, and there are no footpads (Figure 1.7).

The nature of the haircoat depends on the breed. The normal coat consists of a short soft undercoat protected by longer guard hairs. The only hairless

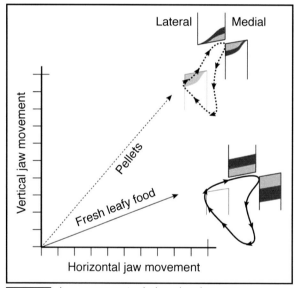

1.5 Jaw movements during chewing vary depending on the food type. The normal lateral power stroke when eating a wild-type diet of grass becomes more vertical in a rabbit on a commercial diet. (Courtesy of David Crossley)

areas are the tip of the nose, part of the scrotum and the inguinal folds.

- In the Rex breed the guard hairs are shortened, so they do not protrude above the level of the undercoat.
- Satin breeds have an altered hair fibre structure that gives the coat a characteristic sheen.
- Angora rabbits have a very long undercoat and guard hairs that are harvested for spinning into wool, and they need regular grooming to prevent matting.

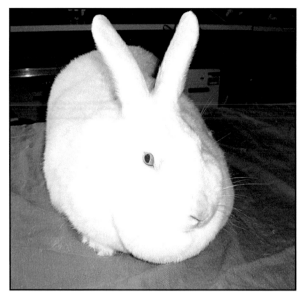

1.6 A prominent dewlap is a normal feature of the doe.

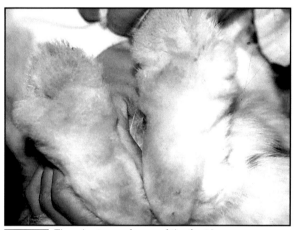

1.7 The plantar surfaces of the feet have no footpads and are covered in hair.

The guard hairs are the first to emerge in newborn kits, followed by the undercoat. By a few days of age this soft baby coat is well developed, and it persists until about 5 or 6 weeks of age. An intermediate or pre-adult coat then replaces this, followed by the adult coat by about 6–8 months of age. Thereafter most rabbits moult approximately twice a year (spring and autumn), but this can vary. Moulting starts at the head and proceeds caudally. Pregnant or pseudopregnant does undergo a loosening of the hairs on the belly, thighs and chest, which are then easily plucked to line the nest and expose the nipples. Does possess four or five pairs of nipples on the ventrum, which are absent from the buck.

Tactile vibrissae are present on the muzzle, which are used to help locate food and when underground.

Scent glands are located on the underside of the chin (submandibular glands), either side of the perineum (inguinal glands) and at the anus (anal glands). Rabbits are strongly territorial and rely heavily on scent for communication. Both sexes will rub their chins ('chinning') to scent-mark territory (see Chapter 5). The size of the glands and frequency of 'chinning' behaviour are under sex steroid control and depend on sexual and dominance status (Melo, 2010). The inguinal glands are large and pouch-like and often contain a yellow/brown oily deposit.

Eyes

The large eyes are located laterally and have a very wide field of vision to aid detection of predators. Rabbits have a 'blind spot' in the area beneath the mouth, so food is detected by the sensitive lips and vibrissae. Rabbits often resent, or are startled by, being touched in this area because they cannot see what is touching them.

The cornea is large and occupies 30% of the globe. The lens is large and almost spherical, and the ciliary body is poorly developed, so accommodation is limited. The retina is merangiotic, i.e. only part of the inner retina is supplied by retinal vessels. The optic disc lies above the midline of the eye and retinal vessels spread horizontally out from it. The optic disc has a natural depression or cup. There is no tapetum lucidum.

The lacrimal gland lies beside the lower eyelid rim and is large, bilobed and pale red, with a bulbous enlargement at the medial canthus.

A third eyelid (nictitating membrane) is present at the medial canthus and the superficial (nictitans) and deep (Harderian) orbital glands are located just behind it. The Harderian gland is encapsulated and has two lobes, the upper being white and the lower larger and pink in colour; the ducts from both lobes converge to emerge behind the third eyelid. This lower lobe is also referred to as the deep gland of the nictitating membrane, and can occasionally prolapse, as in the dog ('cherry eye'; see Chapter 16). The gland is larger and more prominent in males, especially during the breeding season. The normal secretion is milky and lubricates the eyelid edges. This whitish secretion may be noticeable if epiphora is present as a result of blockage of the nasolacrimal duct and should not be confused with a purulent discharge. Rabbits blink spontaneously less frequently than once per minute, on average 10–12 times an hour, and they can go 20–30 minutes between blinks (Maurice, 1995).

The nasolacrimal duct has a single ventral lacrimal punctum in the medial aspect of the lower eyelid. From here there is a short (approximately 2 mm) canaliculus coursing medially and ventrally into a funnel-shaped lacrimal sac, supported medially by the lacrimal bone. The duct then enters the maxilla through a semicircular foramen in the lacrimal bone. The duct has two sharp bends as it courses towards the nose: proximally in the maxillary bone; and at the base of the incisor teeth (see Figure 1.4). The duct narrows at these points, and this, plus the fact that the epithelium of the duct is undulating, and the opening into the nasal meatus is very small, means that the nasolacrimal duct is very prone to blockage in the rabbit.

A large retrobulbar venous plexus lines the back of the orbit and can complicate enucleation surgery.

Engorgement of this plexus and bilateral exophthalmos can occur owing to the presence of a cranial thoracic mass (e.g. thymoma) or severe cardiac disease that impedes or compromises venous return to the heart. Engorgement may also occur in a severely frightened rabbit.

Ears

The ears have a large surface area, are highly vascular with large arteriovenous shunts, and are involved in thermoregulation. Ear size varies among breeds, and those with ears that hang down are referred to as 'lops'. These lop-eared breeds have a narrowed stenotic region in the horizontal canal at the point where the ear folds down that predisposes them to otitis externa. The vertical canal has a natural long diverticulum separated by the cartilaginous tragus. The tympanic bullae are located at the base of the skull in a similar position to those in the dog and cat, and the ventral region extends beyond the level of the occipital bone, but not to the same extent as in the dog and cat. The external acoustic meatus is vertically rather than horizontally oriented and is a prominent bony tube (Figure 1.8). Within the tympanic bulla the rabbit lacks any bony ridge or septum, as found in the dog and cat, respectively.

Respiratory system

Rabbits are obligate nasal breathers, owing to the anatomy of the nasopharynx and larynx and the dorsal location of the epiglottis in relation to the soft palate. Although the rabbit can disengage the epiglottis from the soft palate *in extremis* by extending the neck and raising the head, this is a very poor prognostic sign. The tip of the nose, or rhinarium, is hairless and moves up and down in a normal rabbit ('twitching') 20–120 times a minute depending on the level of excitement or apprehension, but this will stop when the rabbit is very relaxed or anaesthetized.

The glottis is small and visually obscured by the back of the tongue. Reflex laryngospasm is common in the rabbit, which can complicate endotracheal intubation. The left lung is smaller than the right and has three distinct lobes (cranial, middle and caudal). The right lung has four lobes (cranial, middle, caudal and accessory). Both cranial lung lobes are small (left smaller than right). Rabbits do not have lung lobules. The thoracic cavity is relatively small compared with the abdominal cavity (Figure 1.9), and breathing is largely diaphragmatic, with visible chest excursions being minimal in a healthy rabbit. Large amounts of intrathoracic fat are often present. The triangular thymus remains large in the adult rabbit, and lies cranioventral to the heart, extending into the thoracic inlet. It has three lobes, one left thoracic lobe and dorsal and ventral right thoracic lobes.

Cardiovascular system

The heart is relatively small (0.3% of the bodyweight) and lies cranially in the thoracic cavity between ribs 3 and 6. The right atrioventricular valve has only two cusps, rather than three as in other mammals. The rabbit aorta shows neurogenic rhythmic contractions and the pulmonary artery is thicker and more muscular than in other species. There is a limited collateral coronary circulation which can predispose to cardiac ischaemia if coronary vasoconstriction occurs.

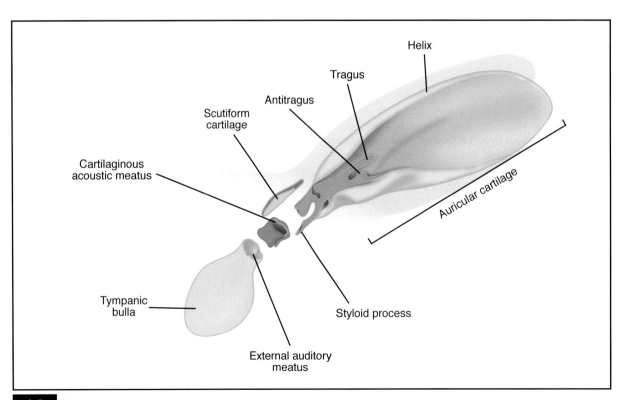

1.8 Diagram of the tympanic bulla.

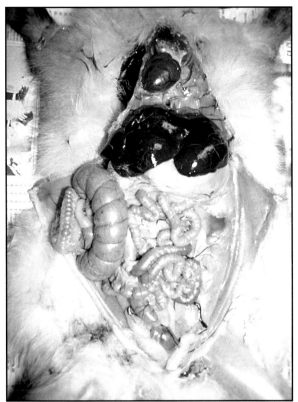

1.9 The thorax of the rabbit is small in comparison to the abdomen and the thymus remains prominent in the adult animal.

Urinary system

Rabbit kidneys are unipapillate, and in wild rabbits they have been shown to be able to adapt to differing environmental and geographical conditions over generations, developing a long medullary region in arid environments and a short medulla in lush environments. Renal function is discussed further in Chapters 9 and 13. Urine is the major route of excretion for calcium. Serum calcium levels in rabbits are not maintained within a narrow range, but are dependent largely on dietary intake, with excess excreted via the kidney. Rabbit urine is often thick and creamy, owing to the presence of calcium carbonate crystals. It can also vary in colour from pale creamy yellow through to dark red (often mistaken for haematuria by owners), as a consequence of the presence of endogenous and exogenous pigments that are influenced largely by diet, such as bile pigments and plant porphyrins.

Adrenal glands

The adrenal glands lie craniomedial to the kidneys against the dorsal body wall. The left adrenal is caudolateral to the cranial mesenteric artery and the right lies in close proximity to the caudal vena cava.

Reproductive system

Does have no uterine body but have two separate coiled uterine horns and two cervices opening into the vagina. The ovaries are elongated. The vagina is large and flaccid. The mesometrium is a major site of fat deposition, which can make location and identification of the ovaries and blood vessels for ligation challenging during surgical neutering. The placenta is haemochorial, i.e. the maternal blood comes in direct contact with the fetal chorion, as in humans. Rabbits are induced, or reflex, ovulators and do not have an oestrous cycle. Ovulation occurs about 10 hours after copulation in response to a surge in luteinizing hormone.

Bucks have two hairless scrotal sacs, either side of and cranial to the penis. There is no os penis. The inguinal canals remain open throughout life. Vesicular, proprostate, prostate, paraprostate and bulbourethral accessory sex glands are present (see Chapter 4).

Digestive tract and associated organs

An understanding of the unique anatomy and physiology of the rabbit's gastrointestinal (GI) tract is fundamental to an appreciation of its nutritional and feeding requirements (see Chapter 3; Figure 1.10).

Rabbits are hindgut fermenters, adapted to digest a high-fibre diet consisting mainly of grass. The abdominal cavity is large and the GI tract makes up 10–20% of bodyweight; the rabbit has – relative to its size – the largest stomach and caecum of any monogastric animal. Gut transit time is rapid so that fibre is eliminated from the digestive tract very quickly, unlike other hindgut fermenters such as the horse (colon fermenter) and ruminants. Gut retention time in the rabbit has been measured at 17.1 hours, compared with 68.8 hours in cattle. This permits the body size and weight to remain low, which is advantageous in a prey species.

Stomach

The stomach is large, thin-walled and poorly distensible with a well developed cardia and pylorus. Vomiting is not possible in the rabbit. Food, caecal pellets and ingested hair are normally present in the stomach, in a loose latticework. Stomach pH is 1–3 in the adult rabbit, and the ingesta are effectively sterilized. Prior to weaning, rabbits have a stomach pH of 5–6.5, but the presence of 'milk oil' prevents growth of microflora. Milk oil is an antimicrobial fatty acid produced from an enzymatic reaction with ingested milk. Protective milk oil is lost at 4–6 weeks, the stomach pH drops and the gut is inoculated with microorganisms, to establish the normal hindgut flora. Weaning is a critical time and can often be associated with GI disease.

Small intestine

The small intestine is approximately 3 metres long. The duodenum and jejunum are narrow, and at the end of the ileum there is the rounded sacculus rotundus, which is unique to the rabbit and is rich in lymphoid follicles, giving it a fine honeycombed serosal appearance. It is also known as the ampulla ilei or ileocaecal tonsil. Peyer's patches (aggregates of lymphoid tissue in the lamina propria) are only present in the jejunum and the distal half of the ileum.

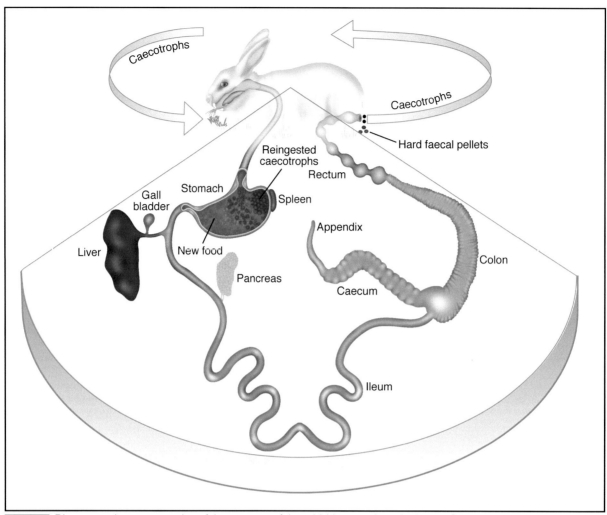

| **1.10** | Diagrammatic representation of the anatomy of the rabbit's gastrointestinal tract. Caecotrophs are reingested to maximize the use of nutrients. |

Large intestine

The colon can be divided into two parts, proximal and distal. The proximal colon is approximately 35 cm long and can be further subdivided into three segments. The first has three taeniae (longitudinal muscular bands) with multiple haustrae (sacculations). The second has a single taenia covering half the circumference of the colon and fewer haustrae. The third segment has no taeniae or haustrae but has a thickened mucosa and is known as the fusus coli. It is a highly innervated and vascularized muscular structure 5–8 cm long and, under the influence of aldosterone and prostaglandins, acts as a pacemaker for peristaltic movements of the large intestine. It is responsible for the mechanical separation of liquid and solid ingesta and has an important role in the formation of both hard and soft faecal pellets (Ruckebusch and Hörnicke, 1977).

In the proximal colon, contractions separate fibrous from non-fibrous particles, and fibre moves rapidly through the centre of the colonic lumen for excretion as hard faecal pellets. The production of faecal pellets coincides with feeding activity. A 2.5–3 kg rabbit typically passes about 150 faecal pellets a day. Antiperistaltic waves move fluid and non-fibrous particles back along the luminal walls within the sacculations, and into the caecum for fermentation. This process is aided by secretion of water into the proximal colon. Three to eight hours after eating, soft mucus-covered caecal pellets are expelled in clusters and eaten directly from the anus (a process known as caecotrophy, coprophagy, refection or pseudorumination). This type of 'colonic separation mechanism', or CSM, in lagomorphs is known as a 'washback' CSM, as distinct from the 'mucus-trap' CSM that is found in rodents, which also practise coprophagy but do not produce two such distinct types of pellets. Although rabbits have a lower capacity for fibre digestion than herbivorous rodents such as guinea pigs, their washback CSM has been demonstrated to be more efficient and requires a relatively less capacious colon and lower gut fill (Franz et al., 2011). Caecotrophs are also referred to as caecotropes, soft faeces or night faeces, and are rich in nutrients for reingestion. Arrival of the caecotrophs at the anus triggers a reflex licking of the anus and ingestion of the caecotrophs, which are swallowed whole and not chewed. The fusus coli acts to regulate colonic contractions and controls production of the two types of pellet. The separation of materials described above does not occur during caecotroph excretion. The separation of caecotrophs and faeces is principally achieved as a result of their entering the colon at different times.

The distal colon runs from the fusus coli to the rectum and is approximately 80–100 cm long.

Caecum

The caecum is very large (40% of the GI tract volume), thin-walled and has many sacculations (18–22). It folds on to itself three times (three gyri) and terminates in the vermiform appendix, which is also rich in lymphatic tissue and has a honeycombed serosal appearance like the sacculus rotundus. The caecum lies on the right side of the abdomen, and the caecal contents are normally semifluid.

The caecal microflora plays a major part in the digestive efficiency and the health status of the GI tract of the rabbit (Michelland et al., 2010). There are an estimated 400 different species of bacteria inhabiting the rabbit caecum, of which 25 are considered the most abundant (Straw, 1988). However, several factors such as physiological parameters, age, environment, diet and diseases can change the composition of the microflora. The rabbit gastrointestinal microflora increases and evolves during the first weeks after birth and stabilizes at around 28 days of age, during the weaning period (Bennegadi et al., 2003). In utero the fetus is sterile; it becomes contaminated by bacteria found in the birth canal and environment. The caecum is generally considered sterile in the rabbit until 3 days of age. It is then colonized by anaerobic bacteria, and 1 week after birth the caecal bacteria have already increased to 10 million (10^7) bacteria per gram of ingesta (O'Malley, 2005). After 2 weeks of age, rabbits start to acquire further non-pathogenic bacteria to add to the gut microflora by eating the doe's caecotrophs (O'Malley, 2005) and in an adult animal more than 10^{11} bacteria/g are present (Straw, 1988).

Organisms that have been identified in the caecal microflora include a variety of Gram-positive and Gram-negative anaerobes, protozoans and fungi (Straw, 1988; Bennegadi, 2003; O'Malley, 2005). The predominant organisms in young rabbits are streptococci and enterobacteria, whereas in adult rabbits, strict anaerobes are the most prevalent bacteria, and among these Gram-negative Bacteroides is considered dominant. This is due to the change in the pH of the stomach, which decreases from pH 6 in juveniles to pH 1–3 in adults, and also to the changes in the diet of the animal. Gram-negative coccoids, fusiform rods, large ciliated protozoans (Isotricha) and yeasts (Saccharomyces (Cyniclomyces) guttulatus) are also present.

The mucus covering protects the bacteria in the caecal pellets from the low pH of the stomach. Caecotrophs remain in the stomach for up to 6 hours, with continued bacterial synthesis and fermentation. Caecotrophs provide microbial protein that accounts for 15–25% of total amino acids and 9–15% of the digestible energy (DE) requirement. They also provide all of the B group and K vitamins and a certain amount of volatile fatty acids. VFAs produced by the fermenting action of the caecal bacteria are absorbed across the caecal epithelium and used as an energy source. Acetic acid (60–80%), butyric acid (8–20%) and propionic acid (3–10%) are produced, the proportions varying according to the time of day, developmental stage of the rabbit and diet. Butyric acid is the preferred substrate for colonocytes and the liver is the main organ for metabolizing propionic and butyric acid. Acetic acid is available for extrahepatic tissue metabolism. It is estimated that the rabbit obtains up to 40% of its maintenance energy requirement from VFAs produced by caecal fermentation.

The degree of caecotrophy is affected by energy and protein levels in the diet. If it is energy-deficient, a rabbit will consume all the caecotrophs produced. During ad libitum feeding, caecotroph intake depends on the protein and fibre content of the diet, and is greater if the diet is lower in protein or higher in fibre.

Gastrointestinal motility

Control of GI motility is complex in the rabbit. Motility is under the influence of the autonomic nervous system, prostaglandins and other hormones, but is also largely stimulated and maintained by a high throughput of indigestible fibre (lignocellulose). Aldosterone levels are known to be lowest during the period of caecotroph production. Motilin is a polypeptide hormone secreted by enterochromaffin cells of the duodenum and jejunum that stimulates GI motility. Fat stimulates its release and carbohydrate inhibits it. In the small intestine, motilin activity decreases as distance from the stomach increases. Activity is absent in the caecum but reappears in the colon and rectum.

Pancreas

The pancreas is associated with the duodenum and is very diffuse and difficult to differentiate from the surrounding mesentery in the rabbit. The single pancreatic duct enters the duodenum at the junction of the ascending and transverse portions. There is only modest production of pancreatic amylase. Insulin appears to have a minor role in rabbits and they can survive for long periods following pancreatectomy. Spontaneous diabetes mellitus has only been reported in one laboratory colony of New Zealand White rabbits.

Liver

The liver lies largely within the caudal ribcage and has a total of six lobes. There are two major lobes, left and right; the left is subdivided into lateral and medial lobes. The right is also divided into lateral and medial lobes plus a smaller quadrate lobe and a caudate lobe, which is attached by a narrow stalk to the dorsal hilar liver region. A gallbladder is present between the right medial and quadrate lobes, and rabbits secrete biliverdin as the primary bile pigment, rather than bilirubin. The bile duct is separate from the pancreatic duct and opens into the proximal duodenum. On a weight-for-weight basis, a rabbit secretes approximately seven times more bile daily than a dog.

Lymphoid tissue

Of the lymphoid tissue in the rabbit, 50% is associated with the gut (sacculus rotundus, vermiform appendix, Peyer's patches). The thymus has been described above. The spleen is relatively small and elongated and lies along the greater curvature of the stomach. Lymph nodes and their locations are similar to those in other mammals; only the popliteal nodes are usually easily palpable in normal rabbits.

Calcium metabolism

Rabbits have a 30–50% higher serum calcium concentration and a wider normal physiological range than other mammals. This is associated with an elevated set point for Ca^{2+}-regulated parathyroid hormone (PTH) release compared with other mammals, i.e. in this species a higher concentration of blood calcium is required to turn off the production of PTH (Warren *et al.*, 1989). Excess calcium is excreted in the urine and the fractional excretion is around 44%, compared with <2% in most mammals. The rabbit maintains serum ionized calcium concentration within its physiological range and protects against hypo- and hypercalcaemia by rapid changes in secretion of PTH and calcitonin. Dietary calcium is absorbed from the GI tract by passive diffusion or active transport. Active transport requires a carrier protein that is synthesized in the intestinal mucosa in response to 1,25-dihydroxyvitamin D3; however vitamin D is not required for absorption if dietary levels are adequate. The kidney is important for preserving or excreting calcium; these functions are mediated by PTH and vitamin D3.

References and further reading

Abdalla KEH, Abd-El-Nasser M, Ibrahim I A, *et al.* (1992) Comparative anatomical and biochemical studies on the main bones of the limbs in rabbit and cat as a medicolegal parameter. *Assiut Veterinary Medical Journal* **26**, 142–153

Barlet JP (1980) Plasma calcium, inorganic phosphorus and magnesium levels in pregnant and lactating rabbits. *Reproduction, Nutrition and Development* **20**, 647–651

Bennegadi N, Fonty G, Millet L, Gidenne T and Licois D (2003) Effects of age and dietary fibre level on caecal microbial communities of conventional and specific pathogen-free rabbits. *Microbial Ecology in Health and Disease* **5**, 23–32

Buss SL and Bourdeau JE (1984) Calcium balance in laboratory rabbits. Minor Electrolyte Metabolism 10, 127–132

Carabaño R and Piquer J (1998) The digestive system of the rabbit. In: *The Nutrition of the Rabbit*, ed. C de Blas and J Wiseman, pp.1–16. CABI, Wallingford

Franz R, Kreuzer M, Hummel J, Hatt J-M and Clauss M (2011) Intake, selection, digesta retention, digestion and gut fill of two coprophagous species, rabbits (*Oryctolagus cuniculus*) and guinea pigs (*Cavia porcellus*), on a hay-only diet. *Journal of Animal Physiology and Animal Nutrition* **95**, 564–570

Gondret F, Hernandez P, Remignon H and Combes S (2009) Skeletal muscle adaptions and biomechanical properties of tendons in response to jump exercise in rabbits. *Journal of Animal Science* **87**(2), 544–553

Greenaway JB, Partlow GD, Gonsholt NL and Fisher KR (2001) Anatomy of the lumbosacral spinal cord in rabbits. *Journal of the American Animal Hospital Association* **37**(1), 27–34

Kennedy A (1965) The urinary excretion of calcium by normal rabbits. *Journal of Comparative Pathology* **75**, 69–74

Marty J and Vernay M (1984) Absorption and metabolism of the volatile fatty acids in the hindgut of the rabbit. *British Journal of Nutrition* **51**, 265–277

Maurice DM (1995) The effect of the low blink rate in rabbits on topical drug penetration. *Journal of Ocular Pharmacology and Therapeutics* **11**, 297–304

Melo AI and González-Mariscal G (2010) Communication by olfactory signals in rabbits: its role in reproduction. *Vitamins and Hormones* **83**, 351–371

Michelland RJ, Combes S, Monteils V, *et al.* (2010) Molecular analysis of the bacterial community in the digestive tract of the rabbit. *Anaerobe* **16**(2), 61–65

Munoz ME, Gonzales J and Esteller A (1986) Bile pigment formation and excretion in the rabbit. *Comparative Biochemistry and Physiology* **85A**, 67–71

O'Malley B (2005) Rabbits. In: *Clinical Anatomy and Physiology of Exotic Species*, pp.173–195. Elsevier Saunders, Philadelphia

Roth SI, Conaway HH, Sanders LL, *et al.* (1980) Spontaneous diabetes mellitus in the New Zealand white rabbit: preliminary morphologic characterisation. *Laboratory Investigation* **42**(5), 571–579

Ruckebusch Y and Hörnicke H (1977) Motility of the rabbit's colon and caecotrophy. *Physiology and Behaviour* **18**, 871–878

Schumacher M (2011) Measurement of clinical crown length of incisor and premolar teeth in clinically healthy rabbits. *Journal of Veterinary Dentistry* **28**(2), 90–95

Shadle AR (1936) The attrition and extrusive growth of the four major incisor teeth of domestic rabbits. *Journal of Mammalogy* **17**, 15–21

Stevens CE and Hume ID (1995) *Comparative Physiology of the Vertebrate Digestive System, 2nd edn.* Cambridge University Press, Cambridge

Straw TE (1988) Bacteria of the rabbit gut and their role in the health of the rabbit. *Journal of Applied Rabbit Research* **11**, 142–150

Verde MT and Piquer JG (1986) The effects of stress on the corticosterone and ascorbic acid content of the blood plasma of rabbits. *Journal of Applied Rabbit Research* **9**, 181–185

Warren HB, Lausen NCC, Segre GV, El-Hajj G and Brown EM (1989) Regulation of calciotropic hormones in vivo in the New Zealand White rabbit. *Endocrinology* **125**, 2683–2690

Weijs WA, Brugman P and Grimbergen CA (1989) Jaw movements and muscle activity during mastication in growing rabbits. *Anatomical Record* **224**(3), 407–416

2

Husbandry

Richard Saunders

Pet rabbits are prone to a number of disease conditions that are due, totally or in part, to incorrect husbandry. Correct husbandry (Figure 2.1) is highly important for preventing and treating such conditions. The veterinary surgeon may be called upon to recommend suitable rabbit housing, or to assess it in order to suggest changes that may improve the quality of life of the rabbit, and should be able to do so.

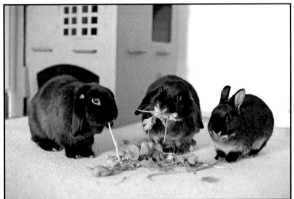

2.1 Rabbits in a good welfare situation. They are living in a group, with plenty of space to exercise, showing relaxed confident body posture and eating good-quality greens. (Courtesy of Marit Emilie Buseth)

Purchase and acquisition

Proper husbandry of the rabbit starts even before acquisition, and a suitable environment should be created before the rabbit is sourced. The environment available may influence the choice of rabbit(s) to be acquired, e.g. prospective numbers, age, breed and eventual body sizes. The source from which to obtain rabbits is a personal decision. A suitable travelling container is required to convey rabbits from the source to the home environment. Veterinary checks should be scheduled and attended at the earliest possible point to confirm the gender, and arrange preventive healthcare (see Chapter 6).

Sources

Breeders

One major advantage of obtaining rabbits directly from a breeder, of whatever type, is that the rabbit(s) may be transported straight from one environment to another with no mixing with other rabbits or intermediate steps in between. This reduces exposure to different pathogens and prolonged stressful situations, and thus minimizes the chances of post-acquisition disease problems. It is worth noting, for example, that the Defra (Department for Environment, Food and Rural Affairs) code of recommendations for livestock (PB7949) states: *'To reduce the risk of disease, wherever possible you should make arrangements to transfer the calves directly from farm to farm rather than through a market'*, and this advice is equally applicable to rabbits.

Professional breeders: These generally sell pure-bred rabbits of various breeds. It should be possible to see the parents (helpful in assessing likely temperament and pre-existing health issues) and thus to obtain a very good idea of the eventual size of the rabbit. The rabbit may or may not be used to being handled, and may be sold along with a litter-mate as a bonded pair. Such rabbits are likely, owing to the experience of the breeder, to have been correctly identified with regard to sex, although checking is wise.

The collections of some breeders are affected by endemic respiratory, neurological, dermatological or gastrointestinal diseases. It should be possible to see what food the rabbits have been weaned on to, and to continue with this diet for a changeover period. Medicated food may have been used (containing antibiotics and/or anticoccidials), and this should be ascertained. Breeders may also sell rabbits that are not suitable for showing, which is of little concern if this is for reasons of coat colour, but may be an issue if they have health-related problems, such as poor conformation, growth, skin or fur. Breeders who also breed for show purposes will almost always place rings on one hindlimb of each young rabbit at approximately 2–4 weeks (Figure 2.2); this should be removed, to avoid potential trauma in later life, at the earliest suitable opportunity.

Non-professional breeders: Unwanted litters resulting from mismating (typically due to incorrect sexing of two adult pair-bonded rabbits) are a common occurrence. It is usually possible to see the parents of such litters, although sometimes the sire

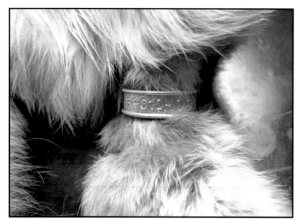

2.2 An identification ring on the hindlimb of a rabbit. This should be removed from pet rabbits as it is not required for identification and may cause trauma to the limb if the rabbit continues to grow or becomes obese.

may be a stray or wild rabbit. The health of the dam and litter may be assessed, and some idea of the likely future size of the rabbit obtained. Health status is variable, depending on the quality of husbandry of the owner, and the health of the stock. These rabbits may or may not be used to being handled, and may be sold along with a littermate as a bonded pair. Veterinary surgeons examining such rabbits should pay particular care to identifying the gender of the rabbit(s), regardless of the stated gender, and offer a re-examination at a suitable interval if it is not possible to be certain at first viewing. It should be possible to see what diet the rabbits have been weaned on to, and to continue with this for a changeover period. Such rabbits are unlikely to have been fed medicated food.

Pet shops
Pet shops usually source their rabbits from a small number of breeders. The rabbits may be obtained locally from a single source, and managed on an 'all in, all out' basis, which is ideal. Conversely, they may be sourced from multiple breeders, all potentially with particular disease issues present, and on different feeding regimes, and mixed either on or off show. With multistore chains, rabbits may potentially be transported from a central holding point to individual stores, which is not conducive to good health and welfare.

Rabbits may be kept in housing of varying standards, and on diets of varying quality. Whilst 'on show' accommodation may be stressful for the rabbit, it may be possible to observe the rabbit's behaviour and demeanour prior to purchase. Although it is rarely possible to see the parent rabbits, it is often possible to acquire two rabbits from the same source which have already been housed together. Gender should be checked by the veterinary surgeon, as above, because mistaken identities and gender are not uncommon.

Rescue centres
All the above options have the advantage of allowing a prospective owner to obtain a rabbit of known, young age, which is often preferred, and may also

provide information on their prior health history. The same cannot be said for rabbits obtained from rescue centres.

Rescue centres (Figure 2.3) vary widely in quality and nature. Rabbits obtained from such centres are often abandoned there, so their prior health status is commonly unknown. Indeed, rabbits may be discarded as a consequence of behavioural or health problems, and therefore their health may potentially be less good than those sourced at a young age. Rescue centres take in rabbits of unknown transmissible disease status all the time, and pathogens may be endemic. It is not possible to see the parents, unless litters have been admitted together with the parents, or pregnant does have subsequently given birth. Likewise, it is not always possible to source young rabbits from centres.

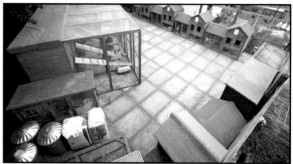

2.3 A rabbit rescue centre. These rabbits have been provided with a good-sized hutch with a large run attached. Their carrier boxes are being used as hides in their outdoor enclosure. They can see the other rabbits, although housing in pairs might be better. (Courtesy of N Constance)

The more knowledgeable centres will have accurately sexed the rabbits, assessed their health, and obtained veterinary diagnosis and treatment where possible. When seeing such rabbits for the first time, the veterinary surgeon should check both gender and health status, and in particular, should assess dental health, as it is extremely common to find dental disease in such rabbits.

It may be argued that with the large number of abandoned rabbits (67,000 in the UK in 2010; Todd and Mitchell, 2012), obtaining a new rabbit or rabbits from a rescue centre is the only truly ethical route. Many centres neuter and pair-bond rabbits prior to rehoming, and this removes two of the initial potential problems for the new owner. Many centres can also help to pair-bond an existing pet rabbit with a rescue rabbit, and this may avoid significant stresses later at home.

Breed selection with regard to the environment
Smaller breeds of rabbit tend to be nervous and have a greater tendency to 'jumpiness'. The particularly small breeds (e.g. Polish, Netherland Dwarf) may be unsuitable for a household with small children who may wish to pick them up, because jumping out of a person's arms is a major cause of injury. Conversely, the larger breeds (e.g. French Lop, Continental Giant) may be too big for a child to pick up.

Larger breeds require more space provision, and may struggle with certain configurations of runs, tunnels and climbing apparatus. It is therefore helpful to know the estimated adult size of the rabbit(s) when planning housing for them (floor space; height of enclosures; need for any roofs to minimize the risk of escape; width and strength of any flights of steps or climbing ramps; diameter of entry holes, tunnels or tubing placed in the environment for shelter and/or environmental enrichment, etc.).

Rex breeds are particularly susceptible to pododermatitis lesions and require care with selection of substrate (see below), and regular checking of the feet. They may pose a challenge to maintain free of foot health problems if the substrate cannot be altered to suit them (e.g. indoors). Meat breeds, e.g. New Zealand White, Californian, Sussex, are particularly prone to obesity, and should be carefully monitored for excessive weight gain. Breeds with excessive fur (e.g. Cashmere, Angora) are high-maintenance pets, requiring regular grooming (see below) and should be avoided by those unable to provide this.

It is more difficult to predict the future size of mixed-breed rabbits, but they may be less likely to exhibit certain breed-specific health problems, and may benefit from hybrid vigour.

Age at acquisition

After taking into account the above considerations, the age of the rabbit at acquisition is a personal choice. It should be remembered that older rabbits may have pre-existing health or behavioural issues, and a full history should be obtained where possible. However, adult rabbits have reached their full size, and are unlikely to undergo significant changes in temperament once past adolescence, especially if they are neutered.

Initial introduction to the new environment

Regardless of the quality of the current diet, a supply sufficient for 7–14 days should be obtained along with the rabbit(s), and they should be gradually converted from the old to the new diet. If a new rabbit is obtained in order to provide a pair-bond with an existing rabbit, bonding is required (see below).

Sudden changes of temperature should be avoided, and if a rabbit that has previously been housed indoors is placed outside, good protection against extremes of temperature should be provided. Rabbits previously housed outdoors should undergo a similar period of acclimatization if moved indoors.

Basic husbandry requirements

Provision of food

Rabbits feed throughout the day and night, and should not be confined to hutches or shelters overnight without allowing access to food and water, including fibre-rich forage such as hay, and including access to grass in their runs. Forage items should be available at all times, and in multiple locations that are easily accessed by all the rabbits within the group. A variety of methods may be used to provide forage, such as hay racks, hanging baskets, wall-mounted baskets, 'hay hedges', and willow or other lattice feeders which also provide environmental enrichment. However, rabbits naturally feed from the ground and feeding options that allow this should be provided for preference, even if this is by allowing rabbits to pull food from a hay rack on to the floor. See Chapter 3 for further details on nutrition.

Provision of water

Water should be accessible at all times, in a manner that allows all rabbits to drink *ad libitum*. Bottles are convenient, and avoid contamination of the water with faeces or urine. Also, rabbits may pick up and turn over bowls, losing and wasting water. However, water bowls encourage greater water intake in rabbits, and this may be helpful in avoiding urinary tract diseases.

Multiple water bowls and/or bottles should be provided, to allow the rabbits to maintain their water intake in the event of failure, emptying or guarding of a source by a dominant rabbit.

Exposure to ultraviolet light

The rabbit's need for ultraviolet (UV) light exposure, in order to produce vitamin D in the epidermis, is controversial. Fairham and Harcourt-Brown (1999) demonstrated a link between exposure to UV light and serum vitamin D levels. However, no further exploration of this link has been reported.

Standard window glass does not permit UV light to pass through it. Specialist plastic or glass must be used, or direct exposure to unfiltered sunlight (i.e. in outdoor areas) is required. Given that house rabbits are increasingly commonly kept in the UK, and that this is the most common method of husbandry in the USA, this may be of concern.

Vitamin D is present in concentrate feeds, and in sun-dried vegetation (e.g. sun-dried rather than barn-dried hay). If these are present in sufficient quantity, UV exposure may be less important.

Husbandry requirements and the law

The husbandry of rabbits in England and Wales is covered under the Animal Welfare Act 2006 and in Scotland by the Animal Health and Welfare (Scotland) Act 2006. These state that all animals shall be provided with an environment that fulfils all their needs, which does not create or have the potential to cause welfare problems. This leaves the onus on the owner to provide the correct environment, and there is some uncertainty in defining whether husbandry is appropriate or not. The assessment has been based on the concept of the 'Five Freedoms'.

Under the Animal Welfare Act 2006, rabbits require:

- Somewhere suitable to live
- A proper diet, including fresh water
- The ability to express normal behaviour
- To be housed with (or apart from, if required) other animals
- Protection from, and treatment of, illness and injury.

Specific husbandry guidelines have not been formalized for England and Scotland but are available for Wales (http://wales.gov.uk/docs/drah/publications/110817rabbitcodeen.pdf); while these are not prescriptive, they provide a useful guide to what rabbits require.

Space

Hutches

- The minimum hutch dimensions for a single rabbit or pair of rabbits is often suggested to be 0.68 m wide x 0.8 m long x 0.75 m high (Boers *et al.*, 2002).
- Alternatively, the hutch should be large enough to allow the rabbit to stretch out comfortably in all directions and stand up without its ears touching the ceiling (PDSA and YouGov, 2011).
- The RWAF (2012) suggested minimum dimensions are 1.8 m x 0.6 m (i.e. 1.08 m²) and high enough to stand up in, as above.
- The RSPCA guidelines suggest a minimum height of 0.75 m.

Runs

The most widely quoted guidelines recommend providing enough space for the rabbit to take three hops in a straight line (1.5–2.0 m for an adult New Zealand White), with sufficient space for the rabbit to stand upright without its ears touching the ceiling. These derive from laboratory animal welfare guidelines (Morton *et al.*, 1993) and should be considered an absolute minimum, because they do not permit normal exercise.

Rabbits should have sufficient space to be able to run, rather than simply hopping. Even this minimal amount of space is often not provided (PDSA and YouGov, 2011), as shown in Figure 2.4. The RWAF (2012) guidelines suggest 2.4 m x 1.2 m as a minimum floor area for a run attached to a living area.

Total space requirements

The home range of domestic rabbits in a free-ranging environment is similar to that of wild rabbits (Vastrade, 1987), approximately 2185 m² for entire males and 1580 m² for entire females (Myers and Poole, 1958, 1961). This highlights the fact that rabbits will utilize large amounts of space when provided with it, and that run sizes should be considerably larger than those typically provided. Free range access to a garden or a fenced-off section of it allows greater space that the average run.

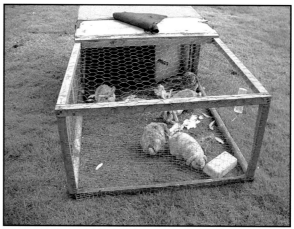

2.4 The rabbits in this set-up of a hutch (approx. 1.2 m x 1.2 m) with a run (approx. 1.5 m x 1.2 m) attached have limited space and are unlikely to be able to run.

Companionship

Rabbits are a social species (see Chapter 5 for further details). Pairs of rabbits are the most widely kept grouping, with trios and quads less common. Single rabbits are not uncommon: 44% of rabbits in one study were not kept with rabbit companions (Mullan and Main, 2006), and 67% in another (PDSA and YouGov, 2011). Some are kept entirely alone, and some with guinea pigs and/or other animals.

Pair bonding in rabbits is discussed later. Bringing siblings up together and then keeping them together is one method, but different gender pairings will behave differently upon maturity.

Gender combinations in paired rabbits

The following combinations are possible in pair-bonded rabbits.

Entire male with entire male

This pairing becomes untenable at adolescence, especially in the breeding season, and particularly if a female rabbit is also present in the area. Previously amicable males will become extremely aggressive towards one another, biting and kicking/scratching each other. Aggression often seems to be directed towards the genital region, and results in variable, but often severe, scrotal and preputial trauma. This can lead to fly strike, infection, scarring and deformity. Most cases can be treated by debriding the affected area, although the long-term prognosis associated with subsequent urinary problems can be poor. Males should not be housed together after sexual maturity unless they have been neutered. Castrating both rabbits prior to bonding is recommended, as neutering may only reduce the amount of aggression if fighting behaviour has already been established within a pair.

Entire male with entire female

This pairing does not tend to be possible on a permanent basis. In addition to the obvious problems with unwanted litters, and the need to separate the parents from oppositely sexed offspring in future to prevent still further litters, when she is not receptive to the male a female rabbit may be aggressive towards his advances. Entire males kept alongside entire females may become distracted by mating behaviour and lose weight, and if they are unable to mate they will become frustrated and potentially aggressive themselves.

Entire female with entire female
This is a common pairing, because entire females together cannot become pregnant, do not appear to fight, and avoid the expense of neutering. However, the arrangement has drawbacks. In particular, neutering is carried out in female rabbits to avoid the risk of extremely common uterine and mammary pathology (in particular, uterine adenocarcinoma). In addition, unneutered female rabbits may restrict access of subordinate animals to favoured areas or food or water and may be aggressive to one another or to anyone entering their 'safe area'. This behaviour may not develop until sexual maturity, although it may be minimized if large amounts of space are available, which is often impractical in domestic settings.

In laboratory situations, groups of entire females may be kept together because it is generally felt that the advantages of social housing outweigh any aggression among individuals. One study of entire female pairs showed that subordinate animals were not prevented from access to favoured items (Chu et al., 2004). However, with some cage designs, the dominant female may be able to block access to areas or items such as food, water, litter areas or enrichment (RSPCA/UFAW, 2008). Such situations have to be planned carefully. They work better with more placid breeds of rabbit, and may not always be possible to achieve in domestic settings.

Neutered female with neutered female
This combination avoids uterine disease, and neutered paired females tend to be more stable and compatible pairs than entire ones.

Neutered male with neutered male
This combination also works well. It is generally felt that this is a more stable pairing than neutered female–neutered female. However, probably because of the possibility of fighting behaviour between unneutered or only recently neutered males, many rescue centres avoid this combination.

Neutered male with neutered female
This is generally held to be the most compatible and stable pairing.

Entire female with neutered male
The female in this situation is likely to be dominant over, and potentially aggressive towards, the male, as well as being susceptible to future uterine/mammary pathology.

Entire male with neutered female
The male in this situation is likely to attempt mating with the female, even though she will not be receptive, which is likely to be a source of disharmony between the pair.

Combinations other than pairs
Trios, quads and larger groupings become progressively more complex, and it is impractical to discuss all the potential combinations here. As a general rule, while they can be extremely stable groupings, with greater numbers comes greater opportunity for conflict. The temporary removal of one animal (e.g. for veterinary attention), or illness causing a rabbit to change position in the dominance hierarchy, may lead to disturbance and fighting, not necessarily involving that individual. All individuals must be neutered in such groups, because intra-gender aggression is much more likely in the presence of the opposite sex.

Greater space and environmental complexity is required to minimize these possible issues, and more feeding, watering and litter points need to be provided to avoid conflict. Hides or shelters require multiple exits (preferably more than two when large groups are housed together), to avoid 'guarding' by dominant individuals.

Controversy exists as to whether two males plus one female are a more suitable grouping than two females and a male. It is likely that environmental factors and the individual nature of the animals are more significant than the genders in any such rabbit grouping.

Housing with other species
Rabbits are often co-housed with other species. This most frequently involves otherwise lone rabbits, in order to provide companionship but without the risks of unwanted pregnancy where the owners have elected not to neuter the rabbit. In other cases, it may be due to provision of outdated information, or because previous attempts at bonding the rabbit with other rabbits have failed.

Guinea pigs
The most common species kept in direct contact with rabbits (as opposed to merely sharing a house with them) is the guinea pig. This has historically been a common husbandry system, pre-dating the routine neutering of rabbits, and persists for traditional reasons. However, several factors mean that it is not ideal:

- Rabbits may bully guinea pigs, owing to their larger size
- Guinea pigs may bully rabbits; it is not uncommon for guinea pigs to sit on rabbits and barber the fur of the head and back
- While pair incompatibility may also be seen between rabbits, and is an important factor in the animals' lifelong welfare, this may be addressed more successfully in rabbit groups
- Rabbits and guinea pigs have different dietary requirements. Guinea pigs have a higher protein requirement than rabbits, and are also unable to synthesize vitamin C and require a dietary source of this vitamin

- Both rabbits and guinea pigs are unable to express a full range of interactive behaviours unless kept with their own species
- Rabbits have been thought to carry *Bordetella* spp. in the respiratory tract as a commensal organism. This bacterium is pathogenic to guinea pigs. However, *Bordetella* has been identified as both a primary and a secondary pathogen in the rabbit also, and its presence should be addressed in either species.

Birds

Rabbits are occasionally housed with birds. For example, the rabbits may occupy the floor and lower areas of an aviary. In most cases there is almost complete effective separation of the two species. Large psittacine birds may cause trauma to rabbits, but most outdoor aviaries in which rabbits are also present tend to hold smaller psittacine and passerine birds without any problems of interspecific aggression. However, food dropped by birds may be ingested by the rabbits. This may lead to nutritional imbalances and obesity where these foodstuffs are low-fibre high-energy items such as fruit or seeds and nuts. Spoiled food is unlikely to be eaten by rabbits unless no other food is present, but it may give rise to enteric disturbances, or be a source of fungal upper respiratory tract disease. Rabbits and hens are occasionally kept together; the coccidian species affecting each animal are different and are non-pathogenic to the incorrect host.

Cats, dogs and other species

Rabbits may share house space, either at the same time or indirectly, with other indoor or indoor/outdoor pets such as cats and dogs (and potentially more exotic species such as reptiles). The main health and welfare concerns in such cases are adverse behaviour and aggression/trauma from the other animals towards the rabbits. Although there are many cases of rabbits coexisting peaceably with dogs or cats, these species are natural predators, potentially capable of injuring or killing a rabbit before human intervention is possible. While cats and dogs often seem not to be aware of a rabbit's prey status, they may suddenly see the rabbit as a foodstuff and change their attitude almost instantly. Owners should be made aware of this, and advised not to allow such access without strict supervision.

Rabbits may act as transient hosts for ectoparasites such as cat and dog fleas, and may require treatment for these as part of a general household flea control regime. Such fleas rarely cause any significant problems in rabbits, although transient minor pruritus may be noted.

Companionship with humans

Some rabbits are kept as sole pets, with only human companionship. This is not ideal, because rabbits are not able to express a full range of social behaviours unless they are kept with members of their own species.

If sole pet rabbits are kept, females should still be neutered, to reduce the chance of future uterine/ mammary pathology, aid in litter training and reduce hormonally induced territorial aggression. Males may be neutered or left entire, because the health benefits of neutering are not as significant, although urine spraying may be an unwanted natural behaviour in entire males. Every effort to provide a stimulating environment and as much interaction as possible should be made.

Children and rabbits

Rabbits generally do not like to be picked up, and may exhibit fearful behaviour, jumping away, kicking out or even biting in order to avoid such situations. Children like to pick animals up, and therefore they should not have unsupervised access to rabbits until they are old enough to understand the rabbit's behaviour. They should be encouraged to handle and stroke rabbits on the floor.

'Antisocial' rabbits

There are a very small number of rabbits that appear incompatible with others. These require behavioural and medical investigation, but if they are truly unable to spend time with other rabbits, spending as much time as possible interacting with humans and other animals may be the best option (see Chapter 5).

Bonding

Bonding is the term used to describe the establishment of a suitably socially housed pair or group in a stable and amicable relationship. It does not automatically occur on placing rabbits together, requiring a bonding process, as described below, to be carried out. Some pairings may prove to be permanently incompatible. Both rabbits in a pair should be neutered, regardless of gender (see above). If only one is neutered, the other will still attempt mating behaviour, which will provide a poor foundation for a permanent bond. Residual hormones after neutering may affect behaviour in both sexes for up to 4 weeks. It is therefore recommended to postpone the introduction until this point.

Two singly housed rabbits have different environmental requirements from a bonded pair housed together. In a pair, each animal must have the opportunity to choose whether to lie with its companion or be apart. They are also dependent on the ability to chase and run from each other to establish and maintain a hierarchy. A hutch is never adequate on its own, but extremely large environments, such as a garden, may lead to a situation where the rabbits are not truly bonded but simply have sufficient space not to need to interact.

Bonded rabbits should not be separated unless absolutely necessary, such as for medical reasons. Their cohabitation is dependent on stability, and they communicate and orientate themselves mainly by scent. Given this, both rabbits in a pair should be taken together to the veterinary surgery if one of them has an appointment. Relocation and other changes in the environment may also lead to temporary quarrels, caused by the necessity to re-establish rank in the new area.

The bonding process

It is important that rabbits are introduced in a neutral area. The species is highly territorial, so they should meet in a novel environment, such as a new pen, or an indoor room that neither animal has inhabited previously (e.g. a bathroom). Using the territory of other rabbits may be successful in some cases, because each rabbit will be confused by the alien scents and the pair will bond together.

Fighting rabbits may be dangerous to separate, and hand protection is necessary (e.g. thick gloves). The rabbits may injure each other severely, particularly if attempting to mount the head area, and this must be prevented.

There are many different ways to bond rabbits, and many different opinions on which method is best (see also Chapter 6).

Bonding process: Method 1

It is commonly advised that rabbits should be introduced in a gradual fashion. The idea is that they should be accustomed to each other's smells and become familiar with one another under controlled conditions.

The rabbits are often placed in nearby enclosures, so that they can sniff each other and consequently be more familiar when they first meet. Exchange of litter trays may also help the rabbits to get used to each other's scent. After a while, short and frequent meetings in a neutral territory are arranged, and the rabbits are separated if there is any sign of tension between them. This is repeated until the rabbits accept each other. The rabbits are not left alone before they are happy to groom each other. This process, depending on the individual rabbits, can take anything from hours to a couple of months.

This method may prolong the process unnecessarily, causing more frustration and stress in the long run to both rabbits and owner. The rabbits do not get the opportunity to establish their hierarchy when separated repeatedly and, owing to the importance of stability, this may be crucial.

Bonding process: Method 2

Both rabbits are taken separately to a new location and released simultaneously. It is normal for them to run after each other, chasing, nipping and perhaps tearing some fur from one another, and this is an important step in establishing the necessary rank order. Owners should be advised not to be concerned if they see mounting behaviour directed to the other's head and back in an attempt to dominate; this can continue for a period after the initial introduction in their shared enclosure at home. It may look dramatic to the owner, but as long as the rabbits do not actually bite each other, they should not need to be separated.

After a while the rabbits might rest, eat or groom themselves near each other. This is a sign of progress, and the rabbits can be put together in their permanent shared enclosure. If they have been transported, the additional mild stress of a car trip will cause them to look to each other for reassurance and become closer. Such mildly stressful situations may also help to re-bond rabbits after separation or a change in the hierarchy develops, e.g. as a result of one becoming ill. The use of highly stressful experiences, such as being placed on or near to noisy machinery (e.g. a washing machine) or in an empty bath has been suggested. The effects of these are partly due to the neutral environment and partly that the surface of a bath is smooth, difficult to stand on, and may smell strongly, which are all sources of stress. However, there are welfare implications to inducing excessive stress, which must be balanced with the importance of bonding.

Finally, the rabbits can be released at home into their joint living area, which should again be a neutral location, or one from which the scent of the existing rabbit should have been removed as thoroughly as possible. They should be provided with plenty of cardboard boxes or other hiding places, and several feeding and drinking stations, in a sufficiently large area. The rabbits should be supervised until they are eating and lying together with no signs of negative behaviour.

Bonding may be achieved in larger groups by placing all the rabbits together as above, or adding one new rabbit to a pair, to replace a companion in a group. It appears that individual personalities are more important than gender because all combinations are capable of working (see earlier), although neutering and allowing sufficient time after neutering for the levels of sex hormones to decrease are vital. Sufficient space for the larger group must be made available.

New rabbit arrivals should be temporarily confined to their smaller 'safe' area, before being allowed out under supervision. This develops a feeling of safety in that area first. They should always be allowed to return to the safe area at will.

Positive signs during bonding:

- Self-grooming
- Mutual grooming (Figure 2.5)
- Lying alongside each other
- Eating.

Neutral signs during bonding:

These indicate that the process is taking place, but is not completed:

- Ignoring each other
- Mounting each other
- Chasing each other
- Pulling fur and nipping but not breaking the skin.

Negative signs during bonding:

- Lunging at one another
- Biting deeply, grabbing hold of skin and deeper tissues rather than fur only ▶

- Obsessive/excessive grooming of one rabbit by the other, which initially appears positive, but may be very likely eventually to result in severe fighting
- Immediate fighting behaviour, e.g. within the first minute of introduction.

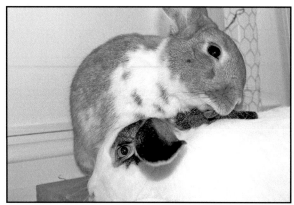

2.5 Mutual grooming is a positive sign during the bonding process. (Courtesy of Marit Emilie Buseth)

Expression of natural behaviours

It is vital that, whatever husbandry system is employed, rabbits can express their natural behaviours safely, as shown in Figure 2.6. This is covered in greater detail in Chapter 5.

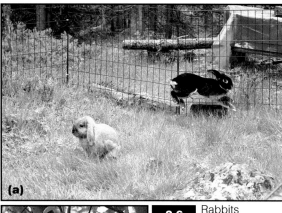

(a)

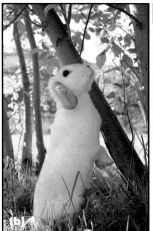

(b)

2.6 Rabbits displaying normal behaviour. **(a)** One rabbit is jumping up in the air, and the other is sitting up and looking around. **(b)** This rabbit is displaying normal investigative behaviour standing on its hindlimbs. (Courtesy of Marit Emilie Buseth)

Environmental enrichment

The best environmental enrichment is an appropriate social group (see above). Environmental enrichment items that may be provided include:

- Boxes of shredded paper, hay or earth to dig in
- Cardboard boxes or tubes, or paper bags stuffed with hay, with or without pelleted food inside
- Newspapers or telephone directories, for chewing and shredding
- Straw baskets or straw brooms, for the rabbits to pull/throw around or chew
- Edible tree branches (e.g. fruit or willow) large enough to be pulled around the floor, or just for chewing
- Willow, straw or twig balls, baskets or other shapes, with or without hay inside (Figure 2.7)
- Hollow toys in which food pellets can be placed, to drop out when they are moved around.

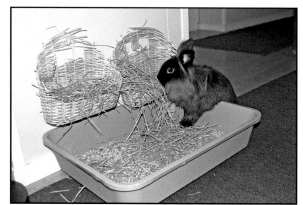

2.7 Straw baskets can be chewed, rubbed against for scenting and also used as hay racks. (Courtesy of Marit Emilie Buseth)

Exercise

Rabbits must have space and time to exercise. Studies at the University of Bristol have shown that the timing of access to exercise areas is at least as important as their size. It is recommended that sufficient space to run around in is provided for at least 4 hours a day, and at least partly at times of day when rabbits are normally active (dawn and dusk), though ideally it should be available *ad libitum*. If exercise is provided only at times other than dawn and dusk, rabbits may have increased stress levels, as indicated by behavioural studies, although they may use the exercise areas at other times if that is their only option (Held, personal communication).

Rabbits are not likely to run on slippery floors, or to use areas where they fear predation.

Encouragement through the provision of toys to push, pull and carry around, interaction and games with humans, and training can all help to promote exercise.

Hiding places

Rabbits require both hiding places and lines of sight with escape routes to feel comfortable in an environment. A balance between provision of hiding spaces and open areas to run, jump and feed can generally be achieved, indoors or outside, by providing sufficient hiding areas within the environment, such as boxes, tunnels or tubes. These should have more than one entrance, to avoid the rabbit feeling trapped (Figure 2.8).

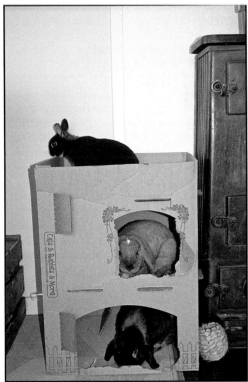

2.8 This cardboard hide has more than one entrance, to avoid the rabbits feeling trapped. (Courtesy of Marit Emilie Buseth)

Rabbits also appreciate being able to stand on top of things, so such items should be robust enough to take their weight. They should be deployed with care so that rabbits cannot use them to gain sufficient extra height to jump over fences and escape.

Scent
A balance between hygiene and disruption of security is important. Cleaning out an environment totally, especially where disinfectants are used, can remove the rabbits' scent and lead to stress. This is particularly an issue where this is carried out repeatedly, and frequently. The rabbits may then begin to scent mark to re-establish their territory, which may be confused with urinary incontinence, or facial pruritus. Leaving some substrate in the environment each time it is cleaned helps to maintain the scent markers.

House rabbits

Rabbits may be housed indoors in various systems and for various reasons: actual or perceived outdoor risks such as predators may be a concern; lack of available outdoor space is commonly an issue in an urban environment; or owners may simply wish to spend more time in contact with their rabbit(s).

In addition to the closer bond between the owner and companion animal, indoor rabbits also benefit from the fact that their owners can more easily detect behavioural changes and subtle symptoms of disease or injuries, as they live in close proximity. House rabbits are often presented much earlier in the course of a disease than outdoor rabbits. However, the rabbits' indoor environment must still permit expression of natural behaviours.

Requirements
The main requirements for indoor rabbits are sufficient space, a suitably complex environment with appropriate environmental enrichment to enable most natural behaviours to be safely expressed, a suitable shelter area and an absence of hazards (Figure 2.9).

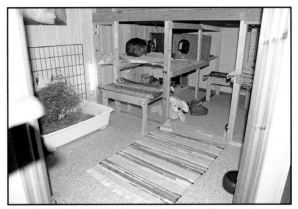

2.9 A suitable indoor environment. Hay and water have been provided, multiple hides can be seen, suitable toys have been provided (cardboard tube, ball, teddy, basket), and there is plenty of space. (Courtesy of Marit Emilie Buseth)

Enclosures
Various materials or pre-constructed items can be used to make indoor enclosures, such as child play pens, puppy pens and compost heap fencing. They can be used to enclose an area for the rabbit, or to protect items within a space.

Such materials are not intended to enclose small animals, however, and the holes may be large enough for young or small-breed rabbits to crawl through or to get stuck in and injured. For tiny rabbits, it is therefore recommended to secure the lower part of fencing with a finer metal mesh.

Cages designed specifically for rabbits are generally unsuitable for anything other than to form a base for litter trays and hay, and an area to retreat into at will. They have no space for enrichment or room for exercise and thus are not suitable as permanent residences. All rabbits confined to such a cage must have an attached exercise run, constructed as above, if they do not have free range of the room or house. They should have permanent access to this run, or have access to it for a minimum of 4 hours a day, preferably at times when the rabbit is naturally active.

Whether the rabbits are free ranging or kept in an enclosure, the environment in which they live must be made safe for them, with the necessary space and 'furniture' available. Water bowls and/or bottles, a food bowl (although the rabbits may be scatter-fed pellets to increase foraging time and provide enrichment) with accompanying hay provision, and a large litter tray, are required.

Rabbits need some private areas, to enable them to get away from each other, humans and other animals, and to feel secure in, and they must have access to hiding places such as cardboard boxes, tunnels or tubes. These should be placed within all rooms and areas to which the rabbit has access.

Substrate

The substrate must be suitable for running and jumping. Large non-slip carpets should be used so that rabbits do not potentially injure themselves trying to jump or run on slippery floors (e.g. laminate, polished wood).

Some carpets contain stiff or irritant fibres, however, which can lead to contact irritation of the plantar and palmar surfaces of the feet. A carpet with a pile depth that is insufficient for claws and toes to sink into will stop rabbits bearing sufficient weight on their toes, resulting in increased contact time and pressure on the hocks. These factors increase the risk of pododermatitis.

Hazards

Potential indoor hazards include electric wires, toxins and a risk of falling. Preventing access to these by providing a safe enclosure within the house is the easiest option. It is possible to supervise the rabbit closely when it is out of its enclosure, but 'rabbit-proofing' any areas to which the rabbit has even occasional unsupervised access is wise (Figure 2.10).

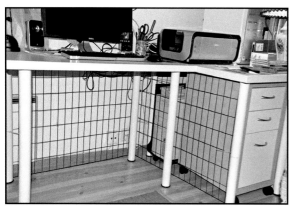

2.10 It is wise to 'rabbit-proof' any areas to which the rabbit has even occasional unsupervised access. A simple panel of plastic-coated wire can be used to prevent access to electrical cables. (Courtesy of Marit Emilie Buseth)

- Much is talked about the potential toxicity of various indoor plants. However, there is controversy about the actual toxic nature of many plants, because there are conflicting lists available. The main indoor houseplant concerns are chrysanthemums and *Dieffenbachia* (dumb cane), although it is worth noting that the bulbs of many other plants are toxic, and it is best to check the safety of any plants in the house specifically. In general, rabbits avoid toxic plants and there are no published reports of plant toxicity in pet rabbits.
- Other toxins include heavy metals, of which the most common is lead. Lead is present in very old toys and paints, as well as leaded glass windows, wine bottle cork coverings, curtain weights, air gun pellets and fishing weights.
- Electrocution is probably the most common – and most preventable – of the hazards faced by rabbits in the home. Rabbits have a behavioural drive to chew long thin items such as wires that resemble young plants and trees. This can cause oral burns and non-cardiogenic pulmonary oedema.
- Poor air quality is less of a concern for rabbits cohabiting with humans than those outside in small confined areas or housed in groups. Ammonia and dust levels may be higher at rabbit level than at human head height, but otherwise the human inhabitants will notice any issues of poor air quality. Tobacco smoke appears to be a risk factor in the development of cardiorespiratory disorders in rabbits, in particular atherosclerosis and chronic obstructive pulmonary disease, and smoking should be avoided in the house (Du, 1991; Zhu *et al.*, 1993).

Litter trays

Litter tray training is mainly relevant to indoor rabbits, as outdoor-housed rabbits generally use a 'latrine' area in an outdoor run or indoor shelter (see below). However, there are similarities between litter tray training and encouraging a rabbit to use a suitable latrine area that are worth being aware of, and owners of outdoor rabbits may benefit from providing litter trays, in terms of improved hygiene and ease of cleaning.

Rabbits urinate, both as elimination and for scent marking, on to objects or other individuals. They defecate for elimination, but faeces are also used for scent-marking purposes. Both urine and faeces are used as subtle chemical signals in the wild, to convey information to rabbits from their own and other warrens. Dominant males tend to have a more marked odour, to scatter their faeces more widely and to urinate on a wider range of objects, in order to mark the limits of their territory, although rabbits generally use a latrine area or areas near the burrow.

There should be sufficient litter trays for all rabbits:

- Generally, at least one per rabbit is needed (although rabbits are more sociable in sharing litter trays than cats are, and one large litter tray per rabbit pair may be better)
- Additional trays may be needed in multi-floor dwellings, or to allow urination in areas where the rabbit might otherwise urinate inappropriately
- At least one tray must be present in any area in which the rabbit is confined for part of the day.

Rabbits that kick litter around may benefit from a slatted base to the tray, under which the litter substrate is placed. Otherwise, suitable litter substrates include shredded paper, hay, soft straw, compressed woodchip or newspaper pellets. *Clay-based clumping cat litter or corn-cob bedding is not advised, unless the rabbit is unable to gain access to it, because ingestion may lead to caecal impaction.*

Hay, placed in an adjacent hayrack, in one corner or in the whole tray, encourages the rabbit to use the tray; in contrast to cats, rabbits will eat and defecate at the same time and in the same location. If the hay becomes contaminated with faeces or urine it must be replenished immediately.

Many rabbits, especially older ones, who are generally more predictable in their urination habits than younger ones, will simply take to using a litter tray. It may take some time to locate the best location for the trays, depending on the rabbits' preferences. Placing faeces and urine from the rabbit in the tray, collected from wherever they currently deposit them, may be useful in establishing it as a latrine area. Initially confining the rabbit to a smaller area within the house, with a litter tray, can be a useful method of establishing the tray as the place for elimination, and can create a sense of safety and security in the rabbit's new environment. This area may be created using human play pens or puppy crates. Once the rabbit has free range of a room, or part or all of the house, it is more likely to return to the established litter area.

Rabbits of both sexes, once mature, are considerably easier to train to use a litter tray if they are neutered, because this reduces the desire to spread their urine and faeces widely over a territory.

Failure of litter tray training: This may be due to inappropriate urination or to scent marking.

- In suspected or actual cases of scent marking, a full medical work-up to exclude urinary tract disease and neuromusculoskeletal problems, and appropriate treatment, are advised.
- If a scent-marking rabbit is entire, neutering is advised. If the rabbit is already neutered, it is likely that it is responding to subtle changes within the environment, which should be addressed.
- Confining the rabbit to a smaller area again, and re-establishing litter training before gradually allowing full access, may be the easiest solution.
- If a specific area is targeted, it is necessary to eliminate (not just cover up) the scent, by using a biological washing liquid and wiping with surgical spirit, or cleaning with white wine vinegar. Alternatively, placing another litter tray in that area, or completely preventing access to that area, may be necessary. Excessive cleaning of the litter tray may stop the rabbit from recognizing it, and therefore following cleaning with replacement of a small amount of soiled litter may be helpful.
- Litter tray training may break down after new animals are added to the social group, or

individuals die or are moved away. Such problems are usually transient and resolve once new groups become established. If multiple groups of rabbits are housed separately within a house, urination and defecation at the boundaries is likely.

Outdoor housing

The typically sized commercially available 'rabbit hutch', by itself, is unsuitable as the sole accommodation for a rabbit or rabbits, although it provides a good secure safe area for sleeping in and retiring to for rest and shelter. Larger hutches, sheds or other shelters allow rabbits to get far away, out of sight of predators, provide more space in inclement weather, and are less susceptible to excessive heat build-up in hot weather. A well insulated nest box within the hutch offers good protection against low temperatures. Ideally, a larger than standard hutch or other area, such as a shed or child's play house, should be combined with a permanently attached secure run, as shown in Figure 2.11. Ideally, rabbits should have permanent access to an outdoor run, so that they are not dependent on being allowed into the run by their owners at limited times.

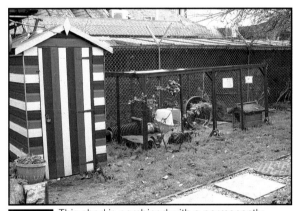

2.11 This shed is combined with a permanently attached and secure run to allow both indoor and outdoor access. (Courtesy of Wood Green Animal Charity)

Temperature

Rabbits are ideally kept at 15–20°C. In the wild they remain mainly in sheltered underground runs during temperature extremes. However, rabbits tolerate temperatures *below* the ideal range relatively well, especially if they are kept free of damp and draughts, are in good body condition, and have a close companion to share body heat with and sufficient bedding. At ambient temperatures below freezing point, rabbits may need supplementary heating. Fresh water must be available at all times; this requires regular replenishment and the use of insulating jackets around bottles.

Even in the UK, the temperature in a shed may exceed the comfortable limit for rabbits. Rabbits tolerate temperatures *above* the ideal range poorly, especially with high humidity. They should be sheltered from direct sun, and not placed in confined spaces such as hutches that they cannot escape from to find cooler areas.

Bringing rabbits inside the home or into outhouses during colder weather may be the best option, but they should not be taken back and forth excessively, because they will struggle to adapt to the differing conditions. If they are brought inside during winter, use of a cooler area of the house is best, to minimize sudden changes of temperature. Garages and sheds may reduce exposure to fresh air and natural light, and may not therefore be ideal, or may require adaptation first. Exercise is still required, and access should be provided to a run during the warmer, drier parts of the day.

Substrates and materials

Grass is the ideal substrate for rabbits kept outside, and should cover at least part of the run area. Excessive time spent standing on concrete may lead to sore hocks. Inside the hutch, bedding may be of hay or soft straw, or dust-free wood shavings.

Hutches are generally made of wood, which has more thermal insulation, is softer on the feet and deadens sound better than metal or plastic, but is difficult to clean thoroughly. Marine ply is less porous and easier to clean, although the edges and joints may need sealing to prevent urine leaking into the wood or damp rising through.

Some hutches are held off the ground, with a ramp to the floor for access. This reduces exposure to damp and cold floors, and offers some protection from predators. Mesh-fronted hutches otherwise offer no protection at night to prevent predators getting extremely close to the rabbit, with potentially fatal stress resulting. The 'Morant' hutch (Figure 2.12) is a moveable hutch/run with a triangular cross-section, which can be carried to an area of fresh grass. While it is practical, by itself it does not offer sufficient space or usable height for the rabbits to sit up on their hind limbs.

Weather protection may be provided by shades (tarpaulin, parasols, etc.) to keep excessive sun or wind and driving rain from the hutch. Plastic sheeting on the front prevents driving wind and rain, but dramatically reduces ventilation. Air quality may become extremely poor, with high ammonia levels in such confined spaces.

Security

Escape must be prevented so that rabbits cannot be caught by predators, run over by cars, or become lost. It is not uncommon for intact females to escape, mate with wild rabbits and return to give birth. Alternatively, wild male rabbits may gain access to domestic females, with the same result. As well as unwanted kits, this allows a breach of biosecurity.

- Holes in perimeter garden fences should be closed off, fences should be of sufficient height to prevent the rabbit jumping out, and all gates and doors should be secure.
- As it is generally impractical to keep out cats and foxes (a minimum 2 metre high fence with angled overhang is required to do so), an enclosed run within the garden is safer (see also 'Runaround' systems, below).
- Mesh runs should be firmly fixed to the ground (e.g. using tent pegs) or weighted down, to prevent being overturned by predators.
- Rabbits may dig under runs, unless they have partly buried mesh with an in-turned section to prevent digging alongside the buried portion. Flooring the run area with mesh is possible; as long as the mesh rests on the ground and grass grows through it, this allows access to grass and is escape-proof, whilst avoiding the rabbit's weight being taken on the wire itself. Generally, female rabbits are more likely to attempt to dig out than males, and neutering reduces this impulse.

Rats and other wild rodents may gain access to almost any outdoor environment, and keeping food securely shut away in closed containers will help minimize the risk of rodent infestation, disease spread and trauma.

Group housing

Some rabbits, typically those in breeding or showing establishments, are housed in stacked (Figure 2.13) or other multiple hutches outdoors, or in sheds (see Figure 2.11). The main problems with this are lack of space (both total space and access to outside runs), lack of social interaction, and problems with maintaining adequate biosecurity and achieving a balance between good hygiene, temperature control, humidity and ventilation.

Sheds may easily overheat, and therefore excellent ventilation is necessary, with windows covered with mesh rather than glass during the summer months and good airflow to create secondary ventilation rather than direct draughts on to the hutch fronts. This may require creation of holes or removable sections of the walls and eaves, which also helps to maintain an acceptable level of humidity and reduce irritant particulates, ammonia and pathogen loads in the air. Further cooling can

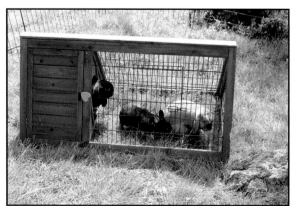

2.12 The 'Morant' hutch. This triangular hutch and run design reduces the amount of vertical space the rabbit can use for sitting, hopping, grooming and standing. The Morant hutch can readily be moved to fresh grass but is otherwise a poor design. (Courtesy of Marit Emilie Buseth)

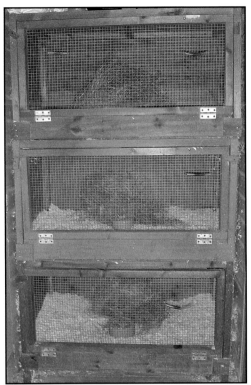

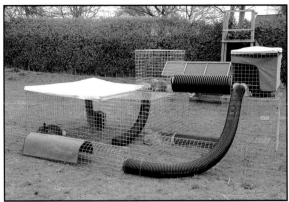

2.14 The 'Runaround' system of housing with attached runs. (Courtesy of Caroline Lord)

2.13 A stack of hutches. The main problems with this are lack of space (both total space and access to outside runs), lack of social interaction, and problems with maintaining adequate biosecurity and achieving a balance between good hygiene, temperature control, humidity and ventilation. These hutches also do not provide any visual security in the form of a hide.

be provided by using fans to move cooler air in, air-conditioning units and reflective panelling surfaces on roofs to reduce the heating effect of the sun. In the winter, the temperature should not be maintained at the expense of a significant reduction of ventilation, because this increases humidity and decreases air hygiene.

Combination housing

Rabbits may be moved between indoor and outside areas; for example, they may be kept predominantly indoors with provision of an outdoor run when weather permits. As long as frequent changes of temperature and exposure to extremes are avoided, and the run is not the sole source of adequate space for exercise, or of grass/hay for forage, this is a good combination.

Tube/tunnel connectors for hutch and run systems

Flexible systems of solid or mesh tubes and tunnels that fit securely to wire mesh runs are commercially available (e.g. Runaround; Figure 2.14). The elements can be set up in any configuration in order to create a secure environment for rabbits, preventing predator attacks, escape and access to poisonous plants or other hazards. The systems can be adapted to any group of rabbits, and the connecting tunnels moved as required. Similar systems can be home-made. This permanent set-up allows

the rabbits to come and go as they please, rather than when the owners are able, or inclined, to lift them from hutch to run, which can be a limitation. A study at the University of Nottingham (Barton and Redrobe, personal communication) showed that rabbits in this system, or in hutches with permanently attached runs, demonstrated more normal behaviours than those kept in hutches only.

Travelling

Travelling stress may be minimized by keeping rabbits in their social groups when transporting them (Figure 2.15). They should be habituated to their travelling box or, if this is not possible, the box should be filled with hay from the rabbit's environment. Food and water should be provided *en route*, in non-spill containers. Boxes should have a non-slip floor substrate. Those made entirely out of open mesh allow excellent ventilation, but rabbits will feel exposed to predators, and the boxes should be covered where necessary. Boxes should be placed sideways on to the direction of transport to minimize the occupants sliding about inside. *Rabbits should not be left in parked cars during warm weather.*

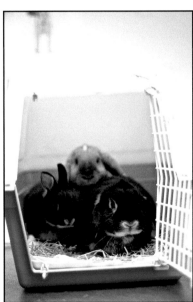

2.15

Travelling stress may be minimized by keeping rabbits in their social groups. (Courtesy of Marit Emilie Buseth)

When owners are away

Rabbits may be boarded or kept in their own environment. The latter is preferable, as long as adequate attention can be paid to them. Transportation of rabbits to boarding facilities is a transient stress, but housing them in unfamiliar surroundings is a greater, more chronic stress, and exposure to disease is a major concern. Access to grass is preferred, but this is difficult to disinfect between rabbits, and infectious diseases may be spread by this route.

Acknowledgements

Many thanks to Rae Todd for reading and commenting on earlier drafts of this chapter, and also to Marit Emelie Buseth for comments, and for supplying many of the illustrations.

References and further reading

Boers K, Gray G, Love J, et al. (2002) Comfortable quarters for rabbits in research institutions. In: Comfortable Quarters for Laboratory Animals, 9th edn, ed. V Reinhardt and A Reinhardt, pp.43–49. Animal Welfare Institute, Washington DC

Chu LR, Garner JP and Mench JA (2004) A behavioral comparison of New Zealand White rabbits (Oryctolagus cuniculus) housed individually or in pairs in conventional laboratory cages. Applied Animal Behaviour Science 85, 121–139

Du BY (1991) The effects of passive smoking on health. Zhonghua Jie He He Hu Xi Za Zhi 14(2), 76–78, 126 [in Chinese]

Dykes L and Flack H (2009) Living with a House Rabbit. Ringpress Books, Dorking

Edgar JL and Mullan SM (2011) Knowledge and attitudes of 52 UK pet rabbit owners at point of sale. Veterinary Record 168, 353

Fairham J and Harcourt-Brown FM (1999) Preliminary investigation of the vitamin D status of pet rabbits. Veterinary Record 145, 452–454

Isbell C and Pavia A (2009) Rabbits for Dummies, 2nd edn, pp.71–92. John Wiley & Sons, New Jersey

Morton DB, Jennings M, Batchelor GR, et al. (1993) Refinements in rabbit husbandry. Laboratory Animals 27, 301–329

Mullan SM and Main DC (2006) Survey of the husbandry, health and welfare of 102 pet rabbits. Veterinary Record 159, 103–109

Myers K and Poole WE (1958) A study of the biology of the wild rabbit Oryctolagus cuniculus in confined populations. I. The effects of density on home range and the formation of breeding groups. CSIRO Wildlife Research 4, 14–26

Myers K and Poole WE (1961) A study of the biology of the wild rabbit Oryctolagus cuniculus in confined populations. II. The effects of season and population increase on behaviour. CSIRO Wildlife Research 6, 1–41

PDSA and YouGov (2011) PDSA Animal Wellbeing (PAW) Report. [available at www.pdsa.org.uk]

RSPCA (2012) Companion Animals Pet Care Factsheet. [available at www.rspca.org.uk]

RSPCA/UFAW (2008) Refining Rabbit Care – A Resource for Those Working With Rabbits in Research. [available at www.rspca.org.uk]

RWAF (2012) Hop To It: The RWAF guide to rabbit care. Rabbit Welfare Association and Fund, Horsham

Todd R and Mitchell A (2012) Rabbit Welfare Association and Fund Rabbit Rehoming Survey. Rabbit Welfare Association and Fund, Horsham

Vastrade FM (1987) Spacing behaviour of free ranging domestic rabbits, Oryctolagus cuniculus. Applied Animal Behaviour Science 18, 185–195

Welsh Government/Llywodraeth Cymru (2011) Code of Practice for the Welfare of Rabbits. [available at http://wales.gov.uk]

Zhu BQ, Sun YP, Sievers RE, Isenberg WM and Parmley WW (1993) Passive smoking increases experimental atherosclerosis in cholesterol-fed rabbits. Journal of the American College of Cardiology 21(1), 225–232

3

Nutrition and feeding

Jenny Prebble

The diet of wild rabbits consists predominantly of grass, with legumes and other wild plants making up a smaller proportion of the diet. Young tree shoots, branches and bark are consumed as grass availability falls. Fruits and cereals are consumed in small quantities when they are available. Ideally the diet of pet rabbits should mimic that of their wild counterparts; however, many are fed a low-forage high-concentrate diet.

Published nutritional requirements for rabbits (NRC, 1977) are outdated and are based on research done predominantly on commercial farmed rabbits, which have a lifespan of 12–14 weeks during which rapid growth and attainment of meat quality are desirable. In contrast, rapid growth and weight gain are detrimental to pet rabbits, where quality of life and a longer lifespan are required. Feeding an appropriate diet to pet rabbits is key in maintaining good health and promoting welfare.

Nutrient requirements

Fibre

Fibre is the type of carbohydrate that forms plant cell walls, and includes cellulose, hemicelluloses, pectins and lignin. These cannot be digested by mammalian enzymes, requiring instead a population of suitable microbes within the gastrointestinal tract. The ability of rabbits to digest fibre is low in comparison to other herbivores. For example, alfalfa hay has a digestibility of 14% in rabbits compared with 44% in cattle and 41% in horses (McNitt *et al.*, 1996). Both the chemical and the physical nature of fibre are important. It can be divided into digestible/fermentable (soluble) and indigestible (insoluble) components, according to particle size. Fibre is separated into its digestible and indigestible components within the proximal colon.

Large particles (>0.3 mm in diameter), made up largely of the secondary cell wall (mainly lignocelluloses), are moved into the colon and rapidly excreted as hard faecal pellets. Whilst it provides no nutritional value to the rabbit, indigestible fibre is an essential component of a rabbit's diet, because it plays a key role in maintaining gut motility and in dental health (see the *BSAVA Manual of Rabbit Surgery, Dentistry and Imaging* for further details). Many commercially available rabbit diets contain inadequate levels of indigestible fibre. Small particles (<0.3 mm in diameter), made up of the primary cell walls of plants, are moved into the caecum. The ease of digestibility of these particles is dependent on their chemical nature. Hemicellulose and pectins are more digestible than cellulose, while lignin is almost completely indigestible. Fermentation of digestible fibre results in the production of volatile fatty acids, which provide up to 40% of the rabbit's maintenance energy requirement.

Fibre measurement is complex and the terminology can be confusing and inconsistent. The level of crude fibre (CF) is legally required to be declared on the packaging of foods. It is a poor measure of total fibre levels, however, because not all fibre types are included and some non-fibre components may be included. It also gives no indication of the ratio of digestible to indigestible fibre. Whilst not frequently reported on packaging, the levels of neutral detergent fibre (NDF) and acid detergent fibre (ADF) give a better indication of the fibre content of feeds. The NDF level is close to the total fibre content of a food, whilst ADF equates to the cellulose and most of the lignin, giving the best indication of indigestible fibre content. The difference between the two is the digestible component.

Grinding during manufacture has a direct impact on the size of fibre particles. Fine grinding of fibre particles leads to prolonged gut transit time and caecal retention time, and increases the potential for caecal dysbiosis (Fraga *et al.*, 1991; Lebas and Laplace, 1997).

The ratio of digestible and indigestible fibre is important in the maintenance of gut motility and providing nutrition to the microbial flora. Low-fibre diets predispose to enteritis and increased mortality, especially in young rabbits. Adequate fibre levels will be reached if *ad libitum* forage (grass or hay) is provided and consumed by the rabbit. When choosing concentrates, foods with a CF level above 18% should be selected. Attention should also be paid to the size of the particles within the food. Pellets/extruded nuggets with no particles above 0.5 mm should be avoided. An NDF above 30% and an ADF above 17% are also advised. The CF level in the overall diet, including forages and concentrates, should exceed 20–25%. Concentrates with a CF level >16% are preferred.

Other carbohydrates

Sugars and starches are an important energy source. They are digested and absorbed in the stomach and small intestine. High-starch diets may be incompletely digested because the rabbit has a rapid intestinal transit time. Residual starch passes into the caecum and is fermented by the microbial population. This is referred to as 'carbohydrate overload' and is thought to be a predisposing factor in the development of diarrhoea in young rabbits. High starch levels alter the microbial population, allowing overgrowth of pathogenic species. High starch levels also predispose to enterotoxaemia as glucose produced from starch digestion is required by *Clostridium spiroforme* for production of iota toxin (Cheeke, 1987). However, as starch and fibre levels are generally inversely related (i.e. low-fibre high-starch), the relative importance of each nutrient is unclear.

Starch digestion appears to be age-related; digestion is less efficient in young rabbits, making them susceptible to carbohydrate overload. Digestion of starch in adult rabbits is more efficient and starch digestion occurs proximal to the caecum (Blas and Gidenne, 2010). The role of high-starch diets in digestive disease in the adult is therefore controversial (Lowe, 2010).

Carbohydrates are found in abundance in grains, roots, seeds, vegetables and concentrate foods. Starches vary in their level of digestibility: those found in cereals are more digestible than those in roots and tubers. Heating starch during the manufacturing process increases starch digestibility.

Protein

Proteins are composed of amino acids, which can be separated into essential and non-essential amino acids. Essential amino acids (Figure 3.1) cannot be synthesized by the rabbit and are required either in the diet or from microbial synthesis within the caecum. Methionine (and/or cystine), lysine and threonine are the most limiting amino acids in rabbit diets (Lowe, 2010).

• Isoleucine
• Leucine
• Lysine
• Methionine
• Phenylalanine
• Threonine
• Tryptophan
• Valine

3.1 Essential amino acids required by rabbits.

Optimum protein levels of 16% for growth and 18–19% for lactation have been suggested. However, these levels are likely to be excessive for pet rabbits, which are prone to obesity, and levels of 12–17% are adequate. The amino acid composition of this protein is important, along with its digestibility. Generally, cereal proteins are rich in non-essential amino acids while those in legumes and peas contain higher levels of essential amino acids. The digestibility and protein composition of forages varies with plant age and the drying process (Lowe, 2010). Protein levels in mature plants are lower and less available because higher proportions are bound to lignin.

Fats

It is generally considered that the essential fatty acid requirements of the rabbit are met by plant materials, and this can be achieved with a diet containing 2.5% fat (Lowe, 2010). As obesity is of concern in pet rabbits, dietary fat levels of 2.5–5% are therefore recommended. Fats within the raw materials should meet the rabbit's requirements; however, oils may be used to coat pellets to increase palatability (Cheeke, 1974).

Vitamins and minerals

Natural vitamins are largely unstable and quickly become oxidized in the presence of light, heat or moisture. Levels in foods can be highly variable. Supplemented compound foods contain protected vitamins and antioxidants to slow vitamin degradation. Current labelling legislation requires the level of vitamins added to the diet to be declared on the packaging, not the vitamin content of the final product. Given that significant quantities of vitamins are lost during the manufacturing process, high levels of vitamins are added to ensure that the final levels meet the animal's requirements. Therefore many commercially available diets appear to contain levels above those recommended. The vitamin requirements and reported deficiencies are outlined in Figure 3.2. As the B complex vitamins and vitamin K are formed by caecal microbes and ingested through caecotrophy, if caecotrophy is not being performed for any reason additional supplementation of these vitamins may be beneficial. Supplementation of vitamins A and K should be considered in cases of hepatic coccidiosis.

Macro-mineral and trace element deficiencies and toxicities are also reported (Figure 3.3). Dietary calcium and phosphorus levels are particularly important. Rabbits have a unique calcium metabolism which is interlinked with that of phosphorus. Calcium absorption from the gut is unregulated, although vitamin D increases calcium absorption when calcium-deficient diets are fed, while phosphorus absorption is regulated by vitamin D. Excess calcium and phosphorus are excreted in the urine. Serum and urinary calcium levels are related to dietary intake. Calcium:phosphorus ratios of 1:1–2:1 are recommended for pet rabbits and are more important than the absolute values of either mineral.

Calcium bioavailability is reduced by compounds that form complexes with calcium, including phytates, oxalates, acetates and phosphate. Phytates are present in high levels in grains and beans. Oxalates are present in many plants including swede, spinach and alfalfa. Plants low in oxalates include kale, broccoli, turnip, collard and mustard greens. Phosphorus bioavailability is influenced by the presence of phytates and phytases. Phytates are phosphorus-rich compounds which cannot be degraded by mammalian systems, but are hydrolysed by plant and microbial phytases. In rabbits phosphorus in phytates is well utilized through phytase production by caecal microflora. Excess levels of either mineral reduce absorption of the other and can induce hypocalcaemia or hypophosphataemia.

Vitamin	Role	Sources	Recommended levels	Deficiency	Toxicity
A (Retinol)	Vision; bone development; reproduction; immune function	Formed in the intestinal mucosa from β-carotene and stored in the liver. Grass and fresh vegetables are good β-carotene sources. Levels in cereals (except maize) and hay are low	10,000–12,000 IU/kg	Deficiency may occur if cereal-based muesli foods are fed because selective feeding may reduce consumption of the vitamin supplemented pellets. Growing rabbits: enteritis; reduced growth; hydrocephalus; cerebellar herniation. Adult rabbits: keratitis; iridocyclitis; hypopyon; permanent blindness	Poor reproduction; birth defects; hypervitaminosis resulting in hyperostotic polyarthropathy has been reported in a rabbit fed exclusively carrots (Frater, 2001)
B complex		Caecal microflora. Needs are met by caecotropy but most rabbit foods are supplemented	Not required	Not reported. B12 deficiency may occur if a low cobalt diet is fed	Not reported
C (ascorbic acid)	Maintenance and repair of connective tissue	Endogenous synthesis from glucose in the liver. It is not required in the diet but supplementation is beneficial in times of stress and illness	Up to 400 mg/kg	Not reported	Not reported
D	Calcium and phosphorus absorption; bone mineralization	Synthesized in the skin in the presence of UVB light. Variable levels present in hay. Converted into its active form in the kidney in response to parathyroid hormone release when serum ionized calcium levels fall	800–1000 IU/kg	Hypophosphataemia. Osteomalacia. Deficiency has been suggested to contribute to dental disease (Harcourt-Brown, 1996). Low vitamin D levels are reported in rabbits kept in hutches compared to outdoor rabbits; however, no clinical abnormalities were reported (Fairham and Harcourt-Brown, 1999)	Soft tissue calcification; fetal mortality; reduced appetite; diarrhoea; ataxia; paralysis; high vitamin D levels may contribute to dental disease (Jekl et al., 2011)
E (tocopherol)	Antioxidant (synergistic with selenium)	Green forages (especially young grass). Cereals. Low levels in hay. Levels rapidly decline in grains stored in moist conditions	50–160 mg/kg	Muscular dystrophy. Poor reproductive performance. Increased incidence of coccidiosis	Not reported; unlike other fat-soluble vitamins, vitamin E does not accumulate to toxic levels; excesses are rapidly excreted in the bile and urine
K	Blood coagulation	Caecal microflora. Grass	1–2 mg/kg	Impaired blood clotting. Deficiencies are unlikely if caecotrophy is being performed	Not reported

3.2 Vitamin requirements of rabbits.

Mineral	Role	Requirement	Deficiency	Toxicity
Calcium	Bone component; tooth component; muscle contraction; nerve conduction; cardiac function; blood clotting	0.4–1%. Minimum for growth 0.22% and 0.44% for maximum bone density (Chaplin and Smith, 1967)	Reproducing does: reduced appetite; tetany; muscle tremors; death. A link between calcium deficiency and dental disease has been suggested	Soft tissue calcification; excess calcium can contribute to the development of urolithiasis in rabbits; however, high calcium diets alone do not cause urolith formation (see Chapter 13)
Phosphorus	Bone component; tooth component; energy storage (ATP)	0.4–0.8%	Growing rabbits: rickets. Adults: osteomalacia	Reduced bone mineralization; a link between excess phosphorus and dental disease has been suggested
Magnesium	Bone component; enzyme cofactor	0.3–3%	Poor growth; alopecia; altered fur texture; hyperexcitability; convulsions; fur chewing; myocardial infarction	Excess excreted in the urine

3.3 Mineral requirements of rabbits. (continues) ▶

Mineral	Role	Requirement	Deficiency	Toxicity
Potassium	Maintaining osmotic pressure; acid–base balance; cardiac function; enzyme cofactor	0.6%	Muscle weakness; paralysis; cardiac abnormalities; respiratory distress; under conditions of stress potassium excretion increases and may result in temporary hypokalaemia; the value of potassium supplementation in periods of stress has not been studied	Higher incidence of nephritis; reduced growth rates
Sodium	Regulation of pH; maintenance of osmotic pressure; nutrient transport	0.2–0.25%	Not reported but may result in reduced efficiency of digestive processes and amino acid absorption	Reduced growth
Chloride	Acid–base balance; hydrochloric acid in stomach	0.17–0.32%	Not reported	Excess (0.4%) does not impair performance
Iron	Component of pigments (haemoglobin, myoglobin) and enzymes involved in oxygen transport and metabolism	30–400 mg/kg	Anaemia; unlikely owing to supplementation in pet diets	Acute: sudden death; decreased myocardial contractility. Chronic: reduced food intake; reduced growth
Copper	Enzyme component	5–20 mg/kg	Can occur if high levels of molybdenum are consumed; decreased growth; grey hair; bone abnormalities; anaemia	Excess copper accumulates in the liver; sudden death; anaemia; depression
Manganese	Amino acid metabolism; cartilage matrix formation	8–15 mg/kg	Poor brittle bone; leg problems	Encephalopathy can be induced experimentally following chronic overexposure
Zinc	Enzyme component; cell division	50–200 mg/kg	Immune suppression; poor weight gain; increased mortality	Not reported
Selenium	Antioxidant; rabbits are more dependent on vitamin E than selenium to reduce oxidative load (Jenkins et al., 1970)	0.05–0.32 mg/kg	Not reported	Not reported
Iodine	Thyroid hormones	0.4–0.5 mg/kg	Goitre may occur if high levels of goitrogens are fed; goitrogens are found in brassicas such as cabbages and turnips	Increased fetal mortality
Cobalt	Component of vitamin B12 synthesized by caecal microflora	Up to 1 mg/kg	Reduced B12 production	Polycythaemia

3.3 (continued) Mineral requirements of rabbits.

Abnormalities in calcium and phosphorus levels have been implicated in the development of dental disease. Calcium-deficient diets (0.11–0.34%) with an inverse Ca:P ratio have been reported in rabbits selectively fed muesli-type diets (Harcourt-Brown, 1996). This study concluded that a low-calcium diet may be a contributory factor in the development of dental disease; however, the calcium content of other dietary components was not reported. High levels of phosphorus fed alongside normal calcium levels in a Ca:P ratio of 1:1 are associated with reduced bone mineralization and with dental disease (Jekl et al., 2011; Gumpenberger et al., 2012; see the BSAVA Manual of Rabbit Surgery, Dentistry and Imaging for further details).

Recent research has also demonstrated that muesli diets with normal calcium levels and Ca:P ratios, even when selectively eaten, are associated with the development of dental disease (Prebble, Shaw and Meredith, unpublished).

Pre- and probiotics

Pre- and probiotics are added to diets with the aim of reducing the incidence of digestive disease. Probiotics are live organisms that are thought to colonize the gut and contribute to the maintenance of a healthy gut flora. Probiotics, including Bacillus spp. (Maertens et al., 1994; Nicodemus et al., 2004) and *Saccharomyces cerevisiae* (Onifade *et al.*, 1999; FEEDAP, 2012), have been used in rabbits with mixed success. Some studies report decreased mortality in treated groups whilst one noted increased mortality (Maertens *et al.*, 1994), and inconsistent improvements in weight gain and feed conversion ratios have been recorded. *Lactobacillus* spp. are not normally found in the rabbit caecum and therefore are not likely to be effective as a probiotic in rabbits. The benefits of probiotics in pet rabbits are unclear. One study investigating the effects of *Enterococcus faecium* and *S. cerevisiae* in healthy rabbits found some evidence that these probiotics can modify body-weight and levels of certain gastrointestinal bacteria (*Bacteroides* spp., *E. faecium*, *Fibrobacter succinogenes* and *Clostridium spiroforme*) when compared with a placebo and given for 14 days (Benato *et al.*, 2012).

Prebiotics are non-digestible ingredients that selectively stimulate beneficial species of bacteria with potential benefits for the health of the rabbit. Various oligosaccharides are currently added to rabbit feeds. In commercial rabbit production reduced mortality, improved feed conversion rates and improved performance have been reported following the addition of oligosaccharides (Mourao *et al.*, 2006; Mateos and de Blas, 2010). The benefits of prebiotics for pet rabbits are unclear.

Energy requirements

The energy requirements of rabbits are affected by age, breed, sex, reproductive status, exercise levels and environmental factors (temperature, humidity, air movement).

- The maintenance requirements of non-reproducing adult rabbits can be calculated using the equation: 400 kJ/day/kg $LW^{0.75}$
- For growing, pregnant or lactating rabbits the energy requirement is 430 kJ/day/kg $LW^{0.75}$

where LW = live weight (Xiccato and Trocino, 2010).

Feeding behaviour

Wild rabbits

Wild rabbits spend 70% of their active time eating, consuming large volumes of low-energy foods. The rabbit is adapted efficiently to make use of a low-energy high-fibre diet, both through the specialized digestive tract and through the selective consumption of young plants of the highest nutritive value. Rabbits also successfully avoid toxic plants within their environment. They are very selective in their preferences and can distinguish between fertilized and unfertilized ground (Miller, 1986), and among hays cut at different times of day (Maryland *et al.*, 2005). The choice of plant species varies with seasonal changes in local flora, which can be very sparse during winter months. While grasses dominate the diet, other plants, leaves, tree saplings and bark also contribute, particularly in winter when grass is limited.

Regulation of food intake

Food intake is regulated by both appetite and hunger. *Hunger* is a physiological state based on energy needs. It is triggered by blood glucose, amino acid, lactic acid and volatile fatty acid concentrations and by stomach contractions. *Appetite* is subjective, made up of acquired preferences and habits related to feeding time.

The volume consumed depends on the nutritional composition and physical nature of the diet. Increasing fibre level and reducing digestible energy content increase the volume consumed. Production rabbits are reported to alter their feed intake as digestible energy changes, to maintain growth rates. This does not appear to be true of pet rabbits, which can become overweight as a result of consuming excess calories. However, if very low-energy, low-protein diets are offered to small breeds they may be unable to maintain body condition.

Rabbits feed selectively, choosing foods that are high in energy and protein, and will eat concentrate foods in preference to forage; if the former are offered in unlimited quantities very little hay will be consumed. When offered in limited quantities concentrates are usually consumed rapidly. Food preferences are influenced early in life by the mother's diet. Kits prefer the diet that was consumed by their mother during pregnancy and lactation (Bilko *et al.*, 1994). It may be difficult to persuade some rabbits to eat new food items (particularly hay) when they are accustomed to a certain diet. This is especially true if they were not offered the food when young. However, if concentrates are fed in restricted amounts, most rabbits will increase their hay intake if good quality hay is offered.

Growing rabbits may consume up to twice as much as adults at maintenance. Lactating does consume three times as much, and may be unable to consume sufficient amounts and consequently lose weight. Neutered rabbits have lower energy requirements than entire rabbits and are more likely to become overweight. Disease states usually decrease food intake, while nutritional requirements are increased. Limiting access to fresh water decreases dry matter (DM) intake (Prud'hon *et al.*, 1975). House rabbits kept in warm ambient temperatures may require less energy than outdoor rabbits (depending on activity levels).

Diet components

Forages

Grasses form most of the diet of a wild rabbit. Grass provides a balanced source of protein, indigestible and digestible fibre, vitamins and minerals. It has fibre levels of 20–40% and protein levels of 15–19%. Young grass has lower fibre and higher protein (up to 30%) levels. As the plant matures, fibre levels increase and protein levels decrease (to as low as 3%).

Ideally, pet rabbits should be able to graze an area with a variety of grass and plant species (Clauss, 2012); however, for the majority of rabbit owners this is impractical. Whilst grazing is preferred, grass can be cut and offered fresh. **Lawnmower cuttings should never be offered because they ferment rapidly and can cause digestive disturbances.**

Hay can be used as a substitute for grass or alongside it. If constant access to good quality grazing is not possible, hay should be provided *ad libitum*. A variety of grass species are used in hay-making, including timothy, ryegrass, fescues and cocksfoot. Meadow hay contains a variety of grasses and often some clover. Alfalfa (lucerne) hays are commonly grown in the USA but are less common in the UK. Legume hays, including alfalfa, are higher in protein (16.5%) and calcium (1–1.5%) with a Ca:P ratio of 5:1 and should not be fed in large quantities to adult rabbits.

The nutritional content of hay varies widely among grass species and with time of cutting. The drying process destroys many of the vitamins present, particularly vitamins A and E. Vitamin D is formed in the presence of ultraviolet (UV) light; however, the quantities are variable and can be low, even in sun-dried hay. Hay stored over long periods may be subject to significant losses, especially of any remaining vitamins. Hay cut before flowering provides the best quality. Second- or third-cut hays are from more mature grass containing higher levels of fibre (especially lignin) and lower levels of protein.

There are many reasons a rabbit may not eat hay, including over-feeding of concentrates, offering poor quality or mouldy hay, soiling of hay when used as bedding, not offering hay to young rabbits, and dental disease. Hay intake can be encouraged by gradually reducing concentrates. It may take several weeks for hay intake to increase as the rabbit adapts to the change in diet. Good quality hay should be provided away from bedding to prevent soiling. Toilet rolls, hay racks, paper bags, cardboard boxes and toys made to hold hay can all be used (Figure 3.4). Rabbits often defecate where they eat, so providing fresh hay near to the litter tray may be beneficial. Experimentation with hay made from different grass species is effective in some rabbits. Concentrates, dried herbs and treats can be mixed into the hay to encourage foraging. If hay is continually rejected a full dental examination (including radiography if necessary) to rule out dental disease is indicated (see *BSAVA Manual of Rabbit Surgery, Dentistry and Imaging*).

Straw has little nutritional value and although rabbits may eat it, it is not suitable as a foodstuff and will cause deficiencies if fed in large quantities. The feeding of silage is occasionally reported but is generally impractical. The high moisture content restricts DM intake and reduces growth rates in farmed rabbits (Partridge *et al.*, 1985).

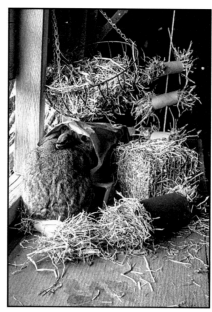

3.4 A variety of everyday and purpose-made items can be used to prevent hay becoming soiled and to provide enrichment.

Concentrates

Coarse mixes containing cereals, legumes, extruded biscuits and pellets are commonly fed. Alfalfa stalks may be added to increase fibre levels. Locust bean hulls may be included as they are very palatable but they can cause intestinal obstruction if swallowed whole (Harcourt-Brown, 2007). Selective eating of these diets is common, with pellets and whole grains frequently rejected (Harcourt-Brown, 1996). This can lead to an unbalanced diet, particularly if pellets containing vitamin and mineral supplements are not consumed. If fed, concentrates should be offered in limited quantities (15–25 g of high-fibre pellets per kg bodyweight per day) and the next meal only provided when the previous one has been consumed. In the author's experience some components can be so unpalatable that they will never be consumed. The feeding of muesli-type diets cannot be recommended because they are associated with the development of digestive and dental disease.

Extruded and pelleted foods can overcome the issue of selective feeding and ensure consistent nutrition. Extruded foods can contain long fibre particles and have increased starch digestibility as a result of heat treatment during the extrusion process.

Edible plants

Green plants provide variety, moisture, micronutrients and dental wear. As water content is high and fibre levels relatively low, consumption of large quantities would be required to meet the rabbit's requirements. The amount offered daily should therefore be limited. New greens should be introduced gradually to allow the caecal flora to adapt. Both commercially available and wild plants can be fed to rabbits (Figure 3.5). Suitable commercially available vegetables include broccoli, cabbage, chicory, chard, collard, parsley, watercress, celery leaves, endive, radicchio, rocket, bok choi, basil, romaine lettuce, kale, carrot and beet tops. Wild

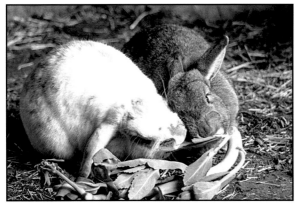

3.5 Greens are well liked by rabbits; a variety of suitable greens should be offered daily.

plants include brambles, dandelion, chamomile, chickweed, clover, comfrey, goosegrass, lavender, plantain, sunflower, nettle, wild strawberry, dock and yarrow.

Treats

Many treats available commercially are high in sugar, fat and/or starch, and are not suitable for rabbits. Human foods, including bread, breakfast cereals, crisps, biscuits and chocolate, are not appropriate. Suitable treats include commercially available high-fibre treats, dried herbs and small quantities of fruits or root vegetables, which contain too much sugar to form a regular part of the diet.

The diet

Feeding the correct diet is essential to maintain health and welfare and prevent diet-related disease. The best diet for rabbits is one that mimics as closely as possible the grass-based diet that wild rabbits evolved to eat. Grass and/or hay should form the bulk of the diet (Figure 3.6) and be available at all times. Green foods (commercially available or wild) should be fed daily and washed prior to being offered. Whilst it is possible to maintain many pet rabbits on hay and fresh greens alone, ensuring that the rabbit receives adequate micronutrients can be challenging (Clauss, 2012). Feeding a limited quantity of a mono-component food provides additional vitamins and minerals to balance the diet, particularly if hay is fed, as its vitamin content is low. All concentrates should be considered complementary; although some are labelled complete they should not be fed alone and muesli-type diets should be avoided completely. Grass/hay intake will be reduced if *ad libitum* concentrates are offered, and this leads to obesity, dental and GI disease, boredom and behavioural problems. The quantity fed should not exceed 25 g/kg of a high-fibre (>16%) pellet/extrudate. Neutered rabbits and those with limited exercise opportunities can require considerably less than this. Body condition score should be monitored frequently and the quantity of concentrates adjusted to maintain ideal weight. If the correct diet is fed, vitamin and mineral supplementation is generally not required.

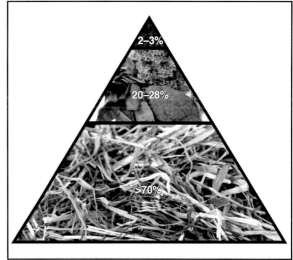

3.6 Pelleted/extruded foods should form only a small portion of the diet. It is essential for rabbits to receive a diet made up of more than 70% hay.

All changes in diet must be made gradually; new items should be introduced over a period of 7–14 days. Several weeks may be required for rabbits, which are particularly sensitive to dietary changes, to adapt. If concentrate diets are being changed, the amount of the new diet should be gradually increased while that of the previous diet is gradually reduced. Sudden changes in diet alter the caecal microflora and can allow the overgrowth of pathogenic bacteria. This may be a factor in the development of gut stasis and reduction in the consumption of caecotrophs.

Feeding for life stages

Feeding kits (including hand-rearing)

Does feed their kits once a day and may ignore them the rest of the time, leading owners to assume that the kits have been rejected (see Chapter 4). Unfed kits have thin abdomens and wrinkled skin as a result of dehydration. Hand-rearing kits is time-consuming and challenging, especially if the kits are under 7 days old. They commonly suffer from aspiration pneumonia and diarrhoea as a result of the lack of protection from milk oil, failure to establish a normal gut flora and overgrowth of pathogenic bacteria.

Kits should be placed in a box containing hay, maternal fur (if available), soft cloths or fleece veterinary bedding. Those under 7 days old should be kept in an incubator or airing cupboard. Above this age, the temperature can be reduced if the kits are thriving. Rabbit milk is concentrated (30–40% DM), high in fat (40–50%) and protein, and low in lactose (5–10%). Milk substitutes close to these values are recommended; those produced for kittens or zoo animals are suitable. Cow's milk should be avoided. Full cream goat's milk and evaporated milk diluted 50:50 with water with the addition of egg yolk and corn syrup have been used. Commercial milk substitutes are recommended and should be made up according to the instructions and fed at body temperature. Made-up milk can be kept refrigerated for 24 hours and warmed for feeding.

Syringes or bottles with teats designed for kittens can be used. Teat-feeding carries a reduced risk of aspiration of milk and is preferred. Weak kits may require nasogastric feeding.

The kit's head should be gently restrained between the thumb and second finger and the first finger placed on the head if necessary. If using a syringe, it should be gently inserted behind the incisors and the plunger gently depressed; milk must be given slowly to minimize the risk of aspiration. Kits should be allowed to swallow between mouthfuls. Once syringe-feeding has begun, it is usually not possible to revert to teat-feeding because the sucking reflex is lost. Once they are accustomed to feeding, kits refuse further milk when they are full.

Feeding regimes vary between three and six times a day; four times a day is usually adequate. Approximate volumes are outlined in Figure 3.7.

Age	Volume (ml/day)	Solid foods
Newborn	2	
1 week	13	
2 weeks	20	Feed caecotrophs from a healthy adult
3 weeks	25	Offer fresh hay and water
4 weeks	30	
5 weeks	20	Limited quantities of concentrates and greens can be introduced if eating hay well
6 weeks	Weaned; gradually reduce the amount offered	

3.7 Suggested volumes of milk replacer for kits that are being hand-reared.

A water bottle can be provided at 3 weeks old. Rabbits need to establish a normal gut flora to prevent digestive disease; this can be achieved by feeding them caecotrophs from a healthy adult rabbit. These can be fed directly to kits or mixed with milk and provided once their eyes are open, but before solid foods are offered. If caecotrophs are not available probiotics are an alternative but their efficacy has not been demonstrated. Probiotics (including yoghurt preparations) made for humans are not suitable because lactobacilli are not a normal part of the rabbit's GI flora. Preparations for animals are available. Initially only hay should be offered, and only once hay intake is well established should concentrates and greens be introduced gradually. Young rabbits are not as efficient as adults at digesting starch, and providing concentrate foods and greens too early or in large amounts can result in alterations in caecal pH and microflora, leading digestive disorders, diarrhoea and death. Feeding a hay-based diet will prevent this.

Frequent weighing is essential; if weight gain is poor, higher volumes or more frequent feeding will be required. For kits of up to 10–14 days old, urination and defecation should be stimulated after feeding by wiping the perineum with a damp clean cloth or cotton wool.

Growing rabbits

After weaning, kits should receive a hay-based diet. Commercial pellets should be fed in a measured quantity and not provided *ad libitum*. Commercial pellets labelled as 'junior foods' contain higher levels of energy, protein and calcium than adult diets but, as they are complementary to the diet, 'junior foods' may not be more beneficial than 'adult foods'. Greens can be fed from weaning and should be introduced one type at a time and initially in small quantities. Adult foods can be introduced from 4–6 months, as the rabbits reach maturity. Following neutering, transition on to an adult diet (if not already done) is recommended because neutered rabbits are prone to weight gain.

Pregnancy/lactation

The pregnant rabbit should remain on a diet of hay/grass and concentrates. Food intake will increase during pregnancy to meet the higher energy and protein requirements. Levels of concentrates can be in-creased but should not exceed 25 g food per kg bodyweight per day. They should not be offered *ad libitum* because this may predispose to diseases caused by reduced forage intake. Introduction of some alfalfa hay into the diet can boost energy intake while maintaining fibre levels. During lactation, weight loss is common because energy expenditure exceeds intake.

Senior rabbits

The point at which a rabbit is considered mature is unclear and varies with breed. Larger breeds will reach maturity at an earlier point than smaller breeds. No research has been performed to assess the nutritional requirements of older rabbits. Commercial pellets labelled as 'mature diets' for rabbits generally have reduced calorie content to limit weight gain and lower protein to reduce the load on the kidneys. They are also often supplemented with compounds such as glucosamine which may aid health, although there is little evidence demonstrating their efficiency. *Ad libitum* hay should be provided alongside these diets. Older rabbits that are unable to maintain weight require veterinary examination but may also benefit from the provision of a higher-energy diet.

Water intake

Fresh water should be available at all times. Vitamin supplements should not be added to water because they may reduce intake, and vitamin requirements should be met if an appropriate diet is fed. Water intake can be increased by feeding a higher proportion of greens and/or grass, as a higher fibre diet promotes a higher intake of water. Most rabbits prefer to drink from bowls rather than from bottles.

Uneaten caecotrophs

Rabbits that are not consuming caecotrophs should be examined for conditions that may prevent caecotrophy (see Chapter 12). If such conditions are found to be absent, dietary alteration can increase caecotroph consumption. Gradual reduction of concentrates encourages hay intake. Higher fibre levels and lower protein levels reduce the number of caecotrophs left uneaten. A hay-only diet may be required initially, before the gradual reintroduction of other foods. If a specific food triggers recurrence the offending item should be eliminated from the diet.

References and further reading

Benato L, Hastie P, Shaw D, Murray J and Meredith A (2012) The semi-quantitative effect of probiotic *Enterococcus faecium* NCIMB 30183 and *Saccharomyces cerevisiae* NCYC Sc47 on the faecal microflora of healthy adult rabbits (*Oryctolagus cuniculus*) using real time PCR. [Clinical Research Abstract] *BSAVA Congress 2012 Scientific Proceedings: Veterinary Programme* p.460

Bilko A, Altbacker V and Hudson R (1994) Transmission of food preference in the rabbit: The means of information transfer. *Physiology and Behaviour* 56, 907–912

Blas E and Gidenne T (2010) Digestion of sugars and starch. In: *Nutrition of the Rabbit*, ed. C de Blas and J Wiseman, pp.17–38. CABI, Wallingford

Chaplin RE and Smith SE (1967) Calcium requirement of growing rabbits. *Journal of Animal Science* 26, 67–71

Cheeke PR (1974) Feed performances of adult male dutch rabbits. *Laboratory Animal Science* 24, 601–604

Cheeke PR (1987) Nutrition–disease interrelationships. In: *Rabbit Feeding and Nutrition*, pp.176–200. Academic Press, London

Clauss M (2012) Clinical technique: Feeding hay to rabbits and rodents. *Journal of Exotic Pet Medicine* 21, 80–86

Fairham J and Harcourt-Brown F (1999) Preliminary investigation of the vitamin D status of pet rabbits. *Veterinary Record* 145, 452–454

FEEDAP (The Panel on Additives and Products or Substances used in Animal Feed; European Food Safety Authority) (2012) EFSA panel on additives and products or substances used in animal feed. Scientific opinion on the safety and efficacy of actisaf sc47 (Saccharomyces cerevisiae) as a feed additive for rabbits for fattening and non food-producing rabbits. *EFSA Journal* 10, 2531.

Fraga MJ, Perez de Ayala P, Carabano R and de Blas JC (1991) Effect of type of fiber on the rate of passage and on the contribution of soft feces to nutrient intake of finishing rabbits. *Journal of Animal Science* 69, 1566–1574

Frater JL (2001) Hyperostotic polyarthropathy in a rabbit – a suspected case of chronic hypervitaminosis A from a diet of carrots. *Australian Veterinary Journal* 79, 608–611

Gumpenberger M, Jeklova E, Skoric M, et al. (2012) Impact of a high phosphorus diet on the sonographic and CT appearance of kidneys in degus, and possible concurrence with dental problems. *Veterinary Record* 170, 153

Harcourt-Brown F (1996) Calcium deficiency, diet and dental disease in pet rabbits. *Veterinary Record* 139, 567–571

Harcourt-Brown F (2007) Gastric dilation and intestinal obstruction in 76 rabbits. *Veterinary Record* 161, 409–414

Jekl V, Gumpenberger M, Jeklova E, et al. (2011) Impact of pelleted diet of different mineral composition on the crown size of mandibular cheek teeth and mandibular relative density in degus. *Veterinary Record* 168, 641

Jenkins KJ, Hidiroglou M, Mackay RR and Proulx JG (1970) Influence of selenium and linoleic acid on the development of nutritional muscular dystrophy in beef calves, lambs and rabbits. *Canadian Journal of Animal Science* 50, 137–146

Lebas F and Laplace JP (1997) Le transit digestif chez le lapin: IV. Influence de la granulation des ailments. *Annales de Zootechnie* 26, 83–91

Lowe JA (2010) Pet rabbit feeding and nutrition. In: *Nutrition of the Rabbit*, ed. C de Blas and J Wiseman, pp.309–332. CABI, Wallingford

Maertens L, Van Renterghem R and De Groote G (1994) Effects of dietary inclusion of paciflor (bacillus cip 5832) on the milk composition and performances of does and on caecal and growth parameters of their weanlings. *World Rabbit Science* 2, 67–73

Maryland H, Mertens D, Taylor B, et al. (2005) Diurnal changes in forage quality and their effects on animal preference, intake and performance. In: *Proceedings, 35th Californian Alfalfa and Forage Symposium, Visalia, California*, pp.223–230

Mateos GG and de Blas C (2010) Minerals, vitamins and additives. In: *Nutrition of the Rabbit*, ed. C de Blas and J Wiseman, pp.145–176. CABI, Wallingford

McNitt JI, Cheeke PR, Patton NM and Lukefahr SD (1996) *Rabbit Production*. Interstate Publishers, Danville, IL

Miller GR (1986) Evidence for selective feeding on fertilized plots by red grouse, hares, and rabbits. *The Journal of Wildlife Management* 32, 849–853

Mourao JL, Pinheiro V, Alves A, et al. (2006) Effect of mannan oligosaccharides on the performance, intestinal morphology and cecal fermentation of fattening rabbits. *Animal Feed Science and Technology* 126, 107–120

Nicodemus N, Carabano R, Garcia J and De Blas JC (2004) Performance response of doe rabbits to toyocerin (*Bacillus cereus* var. Toyoi) supplementation. *World Rabbit Science* 12, 109–118

NRC (1977) *Nutrient Requirements of Rabbits, 2nd edn*. National Reseach Council, Washington, DC

Onifade AA, Obiyan RI, Onipede E, et al. (1999) Assessment of the effects of supplementing rabbit diets with a culture of *Saccharomyces cerevisiae* using growth performance, blood composition and clinical enzyme activities. *Animal Feed Science and Technology* 77, 25–32

Partridge GG, Allan SJ and Findlay M (1985) Studies on the nutritive value of roots, cabbage and grass silage for growing commercial rabbits. *Animal Feed Science and Technology* 13, 299–311

Prud'hon M, Cherubin M, Carles Y and Goussopoulos J (1975) Effets de differents niveaux de restriction hydrique sur l'ingestion d'aliments solodes par le lapin. *Annales de Zootechnie* 24, 299–310

Xiccato G and Trocino A (2010) Energy and protein metabolism. In: *Nutrition of the Rabbit*, ed. C de Blas and J Wiseman, pp.103–132. CABI, Wallingford

4

Reproduction

Sarah Elliott and Brigitte Lord

Veterinary surgeons with a good understanding of the reproduction and breeding of rabbits will be able to support their clients, and this is an important component of the provision and development of a rabbit-friendly practice (see Chapter 6). An appreciation of how the modern rabbit breeder rears and breeds their stock (including the effect of seasonal influences, and the relevance of rabbit shows) is essential, as is an understanding of basic rabbit genetics, selective breeding for desired characteristics and how to avoid common genetic diseases.

Reproductive anatomy and physiology

In the male rabbit ('buck'), the testes descend at 10 weeks of age into the hairless scrotal sacs but may be withdrawn back into the abdomen, through the permanently open inguinal canals, outside the breeding season, at times of fear or during hierarchical disputes. The penis (Figure 4.1) can be easily extruded from the age of 8 weeks by digital pressure at its base. Male rabbits have several accessory glands: the vesicular; prostate; proprostate;

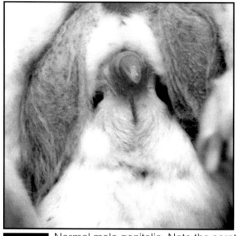

4.1 Normal male genitalia. Note the scrotal sacs lying cranial to the penis, and the close proximity of the anus. Inguinal glands can be seen adjacent to the anopreputial junction.

paraprostate; and small paired bulbourethral glands (Figure 4.2). The vesicular and prostate glands lie in the dorsal wall of the seminal vesicle. The proprostate and paraprostate glands are variable in number and are minute.

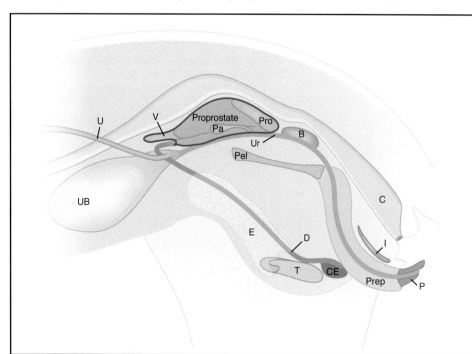

4.2 Diagram of the lateral view of the reproductive tract of the buck. The purple line indicates the seminal vesicle wall which is attached to the vesicular gland, prostate, paraprostate and proprostate glands. B = bulbourethral gland; C = colon; CE = cauda epididymis; D = deferent duct; E = epididymal fat pad; I = inguinal gland; P = penis; Pa = paraprostate gland; Pel = pelvis; Prep = prepuce; Pro = prostate; T = testis; U = ureter; UB = urinary bladder; Ur = urethra; V = vesicular gland.

In the female rabbit ('doe') the elongated ovaries attached to long suspensory ligaments are located more caudally than in bitches and queens. The paired uterine horns then form two cervices and unite to form a large flaccid vagina (Figure 4.3).

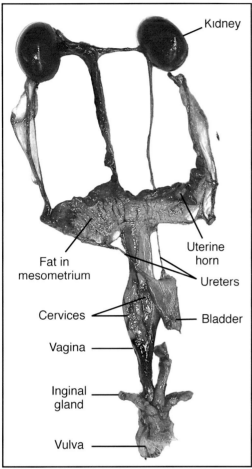

4.3	Normal female urogenital tract removed and displayed during post-mortem examination.

Genetics of rabbit breeding

The European wild rabbit *Oryctolagus cuniculus* is the predecessor of all domestic rabbits. The first clear records of domestic rabbit keeping and breeding, including the existence of various colour forms and sizes, come from the 16th century.

The rabbit has 22 pairs of chromosomes. Each chromosome carries many genes that encode traits such as size, coat colour and hair type (Magnus, 2006). The traditional and current rabbit breeds were initially established by selective breeding based on colour, size and coat type, depending on the personal fancy of the breeder or the intended use of the rabbit (meat, fibre production), and new breeds and varieties continue to be established.

Coat colour

Traits may be dominant or recessive. For example, in a wild rabbit the white-bellied agouti coat pattern allele *A* is dominant over the self-pattern allele *a*, while the recessive tan pattern allele (*at*) produces a tan-patterned animal which looks rather like a self-patterned rabbit but with some tan and a white belly colour.

- *AA* (dominant homozygous), *Aat* (agouti, carrying tan pattern) and *Aa* (agouti, carrying self pattern) rabbits will express the agouti pattern.
- *atat* (tan pattern, carrying tan pattern) and *ata* (tan pattern, carrying self pattern) rabbits will express tan pattern.
- *aa* (recessive homozygous) rabbits will express self pattern.

Genetic disorders

Inbreeding increases the risk of expression of deleterious mutated genes and may be a cause of genetic birth defects. Other factors, including infection of the doe during pregnancy, malnutrition and stress, can also lead to birth defects. Outcrossing, the selective breeding of individuals that are not related, leads to hybrid vigour, which will reduce the occurrence of most genetic birth defects. However, some dominant genetic defects such as the lethal dwarf gene may be difficult to breed out of a line.

Dental defects

A survey of the genetic disorders seen by breeders in the UK suggested that oral and dental defects were the main problems seen in the fancy, fur and lop breeds at 39%, 37% and 31%, respectively (Lord, 2011). Developmental abnormalities such as cleft palate and lack of teeth have also been reported but seem to be rare. Development of fewer than normal teeth is more common than a total absence. The lack of peg teeth is common in some breeding lines, where it can occur as either a dominant or recessive trait. Hereditary mandibular or maxillary length mismatch has been demonstrated to be an inherited defect (Weisbroth and Erhman, 1967). Only a small shortening of the upper maxilla (maxillary brachygnathism) is required to cause severe problems due to primary malocclusion and overgrowth of the incisors (long teeth, 'wolf teeth', 'walrus teeth'). Incisor malocclusion can be seen from as early as 4 weeks of age. As seen in the 2011 survey and reported in the literature, incisor malocclusion occurs more frequently in miniature rabbit breeds, particularly the lop breeds. Abnormal mandibular or maxillary length can also affect the cheek teeth and the effects of cheek tooth malocclusion tend to be seen at an older age than primary incisor abnormalities. These malocclusions may only be clinically apparent after sexual maturity and breeding, and therefore may be perpetuated.

Body size and shape

Body size defects, including under- or oversized kits (Figure 4.4), were seen as the main birth defect in the Rex breed (47%), and in the lop breeds they were seen with similar prevalence to dental disease, at 31%, in the 2011 survey (Lord, 2011). Size inheritance is determined by several general genes, unlike coat colour, and mutations of these genes can lead to birth defects related to size (Fox, 1994).

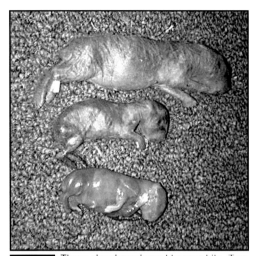

4.4 Three dead newborn Havana kits. Top = oversized; middle = small; bottom = underdeveloped or died *in utero*. (Courtesy of Amanda O'Gorman)

'Peanut' babies are not uncommonly seen in dwarf breeds. These kits are born with abnormally large heads and small bodies. The 'peanut defect' has been seen in the Minilop, Minilion Lop, Netherland Dwarf, Mini Rex, Lionhead and Cashmere Lop breeds.

The 'Max Factor' defect (Figure 4.5) has been seen in Netherland Dwarf, Minilop and Lionhead breeds. Kits with this genetic defect are also known as 'frog' babies; the eyelids are open at birth, the legs may be misshapen, the feet are webbed or clumped and the coat may be longer around the head, giving them a round-headed appearance.

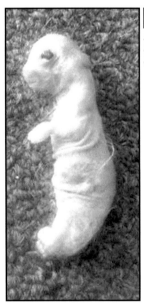

4.5 This dead newborn kit shows 'peanut' and 'Max Factor' deformities. (Courtesy of Amanda O'Gorman)

Ascitic kits (Figure 4.6) are sometimes seen, especially in the Dutch breed.

Selective breeding has been used to manipulate size inheritance to produce a wide variety of breeds from the smallest, the Polish, to the largest, the Continental Giant. The Polish breed was developed by selective breeding of diminutive forms

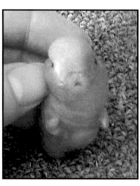

4.6 A dead newborn ascitic kit. (Courtesy of Amanda O'Gorman)

occurring among other breeds, particularly the Dutch. The Polish breed is not only the smallest of the standard breeds but is also a dwarf form. Therefore Polish rabbits have Dutch conformation and, except for the fact that they are albinos, are in reality diminutive (dwarf) Dutch rabbits. However, they vary considerably in size and it has been found that the smaller Polish rabbit individuals transmit a still smaller lethal type of dwarf, entirely different from the normal young of Polish rabbits (Greene, 1940).

The dwarf condition (or 'runts' of the litter) can be identified as various types:

- **Type 1:** The diminutive form; appears to be attributable to size variations of the same genetic order as those that characterize the size variations of standard breeds and have produced animals of the Polish, Netherland Dwarf, Minilion, Mini and Dwarf Lop breeds
- **Type 2:** Those that are small because of the location of the embryo in the uterus. Birth size and weight increase if the embryo is attached to the uterine horn further away from the cervix
- **Type 3:** Small body size due to genetic disease such as the lethal dwarf gene leading to pituitary dwarfs, also known as 'peanuts' and 'Max Factor' babies (see earlier).

The lethal dwarf gene: The primary effect of the dwarfing gene is an inhibition of secretory functions of the anterior pituitary gland in the brain. The acidophilic cells responsible for growth hormone and prolactin are mainly affected, resulting in pituitary dwarfs. As this lethal gene is dominant, it is expressed in both homozygous and heterozygous individuals. In homozygous animals the inhibition is complete and the variation is expressed as a lethal dwarf, which results in a miniature stillborn individual approximately one-third the size of its normal siblings. In heterozygous animals the function of the pituitary gland is altered and some growth hormone is produced, but suppression of the basophilic cells producing follicle-stimulating hormone (FSH) and luteinizing hormone (LH) occurs, causing atrophy of the gonads and partial dwarfism. These undersized animals are typically two-thirds the size of their normal siblings at birth and never attain an equal stature, but may survive for 1–2 months without the full complement of pituitary hormones (Greene, 1940).

Domestic rabbit breeding

Rabbits may be bred for the pet trade, exhibition, or for meat or fibre production. Breeding stock must always be strong, lively, in good body condition and free from disease. It is essential that careful breeding records are kept in order to enable the tracking of any hereditary faults or defects.

In veterinary practice it is most often accidental breeding that is encountered. Figure 4.7 provides a summary of information that can be helpful when addressing the concerns most commonly raised by owners.

Body condition

Rabbits should be lean and muscular, never fat or poorly covered (ideal body condition score (BCS) 3 using a 1–5 scale; see Chapter 7). If breeding for exhibition, those animals that conform most closely to the desired breed standard should be used.

Stock should be housed suitably in a well ventilated area that avoids extremes of temperature, and be cleaned out regularly and fed appropriately (see Chapter 2). Rabbits, especially the doe, should not be bred from whilst in moult because hair growth also places a demand on body resources. The aim with a doe is for her condition to continue to improve throughout pregnancy (Sandford, 1996). The doe should be in firm muscular condition when mated (BCS 2.5–3). The concentrate portion of the food ration should remain the same for the first 3 weeks of gestation; it can be gradually increased over the final 10 days and be double the original amount by the time the kits are a week old. The doe should be offered *ad libitum* hay and water and daily green vegetables throughout this period.

Infection control

The area in which stock is housed should only contain animals free from any signs of infectious disease, especially respiratory problems. Faecal levels of Coccidia within the group should be closely monitored and reduced with an effective treatment (see Chapter 12). Stock should be established as being free of *Encephalitozoon cuniculi*. It may not be practical to test each individual but breeders should understand the risk factors, seek veterinary advice on establishing regimes and remove any animal with clinical signs potentially associated with *E. cuniculi* (see Chapter 15).

Age

The general characteristics of reproduction for the different breeds of rabbit are similar. The larger breeds, such as the New Zealand rabbit, require a longer time to reach puberty and sexual maturity and have larger litters than the smaller breeds such as the Dutch (Figure 4.8).

When determining whether a rabbit is old enough to breed, both physical and behavioural maturity should be taken into consideration. A young doe may be physically capable of conceiving and parturition, but the doe is less likely to produce good quality milk if she is still growing herself, and her offspring will suffer. There is also a higher incidence of scattered litters and poor nesting with very young does.

Puberty in females is defined as the age of first induced ovulation and will occur prior to sexual maturity as indicated in Figure 4.8; therefore it is not desirable to run entire bucks and does together. This will result in untimely and repeated litters.

- **Accidental mating:** If a litter is not wanted, consider spaying in early stages of pregnancy or giving aglepristone.
- **Pregnancy diagnosis:** Via ultrasonography at 6+ days, radiographically at 11+ days or by palpation at 10–12 days by an experienced person.
- **Length of gestation:** Average 31 days, range 30–33 days.
- **Delivery:** Does will often give birth at night or early in the morning, so all that is seen by the owner are a few spots of blood and a moving nest of fur.
- **Re-mating:** The doe is fertile immediately after giving birth so entire male companions should be removed. If they are not the doe will very likely go on to produce a second litter a month later. In rare cases delayed implantation may occur.
- **Difficult deliveries:** It is very unusual to witness a doe in labour. Early signs include pulling fur. A doe observed straining or with visible spots of blood in the absence of kits is likely to be experiencing difficulty. The need for veterinary intervention is indicated.
- **Feeding:** Does feed their kits once or at most twice daily; this is rarely witnessed. For this reason owners often assume that a litter is being neglected.
    - It is not always possible to tell whether kits are being fed in the first 48 hours, therefore they should only be removed from the doe if she is harming them or too unwell to care for them.
    - If after 48 hours the kits are unfed the skin will be wrinkled owing to dehydration, they may feel cool to touch and be weak. Now is the time to decide whether to start supplementary feeding or hand-rearing.
    - Kits 2–5 days old may still be very active and vocal when touched; it is not unusual for them to be hungry at this stage, especially if it is a large litter.
- **Kits:** Altricial, i.e. born blind, naked and helpless.
    - Kits should not be handled in the first few days other than to check they are alive.
    - Eyes open at 10–12 days.
    - Kits start to leave the nest any time after the eyes open. The longer the kits stay in the nest the better fed they are. Some kits will not be seen until nearly 3 weeks of age.
    - Daily handling of kits from the time they leave the nest is good but only for very short periods to begin with.
- **Sexing:** Best done at 4 weeks of age; between 6 and 10 weeks it can be a little more awkward. If an experienced examiner is finding it difficult to determine the sex, the possibility of a buck with hypospadias should be considered. These males will often appear to be female and it can be difficult to be sure of their sex until the testes descend.

4.7 A summary of information that can be used when answering concerns commonly raised by owners.

Breed	Adult bodyweight (kg)	Age of sexual maturity (months)	
		Males	*Females*
Polish	0.9–1.1	4	4
Netherland Dwarf	0.5–1.1	5	4–5
Miniature Lop	1.5	6	6
Dutch	2–2.2	4	6 (puberty from 4)
Dwarf Lop	1.9–2.3	5–6	5–6 (puberty from 3)
Lionhead	1.3–1.7	4	3–4
Rex Standard	2.7–3.6	6	5–6
French Lop	>4.5	8	8 (puberty from 5)
New Zealand White	4–5.4	7–8	8 (puberty from 6)
Continental Giant	>5	10–12	9 (puberty from 6)
Flemish Giant	>4.9	10–12	9 (puberty from 6)

4.8 Age of onset of sexual maturity in bucks and does of common breeds. The age of onset of sexual maturity, i.e. when full reproductive capability is achieved, will vary with strain, husbandry conditions and bodyweight. Puberty in does is defined as the age at the first induced ovulation. (Data from Foote and Carney, 2000; BRC, 2012)

Does may exhibit any of the following behaviour when ready for mating:

- Excessive digging
- Scenting
- Increased aggression
- Becoming more territorial.

Any doe not bred before 12 months of age will be much less likely to conceive and will tend to have smaller litters. Very small litters can include abnormally large kits, leading to dystocia. This can necessitate a caesarean section or lead to maternal and kit fatalities.

When to breed
In the wild the breeding season starts in January and continues until September. Ovarian activity decreases with the shorter day length in late summer to winter; however, the doe can be fertile all year round if conditions are right. Domestic rabbits should be guaranteed a constant diet with adequate nutrition, unlike in the wild. Day length can be extended where rabbits are kept in a building with an electricity supply. Daylight fluorescent tubes mimic natural light and timers can be added so that the lights come on and turn off at a set time each day. Rabbits are reflex ovulators and the doe will ovulate 10–13 hours after mating. Although there is no regular oestrous cycle, there are short periods of 1–2 days every 2 weeks when the doe is not receptive to the buck.

Those breeding for exhibition will plan litters to provide young and adult stock for major shows. Specialist club youngstock shows are held between June and September in the UK and are limited to rabbits between 3 and 5 months old, the exception being Dutch rabbits, which should be 3–4 months old according to the rules of the British Rabbit Council. The breeder will therefore plan matings to provide stock for these shows. Many fur, Rex and a few of the fancy breeds have their best coats between 6 and 10 months of age, so this will also be a consideration in planning because the show life is very short. Other fancy breeds and lops may show until 2–4 years of age. These breeds carry a lot of points for their type and maturity and are less dependent on their coat quality, whilst the fur breeds carry most of their points on coat quality and colour. Those breeding for exhibition tend to have far fewer litters per annum than those breeding for the pet trade. Their focus is to breed stock to show rather than to sell.

Number of litters
Breeders of exhibition rabbits will wish to have maybe two or a maximum of three litters from a doe per year; those breeding for meat will wish to have more. The decision to stop breeding from a doe should not be age-related, though an age of 2.5–3 years is about average. It is more important to stop if there are signs of problems, e.g. late or difficult delivery resulting in oversized or dead kits, or kits failing to thrive.

Mating

Both buck and doe should be checked over to ensure there are no health problems prior to mating. If the doe is overweight and carrying excess body fat, fertilization is much less likely.

It is usual to take the doe to the buck's hutch for mating or to allow the rabbits to mate on a shed floor or running free in a garden. The buck should never be brought to the doe's hutch because she will exhibit territorial aggression. Some breeders supervise the mating process carefully on a table or hutch top, to ensure that no damage befalls their show stock. It is not unusual for a doe to be resistant to being mated and refuse a buck initially. This can result in injury occurring to either or both rabbits. Careful supervision of the mating process also allows the breeder to ensure that mating has occurred.

A receptive doe, ready to be mated, will lift her tail and rear her back end to facilitate the mating process (Figure 4.9). A method of assisted mating may be used when does are reluctant: one hand steadies the doe's front end, while the other hand slides under the belly, raising the hindquarters slightly, the vulva being pressed upwards and backwards with the finger and thumb (Sandford, 1996). After mounting (Figure 4.10), the buck will fall off the doe's back to the rear or side on ejaculation. It is not unusual for the buck to grunt or scream at this point. It is usual to

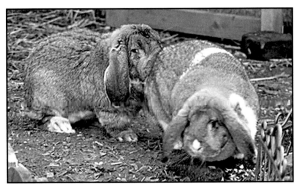

4.9 A French Lop doe lifting her back end and tail, showing that she is receptive to mating. (Courtesy of P Batey)

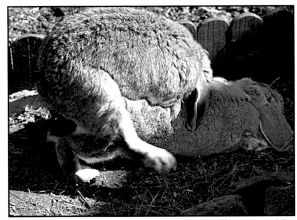

4.10 Mating in a pair of French Lops. (Courtesy of P Batey)

allow the buck to re-mate the doe two to three times before placing her back in her hutch. It is the act of mating which causes ovulation so repeated mating helps to increase the likelihood of conception.

Should unwanted accidental mating occur, pregnancy termination may be performed by ovariohysterectomy in the early stages of pregnancy or administration of the progesterone receptor antagonist aglepristone to prevent early pregnancy, before implantation. A recent study showed that aglepristone 10 mg/kg injected subcutaneously twice 24 hours apart on days 6 and 7 after mating could prevent pregnancy in the rabbit after unwanted mating without any side effects (Özalp *et al.*, 2010).

Pregnancy

Detection
Pregnancy diagnosis is possible from the 6th or 7th day using ultrasonography (Özalp *et al.*, 2010) or from day 11 radiographically (Harcourt-Brown, 2002). Palpation of the abdomen at around 10–14 days is possible; the embryos will be about marble sized, and care should be taken not to mistake faecal pellets for embryos (Sandford, 1996). It is important when palpating the abdomen of a doe that she is relaxed, because tightening of the abdominal muscles will make detection of fetuses more difficult.

Gestation
The date of mating should be recorded, along with the expected date of delivery. The gestation period averages 31 days but can be between 30 and 33 days. Kits born outside of this time frame are often already dead. The signs of pregnancy or pseudopregnancy include behavioural changes such as an increase or reduction in digging, change in temperament and loosening of hair on the dewlap, which is pulled out by the doe to build a nest for the kits. Some does will build a nest well in advance, others will wait until they are in labour and a few will not create a nest at all.

Pseudopregnancy, which lasts 16–17 days, is easily induced in the doe and can be caused by infertile mating, sexual excitement resulting from a doe mounting another doe, or stress.

Does can be allowed to exercise normally for the first 4 weeks of pregnancy but should be left quietly in the hutch for the last few days when they are likely to be nesting, to prevent parturition from occurring in an unsuitable location. The doe should be settled in a familiar environment and protected from any unfamiliar noises or situations. The hutch and enclosure should be large enough not only to allow plenty of room for the doe and her nest but also for the kits until they are at least 8 weeks of age. An ample supply of clean hay or straw should be available from 26 days in addition to a thick layer of wood shavings to absorb urine from the kits. Some breeders prefer straw to hay for bedding because kits may become entangled in hay and lose limbs. Some breeders will provide a nest box for their does but this is not essential. It is inadvisable to disturb the doe for the first few days after delivery. If the hutch does not have a separate nesting area then part of the hutch front may be covered to provide a dark area.

Parturition
Parturition is called kindling. The hutch should be checked each day for signs of nesting and delivery. It is not unusual for the only sign that delivery has occurred to be slight movements in the nest area; however, there may be visible spots of blood on the shavings and occasionally uneaten placentas. These should be removed and disposed of because they will attract flies and are a possible source of infection.

On occasion, kits will have been delivered away from the nest area and be lying exposed in another area of the hutch. It is suggested that the doe be given greens or vegetables to eat while the kits are picked up, checked for signs of damage and then placed into the nest with the other kits. Should any kit be cold it should be warmed up prior to replacing in the nest. This can sometimes be successful even when the kit is stiff with cold and appears dead. Once warm and clearly moving its limbs, the kit can be placed carefully back in the nest and covered with fur and bedding.

Litter size

An average litter size is 4–8 kits. Does of smaller breeds (e.g. Netherland Dwarf, Polish) tend to have smaller litters and those of giant breeds (e.g. British Giant, Continental Giant) much larger litters, with 12–14 kits not being unusual. Litter size is controlled by both heritable and environmental factors (Sandford, 1996). The general health of a doe, her age, nutrition and number of previous litters will all affect litter size. In Dwarf breeds, litters of 1 or 2 kits are not uncommon and it is not unusual for these kits to be very large and to die at 33–34 days' gestation. It is very important with these breeds to select does from lines that produce litters of a good size with no kindling difficulties. Sometimes breeders of giant breeds will unconsciously select for smaller and smaller litters owing to the fact that kits from smaller litters tend to be of greater than average weight (Sandford, 1996). In general a doe's first litter will be smaller than the second and subsequent litters, with older does (>3 years) tending to produce fewer kits.

Care of the doe and new kits

Supplies of hay and roughage should always be plentiful to facilitate gut motility in the doe. It is important to ensure an ample supply of fresh water at all times to prevent dehydration. If a doe usually drinks from a water bottle then putting a bowl of water in the hutch, especially during warmer weather, may increase her water consumption. It is usual to feed a doe with a litter twice daily, morning and evening, ensuring that the quantity is not excessive but allowing for the fact that she will need twice as much concentrate as she ate prior to breeding by the time her litter is a week old. It is important to continue to give fresh vegetables and hay and to keep the water bottle topped up. The doe will increase her fluid intake as lactation increases.

The doe will feed the kits once or sometimes twice daily, going to the nest and uncovering the babies for the time that this takes, usually only a few minutes. It is very common for owners to think that a litter has been abandoned if they do not see the doe with her kits, when in fact many does will rear a litter without anyone witnessing visits to the nest.

It is wise to check the nest daily to ensure that there are no dead or injured kits. If the doe is used to human attention and handling she is unlikely to object. Should the doe be territorial and distressed she can be offered a favoured food item while this is done. Some does will pile excessive bedding on the kits when covering the nest. Copious amounts of straw and fur cause no harm; however, excessive amounts of wood shavings may cause overheating and suffocation, especially in warm weather.

The kits should not be handled unnecessarily in the early days because this can lead to damage or rejection by the doe. Does subjected to loud unexpected noise (e.g. fireworks) or those feeling threatened by other animals are more likely to damage, mutilate or scatter their litters.

Kits can be carefully observed by parting the fur and bedding in the nest (Figure 4.11). The nest should be warm to the touch. In the first 24–48 hours the kits will almost certainly be quite active and vocal because the doe's milk is scarce until the third day. It is only on days 2–3 that it is possible to determine whether the kits are being well fed. Unfed kits will by now be cool to the touch, wrinkled through dehydration and less active or vocal. Well fed kits will be warm, content and have full stomachs. It is however not unusual for many kits at this stage still to be fairly active and vocal, especially in large litters where there may be a limited milk supply per kit.

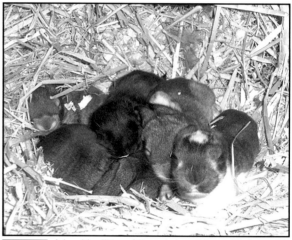

4.11 A healthy litter of French Lop kits at 12 days old, which are well grown and still happily settled in the nest. (Courtesy of H Elliott)

Kits receiving an ample supply of milk will not leave the nest area until 2–3 weeks of age. The eyes open at 10 days or thereabouts. If kits are found outside the nest prior to this, they may have come out when feeding, being latched on to the nipple when the doe jumped off the nest, or just be very hungry, and should be returned carefully to the nest and littermates. Any kit that has not opened both eyes by 12 days old should be picked up and the eyes should be bathed gently open with clean cotton wool and cooled, boiled water. Failure to do this may result in infection, ulceration of the cornea and possible long-term problems such as blindness or entropion.

Caecotrophy starts at about 3 weeks of age, and weaning takes place at 4–6 weeks.

Fostering kits

Breeders will often mate two or more does at the same time, thereby increasing the chances of being able to foster kits if the need arises. This is far more successful than hand-rearing. Kits may be fostered to even out the numbers or if a doe fails to produce enough milk. If a doe dies then her kits should only be fostered if they are disease-free. Kits born by caesarean are generally best fostered, if another doe is available. The kits in both litters should be of similar age and fostering will be most successful during the first 5 days of life. This is simply achieved by letting the foster doe out of her hutch or feeding her to distract her, while placing the young within the nest, underneath the doe's own kits. Care should be taken not to foster more kits than the doe can manage, usually limited to one to two additions. Occasionally the foster doe will recognize and remove foreign kits, but this is rare.

Hand-rearing

This should only be taken on as a last resort and with the knowledge that hand-reared newborn kits rarely survive to become fit, healthy adult rabbits. Before making a decision to interfere, it is essential to ensure that it is necessary. It is unusual to observe a doe suckling her kits and it can be difficult to determine whether kits have been fed for the first 48 hours; therefore they should generally be left alone for this period as long as they are in the nest and not being damaged. Even if the kits appear hungry it does not necessarily mean that the doe is not feeding them; it may just be that the milk is slow to come in or that there is not enough milk. There are two ways to provide extra support.

- Some does, particularly if it is their first litter, are slow to realize what they need to be doing. It may be possible to turn a doe on to her back, cradled in the arms, and for a second person to place one or more kits on her belly and allow it to find a nipple and feed. If the kits are being suckled successfully their abdomens can be seen to fill gradually; when a kit has had enough, it will detach from the nipple and fall asleep. It often happens that after a couple of days the doe will start to mother successfully or her milk quantity will increase and it will be obvious on assessment that the kits no longer need that extra access to milk.
- The second method is to supplement with a bottle feed while still allowing kits to stay with the doe.

Kits should only be completely hand-reared if the doe dies, is too unwell to care for them or is damaging them. The environment should remain as undisturbed as possible, and if the kits are warm and in a nest in a hutch they can be left there during hand-rearing. See Chapter 3 for further details on feeding techniques and regimes for hand-rearing rabbits.

Older kits that have been orphaned (at >2 weeks of age) can be introduced to a rabbit drinking bottle containing milk feed. They would usually learn from the doe how to feed, so it may be necessary to sit each kit in front of the bottle, tap the ball-bearing with a finger to initiate flow and then offer it to the kit. This may require considerable patience but kits will generally start to lick milk from the bottle. Once this is well established, both milk feed and a separate bottle with water can be fixed to the cage. This enables the kit to feed at will and will encourage independence and normal development. This, together with space to exercise and correct feeding, will reduce incidence of gastrointestinal problems. No kit should need bottle feeding after 4–5 weeks of age.

Handling kits

Once the kits start to leave the nest they should be picked up daily by the owner to get them used to being handled. This should only be for very short periods of time, a couple of minutes to begin with. Kits are very quick and likely to make sudden movements at this stage, and should only be handled by experienced individuals. If they are dropped, significant injury may occur.

Breeders of exhibition rabbits will teach a rabbit to pose correctly for its breed from around 4 weeks of age. The rabbit will be removed from the doe and its siblings, placed on a firm non-slip surface and encouraged to sit in the correct position for judging at a show. For example most of the lop breeds are taught to stand square on their fore-limbs to display their deep chests and 'the crown', the basal ridge of the ears which should appear prominent across the top of the skull. Their broad, well furred ears should be carried close to the cheeks, giving a horseshoe-like outline when viewed from the front. This is achieved by lifting the rabbit's head gently until it is in the correct position; the rabbit may then be fed a small treat. Polish rabbits and Belgian Hares are required to stand in digitigrade stance on the forelimbs and plantigrade on the hindlimbs to show off their arched back, with the general appearance of a graceful but racy and alert nature. Himalayans are required to be 'snaky' in type so will be encouraged to lie in sternal recumbency with their head up in a normal prone position.

Health checks and sexing

The kits should be carefully checked at 3 weeks of age to ensure that no damage has occurred to their ears, limbs or tail. Some kits are prone to getting soft faeces stuck around the anus; these should be gently removed. It is possible to sex kits at 3–4 weeks of age (Figures 4.12 and 4.13) and indeed it may be easier than at 6–10 weeks. The kits should also be checked at this time for incisor alignment and occlusion, and for congenital problems such as hypospadias (Figure 4.14). It is a good idea to weigh kits weekly until at least 10 weeks of age to monitor their progress.

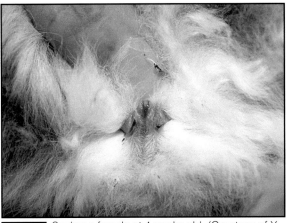

4.12 Sexing a female at 4 weeks old. (Courtesy of Y Bradley)

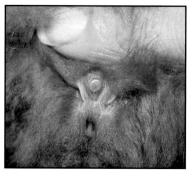

4.13 Sexing a male at 4 weeks old. (Courtesy of Y Bradley)

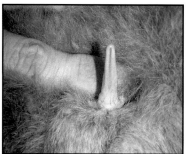

4.14 Hypospadias in a 5-month-old Dwarf Lop.

References and further reading

British Rabbit Council (2012) *Breed Standards.* [available at www.thebrc.org]

Foote RH and Carney EW (2000) The rabbit as a model for reproductive and developmental toxicity studies. *Reproductive Toxicology* **14**, 477–493

Fox RR (1994) Taxonomy and genetics. In: *The Biology of the Laboratory Rabbit, 2nd edn*, ed. P Manning *et al.*, pp.1–19. Academic Press, London

Greene HSN (1940) A dwarf mutation in the rabbit, the constitutional influence on monozygous and heterozygous individuals. *Journal of Experimental Medicine* **71**, 839–857

Harcourt-Brown F (2002) The rabbit consultation and clinical techniques. In: *Textbook of Rabbit Medicine*, pp.52–57. Butterworth-Heinmann, Oxford

Lord B (2011) Genetic diseases seen in the Fancy, Fur, Lop and Rex breed rabbits. *Fur and Feather Magazine* **105**(Feb), 42–43

Magnus E (2006) Genetics, reproduction and breeding. In: *Teach Yourself Keeping a Rabbit*, pp.100–118. Hodder Education, London

Özalp GR, Çalışkan C, Seyrek-İntaş K, *et al.* (2010) Effects of the progesterone receptor antagonist aglepristone on implantation administered on days 6 and 7 after mating in rabbits. *Reproduction in Domestic Animals* **45** (3), 505–508

Sandford JC (1996) Reproduction and breeding. In: *The Domestic Rabbit, 5th edn*, pp.181–193. Blackwell Science, Oxford

Weisbroth SH and Ehrman L (1967) Malocclusion in the rabbit: a model for the study of the development, pathology and inheritance of malocclusion. *Journal of Heredity* **59**, 245–246

5

Normal behaviour and behaviour problems

E. Anne McBride

As with organic disease, the prevention, diagnosis and resolution of behaviour problems requires a deep understanding of the healthy animal and all the potential factors, both intra- and extra-corporeal, that can contribute to the manifestation of problems. Behaviour is the expression of how an animal is feeling, both in terms of its physical state, such as hunger or pain, and its emotional state, be that pleasure, frustration, fear or relief. Behaviour problems may be an indication of underlying organic issues, possibly even before clinical signs are present, as in canine hypothyroidism (Hamilton-Andrews et al., 1999). Alternatively, they may reflect environmental situations that have initiated and/or maintained the behaviour, or result from a combination of both illness and environment. How a particular animal responds to the situation in which it finds itself will be determined by its species, breed, individual genetics and health status, by the environment (both social and physical), and by what the rabbit has learnt through both classical and operant conditioning.

Certainly, a major part of dealing with behaviour problems is to reach an appropriate diagnosis through careful and extensive history-taking, which includes the behaviour of the animal itself and that of others who interact with it, both human and non-human animals. One needs to understand fully not only what the rabbit is doing, but also why. This chapter provides an introduction to normal rabbit behaviour and how this relates to behaviour problems. The basics of taking a behavioural history are described. An understanding of normal behaviour and its associated emotions will assist veterinary professionals in advising owners on prophylactic measures to deter the development of behaviour problems, as well as providing ideas for their resolution.

It is estimated that some 35,000 rabbits per annum are relinquished to rescue centres in the UK, the majority within 3 months of being acquired (Copping, 2009). Rabbits that are properly cared for can have a life expectancy of 5–10 years or more (depending on breed), and will cost some £1500 to keep each year, excluding veterinary treatment beyond vaccinations (RSPCA, 2012). A major reason for rabbits being abandoned or given up to rescue societies, or merely left in solitary confinement in their hutches, is behaviour – in particular aggression towards their owners. Many problem behaviours are the result of misunderstandings between rabbit and owner and thus can be prevented or resolved. Sadly it is still the case that the rabbit that has turned aggressive is more likely to be deemed to have gone 'mad and bad' than to be seen to be fearful, or even sexually aroused (McBride, 2000).

Rabbit ethology and management

The ancestor of all domesticated rabbits is the European rabbit *Oryctolagus cuniculus*. In spite of some 500 years of domestication, studies have shown that the behaviour repertoire of domestic rabbits and wild rabbits hardly differs (McBride, 2000). The rabbit is a medium-sized prey species that is adapted to living in low light conditions. It is crepuscular, spending the daylight hours in narrow underground burrows in the dark, emerging on the surface in the evening and returning below ground soon after daybreak. Living underground means it is not exposed to excessive temperature ranges, as the thick coat, lack of sweat glands and inability to pant mean that rabbits are very susceptible to heat stroke.

Rabbits dig earth and chew obtrusive roots to make their underground burrows. They eat, socialize, play, court and mate above ground. They live in hierarchical groups and are territorial. The wild European rabbit is a successful species with a wide distribution across the European continent, having adapted to habitats ranging from the lush pasturelands and trim golf courses of southern England to the chilly, snowy regions of northern Europe. Yet they originate from the dry landscape of the Iberian Peninsula, notably southern Spain, an area of hot summers and little rainfall, and thus poor quality herbage.

Diet and feeding enrichment

In the wild, foraging takes place mainly overnight, from early evening to early morning, and accounts for some 70% of the night's activity (Myers and Poole, 1961), with caecotrophy occurring during the day, below ground. Natural foraging for this selective feeder means that they travel an area similar to that of two football fields per night whilst feeding.

In contrast, domestic rabbits spend only approximately 5% of a 24-hour period foraging (1.2 hours) (McBride, 1986). This is primarily due to the majority of the diet being presented in the form of commercial pelleted or 'muesli-type' food. The lack of time spent foraging on high-fibre food leads to physical problems, which can be painful, and/or frustration through boredom, both of which may be expressed as aggression or repetitive behaviours such as bar chewing (Figure 5.1).

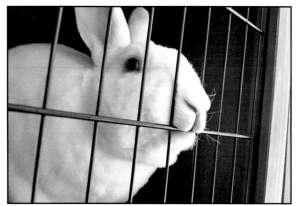

5.1 Bar chewing can be a sign of frustration caused by lack of space and environmental enrichment.

Rabbits require a constantly available *ad libitum* source of indigestible fibre, hay or fresh grasses, herbs, plant and vegetable matter, in order to ensure adequate fibre levels. Just as importantly, this will enable the rabbit to be mentally occupied, and has been shown to prevent repetitive behaviours (Lidfors, 1997; Hansen and Berthelsen, 2000) such as pica, barbering and fur-chewing as well as frustration-induced aggression (McBride *et al.*, 2004), especially if it is provided in more than one location and/or in 'activity feeders'. However, many owners are unaware of, or choose not to follow, such advice. This may be for anthropomorphic reasons, as hay is not the most desirable looking food to human eyes. Schepers *et al.* (2009) found that up to 20% of owners surveyed fed their rabbits bread, treats high in sugar and human snacks, and that 15% of participants did not provide hay.

Owners should be educated about and encouraged to feed an appropriate diet (see Chapter 6). Ideas to stimulate enthusiasm in owners for such food can include advising them on how to make or buy activity feeders for rabbits (Figure 5.2). Guidance on non-poisonous fresh foods that can be grown or picked from the wild can be found in Richardson (2000), and ideas for activity feeders in the Hopping Mad (2011) 'Boredom Busters' video series.

Seeking safety

Rabbits are an important prey species. In their native Spain they make up one-fifth of the diets of more than 20 predators, including animals that attack them on the surface, such as foxes, or underground, including stoats and snakes. The possibility of predation underlies all of rabbit behaviour. Being prey animals, rabbits have a major need for adequate space to run and require constant access to

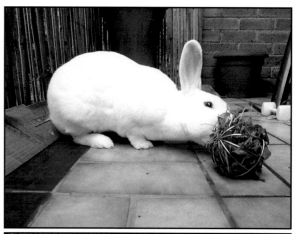

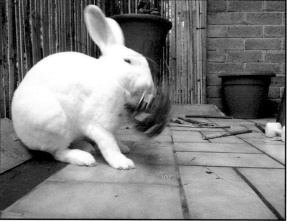

5.2 An activity feeder encourages foraging and physical movement, providing both physical and mental stimulation.

places of safety, such as boxes and pipes (Figure 5.3). Dixon *et al.* (2010) found rabbits in small cages to be less active and less interactive with environmental enrichment items.

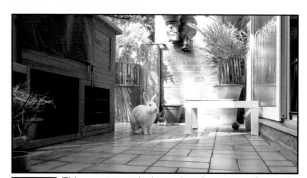

5.3 This apartment balcony has been transformed to provide a freely accessible run, while maintaining the original hutch as a safe retreat and location for a litter tray.

For a prey animal, it is essential for individual survival to be able to detect predators and have good spatial awareness (i.e. to know exactly where you are relative to places of safety, and to have the ability to avoid drawing attention to yourself). Rabbits have acute senses of sight, smell and hearing (Figure 5.4). They are alert, reactive and extremely prone to making fearful associations. Rabbits react adversely to bright lights, sudden movement and to loud or

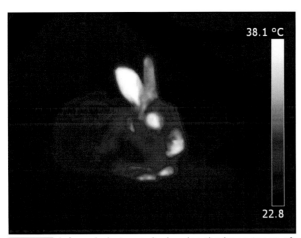

5.4 Infrared photograph showing the importance of the senses, as indicated by higher blood flow (brighter areas).

sudden noises, both sonic and ultrasonic. Their natural response to fear-provoking stimuli is to freeze, and, if the predator comes too close, to flee and seek safety in dark, enclosed spaces. It is essential that rabbits are provided with a number of tunnels, boxes or other places, where they can hide either on their own or as a group.

It is also important that owners are educated about how to behave around rabbits and that children are supervised, especially those under the age of 7 years. Rabbits need to be spoken to softly when approached so they are not startled. This is particularly true for breeds whose senses may be impaired: hearing may be reduced in lop rabbits and sight in those with a lot of fur around the head (e.g. Lionheads and Angoras).

Social grouping

Rabbits are social creatures, living in stable groups of 2 to around 14 individuals. Lisiewicz *et al.* (2009) found faecal corticosterone levels to be significantly higher in rabbits housed alone and concluded that solitary housing is a source of chronic stress for both males and females.

Ideally rabbits should be kept in neutered male–female pairs. Housing two males together can cause problems because male rabbit society is hierarchical and fighting can occur between adult males. Does tend to live in a state of mutual tolerance until their first breeding season when serious, and fatal, fighting can occur (McBride, 2000). Where animals are kept as singletons, the owner must provide sufficient social interaction and/or consider introducing another rabbit if possible. For further information see Jay (2011) and Chapter 2.

Rabbits form bonds with other rabbits (and with people) and these are maintained by behaviours such as resting next to each other in physical contact, and mutual grooming. Grooming bouts are often initiated by the requester lowering its head and pushing it under the chin of the other, and rabbits will push their heads under the hands of trusted humans in the same way. Another means of getting attention is to nip the other gently, or nudge it with the nose or forehead.

Communication

Rabbits do not have flamboyant methods of communication, unlike dogs and cats. They do not indicate when they are scared or in pain by making loud noises or showing obvious overt body language, even when they have a fractured back! To do so would indicate an easy target to a predator. Instead they appear as quiet, stoical creatures, seemingly placid and 'laid back'. This can lead to misunderstanding of how to handle rabbits and lack of early detection of health problems. Different body and ear postures indicate rank, pleasure, pain or fear and behavioural intent. As a general rule, wide eyes, upright ears and tense muscles indicate anxiety, while semi-closed eyes denote relaxation (Figure 5.5). The rabbit whose ears are laid back, and has tense muscles and a crouched body is one that is fearful and may show defensive aggression if it cannot run away.

Likewise, to avoid detection by predators, vocalization is generally used only for close communication and is correspondingly low in volume. Rabbits purr in pleasure, grunt and growl when frustrated or fearful and, in extreme fear, will scream. Perhaps the most obvious auditory signal of anxiety or fear is thumping of the hindlegs on the ground.

Scent, as with cats, is the most highly developed of the rabbit communication channels. Chin-rubbing

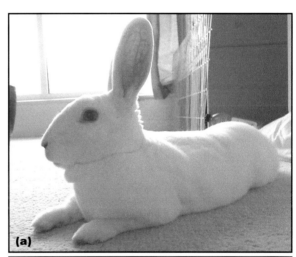

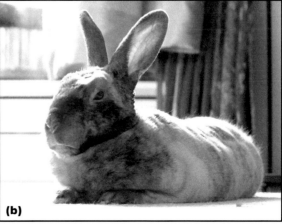

5.5 **(a)** This rabbit is alert and anxious. Note the wide eyes and tense, elongated neck muscles. **(b)** This rabbit is relaxed. Note the semi-closed eyes and head resting back on the shoulders.

on objects, people and other animals denotes territory and identifies group members. While this is performed by both sexes, males tend to be rather more enthusiastic and can have quite damp and sticky chins caused by the secretions from the submandibular gland (McBride, 2000). The role of scent is important to remember should bonded rabbits need to be separated for any reason, such as a veterinary visit. Swapping the body scents of each by rubbing with cloths, and putting used bedding from each into the other's cage prior to reintroducing them in a neutral space will help to prevent rejection and fighting between animals that had previously lived together peaceably (McBride, 2009).

Rabbits also deposit scent with their faeces and will use latrines as boundary markers. The latrines provide both an obvious visual and olfactory signal to other rabbits. To those outside the group they act as a warning that they are about to enter another's territory. It should be noted that while most droppings are deposited in latrines, some are excreted as the rabbits move around their territory.

The third use of scent is through urine spraying and this can be a problem to owners. Unlike cats and dogs, which tend only to spray objects in their environment, rabbits also spray each other, and not infrequently people! Predominately a male behaviour, this is directed at subordinate males or intruders, and it is part of the courtship ritual. Some pet rabbits can learn to spray as an attention-seeking behaviour (McBride, 2000).

Observation – the key to diagnosis

Because rabbits do not show clearly when they are feeling unwell or in pain (Farnworth *et al.*, 2011), owners may not detect a deterioration in physical health until the problem has progressed, sometimes to a point where little can be done to save the animal. It is important therefore to encourage owners to be observant of their rabbit's behaviour so that changes can be spotted early. Rabbits that are ill or in pain are likely to be less active than normal, show reduced grooming, or only groom part of the body, grind their teeth, leave caecotrophs on the ground, drool, sit huddled or appear to be unable to get comfortable. More obvious signs include a lack of coordination, head tilt, or over-grooming of irritating areas such as the ears when they are infected, or displaying aggression towards their owners or companion rabbits.

Likewise, observation can lead to early detection, and thus better prognosis, of behaviour problems. Grunting, growling and avoidance of being handled are early signs of fear or frustration, which if not dealt with appropriately are likely to lead to kicking and biting behaviour. One rabbit chasing another, and perhaps biting and pulling out the other's fur, is indicative of social problems, which may be related to territoriality, lack of recognition, or re-directed fear or frustration. Again, if not recognized early, such behaviours can lead to a complete breakdown of the social relationship and even fatal fighting.

Handling

Most people think that rabbits like to be picked up and cuddled. Actually, being lifted can be very frightening for the animals because the resulting loss of support is a biologically predisposed fear (Seligman, 1971). While rabbits may choose to sit next to their owners and be stroked, that is quite different from being lifted and held either in the air or tucked close to one's body; from the rabbit's point of view both resemble the grip of a predator.

Rabbits need to be socialized to people. Rabbits that have been appropriately handled between 10 and 20 days of age are more willing to approach unknown people when tested at 49 days, a typical age at which rabbits are homed (Der Weduwen and McBride, 1999). Early handling of rabbit kittens needs to be done carefully, so the doe does not abandon them. The person's hands should be rubbed with some of the nest bedding before the kittens are picked up, and ideally the doe should also be stroked, so that the scent profile on both mother and young is similar. Does that are well socialized have been found to be better breeders, and less likely to injure or abandon their young.

Rabbits that are handled gently will enjoy being stroked, particularly in areas where they would normally socially groom each other. This is around the cheeks, forehead, insides of the ears and along the back. Being touched on the nose, feet, belly, tail and lower rump area is more fear-provoking and requires training (see below) if the animal is not going to be fearful, and thus potentially aggressive, when picked up.

Teaching owners how to handle their rabbit is important, because an extremely common behaviour problem is aggression when handled.

Training to be lifted

The principle here is to associate a cue word with being lifted, so the rabbit is not surprised when picked up, and further to make this association pleasant. The first step in this process requires the rabbit to become relaxed when being stroked all over its body, and particularly around the hindquarters. If the rabbit is already showing aggression, then this will need to be done initially using a soft baby brush on a piece of dowel, so the rabbit cannot bite the person. Otherwise, it is possible to start with the hand.

A few mouthfuls of the rabbit's favourite treat, such as fresh herbs, should be provided. Whilst it is eating, the rabbit should be gently stroked along the head, gradually along the back and around the chest, all the time softly saying the rabbit's name and the cue word, such as 'Thumper, lift'. Only continue while the rabbit is eating, and only gradually move to areas where it is less comfortable being touched.

Once the rabbit is relaxed when being touched with a hand, whilst it is eating, the hindquarters can be lifted a few centimetres and let back down again. This should be followed by pushing the fingers gently between the front legs whilst offering the food. When the rabbit is relaxed with this, it is possible to pick the rabbit up, supporting the hindquarters and the chest area (with fingers through the front legs so that the weight is supported and it cannot leap out of the hand; Figure 5.6). Depending on the size of the rabbit, this may or may not need two hands (McBride, 2000).

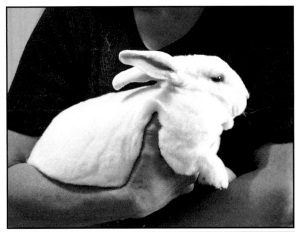

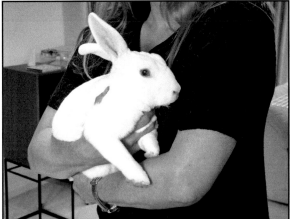

5.6 The appropriate way to hold a rabbit. Note that the bodyweight is supported and forward motion is blocked by placing fingers between the forelegs.

Dorsal immobility response

Laying a rabbit on its back and gently stroking its belly will cause it to become still and apparently relaxed (Figure 5.7); see also Appendix 3. This is a natural response to being caught by a predator and also occurs in some other mammals, amphibians, reptiles and birds. It is a transitory and reversible state of profound motor inhibition and is a behaviour of last resort for an animal that has been caught by a predator. Lying still and 'playing dead' may cause the predator to loosen its grip, possibly moving away or grooming for a moment, giving the prey a final chance of escape. For this to occur the animal would need to be fully alert to all that is going on around it in order to seize the moment. In one study, McBride *et al.* (2006) found that both physiological and behavioural indicators showed that rabbits were highly stressed by this procedure and remained so for at least 15 minutes after they had recovered from the immobile state.

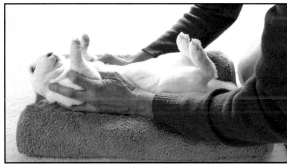

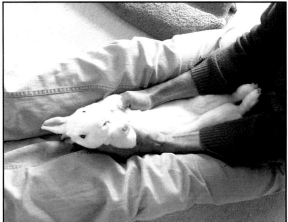

5.7 Dorsal immobility response. Note that this demonstration was conducted at ground level to avoid injury and that support was provided along the whole length of the rabbit's body.

Rabbits may enter the state more quickly over repeated occasions, which may be misinterpreted as habituating. However, research (e.g. Farabollini *et al.*, 1990) shows that it remains very stressful, as would be expected with such a hard-wired, evolutionarily adaptive, predator avoidance behaviour. Therefore, although the dorsal immobility response can be useful for health checks and non-invasive procedures, such as sexing and nail clipping, it should be emphasized to owners that it is not an appropriate means of general interaction with their pets.

Human–rabbit communication and training

Rabbits can be trained to perform behaviours on cue. The most effective way to encourage this is clicker training. Training not only provides mental stimulation for the rabbit and improves bonding with the owner, but also can be useful to help ensure health and better management. For example, training rabbits to accept and enter carry cages reduces the stress of travel, and training them to feed from a syringe will reduce the stress of assisted feeding.

Rabbits can be taught to do various 'exercises' on cue, such as stretching and jumping, and even to do agility courses! These exercises can help to reduce obesity and strengthen bones and muscles. Additional 'tricks' include coming when called, 'leave', and even retrieving named items. For further information see Orr and Lewin (2006) and McBride and Kershaw (2011).

Veterinary visits

Rabbits visiting the veterinary surgery need to be housed in quiet, dark accommodation, away from predators, ideally with their bonded companion or familiar objects that carry the scent of home. Where the companion is not able to be present to pick up the same scents (e.g. in a carrier in the operating room, and in the same recovery accommodation as the patient), the owners must be advised on the need for scent swapping prior to reintroduction.

Rabbit behaviour problems

Rabbit behaviour problems have causes similar to those in other species, including lack of socialization, fear-provoking experiences or the display of normal behaviour that is not understood by the owner or is directed at inappropriate objects. There are also medical reasons, which must be eliminated as the first part of any diagnosis.

Investigation of any behaviour problem needs to identify the underlying emotion that caused the behaviour, such as a fear-provoking or frustrating event, and the outcomes maintaining the behaviour, such as anticipation/acquisition of something pleasurable (positive reinforcement) or anticipation/acquisition of safety and relief (negative reinforcement). In order to do this a comprehensive history of the animal, including its past medical history and current physical status, is required.

While there are more unusual cases, the main areas of rabbit behaviour that are problematic to owners relate to aggression, excretion and chewing:

- Aggression may be directed towards other rabbits (intraspecific) or towards people or other animals (interspecific)
- Excretion problems include not using a litter tray, and spraying urine
- Chewing covers both damage to property and pica, the chewing and ingestion of non-food items. Chewing of the cage or hutch may not be considered a problem by the owners, though such repetitive behaviour may indicate a resolvable welfare issue caused by anxiety and/or frustration.

Behaviour problems may have more than one causal factor. These include:

- Pain
- Fear
- Frustration
- Boredom
- Learned attention-seeking
- Social problems: e.g. resource and territorial issues, incompatibility due to hierarchical problems, sexual status or lack of recognition due to separation.

All of these factors induce stress and thus can have a further impact on physical welfare.

The behaviour consultation

Home visits are preferable for the investigation of rabbit behaviour cases, because environmental details will be more apparent. Where this is not possible, use of diagrams and/or video of the rabbit's accommodation and surroundings is essential. Likewise, video of the behaviour under consideration is extremely helpful. Not only does it provide a record of the behaviour, which may not occur at the time of the consultation, but it also enables closer consideration of the event through slow motion playback.

An example of a history-taking form for rabbit behaviour consultations is provided at the end of this chapter. It covers a wide range of potential factors that can contribute to the initiation and maintenance of unwanted behaviour. This will provide indications of what needs addressing in a modification programme, be that environmental or management changes, and/or re-training of owner and animal, in terms of handling for example. It must be remembered that each behaviour case will be unique, each problem may have multiple aetiologies, and that modification programmes will vary from case to case and must be designed with reference to both the animal and the owner. In terms of the owner, consideration must be given to their willingness and ability to implement a programme. Rabbits that are not pets, i.e. show, laboratory and farm animals, may also display undesirable behaviour that may be ameliorated by consideration of medical, environmental and management factors.

The history-taking form is best given to an owner prior to a behaviour consultation. This enables them to provide more accurate information, especially where this involves recalling events. The questionnaire should not be considered as anything more than a roadmap indicating routes for further investigation, enabling an accurate diagnosis to be reached. It is also important to remember that only one person fills in the questionnaire, but other members of the household may have different perceptions and recollections. Thus, as for any species, it is preferable that all family members, i.e. keepers of the animal, are present at the behaviour consultation, including children. Children should also be included in the fact-finding process.

Veterinary and other behaviour professionals need to understand that eliciting information from owners, especially about behaviour-related issues, requires good counselling and questioning skills. It is more productive to ask owners to *describe* the behaviour: what the animal does; when; where; who/what else is around or happening. Questions such as 'is he aggressive?' may be misinterpreted; what may be perceived as aggression by the owner may actually be a friendly 'attention-seeking' nip from the rabbit. Using terms such as 'aggression' may set up unhelpful attitudes in owners, and cause them to be less willing to try and resolve a problem. It is important to remember that aggression in the majority of cases is based in fear (Jones-Baade and McBride, 1999), whether fear of pain, fear of intrusion into territory or fear of loss of resources such as desired food items.

Likewise, anthropomorphic attitudes may mean that owners do not interpret what is happening objectively. An extreme example of this involved a client whose rabbit had suddenly become agoraphobic and would not come out of the hutch into the adjoining run. The owner had not realized that moving the rabbit's accommodation from the side of the house to the back garden now meant the rabbit was in a state of chronic fear. The reason was that, in the new location, it was surrounded by five birds of prey on their outdoor perches, only some 3 metres from the rabbit run. The lack of owner understanding was simply due to anthropomorphism: they thought that the rabbit would know it was safe behind wire, that the birds were tethered, and that the birds would not hurt a rabbit that was part of the family! This was a simple case to resolve, but anthropomorphism of 'happy animal families' can be an issue when keeping dogs and cats with rabbits, or where two rabbits start fighting, especially if they previously lived together peaceably.

Behaviour modification

Ensuring that the animal has an appropriate environment and management that provides for its physical and psychological needs is essential to any behaviour modification programme. As stated above, rabbits have memory of places, events and of individuals (based on scent). They can learn using both classical and operant conditioning. Thus, desensitization and counter-conditioning can be used for fear-based problems, and behaviours such as coming when asked, going to the hutch/basket, leaving, and being lifted can be trained to cue, ideally in a hands-off manner such as clicker training (Orr and Lewin, 2006). These exercises can be used in behaviour modification programmes, as well as simply providing mental stimulation and enhancing the relationship with the owner. In addition, the use of a commercially available rabbit-appeasing pheromone can specifically help rabbits that are stressed, in the veterinary surgery or when being introduced to a new home, and has been found to assist with production rabbits on farms (Bouvier and Jacquinet, 2008).

While published data are not available, the use of rabbit-appeasing pheromone can be helpful in reintroducing rabbits that have started to fight. The most common reason for this is when animals have been separated and no longer share a common scent profile. As mentioned earlier, this is an important consideration when rabbits visit the veterinary surgery, but is also true when they are separated for other reasons such as being shown or taken to the increasingly popular 'rabbit agility' events. Introducing, or reintroducing, rabbits is not a simple process and the animals need to be closely observed for several hours. Fighting can break out very rapidly and can be extremely bloody, if not fatal, and very distressing for owners. Bonding can take just a few minutes, or more than a week. Assisting the process by scent swapping can reduce fighting. Many recommend that introductions occur on neutral territory, though some evidence using laboratory rabbits suggests that introductions may result in fewer injuries if the newcomers are put into the established recipient group's territory (Graf *et al.*, 2011). However, this study introduced two new animals at the same time into an established group. Likewise, females are introduced to the male's cage for mating, and this can lead to bonding (author, personal experience). Neither situation may be comparable to reintroducing two rabbits whose relationship is damaged, and may not be comparable to the normal pet situation of pairing up two singletons. Further advice is available from a variety of sources including the Rabbit Welfare Association and Fund and Campbell (2010). Local rabbit rescue centres may be able to assist owners with this process.

If not tackled early, behaviour problems can become entrenched and lead to complications. To exemplify this it is helpful to consider a case of aggression towards the owners.

Case example

A baby rabbit was obtained as a pet and housed in a typical commercially available hutch, sold as a superior 'two-tier, with integral run' rabbit hutch. On sunny days, at weekends, it was put out in a run for an hour or two while the children played with it. All was well and the rabbit was happy to be handled. However, about a year later the rabbit started to growl when being picked up and progressed to biting. The rabbit was no longer taken to the run, and the children no longer played with it. The aggressive behaviour worsened, with the rabbit charging at any hand that came towards it. The rabbit was now much larger, but the hutch stayed the same.

Detailed history-taking revealed that the owners had noticed that the rabbit became less active in the run before the growling and biting started. Further, more recently they had seen caecotrophs on the floor of the hutch.

Examination of the rabbit showed that it was not grooming its back and hindquarters particularly well, and radiography revealed arthritis in the back and some deformity. Examination of the hutch, even with its lower level 'integral run' showed that it was too small, and much of the lower area was obstructed by the ramp, litter tray and toys. Indeed, the rabbit was not able to stand, stretch or hop freely.

Pain relief was given and grooming improved, yet the rabbit was still aggressive to people when picked up. The added complication was that the rabbit had acquired a learned association between being handled and pain. This required a process of desensitization and counter-conditioning, training the rabbit to come when called and to be picked up. Additionally, good advice included the need to provide a larger hutch and to combine this with free access, or at least daily access, to the run.

Conclusion

This chapter serves only to introduce the basics of rabbit behaviour. Veterinary surgeons should acquire substantial knowledge of their ethology, nutritional and environmental requirements, as well as an understanding of medical issues that may relate to problem behaviour. Behaviour problems require detailed history-taking, which may not be practical in the time available in a normal veterinary consultation (Roshier and McBride, 2013a). Likewise, design and implementation of a behaviour modification programme can be time-consuming. However, the veterinary profession is in a unique position to advise on the appropriate management of rabbits to prevent problems developing. Further, routine appointments for vaccinations or visits where known physical problems, such as dental issues, are presented enable discussion of behaviour with clients. This can mean that appropriate and timely steps can be taken to resolve any problems, whether directly or via referral (Roshier and McBride, 2013b).

References and further reading

Bouvier AC and Jacquinet C (2008) Pheromone in rabbits: preliminary technical results on farm use in France. *World Rabbit Science Association Congress* [available at http://world-rabbit-science.com/WRSA-Proceedings/Congress-2008-Verona/Papers/R-Bouvier.pdf]

Copping J (2009) Welfare crisis among Britain's pet rabbits. *Daily Telegraph* 4 April [available at www.telegraph.co.uk]

Der Weduwen S and McBride EA (1999) Rabbit behaviour and the effects of early handling. *Proceedings of the 2nd World Meeting on Ethology, Lyon, France*, pp.221–228 [available at http://medical.wesrch.com/Paper/My_papers/display_proceedings.php?proceeding_id=ME1JH88]

Dixon LM, Hardiman JR and Cooper JJ (2010) The effects of spatial restriction on the behavior of rabbits (*Oryctolagus cuniculus*). *Journal of Veterinary Behavior: Clinical Applications and Research* 5(6), 302–308

Farabollini F, Facchinetti F, Lupo C, *et al.* (1990) Time-course of opioid and pituitary-adrenal hormone modifications during the immobility reaction in rabbits. *Physiology and Behavior* 47(2), 337–341

Farnworth MJ, Walker JK, Schweizer KA, *et al.* (2011) Potential behavioural indicators of post-operative pain in male laboratory rabbits following abdominal surgery. *Animal Welfare* 20(2), 225–237

Graf S, Bigler L, Failing K, Würbel H and Buchwalder T (2011) Regrouping rabbit does in a familiar or novel pen: Effects on agonistic behaviour, injuries and core body temperature. *Applied Animal Behaviour Science* 135(1–2), 121–127

Hamilton-Andrews HS, McBride EA and Brown I (1999) Hypothyroidism and aberrant behaviour in the Bearded Collie. *Proceedings of the 2nd World Meeting on Ethology, Lyon, France*, pp.133–138

Hansen LT and Berthelsen H (2000) The effect of environmental enrichment on the behaviour of caged rabbits (*Oryctolagus cuniculus*). *Applied Animal Behaviour Science* 68, 163–178

Hopping Mad (2011) *Boredom Busters* videos: a series of three videos looking at ideas for feeding activities for rabbits by McBride and Robyn [available at www.youtube.com]

Jay (2011) Enrichment and the single rabbit issue. *Hopping Mad e-magazine*, issue 2, July 2011

Jones-Baade R and McBride EA (1999) A biological model for aggression in dogs. *Proceedings of the 2nd World Meeting on Ethology, Lyon, France*, pp.29–42

Lidfors L (1997) Behavioural effects of environmental enrichment for individually caged rabbits. *Applied Animal Behaviour Science* 52(1), 157–169

Lisiewicz NE, Waters M and Jackson B (2009) Social Stress in Rabbits. In: *Proceedings of the 7th International Behaviour Meeting*, ed. SE Heath, pp.85–89. ESCVE, Belgium

McBride A (1986) *Aspects of social and parental behaviour in the domestic rabbit*. Unpublished PhD thesis, University College London

McBride A (2000) *Why does my rabbit...?* Souvenir Press Ltd, London

McBride A (2009) Rampaging rabbits: minimizing stress in the veterinary surgery and rescue centre. *Rabbit Welfare Fund Conference: Rabbit Health Matters, Horsham*

McBride A and Kershaw E (2011) Clicker training for rabbits – a brief introduction. [available at www.rabbitawarenessweek.co.uk]

McBride A, Magnus E and Hearne G (2004) Behaviour problems in the domestic rabbit. In: *The APBC book of Companion Animal Behaviour*, ed. D Appleby, pp.164–182. Souvenir Press, London

McBride A, McNicholas J and Ahmedzai S (2006) Animal facilitated therapy: a practice of welfare concern. In: *Proceedings of VDWE International Congress on Companion Animal Behaviour and Welfare*, pp.95–102. Vlaamse Dierenartsenvereniging, Sint-Niklaas, Belgium

McBride EA, Day S, McAdie T, *et al.* (2006) Trancing rabbits: Relaxed hypnosis or a state of fear? In: *Proceedings of the VDWE International Congress on Companion Animal Behaviour and Welfare*, pp.135–137 Vlaamse Dierenartsenvereniging, Sint-Niklaas, Belgium.

Myers K and Poole WE (1961) A study of the biology of the wild rabbit in confined populations. 11. The effects of season and population increase on behaviour. *CSIRO Wildlife Research* 4, 14–26

Orr J and Lewin TA (2006) *Getting Started: Clicker with your Rabbit.* USA Sunshine Books Inc., Waltham, MA [available at www.clickerbunny.com]

Richardson CG (2000) *Rabbits: Health, Husbandry and Diseases*, pp.7–18. Blackwell Science, Oxford

Roshier AL and McBride EA (2013a) Veterinarians' perceptions of behaviour support in small animal practice. *Veterinary Record* 172(10), 267

Roshier AL and McBride EA (2013b) Canine behaviour problems: discussions between veterinarians and dog owners during annual booster consultations. *Veterinary Record* 172(9), 235

Royal Society for the Prevention of Cruelty to Animals (RSPCA) (2012) The time and costs involved in keeping rabbits [available at www.rspca.org.uk]

Schepers F, Koene P and Beerda B (2009) Welfare assessment in pet rabbits. *Animal Welfare* 18, 477–485

Seligman MEP (1971) Phobias and preparedness. *Behavior Therapy* 2, 307–320

Date of consultation:.. Case number:..

Case diagnosis:.. Video classification:..

Rabbit behaviour questionnaire

Please include as much information as possible. The more detail you can provide, the more able we are to make an accurate assessment of your rabbit's case. Please use additional sheets where necessary.

Owner details:

Your title (Dr/Mr/Mrs/Miss/Ms)   Surname/family name:..

First name or initials:..

Address:...

....Postcode:...

Phone (day):.. (evening):...

Mobile:... Email:..

Are you covered by a Pet Insurance Policy? If so, please give details.

....

....

Referring veterinary surgeon:

Address:...

Tel:...

Patient information:

Name of rabbit:.. Breed/type:...

Age:.. Sex:...

Is your rabbit spayed/neutered and, if so, when was it done?...

Has this rabbit ever been used for breeding?..

How much does your rabbit weigh?...

How long is your rabbit from nose to tail when lying down on its side?..

Early history:

How old was your rabbit when you obtained it?..

Where did it come from? Did it, for example, come from a breeder, rescue centre or pet shop?

....

Medical history:

Does your rabbit have any current medical problems to your knowledge?..

Do you know of any previous medical problems?..

Is it on any current medication?..

Has your rabbit had any teeth problems?..

Does your rabbit have his/her teeth clipped? If so, how often...

Do you clip your rabbit's nails or do you take it to the vet?...

How often are the nails clipped?..

Please ask your veterinary surgeon to provide your rabbit's complete veterinary records.

An example of a rabbit behaviour questionnaire. ▶

Interactions with family members: Please describe other members of your household.

Person's name	Person's age

Who interacts with the rabbit?...

Does the rabbit have a favourite person or people? If so, who?...

Who is responsible for the following tasks:

Feeding the rabbit?..

Cleaning the rabbit's cage/hutch?...

Cleaning the rabbit's run?..

Grooming the rabbit?...

Clipping the rabbit's nails?...

Interactions with other animals:

Other rabbits owned

Does this rabbit live with any other rabbits? If so please give details.

Rabbit name	Breed/type	Age	Sex	Spayed/neutered (yes/no)	How long lived with rabbit patient?

Do you ever see these rabbits lying next to each other? Please give details of who lies with whom.

....

Do you ever see these rabbits licking/grooming each other? Please give details.

....

Do you ever see these rabbits mounting (attempting to mate) each other? Please give details.

....

Do you ever see these rabbits chasing each other? Please give details.

....

Do you ever see these rabbits pulling fur from each other? Please give details.

....

Do you have any other rabbits, besides those described above?

Rabbit name	Breed/type	Age	Sex	Neutered (yes/no)

◄   ►

Other pets

Do you have any other animals? (Please include their type, age and sex):

Type and breed	Name	Age	Sex	Relationship with the rabbit patient (e.g. avoids/no interaction, stalks, stares, grooms, plays)

Cats in the neighbourhood

Do cats come into your garden?...

Have you ever seen them staring at/stalking your rabbit?...

Your rabbit's home:

Please provide a diagram(s) of your rabbit's hutch/cage/run with dimensions including height.

Please indicate where litter trays, water bowls/bottles, food bowls and hayracks are located.

Please indicate where other items such as pipes, boxes are located.

Please give as much detail as possible about where your rabbit lives.

What sort of bedding do you give your rabbit? Please tick all that apply

      Hay ☐   Straw ☐   Sawdust ☐   Blanket ☐

      Other (please state) ....

Outside-living rabbits   If your rabbit lives outside, does it live:

In a cage/hutch? ☐   In a cage/hutch with an attached run? ☐

In a cage/hutch with a separate run, to which you carry your rabbit? ☐

If the run is attached, does it have access to the run:

Always? ☐   Daytime only? ☐   Dry days only? ☐

Other (please describe)..

If the run is separate, when do you put the rabbit in the run?

Every day ☐   Dry days only ☐   Summer only ☐   Weekends only ☐

Other (please describe)..

How long on average does your rabbit have access to the run per week?...

Whether attached or separate, is the run:

On concrete? ☐   On decking? ☐   On tiles? ☐   On grass? ☐

Do you move the run to fresh patches of grass? If so, how often?..

Do you move your rabbit into a shed/garage in the winter? If so please describe any difference in its accommodation in summer and winter ....

....

House rabbits

If your rabbit lives in your home, does it have access to all areas of the house?

Please state which rooms it has access to:...

Does it have a hutch/cage in the house?...

Is it confined to the hutch/cage at night?...

◀   ▶

Is it confined to the hutch/cage during the day? If so, for how long? ....

Does the rabbit ever go outside? If so please describe when and where ....

....

Outdoor run for house rabbits

If your rabbit spends any time in an outdoor run please answer the following:

Is the rabbit's outside run: On concrete? ☐   On decking? ☐   On tiles? ☐   On grass? ☐

Do you move the run to fresh patches of grass? If so, how often? ....

Toiletting:

Does the rabbit use a litter tray? If so, what kind of litter do you use? ....

How many litter trays do you have in the areas the rabbit lives?

Cage/hutch ☐   Run ☐   Your house ☐

How often do you clean the litter trays? ....

How often do you clean the rest of the cage/hutch? ....

How often do you clean the rest of the run? ....

Have you noticed your rabbit spraying inside or outside? (Spraying is when the rabbit runs past and twists its hindquarters, letting loose a jet of urine.) ....

If so, on what items/people does it spray? ....

Have you noticed soft, moist faecal pellets (droppings) on the floor of your rabbit's home? ....

Chewing:

Does your rabbit chew its hutch/cage or run? ....

Does it chew the wooden parts? ....

Does it chew plastic parts? ....

Does it chew metal parts, e.g. wire or bars? ....

If indoors in your home, does your rabbit chew:

Furniture? If so are there any items in particular? ....

Carpets? ....Other? (Please specify) ....

Diet:

What do you feed your rabbit and how often? (Please tick all that apply)

Food	Brand/type	Fed daily	Fed weekly	Fed occasionally
Commercial rabbit pellets				
Commercial rabbit mix (pellets, corn, etc.)				
Commercial extruded pellets				
Hay and straw				
Fresh grass/herbs				
Fruit (please specify)				
Household greens (please specify, e.g. carrot, turnip, broccoli)				
Other (please specify, e.g. bread/milk)				

Do you give any supplements, e.g. salt block? ....

Does your rabbit enjoy their food or would you say it was fussy? ....

Do you give any tit-bits? If so, what and how often? ....

◀   ▶

Do you give any commercial rabbit treats? If so, please give details. ....

Does your rabbit have access to water? Please tick all that apply:

In its cage/hutch: In a water bottle ☐ In a bowl ☐

How often do you change the water?

In its run: In a water bottle ☐ In a bowl ☐

How often do you change the water?..

Please state how many of each item is in the cage/hutch and in the run.

Item	Cage/hutch	Run
Food bowls		
Hay racks		
Water bottles		
Water bowls		

Human interaction:

Does the rabbit have any toys? Please describe...

Do you play with the rabbit? Please describe the games and approximately how long each day

you play with the rabbit ....

....

....

Does your rabbit know any tricks? If so, please give details...

....

....

The problem:

Describe the problems you are having with your rabbit in as much detail as possible. (Please use additional

sheets as necessary.)..

....

....

....

As rabbit communication is very subtle and difficult to describe, it would be EXTREMELY helpful if you could send a video showing the problem you are having with your rabbit. If this is not possible, please describe your rabbit's behaviour in as much detail as possible, e.g. are its ears flat or upright, is it making a noise, struggling, kicking, biting? Please do try, however, to provide a video. Thank you.

What happens immediately before your rabbit displays these behaviours? Try to think both what you/others and

your rabbit are doing when the problem occurs...

....

....

What happens immediately after? Again, think about what you/others do, and what the rabbit does...............

....

....

When did the problem begin? Can you remember the first time it happened? ....

When does the problem occur? Is it in any particular circumstances?..

....

◀ ▶

How frequently, on average, does the problem occur? Do you think it is becoming more frequent, less frequent, or staying about the same? ....

Where does it occur? Is it, for example, always in the same place? ....

Who is usually present at the time, if anybody? ....

When was the last incident, and can you describe this? ....
....

Have there been previous attempts to cure this problem? (If so, please describe.) ....
....
....

Other problems:

Does your rabbit have any other problems? For example, is it nervous of:

Children? ☐　　　Strangers? ☐　　　Any family members? ☐　　　Dogs? ☐　　　All of these ☐

Does it struggle/bite/kick) when you:

Groom it? ☐　　　Stroke it? ☐　　　Pick it up? ☐

If so, please give details: ....
....
....

What sort of brush do you use to groom your rabbit? ....

Are there any other problems with the rabbit that you would like to discuss at the consultation?
....
....
....

Rehabilitation:

How much time do you feel able to commit to working with your rabbit to solve these problems?
....

What would you envisage happening if the behaviour problem persists?
....

Finally, to help us understand more about pet rabbits it is helpful if you can give us information about rabbits that you have owned before.

Breed	Age of rabbit when obtained (if known)	How long was the rabbit owned for?	Were there any behaviour problems encountered? If so, please describe	What was the outcome? (e.g. behaviour improved, someone else in family looked after rabbit (I was a child at the time), rabbit was rehomed/given to a rescue charity, rabbit was euthanased)

Thank you very much for your cooperation in filling in this questionnaire. If you have any queries, please do not hesitate to contact me.

I look forward to meeting you and your rabbit or speaking to you on the telephone.

◄

6

The rabbit-friendly practice

Molly Varga

Veterinary surgeons must make animal health and welfare their first consideration when attending to animals. For several years small animal practices have been working on being 'cat-friendly' in order to promote the reduction of stress in the surgery, and its associated negative impact on the welfare of feline patients. With the increase in numbers of rabbits being presented for veterinary care the same principles should be applied to rabbit patients. Unless careful consideration is put into making a practice less stressful to rabbits, they can suffer significant stress during a visit. This is certainly an issue that concerns most rabbit owners, and the degree of effort that has gone into making a practice rabbit-friendly is likely to be proportional to how many rabbit clients a practice attracts and retains. Recently, schemes have been set up to highlight rabbit-friendly practices (e.g. the Rabbit Welfare Association and Fund (RWAF) and Supreme Petfoods' 'Think Rabbit' initiative).

As a natural prey species, the rabbit is sensitive to both novel situations (particularly where flight is not an option) and the presence of predators. Both circumstances are likely to occur in the veterinary practice. One of the main physiological responses is to produce adrenaline. This can have several consequences:

- Cardiomyopathy
- Gut stasis, caecal dysbiosis and enterotoxaemia
- Increased gastric acidity and ulceration
- Reduced renal blood flow leading to oliguria
- Lymphopenia
- Altered carbohydrate metabolism leading to hyperglycaemia and eventually hepatic lipidosis
- Heart failure and death.

Clearly it is important for the veterinary practice to address potential issues proactively to avoid potentially life-threatening complications.

First contact: reception training and pre-visit advice

The person answering the phone is the primary contact a rabbit owner has with any veterinary practice, and this is where lasting first impressions are made. It is vitally important that the reception staff are well trained in answering rabbit-related enquiries and recognizing rabbit emergencies. Training for reception staff should form an integral part of making a practice rabbit-friendly.

Recognizing an emergency

The reception staff are the first contact with the practice and essentially control the running of the day. This means that when (and whether) patients are booked in depends on the receptionists' experience and training. Because rabbits differ significantly from dogs and cats, specific training is needed.

Rabbit-specific questions to ask should include:

- Is the rabbit eating? If not, how long is it since it last ate voluntarily? *If more than 12 hours, or if the owner is worried, the rabbit should be booked in immediately*
- Is the rabbit passing faeces? If not, when were faeces last noticed? *If more than 12 hours has passed since faeces were passed, or if the owner is worried, the rabbit should be booked in immediately*
- Has diarrhoea been noted? *If so, the rabbit should be booked in immediately*
- If altered faeces have been noted, has the owner checked the rabbit's perineum for soiling and fly strike? *If fly strike is present the rabbit should be seen immediately.*

Rabbit-specific advice to answer common questions should also be forthcoming, for example:

- Rabbits should not be starved overnight prior to surgery
- Rabbits should be vaccinated even if kept indoors
- Where possible, bonded companions should be brought to the surgery for company
- Rabbits do not require routine worming
- Rabbits can be neutered safely and should be unless they are intended for breeding.

There are some situations serious enough to warrant immediate attendance at the surgery. These emergency conditions include:

- Acute collapse
- Head tilt or seizure
- Known trauma/bleeding
- Paralysis

- Bloated abdomen
- Watery foul-smelling diarrhoea
- Fly strike
- Dyspnoea
- Heat stress
- Dystocia.

The owner should be advised to bring the rabbit straight to the surgery.

Travelling to the surgery

There are various ways in which travelling to the surgery can be made less stressful for rabbits.

- Rabbits should always be transported in a secure carrier, not loose in the car.
- The carrier should be familiar to the animal and contain hay, some familiar food and, if the journey is likely to be long, a water bottle.
- A bonded companion can also help to reduce stress.
- Covering the carrier with a towel or blanket can make it appear more secure, thereby calming the rabbit; however, adequate ventilation must be maintained.
- Owners should be advised to minimize the time their rabbits spend in the car, particularly in warm weather.
- Rabbits are sensitive to heat stress and should never under any circumstances be left in a hot car.
- If the weather is warm, the car windows should be opened or the air-conditioning put on, to maintain a suitable ambient temperature (preferably <21°C).
- Rabbits often find car journeys stressful so the less time spent travelling the better.

What to bring

The presence of familiar food and bedding can make time spent in hospital less difficult. While veterinary practices should aim to have a range of foods available for all species, it is not feasible to stock everything. Owners can be asked to bring any unusual diet items as well as some fresh food. Familiar hay and possibly some bedding from home will make a hospital cage less stressful. If the hospital stay is likely to be longer than a few hours, consideration should be given to allowing the bonded companion to accompany the patient. Hospitalization must, however, also protect the welfare of the companion, and the benefits must outweigh the stress of separation. This means that the hospital situation must be optimal for rabbits. Cage furniture, such as a litter tray, is also often brought into the surgery.

Ancillary information

Now that many practices have websites, these are a useful tool for providing advice to owners. What constitutes an emergency, how to transport your rabbit, what to bring to the surgery, general first aid tips and preoperative information can all be posted online. Equally, links to other sites can be helpful (as long as these have been checked), and getting the practice on the Rabbit Friendly Practices list of the RWAF (in the UK) is also a positive step to attracting more rabbit clients.

Staff training

Many rabbit owners are very knowledgeable and will immediately spot any gaps in the knowledge of practice staff. Nursing staff need to be able to give advice on husbandry, feeding, routine medical care and neutering as well as being able to recognize when veterinary input is required. In recent years there has been a dramatic increase in the resources available to provide information on rabbit care. There is a recognized nursing qualification in Nursing Exotic Pets in the UK, as well as the *BSAVA Manual of Exotic Pet and Wildlife Nursing*. Many of the companies producing commercial products such as rabbit food offer continuing education webinars and information sheets or sponsor lectures. Most veterinary conferences now include an exotic pets, or even a rabbit only, series of lectures. Web-based information sites can also be very useful (e.g. Veterinary Information Network (VIN) and the RWAF website); however, discussion forums may not provide reliable advice.

Factual knowledge, while important, is not the only aspect of staff training that needs to be addressed. A nurse's ability to handle a rabbit in a safe and confident manner (and one that will not upset the owner or the rabbit) is also very important. Any nurse undertaking a lot of rabbit work should familiarize themselves with methods of picking up and restraining rabbits, and practise these if necessary.

Equally, veterinary surgeons need to have up-to-date and factually correct knowledge of rabbit medicine, nutrition, reproduction and examination techniques. What is discussed and how a rabbit is handled during a consultation will determine whether an owner is willing to allow a practice to continue treating their rabbit. Training options for veterinary surgeons include the CertAVP in Zoological Medicine (which includes a Small Mammal module), a large variety of webinars available from many different continuing professional development (CPD) providers, a choice of lectures at most veterinary conferences, and an explosion in published literature (both peer-reviewed journal papers and textbooks). For practices interested in rabbits there is a wealth of information available.

The waiting room

The waiting room is the first clinic area to which both rabbits and their owners are exposed. It can be a significant source of stress if the situation is not managed sensibly. Because rabbits are a natural prey species, the presence of other patients (often natural predator species such as cats and dogs, ferrets or birds of prey) will be stressful. Separating rabbits from cats and dogs, even if this just means using different sides of the waiting room, will be helpful. Removing rabbits from the sight, smell and sound of cats and dogs is even better. This means either attempting to separate surgery times or having a separate waiting room (Figure 6.1). Separate surgery times are not always feasible and emergency consultations always make this system unreliable. Having a separate waiting room is not feasible for many surgeries. Reception staff should be trained to manage the situation by separating rabbits from predators as widely as possible, and offering a quiet place for rabbits to be placed in their carriers if a separate room is not available. For all patients reduction of the waiting time as much as possible will reduce stress.

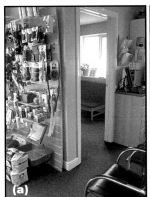 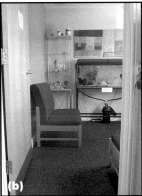

6.1 **(a)** Entrance from reception into the separate 'quiet' waiting area. **(b)** Quiet waiting area. This room leads directly off the reception area. It can be used as a waiting area for rabbits and small exotic pets or as a non-clinical space in which to perform euthanasia. The room has couches and reading material similar to the waiting room; however, there is no clinical equipment.

Most veterinary practices display products for sale in the waiting room. Having a number of good quality rabbit-related products for sale, for example foods, hay, over-the-counter medications and books, reinforces the fact that the practice is committed to serving its rabbit-owning clients. It is certainly worthwhile, both financially and from a client satisfaction perspective, making certain that clients can get what they need at the surgery rather than having to buy food at the pet shop, or another practice. Having rabbit-related magazines for owners to read while waiting is also useful as it will very often reaffirm the advice given during consultations, as will rabbit-related posters and information leaflets.

The consultation room

The initial examination is inevitably one of the stressful events that occurs when a rabbit is presented for treatment. Stress can be reduced in several ways. One way is to avoid examining rabbits in rooms that have been recently used for predator species, in particular ferrets and birds of prey. If separate rooms are not available and consultations cannot be spaced out time-wise, then the consultation room should be cleaned and deodorized prior to examining the rabbit. The veterinary surgeon examining the rabbit should also make certain that their hands have been washed and deodorized between patients.

Handling

Stress can also be reduced by handling rabbits in a gentle and calm manner. Non-slip surfaces on tables and floors help prevent scrabbling and slipping (and often injury to the rabbit). Some rabbit vets advocate leaving the rabbit in its carrier (possibly covered) for a few minutes prior to examination, to allow the rabbit to take stock of the new environment. This gives the veterinary surgeon the opportunity to take a detailed clinical history. The author will often allow the rabbit to sit on the floor or move around the room while the history is being taken. This allows the rabbit to explore its environment, and the veterinary surgeon to assess its general condition, attitude and mobility. Having towels on the floor allows the rabbit to move without slipping. The rabbit can then be picked up gently from the floor. Although some rabbits resist being caught, most do not and can easily be restrained. Rabbits should never be picked up by the ears or the scruff. Placing a hand under the chest and scooping up the bottom, thereby supporting the weight and protecting the back, is the safest and most comfortable method of picking up the rabbit. The rabbit can then be placed on the examination table. Again, the table should have a non-slip surface: either a clean towel or a rubber mat is suitable. In most situations the rabbit's owner can help with handling; however, where a rabbit is struggling or aggressive, enlisting the help of a nurse who is experienced with rabbits may be more appropriate. The rabbit should be placed on the examination table and held there gently. Most rabbits do not resist this and the examination can proceed. If the rabbit struggles even before examination, wrapping it in a towel can be helpful. Covering the rabbit's eyes loosely with a hand can also calm the situation, especially when the rabbit appears to want to jump.

The risks of handling include bite and scratch wounds to the human handlers, and muscular and/or skeletal damage to the rabbit itself. Rabbits occasionally jump over the shoulder of the handler and, if not grasped, can land on the floor, risking long bone fractures. Rabbits that struggle while restrained can also break their own backs. With very reluctant rabbits, using a towel can be helpful, placing the towel underneath the rabbit and wrapping it snugly to form a 'bunny roll' ('bunny burrito') (see Chapter 8). This usually makes the rabbit a lot easier to handle; however, it is important to remember that even rabbits that appear to be restrained well in a 'bunny roll' can contract their lumbar muscles strongly enough to cause spine or hindlimb damage. Sedation should be considered early on when examination is resisted. Having the ability to dim the lights in the consultation room can also help to calm a nervous rabbit.

Equipment

The equipment commonly required for examining rabbits includes:

- Towels
- Otoscope with appropriate cones for dental examination as well as ear examination
- Stethoscope
- Scales
- Nail clippers
- Access to high-speed dental burrs for incisor tooth trimming if required.

The hospital ward

Regardless of whether a practice sees rabbits regularly, it is not appropriate to house rabbits in the same area as dogs and cats. Ideally rabbits should be kept separate from all natural predator species (cats, dogs, ferrets, birds of prey). Auditory, olfactory and visual cues can all be distressing to the rabbit. Although a separate rabbit ward is not always possible, finding a quiet corner where rabbits can be safely housed for short periods is generally possible. The ability to monitor rabbit inpatients properly is also important. Regular checks to assess gut motility and the amount of faeces passed are needed in addition to the more common parameters. Having a member of staff around to watch whether a rabbit is eating voluntarily, is fully mobile or spending most of the time hunched in a corner is invaluable. Behavioural observations are almost as important as physical parameters in rabbit medicine.

Cages

Rabbits can be housed in cages designed for cats. Most cages are large enough to house two average-sized rabbits for a short period. In addition to newspaper lining, plenty of hay should be provided as both a substrate and a food source. Fluffy blankets can be used as a floor covering where a wound requires a non-particulate/non-adhesive bed. However, some rabbits will shred and chew this type of blanket.

All rabbits should be provided with some kind of hide box inside their cage. As a prey species it is stressful for a rabbit to be unable to seek cover. A hide (Figure 6.2) can be as simple as a cardboard box of an appropriate size (this is easily changed if it becomes soiled and costs very little); alternatively, in a suitably sized cage, the carrier can be used as a hide. The advantage of this is that the carrier is a familiar place for the rabbit, containing familiar bedding and food.

Patients staying in hospital for long periods benefit from environmental enrichment within the hospital cage. This can be as simple as scatter feeding (hiding pelleted feed in hay around the cage so the rabbit must make an effort to find it) or stuffing an empty cardboard cylinder with hay and fresh leaves. A bonded companion (Figure 6.3) or familiar toys are also good options.

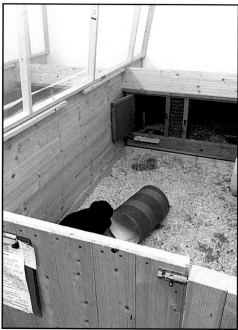

6.2 A boarding cage showing a large cardboard tube used as a hide area. (Courtesy of R Guy)

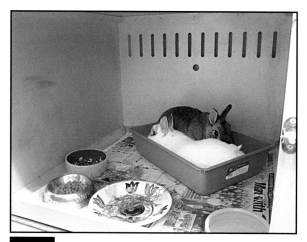

6.3 Bonded pair of rabbits in a hospital cage.

Food and water

Many owners will automatically bring familiar food items with their pets for a planned hospital stay. Even if this diet is inappropriate, hospitalization is not the time to make any sudden dietary changes. It is not unreasonable for even the smallest practices to keep a small amount of common rabbit foods and hay for inpatient use. Food can be offered in heavy ceramic dishes used for cats, or can be scatter fed to provide environmental enrichment. Fresh food will also be needed, especially if the inpatient is not eating reliably. Fresh food is an important tool for stimulating appetite in rabbits. This can be freshly picked grass and dandelions (from a site away from the roadside that has not been sprayed with chemicals, and where dogs do not urinate) or vegetables bought from a shop. Practices that see a lot of rabbits may wish to consider having a vegetable patch to provide fresh food regularly (Figure 6.4).

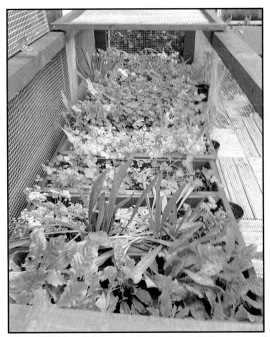

6.4 Vegetables planted in the veterinary practice for rabbit patients. (Courtesy of S Weaver)

It is worth confirming whether a rabbit is used to a bowl or a bottle for drinking water; providing both is a good strategy if this information is not known. Many rabbits used to a bottle will appear to drink excessively when provided with a bowl. This is usually behavioural rather than pathological, and providing water in a bowl can be a good tool for improving hydration. The use of bottles makes more sense in terms of reducing contamination and disease transmission; however, rabbits that are not used to them will not easily learn to use bottles in a hospital environment.

Temperature

One factor that is often overlooked when keeping rabbits in hospital is the ambient temperature. The tendency is to keep hospital wards slightly warmer than normal room temperature. Rabbits do not tolerate high ambient temperatures. In the wild they would usually avoid heat by going down into underground burrows. Temperatures >22°C cause a reduction in feed intake, and severe signs of heat stress are seen at temperatures >27°C. The recommended ambient temperature for rabbits is 18–21°C (Cervera and Fernandez Carmona, 2010). Increasing ventilation and making certain rabbits have shade from direct sunlight will allow them behaviourally to control the temperature more readily. Rabbits recovering from anaesthesia and neonates may require slightly warmer temperatures until they are able to thermoregulate normally.

Cleaning

Many rabbits are house-trained and use litter trays. Small litter trays with non-clumping litter (preferably a familiar type) should also be provided within the hospital cage. Clumps of litter can lead to gut impaction if eaten. Disinfection should be performed in the same way as for dogs and cats. Cages and cage furniture should be cleaned and a proprietary disinfectant applied at the correct concentration for the correct length of time (see Chapter 8).

Infection control

In general, rabbits pose minimal risks for zoonotic infection in hospital, although cases of encephalitozoonosis and pasteurellosis have been reported in immunocompromised humans (Figure 6.5). Rabbits can pass infections to other rabbits while in hospital (myxomatosis, rabbit haemorrhagic disease (RHD), coccidiosis, encephalitozoonosis, pasteurellosis)

Agents	Epidemiology	Clinical signs	
		In rabbits	*In humans*
Cheyletiella parasitivorax	Transmission by contact with infected animal. Mites are usually host-specific but will move transiently to other species	Heavy scurf/dandruff	Non-specific pruritic dermatitis
Microsporum canis, Trichophyton mentagrophytes (dermatophytosis)	Contact with an infected animal allows transmission. May also be transmitted via contaminated fomites. Incubation period is 1–3 weeks	Areas of patchy alopecia, with broken hairs visible. May be pruritic with secondary infection	May cause red scaly lesions, usually categorized with regard to location on the body
Encephalitozoon cuniculi (encephalitozoonosis)	Transmission is by oral intake of spores, usually shed in the urine of infected animals	Many seropositive animals are asymptomatic; however neurological signs and those of renal disease are thought to be associated with infection	Ocular lesions and more disseminated disease in immunocompromised persons
Pasteurella multocida (pasteurellosis)	Direct transmission from inhalation of infected respiratory secretions postulated but unproven. Indirect transmission via contact with infected surfaces, also postulated but unproven. One case proven in a human who was immunocompromised	Many animals carry this bacterium without clinical signs. May see mucopurulent nasal discharge, head tilt due to otitis media/interna, abscesses or evidence of systemic illness	Respiratory infection usually occurs in humans with chronic underlying respiratory compromise. Infected wounds, with a history of a previous bite

6.5 Zoonotic agents and their method of transmission.

and on occasions can be a source of infection to guinea pigs kept in close proximity (bordetellosis is carried by rabbits but can cause significant disease in guinea pigs). Rabbit fleas can spread to other species in the same way as cat and dog fleas can infest rabbits.

Rabbits do not appear to be very susceptible to many of the diseases that humans carry; however, encephalitis secondary to infection with human herpes simplex virus (HSV) has been documented. Staff suffering from cold sores should be advised to avoid close contact with rabbit patients and to practise good hand hygiene if it is necessary to handle rabbits while an active cold sore is present.

Exercise

Just as canine inpatients are usually exercised during their hospital stay, rabbits also benefit from the ability to have some exercise outside their cage. This is particularly important for rabbits that are not eating well, because exercise is one factor that stimulates gut motility. A short supervised period of exercise in the ward is fine; use of an outdoor secure run would be ideal. However, rabbits exercised indoors may chew wires if not watched, and rabbits exercised outdoors may be exposed to the threat of predation and the risk of disease transmission.

Preparation areas and theatre

Many rabbits admitted for a hospital stay will require some kind of medical or surgical intervention. In order for this process to run smoothly some re-organization and additional equipment may be required. The principle of keeping predator and prey species separate (where possible) should extend to the preparation and surgery areas.

Scheduling procedures and postoperative monitoring

From a practical perspective it is sensible to schedule rabbit surgeries early to avoid long waiting periods in a potentially stressful environment. Rabbits can be admitted and then anaesthetized soon after, undergo the surgical procedure and be recovering while the dogs and cats are attended to. This allows a longer postoperative observation period and an opportunity to institute assisted feeding or fluid therapy if required. During the afternoon many of the dogs and cats are likely still to be recovering from anaesthesia and therefore hopefully will be less noisy than usual.

Good postoperative observation of rabbits is essential and, outside of anaesthesia itself, this is the most common period in which perioperative deaths occur. Many of these deaths are preventable and can be avoided if emergent situations are noticed early. Many critically ill patients are monitored in an area where lots of people are working (often the preparation area) and the benefits of immediate action in the event of an emergency must be weighed against the stress of the proximity of staff, cats and dogs.

An ideal sequence of events for a rabbit admitted to hospital for surgery

1. Clinical examination is performed and the rabbit admitted to hospital.
2. The rabbit is weighed and any preoperative blood work completed.
3. Anaesthetic drug doses are calculated and the drugs prepared.
4. Fluid therapy is started and pain medication administered.
5. Anaesthesia is induced, the rabbit is intubated and the anaesthetic monitoring chart started.
6. The procedure is completed and anaesthesia concluded.
7. The rabbit is monitored after extubation until it is able to maintain its position in sternal recumbency and lift its head.
8. Thereafter regular checks are made on clinical parameters, and adjustments to fluid therapy and pain relief made as appropriate.
9. If the rabbit is not seen eating within 1 hour of awakening then assisted feeding should be instituted, providing the animal is able to swallow.
10. Once the rabbit is eating voluntarily, fluid therapy can be stopped and in many cases the rabbit may be discharged from hospital.

Equipment

Additional equipment is useful in the preparation and operating areas of surgeries undertaking rabbit work. This can include:

- Suitably sized endotracheal tubes (preferably clear uncuffed plastic; Figure 6.6) or supraglottic laryngeal devices
- Laryngoscope with a Flecknell or Wisconsin size 0 or 1 paediatric blade
- Suitably sized anaesthetic circuits (Ayres T-piece or Bain with paediatric connections) with the minimum of dead space
- Ventilator
- Sharp fine clippers that are reserved for rabbit use only

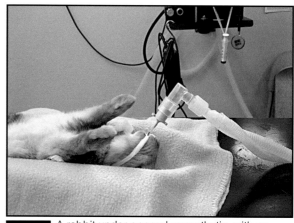

6.6 A rabbit under general anaesthetic, with an endotracheal tube in place.

- Heat mats and insulating blankets
- Suitably sized surgical instruments
- Suitably sized intravenous catheters
- High-speed dental burr
- Rabbit dental kit.

Discharge and follow-up

Once a rabbit has completed its treatment and is discharged from hospital, provision should be made for monitoring its continued recovery. This should start at the discharge appointment. The discharge appointment is an opportunity to communicate to the rabbit's owner what has happened to their animal in terms of treatment, procedures, surgical intervention and supportive feeding. Ideally, everyone involved in the ongoing care should be present at the appointment; however, this is not always achievable.

The appointment should also be used to:

- Discuss ongoing feeding and medication needs
- Demonstrate supportive feeding and medicating to confirm that the owner will be able to accomplish these things at home
- Discuss the criteria for determining whether the recovery is going according to plan (or not).

At the time of hospital discharge an appointment should be made for the next recheck examination. An example of a rabbit discharge sheet can be found at the end of this chapter.

Referrals

Not all cases will be within the competence of the primary veterinary practice. In this case, referral should be discussed. Because so many more rabbits are now insured and/or owned by people requiring or requesting the same service that is accorded to other species, referral is now a fairly common procedure. Referral to a specialist exotics practice may be considered if long-term care for rabbits is outside the practice capabilities; however, for a practice that is rabbit-friendly, referral for specific expertise and care (e.g. orthopaedic services) may be more appropriate. The *RCVS Guide to Professional Conduct* requires that referral be offered to a suitably qualified colleague should the diagnosis or treatment of a condition be outside the veterinary surgeon's area of competence. It is incumbent on the veterinary surgeon to assess the facilities and care provided within their practice and offer referral appropriately.

Preventive healthcare

Most animals under veterinary care have a preventive healthcare programme designed for them and rabbits should be no exception. Vaccination, neutering and parasite control are all common procedures in other species, yet in many areas of the UK fewer than 30% of rabbits registered with veterinary surgeons are vaccinated, and many are left unneutered. A rabbit-friendly practice should be able to advise on and undertake a comprehensive preventive healthcare programme for their rabbit clients.

Vaccination

Rabbits in the UK should be vaccinated against myxomatosis (see Chapter 17) and rabbit haemorrhagic disease (RHD; also known as viral haemorrhagic disease, VHD). At the time of writing (2012) there are two single vaccines against RHD available in the UK (Lapinject, CEVA; Cylap, Pfizer) and a combined myxomatosis/RHD vaccine (Nobivac Myxo-RHD, MSD Animal Health). There is currently no monovalent myxomatosis vaccine available in the UK; however, this position may change in the near future. Myxomatosis and RHD can both be spread by direct contact with infected rabbits, but contact is not the only method of transmission. Myxomatosis is spread by biting insects such as mosquitoes and midges, while RHD can be spread by fomites such as contaminated hay or vegetables. Clearly, even house rabbits that never have access to the outdoors should be vaccinated.

The incidence of myxomatosis varies yearly and also geographically; however, it is endemic in the UK and protection against this disease is always recommended. RHD has often been felt to be less common because clinical cases are seen much less frequently. However, outbreaks have been reported regularly in wild rabbits and the likelihood is that RHD is under-reported in both wild and domestic rabbits. This is because death often occurs rapidly without preceding clinical signs. Wild rabbits with RHD often die inside their burrows and the bodies are not found or examined. Pet rabbits dying from RHD are also often not presented or reported to veterinary surgeons; RHD that affects meat or breeding rabbit colonies is much more likely to be reported. Many rabbit owners will vaccinate against myxomatosis but not RHD because the perception is that RHD is not prevalent in the UK.

As stated above, the recommendation is to vaccinate all rabbits against both myxomatosis and RHD. With the currently available vaccines this means that the combined myxomatosis–RHD vaccine is indicated in all cases. The combined vaccine contains recombinant myxomatosis–RHD that comprises RHD capsid protein that has been inserted into the myxoma virus genome. The vaccine may be used in rabbits from 5 weeks of age and has a duration of immunity of 12 months. The vaccine is administered as a single subcutaneous injection, and a single primary injection is sufficient. Few side effects are reported subsequent to vaccination; however, a mild febrile response (an increase in temperature of 1–2°C) and a small subcutaneous swelling may be noted. The skin swelling should resolve within 3 weeks of vaccination. Rarely, skin scabs around the eyelids and face have been reported. These do not affect the health of the animal and resolve quickly. While no vaccine is 100% effective, the combined vaccine has shown good efficacy against both myxomatosis and RHD, and has been used successfully in the face of a myxomatosis outbreak (A. Meredith, personal communication).

One drawback of this vaccine is that the RHD portion may not be effective in rabbits that have been previously vaccinated using a myxoma virus-based myxomatosis vaccine (i.e. rabbits vaccinated against myxomatosis in continental Europe or the USA; the monovalent myxomatosis vaccine in the UK was based on Shope fibroma virus), or in those that have suffered from clinical myxomatosis and recovered. The recommendation in this case is to vaccinate the individual with a single dose of stand-alone adjuvanted RHD vaccine, prior to using the combined vaccine.

Routine neutering

Neutering is advised for all rabbits not intended for breeding. It reduces the possibility of unwanted pregnancies, transmission of venereal diseases such as treponematosis, sexual frustration, territorial aggression and urine spraying. Females left unneutered can develop uterine changes that lead to uterine adenocarcinoma. Early neutering avoids this issue, and neutering even when changes have begun within the uterus can be curative.

Neutering at or after puberty has been advocated; however, many practitioners feel that neutering earlier is technically easier, particularly in females. While prepubertal uteri are tiny and can be difficult to find (possibly making the risk of post-surgical adhesion formation greater), there is far less fat in the broad ligament and the procedure is far quicker and technically simpler. What is not known is whether early neutering results in an increase in the incidence of adrenal disease in the same way as it does in ferrets.

Depending on breed (smaller breeds mature earlier) neutering can be accomplished from 4 to 6 months of age (possibly up to 8 months in giant breeds). The individual should ideally be large enough to intubate, and in males the testicles should be descended. Female rabbits are immediately sterile while in males a period of 6 weeks must pass before sterility can be guaranteed. This is because viable sperm remain in the spermatic cord for a period of time after removal of the testicles.

Neutering procedures are described and illustrated in the *BSAVA Manual of Rabbit Surgery, Dentistry and Imaging*.

Routine worming

Rabbits in the UK do not often develop nematode worm burdens that require routine worming treatment. The rabbit is the intermediate host for several tapeworms that affect dogs and cats, and pet rabbits that graze in gardens inhabited by pet dogs or visited by foxes can become infected. The incidence of these parasites is not high because most pet owners now worm their dogs with preparations that are effective against tapeworms. The rabbit can

also be a primary host for tapeworms; cestode species vary in wild rabbits from different parts of the world. There are various intermediate hosts, some of which are invertebrates. There are no routine worming treatments advocated for prevention of cestode infection (either primary or secondary). Routine worming of in-contact cats and dogs, and prevention of build-up of faecal matter on grazing land, are secondary strategies.

No species of trematode has been reported in rabbits.

Nematodes

The commonest intestinal nematode found in pet rabbits is *Passalurus ambiguus*. This worm is thought to be non-pathogenic in adult rabbits and may have a role in mechanical mixing of ingesta in the caecum. Heavy infestations in young animals may cause clinical signs requiring treatment and may contribute to the enteritis complex seen in this age group. Unless clinical signs are noted, routine worming is not required. The small, thread-like worm is seen in the faeces of affected animals. The life-cycle is direct. *P. ambiguus* is susceptible to most anthelmintics, e.g. piperazine and fenbendazole. Ivermectin is ineffective at 0.4 mg/kg (Tsui and Patton, 1991). It is unlikely that *P. ambiguus* would require treatment in the adult rabbit. Control strategies in the environment involve restricting access to potentially infected faeces, for example by regular cleaning of hutches, and pasture rotation, particularly where young rabbits are kept.

There are other nematodes that principally affect wild rabbits. These include *Graphidium strigosum* and *Trichostrongylus retortaeformis*. *Obeliscoides cuniculi* occurs in wild rabbits in various parts of the world and in domestic rabbits in the USA. Clinically it causes haemorrhagic diarrhoea.

Cestodes

Cysticercus pisiformis is the larval stage of *Taenia pisiformis*, which is a tapeworm that affects dogs and foxes, with rabbits acting as the intermediate host. Tapeworm segments packed with eggs are shed in faeces and contaminate pasture. Grazing rabbits ingest eggs that pass into the small intestine where the onchosphere emerges and migrates to the peritoneal cavity via the liver. Multiple oval cysts are found in the mesentery. The cysts contain the inverted scolex of the tapeworm. Heavy infections cause abdominal discomfort and distension. In severe cases, they can cause intestinal obstruction. Migration through the liver results in the development of fibrous tracts and necrotic foci.

Coenurus serialis is the larval stage of *Taenia serialis*, which is a tapeworm that affects dogs and foxes. A variety of mammals can act as intermediate hosts; these are usually wild rabbits and hares, but primates and even humans can host the intermediate stages. Onchospheres from this tapeworm migrate to the subcutaneous tissue where they form cysts that are palpated as soft swellings under the skin. Occasionally a cyst may be found in the orbit where it causes a retrobulbar swelling.

Echinococcus granulosus affects dogs and foxes. Most mammalian species, including humans and rabbits, can act as intermediate hosts. Huge cysts that are able to produce secondary buds develop. The daughter cysts can, in turn, produce granddaughter cysts with the result that a huge cyst full of smaller cysts develops. Rupture of the cyst seeds the surrounding tissues with smaller cysts, all of which are capable of developing. The clinical result is abdominal swelling (due to palpable masses), abdominal pain and anorexia.

Routine treatment for ectoparasites

Rabbits can host a variety of ectoparasites, and owners may request routine treatment. Dog and cat fleas from other animals in the household, rabbit fleas, lice and mites may all be found. Imidacloprid and selamectin preparations are both safe and effective for the treatment of most ectoparasites. With all ectoparasites it is important to be aware that there may be an underlying reason for the rabbit to be infested, for example dental pain reducing grooming. Any rabbit presented for ectoparasitism should be thoroughly examined for underlying disease. See Chapter 17 for further detail.

Routine control of *Encephalitozoon cuniculi*

E. cuniculi is a microsporidial organism that is commonly found in rabbits in the UK and is a cause of both neurological signs and renal failure, although many infections are subclinical. Infection usually results from ingestion of infective spores passed in the urine and faeces of infected animals. Spores can remain viable in the environment for 4–6 weeks, although they can easily be inactivated by most disinfectants. Infection *in utero* can also occur. Control of this disease should be aimed at control of the spread of the organism within the host and minimizing contact with spores in the environment. This is achieved by using fenbendazole to clear the organism from the host, and strategies such as elevating feeding bowls, using hay nets rather than hay as bedding, maintaining good standards of hygiene and separating seropositive from seronegative individuals. See Chapters 9, 13 and 15 for more detail.

There are now products commercially marketed for prevention and treatment of encephalitozoonosis under the Small Animal Exemption Scheme. The recommendations made include a 28-day course of fenbendazole for treatment of the disease, and a 9-day course every 6 months for prevention. More than 50% of rabbits in the UK are seropositive for *E. cuniculi*; however, many of these rabbits never become clinically ill. A positive antibody titre does not confer resistance to infection, and neither does regular treatment.

Routine *E. cuniculi* control should be based on risk of exposure, knowledge of serological status and perceived risk of administering the medication.

Grooming procedures

There are various grooming procedures that may be requested by rabbit owners.

Nail trimming

This is similar to the procedure in dogs and cats. One caution is that once a rabbit's nails are clipped the edges can be very sharp, so if the nails are being clipped because the rabbit tends to kick and scratch then this may make the risk of injury higher. Occasionally rabbits that are struggling will lose a nail. The keratin portion separates from the nail bed; this may bleed and become painful. Keeping nails short or well worn down will help alleviate this problem. Rabbits that are ageing or overweight may develop rotation of the digits so that their toes appear twisted. These nails will require regular trimming or they will overgrow and twist, possibly digging into the adjacent toe.

Fur trimming

Asking for a nurse to trim matted fur, particularly in long-haired breeds, is a common request from rabbit owners. It is important to recognize that in many cases there is an underlying clinical reason for fur to be matted, and this should be explained to the owner and the cause investigated. Possible reasons include: urine sludging; failure to eat caecotrophs; back pain; abdominal pain; dental pain; and lack of balance due to middle ear disease or encephalitozoonosis. Rabbit skin is fragile and their fur is dense, so often clipping poses a risk of damaging the underlying skin unless it is performed carefully. A dedicated pair of rabbit clippers with sharp blades should be used. The skin should be held taut and the fur clipped away in the direction of its growth. If the area is painful or the rabbit fractious, sedation should be used.

Tooth trimming

Requests for dental trimming should be dealt with by a veterinary surgeon in the first instance. Overgrowth of incisors is rarely an isolated problem, and the cheek teeth should be checked at the time of incisor coronal reduction. Incisor trimming should never be done using nail clippers, as this can result in the teeth shattering, sharp edges that can damage the oral soft tissue, and vertical cracks that can result in apical abscessation. Some rabbits tolerate manual restraint for incisor trimming using a dental burr. The rabbit is restrained and the oral soft tissues pushed back using a tongue depressor placed behind the incisors. The burr is then used to shorten the incisor crowns. There is a risk of soft tissue damage from a spinning burr if the rabbit struggles. In this event sedation should be used. Options for tooth trimming are discussed in detail in the *BSAVA Manual of Rabbit Surgery, Dentistry and Imaging*.

Nursing clinics

Offering nursing clinics to rabbit clients is a great way to bond these clients to the practice, increase footfall and showcase the knowledge and competence of the rabbit nurses. Various clinics can be offered (see also Chapter 8).

Growing-up clinics

Once a young rabbit is vaccinated at 6 weeks old there is a long period prior to neutering where there is little contact with the surgery. Growing-up clinics are designed to cover issues such as litter training, rabbit-proofing and when to neuter, and to address any nutritional or health issues that may arise. Getting the rabbit into the surgery for a non-stressful appointment and giving the owner an opportunity to ask questions at their leisure without a time constraint can be very valuable.

General new pet clinics
New rabbit clinics can be held just prior to or just after obtaining a new rabbit. They are an opportunity to give advice on routine healthcare, neutering, diet, housing, exercise, environmental enrichment and companionship.

Geriatric clinics
Many rabbits are now living significantly longer and geriatric problems are being recognized more commonly. Geriatric clinics are a good way of ensuring that these rabbits are checked more than once a year at the vaccination appointment. Routine weighing, blood tests, blood pressure monitoring and dental checks can all be accomplished (see Chapter 20).

Weight management clinics
Obesity is an increasing problem in pet rabbits and having support during the weight loss process can help the owners comply with the dietary modifications (see also the *BSAVA Manual of Exotic Pet and Wildlife Nursing*).

Dental clinics
A 6-monthly routine dental check can be very helpful in assessing oral health, and can lead to dietary advice or modification and initiation of veterinary dental procedures. For most rabbits a year between routine consultations is too long to keep a proper watch on dental changes.

Client information sheets
Clients will retain only around 30% of what is said to them during a consultation. It is very useful for a rabbit-friendly practice to have a variety of information sheets available that owners can take home and read at their leisure. Many information sheets are produced by food or drug companies and contain a wealth of good information as well as advertising. Purpose-written sheets reinforce the commitment of the practice to serving their rabbit clients and display the level of knowledge and experience available from the clinic. Several examples of rabbit information sheets are included at the end of this chapter.

A natural extension of providing information sheets is the compilation of packs that provide a range of information to the owner. These can be themed to different life stages (e.g. juvenile rabbits, geriatric rabbits) or to specific disease conditions (e.g. a rabbit dental disease pack).

Insurance
At the time of writing there are at least three large pet insurance companies in the UK offering policies for rabbits. Availability in other countries may vary. One company offers a free 4-week cover note for all young rabbits presented for vaccination, alongside those offered for puppies and kittens. While the policies vary in their particulars, they generally cover unexpected illness or traumatic injury. They do not cover vaccination, routine preventive treatments or the full cost of dental work. All policies require that routine preventive care is undertaken, including but not limited to routine dental examinations. Owners should be encouraged to consider what they need from an insurance policy and compare the policies available.

Insurance for rabbits should be supported in the same way as insurance is advised for cats and dogs. The obvious benefit is that owners do not need to make a financial decision if their pet becomes ill; the less obvious but more important welfare benefit is that all insured rabbits should be seen regularly and receive routine preventive care.

Euthanasia

Euthanasia is always an emotive subject, and the decision to euthanase a pet rabbit is as difficult as it is in other species. Rabbits are perhaps unusual in that, while some are treasured family pets, others may be thought of as 'disposable' children's pets. This can mean that the reasons for requesting euthanasia are different from those we are comfortable with in other pet species. While euthanasia itself is not a welfare issue (failure to euthanase in a timely fashion can be), it is an ethical one. It is not uncommon for euthanasia to be requested for young rabbits with treatable conditions. The *RCVS Code of Professional Conduct* states: 'No veterinary surgeon is obliged to kill a healthy animal unless required to do so under statutory powers as part of their conditions of employment. Veterinary surgeons do, however, have the privilege of being able to relieve an animal's suffering in this way in appropriate cases'. Variations in how owners think of their pets dictate how and when euthanasia takes place. Some owners may not be aware of appropriate treatment options, while others have discounted them for whatever reason. In some circumstances rehoming the rabbit may be a welcome option. In all circumstances the welfare of the rabbit must be protected and undue fear, pain and distress avoided.

Location
Where euthanasia is to take place should be carefully thought through. Some practices are lucky enough to have a separate room (i.e. not a consulting room) that can be used for this purpose. This allows the owner enough time to experience the process without the added stress of being rushed. In the author's practice this room contains couches, but no consultation table, firmly removing it from the more clinical areas of the surgery. Owners are encouraged to spend as much time as they need both before and after the euthanasia, in order to process the event. In situations where this sort of

accommodation is not practical then a consultation room can be used, as long as some thought is given to reducing the impact of dogs and cats being in proximity. Ideally euthanasia should be scheduled at a quiet time of the day, and plenty of time allowed so that the consultation room is not needed for other routine work. Making certain that a chair is available and having blankets or towels placed over the examination table or on the floor to reduce slipping and struggling is helpful. The idea is to make the room more comfortable for both the rabbit and the owner.

Increasingly owners are requesting euthanasia in their own homes. This is often less distressing for both the rabbit and the owner. The visit can be planned at the owner's convenience and can take place in surroundings that are familiar to the rabbit. The downside is that veterinary facilities are not available other than those brought in the visit bag. Good planning is therefore essential and the visit bag needs to be packed to cover all eventualities (e.g. syringes disengaging and leaking sedative or euthanasia solution, the animal requiring intraperitoneal injection rather than intravenous, heparin saline in the event of intravenous catheters blocking). An important consideration for home euthanasia is what will be done with the body afterwards. Often the owners will bury the body (see later) but appreciate their pet being placed on a blanket or in a box in a cosmetic way by the veterinary surgeon. On some occasions the owners request that the rabbit be returned to the surgery for cremation. In this circumstance it is important that the rabbit be treated with respect, and carried away in an appropriate manner. An open carrier or basket, or a blanket, are all suitable and the rabbit can be placed safely in the car or van. This is often a very important moment for the owner as it is the last view of their pet.

Communication

Good communication with the owner is vital at all stages of the euthanasia process. It is worth letting owners know what to expect at each point, from how the rabbit needs to be restrained to how rapidly loss of consciousness occurs. At times where emotions are heightened, keeping up a non-intrusive narrative about everything that is going on can be helpful and often gives the owner something to focus on. Many owners are surprised at how rapidly death occurs once the intravenous agents are given, so it is considerate to prepare them for this.

Techniques

Pentobarbital injection

The most common method of euthanasia of pet animals in the UK is an intravenous injection of a lethal dose of pentobarbital. This is certainly an appropriate method in the pet rabbit. It is not appropriate where the rabbit carcass may thereafter be used as food for other animals, e.g. birds of prey or snakes. Rabbits are not tolerant of intravenous injections unless moribund or sedated. They often respond by struggling or screaming (albeit nearly

silently in many cases). Either situation can be very distressing to the rabbit and also to the owners if they are present. It is preferable to consider placing an intravenous catheter prior to euthanasia to avoid the rabbit reacting to injection of irritant euthanasia solution. The author will commonly use the marginal ear vein for catheter placement. Depending on the size of the rabbit, a 23 or 21 G catheter can be inserted and secured in place. Applying a local anaesthetic cream (e.g. EMLA) to the area first can make catheterization less painful and stressful. Once the catheter is secured in place it should be flushed with heparin saline to prevent blood clots blocking the end and rendering it useless.

In some circumstances sedation of the rabbit prior to euthanasia may be viewed as a good option. The author tends to do this in cases where the owners wish to remain present but the rabbit is not moribund. It depends on the situation and the temperament of the rabbit as well as the degree of discomfort the rabbit is suffering. The sedative combination the author uses most commonly is medetomidine (0.25 mg/kg) and buprenorphine (0.03 mg/kg) combined in the same syringe. The injection can be given either intramuscularly or subcutaneously. In the author's experience this combination produces rapid and reliable sedation (the owners can hold the rabbit while it becomes unconscious) before the peripheral vasoconstriction associated with medetomidine occurs. This means the rabbit is sedated enough to tolerate intravenous injection while there is still elevated blood pressure and peripheral vasodilation, making the veins easier to see and access. Once the owner is ready, the pentobarbital can be injected into the marginal ear vein while the owner holds the rabbit. Other sedatives that are suitable include fentanyl/fluanisone and midazolam.

Other methods

Reports of other methods of euthanasia have been published. Several are acceptable in practice (although perhaps not with owners present). These include the following.

- **An overdose of inhalant anaesthetic:** This method can be rapid; however, many rabbits breath-hold in response to the smell of anaesthetic gases and may struggle or scream. Injectable anaesthetics used as a premedication can make the process smoother; however, it is difficult to understand why this method would be chosen over injection of pentobarbital.

- **Injection of an anaesthetized rabbit with potassium chloride:** This method can be acceptable even with owners present. The rabbit is anaesthetized and potassium chloride is injected intravenously in order to stop the heart. Again it is difficult to think of a circumstance where this would be chosen over pentobarbital injection.

- **Intraperitoneal injection of barbiturates:** This method has been commonly used for the euthanasia of pet rabbits over the years. An overdose of pentobarbital is injected into the peritoneal cavity and the drug diffuses into the circulation, eventually causing death. The injectable pentobarbital solution is fairly irritant, so the action of putting it into the peritoneum causes discomfort. Because the drug must diffuse into the circulation in order to work, the process is fairly slow and some rabbits exhibit an excitation phase that can be distressing both for the rabbit and the owner. This method is not one the author would advocate unless all other options have been explored and discounted.

- **Alternative methods** that may be suitable in a moribund or sedated/anaesthetized rabbit where intravenous access is not possible involve the intrarenal, intrahepatic or intracardiac injection of pentobarbital. This is quicker than using the intraperitoneal route but again the potential for discomfort must be considered.

After euthanasia

Many rabbits are kept in bonded pairs, so it is important to consider the surviving individual's welfare within the euthanasia decision. In some circumstances, particularly where the surviving animal has been very reliant on the one to be euthanased, it may be decided to euthanase both individuals at the same time.

Should the surviving rabbit be healthy then consideration should be given to allowing it to see its companion after it has died. This allows the remaining rabbit to understand what has happened. Rather than perform the euthanasia with the other rabbit within sight, the author usually just allows the companion access to the body for a period of time afterwards. This stems from the feeling that the stress of separation for a short period is less than that of seeing a companion restrained and euthanased. At this point if the owners have strong views on whether the companion rabbit should be present, these are taken into account. Most rabbits will approach their companion, sniff and nudge them and some will lie down and groom the dead animal. Eventually, and usually sooner rather than later, the surviving rabbit appears to understand, lose interest and move away. At that point the rabbit can be taken away from the body. If the owners have any strong feelings regarding how long the rabbits stay together afterwards, there is no harm in letting the surviving rabbit stay with its mate overnight.

Preparing a body for viewing

Where a rabbit has either died unexpectedly or has been euthanased without the owners present it may be necessary to prepare the rabbit for a 'goodbye viewing' with the owners. It is important that the rabbit is presented in a cosmetic manner (blood or discharge must be cleaned off and the fur dried) and most owners prefer that clinical items, such as intravenous catheters, are removed. The rabbit should be placed on absorbent pads to deal with leakage of body fluids (incontinence pads or puppy pads are suitable) and then wrapped in a blanket. The head can be left visible, but able to be covered easily should this be necessary. The eyes can be held shut with skin glue if needed. This visit is often very difficult for the owners as feelings of guilt at not being with the rabbit at the end can surface. This visit should not be rushed, and time should be allowed for the owner both to say goodbye and to talk to staff members about their rabbit and the circumstances of its death.

Grieving

The circumstances of a rabbit's death can have a strong impact on grief. An unexpected or traumatic death is shocking and can bring feelings of anger and guilt to the surface. There are several stages of grieving: denial; weeping; bodily distress; anger; guilt; and eventual acceptance. This process can take a significant amount of time. It is also important to remember that adult owners grieve differently from children. Information on grief counselling and resources for helping children to cope with the loss of a pet can be obtained from the Internet. Books for both adults and children on pet loss and grieving can be obtained and kept in the practice. Many practices send a sympathy card or flowers after the loss of a pet, and this, as much as the treatment owners receive at this difficult time, can help owners cope with the loss of their pet.

The options for disposal of the body after death are the same as for other species. Many local authorities do not condone the burial of animals in their jurisdictions, even on private land. Animals that are buried should be wrapped in plastic and buried fairly deeply to avoid being dug up by local wildlife. Animals euthanased using barbiturates pose a significant risk to any animal excavating and consuming the body. Owners should be advised that cremation is often the better option; ashes can be returned and buried or scattered.

References and further reading

Cervera C and Fernandez Carmona J (2010) Nutrition and the climatic environment. In: *Nutrition of the Rabbit, 2nd edn*, ed. C de Blas and J Wiseman, pp.267–285. CABI International, Wallingford

Harcourt-Brown F (2002) *Textbook of Rabbit Medicine*. Butterworth-Heinemann, Oxford

Tsui TLH and Patton NM (1991) Comparative efficiency of subcutaneous injection doses of ivermectin against *P. ambiguus* in rabbits. *Journal of Applied Rabbit Research* **14**, 266–269

Varga M, Gott L and Lumbis R (2012) *BSAVA Manual of Exotic Pet and Wildlife Nursing*. BSAVA Publications, Gloucester

Online resources

Veterinary Information Network (www.vin.com)

Rabbit Welfare Association and Fund (RWAF) (www.houserabbit.co.uk)

American Association for Laboratory Animal Science (www.aalas.org)

Rabbit discharge sheet

Animal's name:...

Condition:...

....

....

....

....

Supported feeding required?   No ☐

Yes: Food required is:..

Method of feeding advised: ....Demonstrated?   Yes ☐   No ☐

Volume of food:...Frequency..

Current bodyweight:..Target ....

Medications prescribed: Drug, duration and dose:

1.   ....

2.   ....

3.   ....

Methods of administering medication demonstrated?   Yes ☐   No ☐

Recheck required?   No ☐   Yes ☐   Date...

Please call the surgery if your pet:
1.   Does not tolerate the supported feeding.
2.   Fails to swallow food or medication.
3.   Is not passing faeces or urine.
4.   Appears weak or unable to move.
5.   Or if you are otherwise concerned about their condition.

If your pet has had an operation:
1.   Check the surgical wound daily and contact the surgery immediately if it seems red, swollen, smells or is seeping fluid.
2.   Monitor the sutures. These are due to be removed on:...
3.   Signs of pain or discomfort can include: aggressive behaviour, lack of mobility, vocalization, and reduction in food intake. If any of these signs are shown, contact the surgery immediately.
4.   Should your pet have a dressing applied, please make certain this remains dry and is not being chewed by your pet. If the dressing gets wet, smells or has been chewed, please contact the surgery immediately.

Additional information:...

....

....

....

....

Surgery out-of-hours phone number is:

An example of a rabbit discharge sheet.

Client handout examples follow ▶

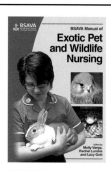

BSAVA CLIENT HANDOUTS: EXOTIC PET AND WILDLIFE SERIES

Introducing a new pet rabbit

Molly Varga

Preparation

- Introducing a new rabbit to your established pet needs to be approached carefully and can be a time-consuming process. Rabbits are territorial in the wild and have a defined social structure so they will need to 'work this out' in the home.
- Before introducing the new rabbit, your existing rabbit should be well and fully up to date with vaccinations. A check-up with your veterinary surgeon is recommended.
- Some pairings work better than others and this will depend on the individual rabbits. A neutered male with a neutered female is ideal, but other combinations can work.
- Before introduction both rabbits should have recovered from their neutering surgery.

First steps

- The first step is to keep both rabbits within sight and smell of each other. Bedding from each cage can be moved into the other cage regularly, so that each rabbit gets used to the smell of the other rabbit within its territory.
- It is also a good idea to feed the rabbits within sight of each other, preferably near the barrier between them. This is because eating is a social activity and it gets the rabbits used to being part of a social grouping.
- Once the rabbits are showing positive interest in each other (having non-aggressive interactions through the barrier, lying down near to each other) then physical introduction can start.

Putting them together

- The rabbits must be introduced to each other on neutral territory, such as in a room where neither rabbit has been previously. A bathroom (or even a bath!) or a pen in a new room is suitable. For rabbits that live outdoors, an area that is neutral must still be chosen. Bringing the rabbits indoors can work, or you can use outside space that neither has had previous access to.
- It is a good idea to scatter food around the area in which the rabbits are to meet. This avoids them having to fight over a single food bowl, and encourages them to forage, an activity they would perform in the wild socially.
- The meeting must be supervised by an adult who is prepared to physically separate the rabbits if they fight. Care must be taken, as rabbits in the middle of a fight will often bite indiscriminately and human injury can occur.
- A short meeting – 5 to 10 minutes – is suitable for the first time. There should be some sniffing and chasing, but the meeting should be stopped if fighting occurs. A good outcome is both rabbits lying down and apparently ignoring each other.
- If fighting does occur, both rabbits should be checked for wounds and must be treated if wounds are found.
- Meetings can be repeated daily for increasing lengths of time.
- Once the rabbits are grooming each other, eating together and lying down peacefully with one another, they can be put together in their original territories (where they are living when they are not being bonded). If this goes well, and the rabbits are behaving positively for hours at a time, then they can be allowed to share a sleeping area and to live together permanently.
- If bonding does not progress as expected, contact your veterinary surgeon who will be able to refer you to a rabbit behavioural specialist.

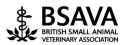

© BSAVA 2012
BSAVA Manual of Exotic Pet and Wildlife Nursing

BSAVA CLIENT HANDOUTS: EXOTIC PET AND WILDLIFE SERIES

Feeding your rabbit a healthy diet

Molly Varga and Lucy Gott

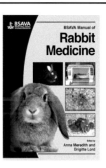

What should I feed my rabbit?

The best diet for rabbits is one that mimics as closely as possible the grass-based diet that wild rabbits evolved to eat. Grass and/or hay should form the bulk of the diet and be available at all times. Grass and hay are essential to keep your rabbit's teeth and digestive system healthy. Grass/hay intake will be reduced if too much commercial rabbit food is offered; this can lead to obesity, dental disease, digestive disease, boredom and behavioural problems. If the correct diet is fed, vitamin and mineral supplementation is generally not required.

1. **Grass-based food.** At least 80% of your rabbit's diet should be made up of good quality hay or fresh growing grass. A rabbit should eat a pile of hay equal in size to its own body (if not more) each day. Hay should be good quality (e.g. timothy); check it is clean, sweet smelling and not dusty or mouldy. Grass should be hand-picked, or the rabbit should be allowed to graze daily. Do not use lawnmower cuttings as the crushing and heat of the grass produced by the lawnmower causes it to start fermenting, which can lead to serious digestive problems and can even be fatal.
2. **Leafy green weeds and vegetables.** Feed a handful once a day. Good leafy greens are dandelions, brambles, dock, cabbage, watercress, rocket, mixed salad leaves (not iceberg lettuce because this has poor nutritional value and may cause diarrhoea), broccoli, carrot tops, kale, basil, coriander, parsley, spring greens and spinach. All green foods must be washed before being fed to your rabbit.
3. **No more than 25 g of commercial rabbit food per kilogram bodyweight per day.** This is about 1 tablespoon a day for dwarf and medium rabbit breeds. Neutered rabbits and those with limited exercise opportunities can require considerably less than this. Feed a good quality high-fibre pellet or nugget. Muesli-type diets increase the risk of dental disease and if the rabbit does not eat all the components it will not have a balanced diet.

How do I know if my rabbit is eating well?

Your vet or vet nurse can show you how to weigh your rabbit regularly and assess their body condition (body condition score, BCS). The quantity of commercial rabbit food should be adjusted to maintain an ideal weight.

Appetite

Reduced eating can be caused by many things, including pain, dental problems or fear (e.g. getting a fright from a neighbour's cat or a fox). If a rabbit stops eating, the gut will slow down and could even stop working, which can be very serious and even life-threatening. Please contact your vet if you notice changes or a reduction in appetite, especially if your rabbit hasn't eaten for more than 12 hours.

Droppings

Your rabbit should pass formed, firm droppings about the size of large peas (slightly larger for large rabbits). These should be passed frequently throughout the day. Any changes in quantity, consistency and frequency of droppings could be a sign of illness and should be addressed as soon as possible. *Please contact your vet if your rabbit has passed few or no droppings in 24 hours, if the droppings are very small, dry and hard or are very runny or sticky.*

continues ▶

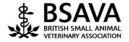
BRITISH SMALL ANIMAL
VETERINARY ASSOCIATION

Feeding your rabbit a healthy diet

continued

Your rabbit will also pass larger, stickier droppings called caecotrophs, which contain partially broken down fibre. Your rabbit will usually eat these so that he/she can fully digest the fibre. This is normal behaviour. Caecotrophs are often eaten as soon as the rabbit passes them, and most often at night, so you may not notice this happening. If your rabbit has difficulty turning around (due to being overweight, stiff or in pain) or has dental problems, it may not be able to eat the caecotrophs. This can lead to clumps of them forming around the rabbit's bottom, which could lead to skin infections and other problems. You should check the area around your rabbit's anus and genitalia for soiling, ideally every day, especially in the summer months.

Preventing 'fly strike'

Any build-up of urine and faeces around your rabbit's bottom or soiled bedding can attract flies, which could lead to 'fly strike' – this is where flies lay eggs that hatch into maggots on the rabbit. Fly strike can be prevented in a number of ways:

- Replace wet and soiled bedding daily
- Use fly screens in the hutch
- Clean off any urine or droppings stuck around the rabbit's bottom using lukewarm water, taking care not to get the whole of the rabbit soaking wet so it doesn't become too cold. Towel dry the fur (hairdryers can become very hot, causing rabbits to overheat or develop burns). ***If you notice that your rabbit has a wet or soiled bottom, an examination by your vet is advised to try and find the underlying reason for this.***

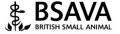
BRITISH SMALL ANIMAL

Should I have my rabbit neutered?

Molly Varga and Lucy Gott

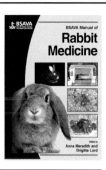

Female rabbits

Neutering (commonly called spaying) your female rabbit (doe) can:

- Prevent unwanted pregnancies
- Allow both sexes to be kept together
- Prevent reproductive tumours of the uterus (womb). These develop in 80% of rabbits by the time they reach 4 years of age. The cancer can spread to other organs, which is often fatal. Removal of the womb is therefore recommended even in older rabbits once breeding is no longer desired
- Help to reduce hormone-related behaviours such as aggression towards owners and other rabbits, scent-marking and mounting (although these may not stop completely).

Ideally, spaying is performed at around 5 months of age. As female rabbits get older, fat develops around the womb. This makes surgery more difficult and may increase the risk of complications.

What does spaying involve?

The operation is performed under general anaesthetic and it involves removal of the womb (uterus) and ovaries.

Your rabbit should be in good health, have a normal appetite and be passing plenty of normal droppings. She will be admitted to the hospital on the morning of her surgery but she can eat right up until her arrival at the practice.

After the operation your rabbit will have a shaved patch on her abdomen and a scar with stitches in the skin (or stitches just under the skin and surgical glue in the skin). There will also be stitches in the muscle layers underneath the skin.

Male rabbits

Neutering (commonly called castrating) your male rabbit (buck) can:

- Prevent unwanted pregnancies
- Allow both sexes to be kept together
- Help to reduce (although may not completely stop) hormone-related behaviours such as aggression towards owners and other rabbits, scent-marking and mounting
- Prevent testicular tumours developing.

Castration can be performed from 5 months of age, or possibly when the rabbit is slightly older, depending on the size of his testicles.

What does castration involve?

Castration is performed under general anaesthetic. It involves removal of both testicles but the scrotum is left.

Your rabbit should be in good health, have a normal appetite and be passing plenty of normal droppings. He will be admitted to the hospital on the morning of his surgery but he can eat right up until his arrival at the practice.

After the operation your rabbit will have a shaved area between his back legs and two small scars, which are closed together with either several small stitches or skin glue.

continues ▶

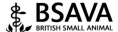

BRITISH SMALL ANIMAL

BSAVA CLIENT HANDOUTS: EXOTIC PET AND WILDLIFE SERIES

Should I have my rabbit neutered?

continued

After the operation

Your rabbit should be able to come home on the same day as the surgery, provided he/she is eating well and passing droppings. Occasionally we need to keep a rabbit in overnight if they are not eating so we can monitor them and give them supportive care.

Your veterinary nurse will explain the postoperative care and pain relief required at a discharge appointment when you come to collect your rabbit.

Once your rabbit is back home:

- Check they are eating and passing droppings:
  - If they are not eating properly and/or they are producing fewer droppings, contact the practice
- Look at the scar and stitches every day:
  - If there is redness, heat, swelling or a discharge, please contact the practice
  - If your rabbit is interfering with the scar, please contact the practice. An Elizabethan collar may be needed but we don't use them on every rabbit, as they can interfere with appetite and eating.

Skin stitches (if applicable) will need to be removed after 10 days, at a re-visit appointment.

> **IMPORTANT NOTE**
> Male rabbits can still have viable sperm for up to 4 weeks after castration and may need to be separated from unneutered females during that time if pregnancy is to be prevented.

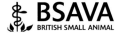 **BSAVA**
BRITISH SMALL ANIMAL

BSAVA CLIENT HANDOUTS: EXOTIC PET AND WILDLIFE SERIES

Housing your rabbit

Molly Varga

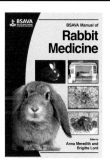

Most rabbits live in hutches; however this traditional form of housing often doesn't give the rabbit enough room to behave normally.

What does my rabbit need?

- Every rabbit should be able to travel three hops in every direction inside their house.
- Every rabbit should have access to a large exercise run, either indoors or out.
- Every rabbit should be able to stand up on its hindlegs without its head or ears being squashed by the ceiling.
- Every rabbit should have shelter from adverse weather (wind, rain and direct sunlight).
- Every rabbit should have access to fresh water at all times.
- Every rabbit should have access to fresh appropriate food at all times.
- Every rabbit should be able to get away from scary situations: a hide box for each rabbit plus one extra is necessary, especially in outdoor runs.

How can I provide what my rabbit needs?

- Provide a large sheltered house: this can be a shed, an inside room or a large hutch if your rabbit is fairly small. Building your own shelter can be a cheaper option and allow you to customize the space to your rabbit's needs.
- Provide some additional exercise space. This enclosure can be inside or out and should be as large as possible. Let your rabbit play in the larger enclosure for at least 4 hours every day, more if possible.
- If the larger enclosure is outside, make certain your rabbit has access to their indoor shelter, or that there is an area in the enclosure that is covered to protect from wind, rain and direct sunlight.
- Outdoor enclosures also need to protect your rabbit from predators, e.g. neighbourhood cats and dogs, foxes and birds of prey. If the enclosure does not have a secure roof, you will need to keep a careful watch while your rabbit is outside.
- Give each rabbit a place to hide and provide one extra one so that each rabbit can run from one hide to another should it choose to. Hides can be pieces of wide-bore plastic drainpipe, cardboard boxes, wooden boxes or even pet carriers.
- Make certain that you check your rabbit has enough food and water twice every day, and more frequently if the weather is very cold or very hot.
- If you use water bottles, make sure these are cleaned regularly and check they are working (they can freeze in cold weather or clog up with limescale).
- Give your rabbits unlimited access to hay. This can be used for food and also bedding in cold weather.

Why is space important?

- Just like humans, rabbits benefit from regular exercise.
- Exercise promotes muscle and bone health, reduces obesity and helps your rabbit's guts stay healthy.
- Rabbits kept in a small hutch are unable to exercise and may suffer from diseases such as sore hocks, arthritis, gut stasis, failure to eat their soft faeces, or urine scalding.
- The larger the space available, the better the opportunity for your rabbit to run around and play. A pair of rabbits will need even more space.
- If your rabbit is usually happy to run and play but suddenly doesn't want to, get him/her checked out by your veterinary surgeon.

continues ▶

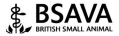

BSAVA CLIENT HANDOUTS: EXOTIC PET AND WILDLIFE SERIES

Housing your rabbit

continued

What if my rabbit seems bored?

- All rabbits enjoy having something to play with. Giving your rabbits toys can give them hours of entertainment.
- There are lots of toys that you can buy for your rabbit, but homemade ones are just as good. Wicker balls, cardboard cylinders stuffed with hay and fresh leaves, sisal mats and even some plastic dog toys are all acceptable.
- If your rabbit is a single rabbit, give serious consideration to getting him/her a companion. Rabbits are very social animals and they benefit from having a rabbit friend. (We DO NOT advise getting a guinea pig to befriend your rabbit, because often the guinea pig gets bullied and they can also catch *Bordetella* from the rabbit. This is a bacterium that causes pneumonia in guinea pigs.)

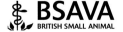

BSAVA CLIENT HANDOUTS: EXOTIC PET AND WILDLIFE SERIES

Looking after your older rabbit

Molly Varga

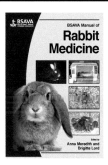

Because more people are keeping rabbits as pets and because they feed them well and seek veterinary care when they are ill, many more rabbits are living well into old age. Rabbits over 7 years of age are considered 'older' or geriatric rabbits. Your geriatric rabbit may have some special requirements as he/she gets older.

What should I look for?

There are some common signs that your older rabbit may be less well than he/she used to be. These include:

- Increased drinking and increased urination
- Loss of litter training
- Changing food preference (e.g. only eating pellets when he/she used to eat hay and vegetables also), or just eating less
- Weight loss
- Dandruff, especially over the back and near the tail
- Not eating all or any of their caecotrophs (soft faecal pellets)
- Getting wet or dirty under his/her bottom
- Being reluctant to get out of the hutch
- Increased aggression to you or his/her companion.

What might be wrong?

Older rabbits get similar ageing problems to other pets, and it is important to recognize and diagnose these. 'Old age' problems can often be treated. Common problems include:

- Chronic renal failure (kidney disease)
- End-stage dental disease
- Osteoarthritis
- Heart disease
- Sore hocks
- Senile changes including blindness, deafness and cognitive dysfunction (reduced ability to understand)
- Tumours.

What should I do?

If you notice any of the changes described above, the first step is to get your rabbit examined by your veterinary surgeon. Your vet may want to run some tests or take some X-rays. This will allow them to diagnose what is causing the changes you have noticed. Your vet will then be able to prescribe medication to treat these changes, or advise you on changes you can make to the diet or environment to make your rabbit more comfortable. It important to remember that many age-related diseases cannot be cured; the treatment is aimed at managing the disease so your rabbit can cope more easily.

Your veterinary practice may run 'Geriatric clinics' supervised by one of the qualified veterinary nurses. Attending these every 6 months or so will allow you to monitor any changes in your rabbit and let your veterinary team act promptly on any problems you or they have found.

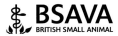

7

Physical examination and clinical techniques

Jenna Richardson and Emma Keeble

Rabbit medicine is a rapidly evolving field, with owners increasingly expecting a high standard of veterinary care for their pets. Veterinary surgeons must be competent and confident with handling, restraint and clinical examination of the rabbit, with all being performed in a safe manner to reduce the risk of injuries to the rabbit. Rabbits are natural prey species and, unless habituated to transportation, handling and restraint, will find these stressful.

Clinical examination of the rabbit has important differences when compared with other common pet species. Many clinical procedures used in rabbits are similar to those in canine and feline medicine, but differences in anatomy, physiology and behaviour result in variations to techniques that are unique to the rabbit patient.

This chapter outlines clinical history-taking specific to the rabbit and describes safe handling techniques, physical examination, common diagnostic techniques and advanced diagnostic procedures in the pet rabbit.

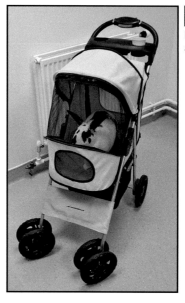

7.1 Rabbits may be brought to the clinic in a variety of carriers.

Before the consultation

A trip to the veterinary surgery should be assumed to be very stressful for the majority of rabbits. This begins before arriving at the practice. Being removed from their regular habitat, placed in a box and then, in most cases, undergoing a car journey are all very unnatural situations.

When a veterinary visit is necessary, steps should be made to reduce the negative effects on the rabbit:

- Owners should be encouraged to bring a bonded rabbit along to provide companionship for the patient
- The transportation box should be filled with hay for familiar scent and to provide the rabbit with something to burrow into and eat
- Other food items can also be placed in the box to act as a distraction and reduce the amount of time the rabbit is not eating.

Owners should be strongly dissuaded from carrying their rabbits loose in hand and should always be encouraged to transport their pets in a secure, well ventilated box (see Chapter 6). Rabbits may be presented in a range of carriers (Figure 7.1).

Clinical history

As with all species, a thorough and accurate history is of key importance. Owing to the rabbit's innate ability to hide signs of disease, subtle changes in behaviour, appetite and faecal output at times of illness can be overlooked by owners. Histories can be time-consuming to obtain; however, the more information gathered, the quicker and more accurate will be the diagnosis. To gain value from answers given by the client, particular care should be taken to avoid asking leading questions. It should also be remembered that levels of client attentiveness can vary widely. In addition, some rabbits are not handled daily and therefore owners may have only recently noticed an ailment that has actually been present for some time.

Thorough histories should not only be obtained at times when the rabbit is presenting with a clinical problem. The rabbit's background and husbandry should be discussed at routine health check and vaccination consultations. Inappropriate diet, housing and general management can predispose to a variety of different diseases. By making the owner aware of this, the veterinary surgeon can advise on changes to be implemented, reducing the likelihood of disease developing. Disease prevention is key to good welfare.

For existing patients, the husbandry may already be known; however, it is still important to check that no recent changes have been made that could account for the presenting signs. A complete review of husbandry is worthwhile once a year in such patients, usually to coincide with the annual vaccination.

A standard history form is often a useful starting point. Although not exhaustive in its questioning, the main topics are covered and a lot of useful information obtained. It can also flag up where further investigation is needed. An example is given at the end of this chapter. Such forms can either be used as an aid in consultations or can be given to the client to fill in prior to being seen by the veterinary surgeon. Priming reception staff and veterinary nurses allows this to be standard procedure before rabbit consultations. Forms can also be posted or emailed to the client before a visit, which, depending on owner compliance, may yield useful information.

As long as the rabbit is not critically ill, the history should be taken before the examination begins. General background and husbandry information should be obtained first, which ideally have already been covered by the form (e.g. housing, diet, exercise, vaccination status), before tailoring the line of questioning to the presenting problem (e.g. duration of illness, presenting signs, demeanour). Examples of specific questions are given in Figure 7.2.

Dental disease

Has there been any:

- Change in appetite?
- Dysphagia?
- Excess salivation?
- Observed bruxism?
- Ocular discharge or epiphora?
- Recent change in food selection?
- Recent weight loss?
- Change in grooming behaviour?
- Reduction in the ingestion of caecotrophs, usually noted as 'dirty bottom'?
- Change in faecal size or quantity?
- Facial swellings noted?
- Incisor abnormalities noted?

Gastrointestinal ileus

Has there been any:

- Inappetence?
- Diet change?
- Recent surgery?
- Any displays of 'pain' behaviour?
- Reduction in exercise?
- Change in companionship?
- Change in housing?
- Contact with predator species?
- General changes in routine?
- Excessive moulting?
- Known concurrent illness?

7.2 History questions for specific clinical presentations. (continues)

Urine scald

Has there been any:

- Polydipsia?
- Changes to urination frequency?
- Incontinence or inappropriate urination?
- Dysuria?
- Urine spraying?
- Change in urination posture?
- Change in activity levels?
- Colour change of urine?
- Calcium deposits noted in urine?
- Change in level of enclosure cleanliness?
- Hindlimb weakness/lameness?
- History of neurological problems?
- History of being neutered?

7.2 (continued) History questions for specific clinical presentations.

Handling and restraint

Being natural prey animals, rabbits are well adapted to hiding signs of disease and this is maintained while they are handled for examination. Extra care should be taken, as rabbits can be very flighty and may react unpredictably in threatening situations with little or no warning. The light skeletal frame (comprising only 8% of total bodyweight) and long powerful hindlimbs mean that spinal and limb fractures are a risk associated with inappropriate handling. The most serious of these are fractures of the lumbar vertebrae, which often result in paresis due to spinal cord compression.

WARNING
It is important that the rabbit is handled securely in the clinic. Transportation, even for short distances between rooms, should be in a carrier. Owing to their unpredictable flighty nature, it is not advisable to carry a rabbit by hand around the practice.

Removal from the carrier

Removing a rabbit from its carrier can be done in a number of ways:

- During the history-taking, the box can be placed on the floor with the door open, to allow the rabbit to emerge and explore the room; this is unlikely to work with nervous rabbits
- The box may be placed on the examination table and, with the owner holding the box steady, one or both arms are then slid along the sides of the rabbit, using a hand to apply gentle pressure on the rump to encourage the rabbit out of the box. Alternatively, a hand can be placed under the thorax, with a second hand supporting the hindquarters
- The clips on the carrier can be opened, to allow the lid to be removed.

Avoiding injury

Rabbits must be handled with care for their own safety. It is also important to realize that they can inflict injury upon those handling them. Along with giving a powerful kick, their claws can be very sharp and can cause deep scratches in a handler's skin. Rabbits have sharp incisors that can give a deep bite if the rabbit feels frightened or threatened.

By following standard protocols, the risk of injury to the handler, and the rabbit, can be reduced:

• The table surface should be non-slip; if this is not the case, a towel can be placed on the table to allow the rabbit to feel more secure
• Movements around the rabbit should be calm, quiet and confident, with sudden movements and loud noises avoided
• The minimum restraint that is safely possible should be used to avoid stressing the rabbit with excessive handling
• At all times during lifting and carrying, the rabbit's spine and hindlegs should be supported
• A rabbit should never be left unattended on the examination table
• Although it is always important to be efficient when performing an examination, it is particularly important when the rabbit is very stressed. Once the examination is complete, the animal should be placed back in the carrier for a 'calm-down' time
• If a procedure is known to be painful or uncomfortable, suitable analgesia or anaesthesia should be provided
• For flighty individuals, examining the mouth reliably may be extremely difficult in the conscious rabbit, and sedation may be required.

Basic hygiene should be followed to prevent transmission of zoonotic infections, including *Pasteurella multocida*, *Campylobacter* spp. and *Encephalitozoon cuniculi*, with immunocompromised individuals being at greater risk.

Restraint for examination

For the majority of the examination, the veterinary surgeon should be able to restrain and examine the rabbit single-handedly. For especially aggressive or nervous rabbits an assistant can be helpful. Correct lifting and handling technique for rabbits is shown in Figure 7.3.

Once on the consulting room table, the rabbit should be allowed to relax and sit in a natural position. One hand should be on the rabbit at all times to prevent any falls from a height. Covering the eyes gently with the other hand can help to calm the rabbit.

When examining the ventral area, the rabbit can either be held in the crook of the veterinary surgeon's arm or an assistant can hold the rabbit in an upright position. The assistant should hold the dorsum of the rabbit against their abdomen, with one hand held around the thorax and the rabbit's rump supported either by the table or the holder's hand (Figure 7.4).

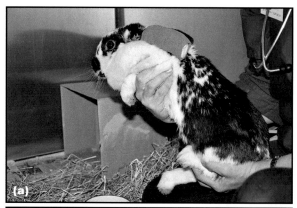

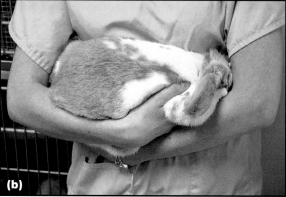

7.3 **(a)** Rabbits can be lifted by sliding one hand under the rump and supporting the thorax with the other hand. Once lifted, the rabbit is cradled into the handler's body for security. **(b)** Again using one hand to support the rump and the other to support the thorax, the rabbit is held with the head tucked into the crook of the elbow of the handler.

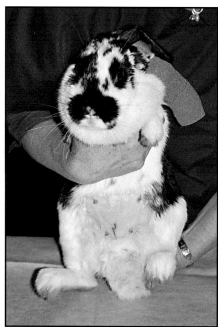

7.4 The correct method of restraint for examination of the ventral area with the help of an assistant.

Very aggressive rabbits may require a towel placed over them prior to being lifted for examination. Keeping the eyes and head covered can help to calm the rabbit, as long as its breathing is not restricted. In extreme cases, uncooperative rabbits may require sedation for examination.

Restraint for medication

With scared or aggressive animals, in order to administer oral, ocular or aural treatments it may be necessary to wrap the rabbit in a towel (the so-called 'bunny burrito'; Figure 7.5). The end result of this is often more manageable, with the limbs all contained and only the head left to control.

Dorsal immobility response

This has often been utilized in the consulting room for examination; however, it is very important to remember that it has been shown to be a highly stressful event for the rabbit. With this in mind, it is advisable to avoid using this method for restraint. If it is used, it should be for as short a time as possible and not for painful procedures. See also Chapter 5 and Appendix 3.

Lateral recumbency

There may be rare occasions when holding a rabbit in lateral recumbency is required. In most rabbits this is possible with gentle handling. A two-person method of restraint is more straightforward, with one person holding around the thorax and front legs, and the other holding around the pelvic area (Figure 7.6). The rabbit should be held in a normal position first, before a synchronized 'rolling' of the rabbit is performed. The rabbit's back should be supported

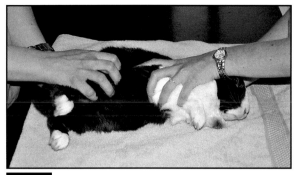

7.6 Two-person restraint in lateral recumbency.

at all times whilst 'rolling', to prevent any twisting action that could result in spinal trauma. It is important that the rabbit does not struggle or kick out. If this occurs, the rabbit should be returned to a natural position.

Clinical examination

There are a number of ways to perform a clinical examination on a rabbit; as long as a systematic approach is applied and all areas covered, there is no 'right' or 'wrong' way. The methodical approach described here is the authors' preference. Rabbits

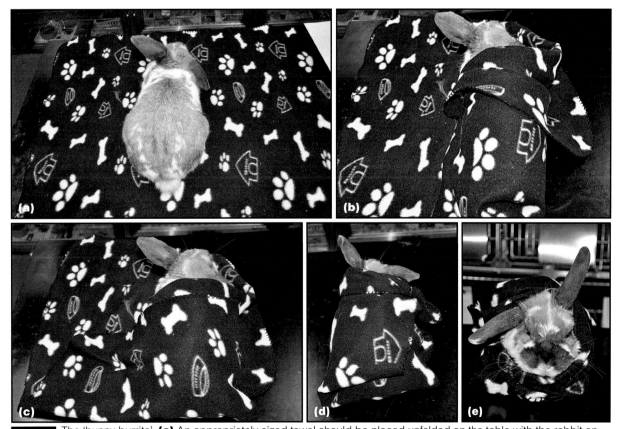

7.5 The 'bunny burrito'. **(a)** An appropriately sized towel should be placed unfolded on the table with the rabbit on top. Do not use too small a towel or the folds will loosen. **(b)** One side of the towel is wrapped over the dorsum and 'tucked in' under the ventrum of the opposite side. **(c)** The towel at the rump area is folded forwards over the lumbar spine region. **(d)** The remaining towel end is folded over the dorsum, tucking in the front feet, before being secured under the ventral area of the opposite side. **(e)** Only the head of the rabbit is visible, which can facilitate examination of the head and also administration of medication.

do not always show obvious signs of illness and owner histories can, at times, be non-specific and vague. A good examination, with appropriate restraint (see Figures 7.3 and 7.4), will yield information to direct further diagnostic testing and treatments.

Initial observation

Before handling the patient, it is advisable to monitor it from a distance. This allows the overall demeanour, awareness of surroundings and posture to be assessed. If observing two or more rabbits, their interactions should also be noted. The respiratory rate and character should be noted at this point, as a marked increase in rate is usually observed following handling. It is important to remember that chest movements rather than nose twitches should be counted.

Vital signs

The more a rabbit is manipulated for examination, the more stressed it becomes. The vital parameters (respiratory rate, heart rate and body temperature; Figure 7.7) may already be elevated as a result of transportation to the practice and time spent in the waiting room. Interpretation of the values obtained should therefore take these factors into account.

Heart rate
154–300 beats/min
Respiratory rate
30–60 breaths/min
Body temperature
38.5–40°C

7.7 Vital parameters: normal ranges.

Heart and pulse rates

A paediatric stethoscope is very useful for auscultation of the heart, which is positioned more cranially than in dogs and cats. The rate and rhythm should be noted, and any murmurs recorded and graded. The location, duration and character of the murmur should also be appreciated.

Pulse rate and quality can be evaluated simultaneously with auscultation of the heart. The femoral arteries can be used in all rabbits, while the central auricular artery (Figure 7.8) can be used for medium- and large-breed rabbits.

Respiratory rate and character

- The respiratory rate should ideally be obtained before the examination begins. If it is not possible to assess it using a 'hands-off' approach, it should be measured at the very beginning of the examination.
- Auscultation of the chest should be performed in quadrants – upper and lower sections on each side (NB the lung field is significantly smaller

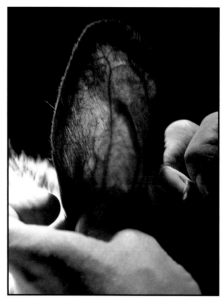

7.8 The position of the central auricular artery, which can be used for pulse palpation, is shown here by transillumination.

than in dogs and cats). Inspiratory noise is a normal finding in a clinically healthy animal. The breaths should be regular and of short duration.
- The respiratory pattern requires assessment. Is the breathing excessively noisy? If so can an upper or lower respiratory tract source be differentiated? Is there increased effort on inspiration or expiration? Is there an abdominal component to the breathing?
- The trachea should also be auscultated. In cases of respiratory disease this can help differentiate between true lower respiratory tract noise and referred upper respiratory tract noise.
- Abnormal noises include wheezes, crackles and absent sounds. The position of sounds should also be noted.
- Percussion of the chest can also be useful; solid lung is audibly duller. This can be a sign of neoplasia, abscess formation or consolidation.

Gut sounds

The final third of the stethoscope examination includes evaluation of gut sounds (Figure 7.9). Both sides of the abdomen should be auscultated.

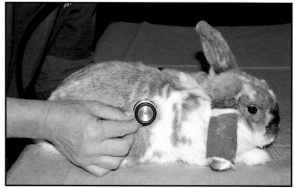

7.9 Using a paediatric stethoscope to auscultate gut sounds.

- In a normal rabbit, periodic gurgles can be heard on both sides of the abdomen.
- Although appreciation of gut sounds is important, colonic motility is known to be influenced by the autonomic nervous system and aldosterone. Stress can therefore reduce gastrointestinal motility. Even in stressed rabbits, however, gut sounds should be audible when listening for 2–4 minutes, although they may be reduced in volume.
- Absent gut sounds, along with clinical signs of gastrointestinal ileus, are grounds for further investigation.

Temperature

Before the rest of the clinical examination is performed, the rectal temperature should be obtained. If it is taken at the end of the consultation, the stress of handling can result in falsely elevated readings.

Physical examination

This can be divided into four sections: head; body; ventrum; and dental examination.

Head

Nose:

- As rabbits are obligate nasal breathers, care should be taken when examining the mouth and nasal area to prevent occluding the nostrils.
- The nares should be examined for any discharge or crusting. If present, its nature should be noted, i.e. unilateral *versus* bilateral, serous *versus* purulent.
- The nasal area should be palpated and examined from the nares to the nasolacrimal duct puncta to detect any swellings or asymmetry.

PRACTICAL TIP

Patency of the nares can be assessed in turn by holding a tuft of fur directly in front of each nostril and looking for airflow, indicated by movement of the fur.

Mouth:

- Mucous membrane colour can be assessed by gently parting the upper lips at the philtrum and examining the gingival surface. The normal colour in a rabbit is pink, but slightly paler than that observed in a dog or cat.
- Capillary refill time can also be assessed in the gingival membranes.
- A brief evaluation of the incisors can be carried out at this point; however, an entire oral examination should be included with the dental assessment at the end of the process.

Eyes:

- The eyes should be bright and alert. Sunken or dull eyes can be a sign of dehydration.

- The corneal surface should be smooth and regular. The position, depth and degree of neovascularization of any ulcers should be noted.
- Ocular discharges (Figure 7.10) should be thoroughly assessed, as they can be indicative of ocular disease or underlying dental problems. The nature of the discharge, whether it is uni- or bilateral and where it originates from, e.g. the nasolacrimal duct, should be recorded.
- The periocular area should be dry, with no areas of crusting or alopecia.
- Eye position and range of movement should be noted.
- Gentle depression of the eyeball should be possible without resistance. Protrusion of the globe can be seen either uni- or bilaterally. Limitations in medial depression unilaterally suggest a retrobulbar abscess or lesion. Bilateral exophthalmos can be indicative of an intra-thoracic mass, e.g. thymoma.
- Rabbits have an unreliable menace response, so this should not be used as a reliable indicator of vision on clinical examination.
- Gently tenting the lower lid laterally allows the nasolacrimal punctum to be visualized (Figure 7.11). By lightly rubbing rostromedial to the duct, this can help milk out fluid in the proximal area of the nasolacrimal duct, allowing more detailed assessment.

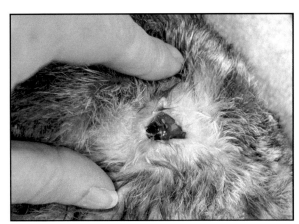

7.10 This rabbit had a chronic ocular discharge with involvement of the nasolacrimal duct, conjunctivitis and severe blepharitis.

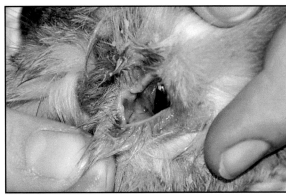

7.11 The slit-shaped opening of the nasolacrimal duct can be seen clearly in the majority of rabbits.

- The eyelids should be free of erythema and swelling, and cilial growth should be in a lateral direction away from the corneal surface.
- The conjunctiva should not be injected or swollen and the sclera should be free of excessive vascularization.
- The nictitating membranes should move with ease with gentle depression of the eyeball. In certain rabbits, they can become prominent when stressed.
- If required, further examination of the globe using an ophthalmoscope can be performed to assess the anterior and posterior chamber, iris, lens and retina.

PRACTICAL TIP

If there are concerns over the patency of the nasolacrimal ducts, fluorescein dye can be used as an aid. One or two drops are added to the inside of the lower eyelid; after 30–60 seconds the dye should be visible at the nostril. Drop administration into each eye can be performed 1 minute apart to identify which side is patent. The eyes should be rinsed with sterile warm normal saline to clear the dye afterwards.

Ears:

- The pinnae should be clean, without scabbing or scaling.
- The ear canals should be inspected with the naked eye and with an otoscope. It is important to check on either side of the tragus: laterally it leads to the inner ear, while medially it is a blind-ending pocket.
- A small amount of wax within the ear is a common finding. Ear wax is pale yellow in colour and should not be confused with pus from the inner ear.
- The tympanic membrane should appear pale and translucent on otoscopic examination.
- The base of the ears should be palpated thoroughly for any swellings, particularly the lateral aspect of the base of vertical canal, where abscesses can be found. Often these can be bilateral.

Jaw:

- Palpation of the ventral mandible, bilateral masseter muscles, lateral maxillae and zygomatic arches is extremely important. Both sides should be symmetrical and any associated soft tissue swellings or bony abnormalities should be noted.
- The cheeks should be palpated to allow the lateral surface of the premolars and molars to be appreciated. Sharp lateral spurs can be detected by this means and affected rabbits are likely to resent palpation.
- Lateral jaw movement can be appreciated (Figure 7.12) by placing a thumb and forefinger of one hand on either side of the mandible, with the opposite thumb and forefinger on the maxilla.

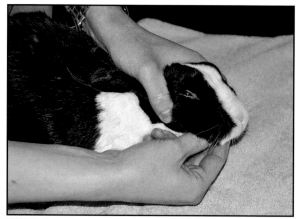

7.12 With gentle pressure, the occlusal surfaces of the cheek teeth should allow smooth lateral movement from one side to the other. If 'sticking' of teeth is noted, this can be a sign of abnormalities of the premolars and molars.

This allows the jaw to be manipulated medially and laterally. In a healthy rabbit this is a natural motion. In rabbits with cheek tooth elongation, or uneven dental wear, the jaw will often have restricted lateral movement or will move one way with ease before appearing to 'stick' going the opposite way.
- The internal oral examination can be performed with an otoscope at the end of the consultation, as rabbits tend to find this stressful.

Body

Body condition:

- Visual assessment and palpation of the soft tissue structures overlying the ribs, dorsal spinous processes and pelvic bones, along with appreciation of muscle masses, allows a body condition score (BCS; Figures 7.13 and 7.14) to be recorded.

Body condition score	Description	Clinical findings
1	Emaciated	Bone structures evident from a distance and obvious poor musculature. Welfare implications
2	Underweight	Minimal fat covering ribs on palpation, with prominent vertebrae and pelvic bones
3	Ideal	Light fat padding palpated over ribcage. Abdomen shapely. Well defined musculature
4	Overweight	Ribs difficult to palpate due to fat deposits. When viewed from above, abdomen appears rounded
5	Obese	Skeletal structures difficult to palpate due to excessive fat accumulation; very rounded and distended abdomen

7.13 Body condition scoring.

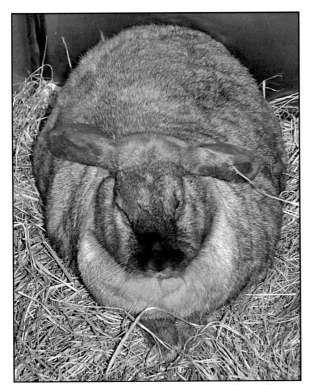

7.14 This obese rabbit had been fed pellets *ad libitum*. It was given a body condition score (BCS) of 5/5.

- It is also extremely important to record the rabbit's bodyweight at every visit, allowing fluctuations over time to be appreciated. The importance of this measurement should not be underestimated. Often obtaining a weight is left to the end of the consultation.

Lymph nodes:

- The main lymph nodes noted are the submandibular, prescapular and popliteal.
- The popliteal lymph nodes are reliably palpable, even at normal size, whereas the submandibular and prescapular are variable. The prescapular lymph nodes can be transiently enlarged after a subcutaneous vaccination injection into the scruff.
- As with other species, local or generalized lymphadenopathy can be associated with disease or injury/wounds.

Thorax:

- Evaluation of chest compliance in a rabbit is generally limited. The ribs of younger animals are more pliable than those of older animals. In some cases, space-occupying lesions of the thorax may be appreciable by this method.

Abdomen:

- Abdominal palpation (Figure 7.15) is extremely important in the rabbit. A systematic approach is very useful to ensure that a complete examination is performed.

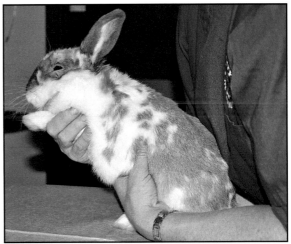

7.15 Abdominal palpation. Elevating the thorax allows structures in the cranial abdomen to be better appreciated.

- The rabbit remains in sternal recumbency and is examined with open, flat hands against either side of the body wall. If necessary, the rabbit's forelegs and chest can be elevated to allow better palpation of structures in the cranial abdomen.
- It is important to remember that structures within the abdomen are often thin walled, and delicate palpation is required.
- The stomach is situated in the cranial left portion of the abdomen. Easily palpable, it extends caudally from the last rib and always contains ingesta. On palpation, the stomach should be doughy and soft with semifluid contents. If it is tympanitic, hard or distended, further investigation and treatment is required.
- Small intestines are mostly palpated cranially and in the mid-abdomen individual bowel loops are palpable if distended with ingesta or gas. Lesions and impactions may also be detected.
- The caecum takes up a large portion of the abdominal cavity. It lies ventrally and either in the midline or on the right side. It is readily palpable and should be soft and filled with semifluid fermenting ingesta. Caecal impaction or gas accumulation can be easily palpated and are abnormal findings.
- The colon is positioned dorsally in the mid-caudal abdomen. Formed fibrous faecal pellets are palpable in the healthy rabbit.
- Both kidneys are easily palpable. They are readily mobile and the right is positioned more cranially than the left. Both are situated further cranially than in the dog or cat.
- Situated in the midline caudal abdomen, the bladder is thin walled. Often surrounded by fat in overweight rabbits, it can be difficult to palpate when empty. Palpation can detect thickening of the bladder wall and the presence of sludge or calculi and is often resented in these cases.
- Detection of a healthy, non-pregnant uterus is rarely possible. Pregnancy can potentially be

detectable by palpation after the first trimester of gestation. In older intact female rabbits uterine neoplasia is easily palpable in advanced cases.
- The liver, pancreas and spleen are very difficult to palpate unless abnormal, as a result of disease processes.

Integument:

- The fur should be dry, clean and free from matting, discoloration and odour. Blowing on the coat or running the hair backwards against the direction of growth allows the skin surface to be seen.
- The skin on the chin, around the dewlap (if present) and around the eyes should be checked, if not already evaluated during examination of the head.
- Any abnormalities of the skin should be noted, including erythema, crusting, scale formation, ulceration, wounds, bruising and wetness. Any lesions should be noted, including their nature and location. Types of lesion include papules, macules, pustules, comedones, alopecic areas, coat discoloration and masses in the cutaneous and subcutaneous areas.

Limbs:

- All limbs should be palpated for abnormalities, and nail length checked in case trimming is required.
- If there is concern over a particular limb, the rabbit should be observed moving. The patient can be placed on the floor to assess gait. To encourage movement, the carrier can be placed at the other side of the room, or a companion rabbit can also be allowed out, to encourage exploration.
- The fur on the medial front legs ('hankies'), which a rabbit often uses to wipe its eyes, nose and mouth, should be examined for staining (Figure 7.16) to ensure that no nasal discharge or excess salivation has been overlooked.

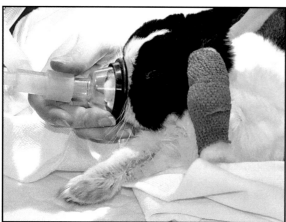

7.16 'Dirty hankies'. The medial aspects of the front legs are often used by the rabbit to wipe nasal, oral and ocular discharges and are referred to as 'hankies' in the rabbit world.

Ventrum

This can be examined with the rabbit restrained to display the ventral area (see Figure 7.4).

- The mammary chain should be palpated bilaterally for any swellings, heat or discharge.
- The skin of the ventral area should be checked, especially around the perineum and inguinal region. Particular attention should be paid to any urine or faecal staining (Figure 7.17).
- The mucous membranes can be further assessed in the genital area.
- The anus should be examined for faecal accumulation and any abnormal growths.
- In both sexes, the skin in the inguinal area can be used to assess hydration status.

If not already known, the sex of the rabbit should be determined.

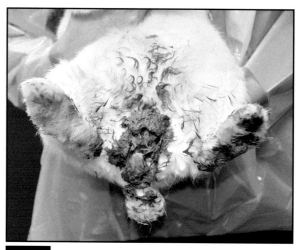

7.17 This rabbit is at high risk of fly strike.

Male genitalia:

- The scrotum and testicles (if present) should be examined (Figure 7.18).
- The scrotal skin can be used to gauge hydration.
- The testicles should be palpated. It is possible for the rabbit to retract them partially into the abdomen. If this happens, gentle rolling pressure

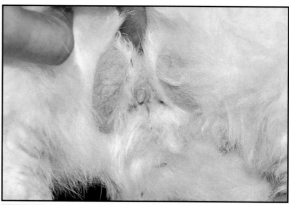

7.18 Male genitalia. In older rabbits the testicles and penis are readily identifiable.

on the abdomen will encourage re-entry into the scrotal sac.
- Testicles should be symmetrical, smooth and non-painful.
- The scent glands present in the skin folds either side of the penis should be checked for impactions.

Female genitalia: The vulva (Figure 7.19) should be examined for any swellings or discharge. NB It is normal in both sexes to find a small amount of glandular secretions in the thin skin folds on either side of the external genitalia.

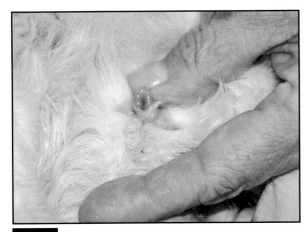

7.19 Female genitalia. The vulva is slit-like.

Feet: Pododermatitis is a very common finding in the authors' experience. The points of the hocks are the most common areas affected (Figure 7.20); however, the lesions can extend linearly along the plantar surfaces of the hind feet. The front feet should also be checked, with the medial digits being most commonly involved.

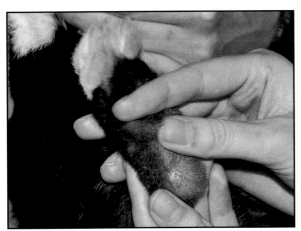

7.20 The point of the hock is the most common location for pododermatitis.

Dental examination

This should always be left to the end of the examination, as the rabbit will often find it stressful. The rabbit should be held firmly in sternal recumbency, with the assistant using their thumbs over both shoulder blades to apply gentle downward pressure

and prevent the rabbit from rearing up. The rump of the rabbit should be held against the abdomen of the assistant, to prevent backwards movement (Figure 7.21).

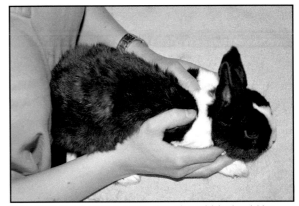

7.21 For dental examination, the rabbit should be held on a non-slip surface with the rump resting against the abdomen of the holder. The handler supports the thoracic area, using their thumbs to apply gentle downwards pressure.

Conscious dental assessment is somewhat limited in the rabbit, owing to the narrow and long oral cavity. Although otoscopic examination is very useful, sedation is required for a complete, reliable oral examination. The use of incisor gags, cheek dilators and a head torch with a sedated rabbit improves visualization greatly (Figure 7.22); however, endoscopic examination yields the best results for full assessment of the dental arcades under sedation. Further information on dental assessment is given in the *BSAVA Manual of Rabbit Surgery, Dentistry and Imaging*.

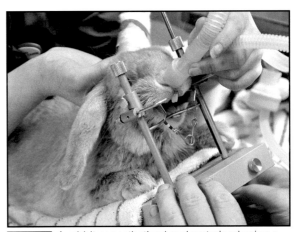

7.22 A rabbit anaesthetized and restrained using a dental frame to aid oral examination.

- Initial dental assessment should begin rostrally, with the incisors and peg teeth being evaluated. Gently parting the upper lips allows visualization of the four main incisors. The presence of upper peg teeth caudal to the main incisors should be noted. Changes to note include: direction of growth; malocclusion; ribbing; discoloration; infection; occlusal angle; and loose, fractured or absent teeth.

- Examination of the cheek teeth, buccal gingiva and tongue is performed with the aid of an otoscope (Figure 7.23). Most rabbits will initially resent placement of the instrument, but quickly become tolerant. In particularly fractious rabbits, it may be necessary to wrap the rabbit in a towel, but this is not common.
- Holding the rabbit's head loosely in one hand, the otoscope with a metal cone attachment (do not use plastic because the rabbit will chew this) is introduced lateral to the incisors and run along the buccal surface. If the rabbit does not chew, viewing of the teeth can be limited to the first two cheek teeth on the upper and lower arcade. Allowing the rabbit to chew while being examined often aids in the visualization of molar teeth further caudally. Once the two arcades on one side have been evaluated, the otoscope can be gently moved over the tongue, between the incisors, to the opposite side, or can be removed and reintroduced on the opposite side.
- Although otoscopic examination has its limitations, a large amount of information can still be gained and no examination should be completed without some evaluation of the dentition.
- Noteworthy abnormalities to consider include: changes to growth angles of cheek teeth arcades; inappropriate occlusal surface angulation; irregularities to crown heights; spike formation; soft tissue trauma; food impaction; excessive saliva accumulation in the mouth; halitosis; absent or loose teeth; and haemorrhage. Ingested foreign material, such as newspaper, is also often seen.
- For rabbits that are uncooperative during the otoscopic examination, sedation may be required to reach a reliable assessment of the severity of the dental disease present.
- It is not possible to age rabbits using their dentition.
- It is important to warn the owner that lesions may be missed using this technique. In cases with suspicious clinical signs, general anaesthesia is required for a full dental assessment.

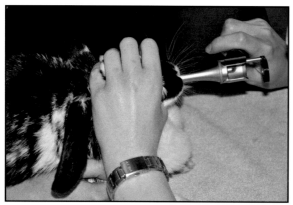

7.23 Otoscopic examination of the mouth is extremely useful and an important part of every examination. Care should be taken when holding the rabbit's head not to occlude the nostrils.

Diagnostic procedures

Venepuncture

Indications

- Blood collection for diagnostic analysis.
- Blood collection for transfusion.

The maximum volume removed should not exceed 10% of circulating blood volume (Figure 7.24). Average blood volume in an adult rabbit is 55–78 ml/kg. This means that between 5.5 and 7.8 ml/kg bodyweight can be safely drawn at any one time (within a 24-hour period). Sample volume is therefore rarely a limiting factor in rabbit medicine, except where large volumes are required for blood transfusion.

Average adult bodyweight (kg)	Average adult blood volume (ml)	Maximum safe sample volume (ml)
1	55–78	5.5–7.8
2	110–156	11–15.6
3	165–234	16.5–23.4

7.24 Safe blood sampling volumes in the rabbit.

Anatomical sites
The jugular, lateral saphenous, marginal ear and cephalic veins are all accessible (Figures 7.25 to 7.28).

Procedure

1. The area is clipped free of hair.
2. A topical local anaesthetic cream (e.g. EMLA) should be applied a minimum of 15–20 minutes prior to venepuncture.
3. The rabbit should be restrained appropriately (see above). Good lighting is essential to aid visualization of the vessel.
4. Rub or tap the area to dilate the vein and swab with alcohol.
5. Use a 23–27 G needle with a 1–10 ml syringe, depending on the chosen site and the volume of blood required. (This may be preloaded with heparin, depending on the sample required.) Alternatively, a butterfly catheter may be used.
6. Insert the needle into the vein (most veins are superficial in rabbits) and withdraw blood using gentle negative pressure on the syringe.
7. It is important to apply digital pressure to the site following withdrawal because haematoma formation is common, particularly involving the lateral saphenous vein.

PRACTICAL TIP
Sedation may be required for sampling from the jugular vein.

Vein	Patient restraint	Comments
Jugular vein (Figure 7.26)	The rabbit is placed in sternal recumbency at the edge of the table. The neck is extended; the forelimbs may be restrained over the table edge	Use a 2.5 ml syringe and 23–25 G needle. Larger syringes can be used if greater blood volumes are required. Difficult in obese animals or those with large dewlaps. Not recommended for fractious or nervous rabbits
Lateral saphenous vein (Figure 7.27)	The rabbit is held in sternal recumbency with the hindlimb extended down over the table edge or with both hindlimbs lying on the table laterally and the upper hindlimb restrained above the stifle. The rabbit can also be held in lateral recumbency, being restrained with one arm over the rabbit holding the forelimbs and one holding the hindlimbs	An appropriately sized syringe (2.5 or 5 ml) and a preheparinized 21 G butterfly catheter are recommended for this site. The vein is prominent but mobile and needs to be stabilized prior to needle insertion. Haematoma formation can be limited if adequate digital pressure is applied for approximately 1 minute after sampling. Restraint and procedure are generally well tolerated by most rabbits
Marginal ear vein (see Figure 7.39)	The rabbit is held in sternal recumbency on a table. The handler uses one hand to raise the vein	Restraint and procedure are generally well tolerated by most rabbits. Small volumes only are possible. Easy to visualize vein
Cephalic vein (Figure 7.28)	The rabbit is held in sternal recumbency with one forelimb extended	Small mobile vessel. Restraint may be resented

7.25 Common sites for venepuncture in the rabbit.

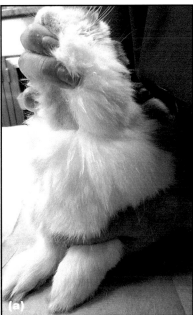
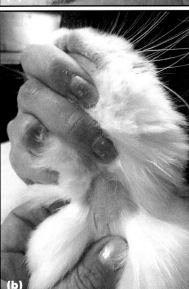

7.26 Blood sampling from the jugular vein. **(a)** Correct restraint. **(b)** With the neck extended, the jugular vein is easily located lying in the jugular groove lateral to the trachea.

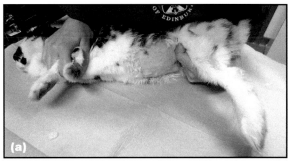
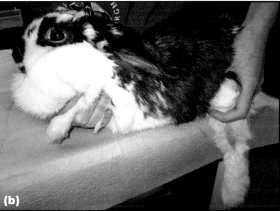
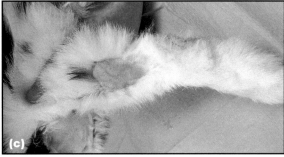
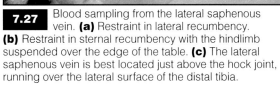

7.27 Blood sampling from the lateral saphenous vein. **(a)** Restraint in lateral recumbency. **(b)** Restraint in sternal recumbency with the hindlimb suspended over the edge of the table. **(c)** The lateral saphenous vein is best located just above the hock joint, running over the lateral surface of the distal tibia.

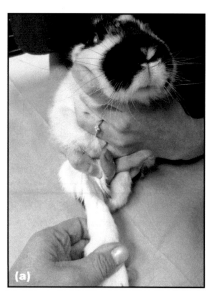

7.28

Blood sampling from the cephalic vein. **(a)** Correct restraint. **(b)** Once raised, the cephalic vein is easily visible on the cranial forelimb.

WARNING
- Use caution when clipping the fur, as rabbit skin is easily torn.
- Long-term repeated use of the marginal ear vein may cause sloughing.
- The jugular vein may be difficult to visualize in obese rabbits or in does with large dewlaps.

Urine collection

Urinalysis is an important and often underutilized diagnostic tool in the evaluation of many rabbit illnesses. A basic urinalysis requested routinely by the authors consists of: macroscopic examination; measurement of specific gravity; semiquantitative chemistry; and microscopic sediment examination. Further analysis may include bacterial and fungal culture and sensitivity testing, and quantitative urine chemistry (including urine protein:creatinine ratio). See Chapter 9 for reference ranges for urinalysis.

Urine samples can be collected by one of four methods in the rabbit:

- Free catch
- Manual expression of the bladder
- Urethral catheterization
- Cystocentesis.

The relative advantages and disadvantages of each technique are highlighted in Figure 7.29. Urethral catheterization and cystocentesis are the authors' favoured techniques for obtaining sterile urine.

Free catch

This is a straightforward technique in rabbits that are trained to use a litter tray. Sterilized pea gravel litter may be used as a substrate to reduce contamination

Urine sampling technique	Advantages	Disadvantages	Comments
Free catch	Least stressful technique for the rabbit as no handling required	Non-sterile sample. Not suitable for culture. Cytology may be limited due to contamination with environmental bacteria and debris. Useful for urinalysis but not culture	If the rabbit has been stressed or has been given alpha-2 adrenoreceptor agonists, glucosuria may be seen
Manual bladder expression	Stressful technique, but does not require sedation	Non-sterile sample obtained. Risk of iatrogenic bladder rupture and haemorrhage, with blood contamination of sample	If the rabbit has been stressed by transport and handling or has been given alpha-2 adrenoreceptor agonists, glucosuria may be seen. Glucose may be falsely elevated due to stress
Urethral catheterization	Sterile sample obtained suitable for full urine analysis. Also useful to rule out urethral obstruction and perform contrast studies	Requires heavy sedation/general anaesthesia	Premedication with a benzodiazepine reduces urethral spasm
Cystocentesis	Can be performed in a calm conscious rabbit that is carefully restrained. Sterile sample obtained suitable for full urinalysis	Iatrogenic damage to viscera, in particular the caecum, is possible if a blind technique is used. In fractious animals sedation/general anaesthesia may be required	Ultrasound guidance is extremely useful and reduces the risk of trauma from this technique

7.29 Techniques for urine sample collection in rabbits and their relative advantages/disadvantages.

of the sample. The sample obtained has limited diagnostic use because it is of poor quality and contaminated. It can, however, be used in the first instance to determine by semiquantitative chemistry (dipstick analysis) whether there are any abnormal values that could indicate the need for further sterile urine sampling. It is useful for the measurement of urine protein:creatinine (UPC) and GGT:creatinine ratios.

Manual expression of the bladder

The bladder may be expressed to obtain a urine sample; however, haemorrhage and potential rupture is common following overzealous palpation. The bladder is palpated in the caudal abdomen and gentle pressure applied on either side. Urine is collected straight into a sterile universal container.

> **WARNING**
> - This technique should not be performed if there is a risk of partial or complete urethral obstruction as indicated by dysuria/stranguria.
> - Some rabbits will resent this procedure.

Urethral catheterization

Indications:

- Collection of a sterile urine sample for urinalysis.
- Treatment of hypercalciuria with urethral catheterization and flushing of the bladder with warm sterile saline.
- Treatment of partial or complete urethral obstruction secondary to calculus formation.
- Administration of contrast material/air into the bladder/urethra for imaging purposes.
- Aspiration of samples for cytology from urethral wall masses identified on ultrasonography.

Procedure:

- The rabbit should be anaesthetized or heavily sedated. Premedication with benzodiazepine drugs (midazolam is routinely used by the authors) and/or metamizole/hyoscine (Buscopan) at 0.25 ml/kg s.c. may be used to reduce the risk of urethral spasm.
- If soiled, the perineal area should be carefully washed with warm dilute antiseptic solution, rinsed and dried.
- A sterile 4–9 Fr feline urinary catheter with stylet should be used. Sterile gloves should be worn and the end of the catheter packaging should be snipped, pushing the sterile catheter out via this opening to maintain sterility.

Bucks are best placed in dorsal or lateral recumbency for this technique:

1. Extrude the penis with one hand while the other carefully introduces the catheter into the urethra. Some resistance is felt as the catheter passes over the pelvic brim.

2. Correct placement is confirmed by urine in the catheter.
3. Connect a three-way tap and syringe to prevent urine flow once in place.

Does are easily catheterized if positioned correctly:

1. The rabbit should be placed in sternal recumbency with the hindquarters elevated slightly using sandbags or foam pads. A towel or absorbent pad should be placed under the rabbit to avoid urine contamination of these items (Figure 7.30a).
2. Introduce a catheter into the vulva and direct it ventrally along the floor of the vagina and into the urethral ostium. Correct placement is confirmed by urine in the catheter.
3. Connect a three-way tap and syringe to prevent urine flow once in place.
4. If resistance is met to catheter placement it should be carefully retracted 1–2 cm and advanced again.

PRACTICAL TIP
- Sterile lubrication of the catheter tip with a local anaesthetic gel will aid passage of the catheter and reduce urethral spasm, particularly in males.
- Gentle flushing of the catheter with a small amount of warm sterile saline may facilitate the passage of the catheter in cases where this technique proves difficult. It acts to lubricate the catheter tip and may help dislodge any material obstructing the urethral lumen.

> **WARNING**
> If resistance is met to catheter placement do not apply increased pressure because this may result in iatrogenic urethral damage, potentially leading to rupture or stricture formation.

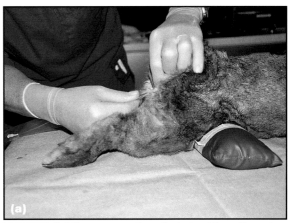

7.30 **(a)** Does are easily catheterized if positioned correctly. (continues) ▶

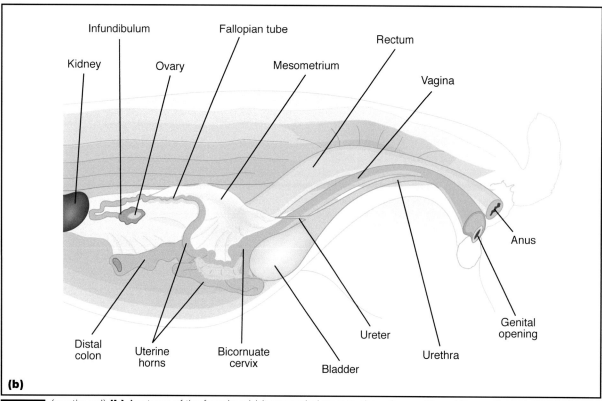

(b)

7.30 (continued) **(b)** Anatomy of the female rabbit urogenital tract to show the position of the urethra, ventral to the vagina. The urinary catheter should be directed ventrally along the floor of the vagina and into the urethral ostium for correct placement. (Reproduced from the *BSAVA Manual of Rabbit Surgery, Dentistry and Imaging*)

Cystocentesis

Indications:

- Collection of a sterile urine sample for urinalysis.
- To reduce bladder size and overdistension in cases with suspected urethral blockage.

Procedure:

1. Calm animals can be conscious for the procedure, but fractious animals may require sedation/anaesthesia.
2. Restrain the rabbit in dorsal or lateral recumbency.
3. Clip and surgically prepare a small area of skin in the midline and cranial to the pubis.
4. The bladder should be palpable cranial to the pelvis in the ventral midline.
5. Isolate the bladder with one hand while the other hand introduces a 23–25 G 1 inch (25 cm) needle attached to a 5 or 10 ml syringe through the ventral midline abdominal wall and into the bladder.
6. Aspirate urine.

PRACTICAL TIP
- Prior to performing this procedure, the bladder should be palpated to assess the degree of filling. If it is empty the technique should be postponed. ▶

- Iatrogenic damage to viscera is possible with this technique and the authors therefore strongly recommend the concurrent use of ultrasonography to visualize the bladder prior to needle puncture.

> **WARNING**
> If blood or gut contents are aspirated, the procedure should be stopped and a new attempt made using a fresh sterile needle and syringe. If gut contents are aspirated systemic antibiotics are indicated.

Faecal collection and analysis
More detail on the interpretation of faecal and caecotroph examination is given in Chapter 12.

Indications

- Visual assessment of size, shape, consistency and amount passed.
- Parasitological examination.
- Faecal culture and sensitivity testing.
- Transfaunation.

Procedure

1. Faeces should be assessed routinely for size, number and fibrous content, as part of any clinical examination.

2. Fresh faeces may be examined microscopically by preparing a wet preparation as a direct smear. Motile protozoans may be identified using this technique.
3. Coccidiosis may be diagnosed using saturated salt flotation techniques, which will also detect helminths and cryptosporidia.
4. *Saccharomyces* yeasts are commonly seen on faecal microscopy. These are normal symbiotic inhabitants of the caecum in healthy rabbits; however, they may be seen in excess and are thought to cause soft stools following oral antibiotics.

PRACTICAL TIP
Caecotrophs may be collected by placement of an Elizabethan collar on the rabbit to prevent caecotrophy (Figure 7.31).

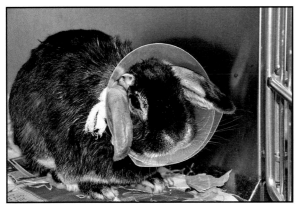

7.31 An Elizabethan collar can be used to prevent caecotrophy if collection is required.

Abscess diagnosis and culture technique
Fine-needle aspiration from rabbit abscesses may be unsuccessful because the pus is thick and caseous. The material at the centre of the abscess is likely to be sterile and the best culture results are obtained by culturing the abscess wall or capsule. Sections of tissue give the best culture results, rather than capsular swabs.

Advanced diagnostic techniques

Arterial blood collection

Indications:

• Monitoring blood gases (particularly under general anaesthesia).
• Measurement of real-time blood pressure.
• Measurement of acid–base status.

Arteries used: The authors routinely use the central auricular artery (see Figure 7.8) for arterial blood gas monitoring under anaesthesia. The procedure is also well tolerated in conscious rabbits. An alternative site is the femoral artery; however, anaesthesia is required for this site.

Procedure:

1. The area is clipped and surgically prepared.
2. It is not necessary to occlude the vessel prior to needle insertion.
3. The procedure is as for blood sampling from a vein. Small volumes only are generally required for blood gas measurement
4. Following arterial puncture it is essential to apply firm digital pressure for several minutes to avoid haemorrhage from the site and haematoma formation, which could result in tissue necrosis.

PRACTICAL TIP
Application of local anaesthetic cream (e.g. EMLA) is recommended prior to arterial blood collection. For repeat sampling, placement of an indwelling catheter is recommended.

WARNING
• Arterial sites are not recommended in rabbits for routine blood sampling nor for administration of medications.
• Risks associated with arterial catheter placement include haemorrhage from the site, blood clots and infection.
• Ischaemic necrosis of the pinna has been well described in rabbits following poor collection technique.

Bone marrow aspiration and biopsy

Indications:

• The most common indications for bone marrow examination in the rabbit are anaemia (particularly non-regenerative anaemias), thrombocytopenia, leucopenia and, less commonly, neoplasia (lymphosarcoma), infectious disease (*Pasteurella multocida*, *Staphylococcus aureus*) and bone marrow dysplasia. (For interpretation of results see Williams, 2000.)
• Aspirates are used to look at cell morphology and the myeloid:erythroid ratio.
• Core biopsy samples should be used to evaluate hypocellular marrow.

Anatomical sites: Potential sites include the proximal femur, proximal humerus and proximal tibia. The authors' preferred site is the proximal femur. The wing of the ilium has also been reported as an alternative site; however, in rabbits this bone is fine and it is easy to penetrate both cortices, so this site is not recommended by the authors.

Procedure: Collection of bone marrow samples (Figure 7.32) is carried out under general anaesthesia with aseptic technique observed.

1. The site is clipped and surgically prepared.
2. Sterile gloves should be worn and a sterile drape applied.

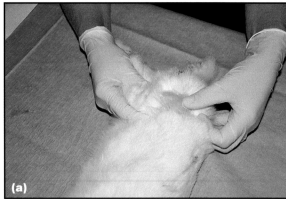

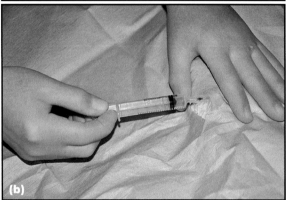

7.32 Bone marrow sampling. **(a)** Holding the stifle, the thumb is moved along the femur until it reaches the fossa between the greater and lesser trochanters of the femur. The needle is then inserted under the thumb into the bone, directed towards the long axis of the bone. **(b)** Suction pressure loosens the marrow particles, which are aspirated into the syringe. See text for more details.

3. Lidocaine 2% is infiltrated into the skin, muscle and periosteum.
4. Premedication with an opiate analgesic should be provided, e.g. buprenorphine at 0.03–0.05 mg/kg i.v. or s.c.
5. A small incision may be made in the skin with a scalpel over the site of needle placement.
6. For aspiration, a needle and stylet (20–22 G, 1.5–3 inch (4–8 cm)) are introduced with a drilling action into the medullary cavity in the direction of the long axis of the bone. Alternatively, a 20–22 G hypodermic needle can be used with a small-gauge sterile surgical wire inserted into the needle bore as a stylet. Correct positioning within the medullary cavity is confirmed by a loss of resistance to drilling.
7. The stylet is removed and a 5 ml syringe attached (containing 1 ml sterile phosphate-buffered saline with 0.24% EDTA).
8. Aspirate 0.5 ml of marrow. Apply suction pressure to loosen marrow particles and obtain a sample. Reposition the needle if nothing is aspirated at first.
9. Samples should be placed on microscope slides and smears made using a crush technique.
10. Core biopsy samples are obtained with the same technique but using a 1.5 inch (4 cm) 18 G needle. Biopsy samples should be placed in 10% formalin for processing.

Anatomical landmarks for placement in the proximal femur: The needle is inserted into the trochanteric fossa just medial to the greater trochanter, between the greater trochanter and the femoral head.

1. Hold the stifle and place your thumb along the femur and into the fossa (Figure 7.32a).
2. Insert the needle under the thumb into the bone and position it in the direction of the long axis of the bone.

Anatomical landmarks for placement in the proximal humerus: Insert the needle into the proximal humerus at the distal end of the greater tubercle.

1. With the rabbit in lateral recumbency, rotate the elbow joint inwards so that the shoulder joint is rotated outwards for increased accessibility. The shoulder joint is found by running your finger down the spine of the scapula to the acromion. The next prominence distal to this is the greater tubercle of the humerus.
2. The needle should be inserted at a 45-degree angle to the long axis of the humerus, to prevent accidental penetration of the joint or bursa.

PRACTICAL TIP
- Rabbits have small bones with thin cortices and therefore sample collection by aspiration is preferred because there is less risk of iatrogenic damage.
- Core biopsy is possible, but greater care must be taken with this technique.

WARNING
A few complications have been reported following bone marrow aspiration in the rabbit, with mild haemorrhage being the most common (Williams, 2000).

Cerebrospinal fluid tap

Indications:

- Cytological analysis and culture of cerebrospinal fluid (CSF).
- Detection of specific pathogens in CSF samples using polymerase chain reaction (PCR) analysis (for example *Encephalitozoon cuniculi* infection) or serology.

See Chapter 9 for reference values for CSF analysis in the rabbit.

Anatomical sites: CSF may be collected in small volumes from either the cisterna magna (atlanto-occipital approach) or the lumbosacral epidural space (lumbar approach).

Procedure: Samples are collected under general anaesthesia with the rabbit intubated.

Collection from the cisterna magna: This is the preferred site for CSF collection in the rabbit.

1. The animal is placed in lateral recumbency and the neck is flexed towards the sternum.
2. An area is clipped and surgically prepared, extending caudally from the occipital protuberance to the third cervical vertebra and laterally just beyond the wings of the atlas (Figure 7.33a).
3. A sterile drape is applied and sterile gloves are worn.
4. The anatomical site for needle placement is first located by palpation of the occipital protuberance and the craniodorsal edge of the dorsal spine of the axis (C2). Needle placement is in the dorsal midline at a point equidistant between these two anatomical landmarks in a site just cranial to the cranial margins of the wings of the C1 vertebra (atlas).
5. A 22 G 1.5 inch (4 cm) spinal needle is inserted at right angles to the vertebral column in the dorsal midline (Figure 7.33b). Alternatively a 23 G 1.25 inch (3 cm) needle may be used.
6. The needle is slowly advanced a few millimetres at a time in the direction of the rabbit's nose, until a slight 'pop' is felt on penetration of the dura and subarachnoid membranes.
7. The stylet is removed and CSF should gather in the hub of the needle. Do not aspirate, just allow the CSF to drip into a plastic container (Figure 7.33c) (glass causes leucocytes to stick to the walls of the container). *No more than 0.5 ml should be collected from an average-sized rabbit.*
8. Analyse immediately (within 30–60 minutes) or refrigerate the sample.

Collection from the lumbosacral space: This procedure is technically more difficult, tends to yield smaller volumes of CSF and has a higher associated risk of blood contamination of the sample. This is also the preferred site for myelography in the rabbit (L5–L6 is typically used).

1. The rabbit is placed in lateral recumbency with foam pads placed between the limbs and under the lumbar area to ensure correct positioning.
2. An area is clipped and surgically prepared over the lumbar vertebrae, cranial to the pelvis. The trunk is flexed and the 6th lumbar vertebra is located.

3. A 22 G 1.5 inch (4 cm) spinal needle is inserted at a slight angle, almost at right angles to the spine in a cranial direction at the cranial aspect of the dorsal spinous process of L6 (Figure 7.34). The position is similar to that in the dog, with the epidural space between 0.75 and 2.5 cm below the skin surface. Alternatively a 23 G 1.25 inch (3 cm) needle may be used.
4. The needle may pass beyond the dorsal subarachnoid space through the spinal cord (causing twitching of the hindlimbs), in which case the ventral subarachnoid space may be sampled.
5. Sample collection is performed as described above; however a smaller volume is obtained from this site.

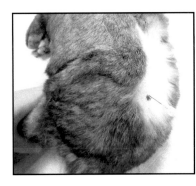

7.34 Needle placement for collection of CSF from the lumbosacral space (shown here on a cadaver). See text for more details.

PRACTICAL TIP
Normal CSF is colourless and clear. If samples are blood-tinged this is most likely secondary to iatrogenic blood contamination or possible previous haemorrhage.

WARNING
- Direct pressure should never be applied to the needle using a syringe, as this could result in herniation of the cerebellum into the foramen magnum.
- CSF taps should not be performed in cases with suspected increased intracranial pressure because there is an increased risk of herniation in these cases.
- In other species ketamine administration can result in an increase in intracranial pressure and it should therefore be avoided.
- Other risks include haemorrhage and trauma to the brainstem or spinal cord.

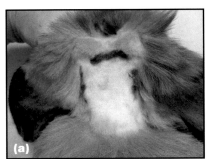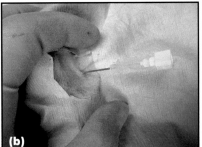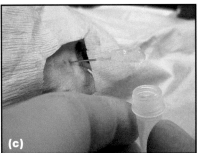

7.33 Collection of CSF from the cisterna magna. **(a)** An area extending caudally from the occipital protuberance to the third cervical vertebra and laterally just beyond the wings of atlas is prepared. **(b)** Needle placement is in the dorsal midline just cranial to the cranial margins of the wings of atlas. **(c)** When the stylet is removed CSF gathers in the hub of the needle and drips into a plastic container. See text for more details.

Deep nasal sample collection

Indications:

* Diagnostic evaluation of nasal discharge or upper respiratory tract disease.
* Sample collection for bacterial and fungal culture and sensitivity.

A pure single culture is likely to be significant, whereas mixed cultures are likely to represent normal bacterial flora. Normal nasal flora in healthy rabbits includes *Moraxella catarrhalis*, *Bordetella bronchiseptica*, *Pasteurella multocida*, *Staphylococcus* spp., *Streptococcus* spp. and *Bacillus* spp.

Procedure: Deep nasal samples for culture should be obtained with the rabbit under general anaesthesia.

1. Application of a local anaesthetic spray to the external nares prior to placement of the swab is recommended by the authors, to provide analgesia on recovery.
2. A fine sterile swab is pre-measured to the level of the medial canthus of the eye from the external nares (Figure 7.35a).
3. Introduce the swab into the ventral nasal cavity and advance it slowly in a ventromedial direction (Figure 7.35b).
4. Both sides should be sampled for comparison.

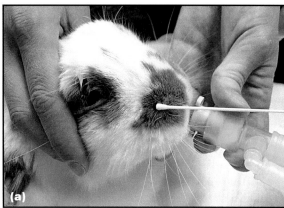

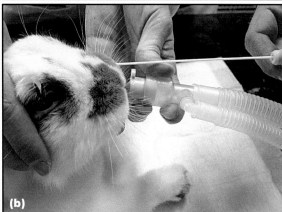

7.35 Deep nasal swab sampling. **(a)** Pre-measuring the swab. **(b)** The swab is slowly advanced ventromedially. See text for more details.

PRACTICAL TIP
Nasal endoscopy is used by the authors to aid visualization; biopsy specimens for histopathological examination may also be taken.

WARNING
* Iatrogenic damage to the nasal turbinates may occur, with mild haemorrhage, particularly in animals with pathological changes.
* Unless care is taken, contaminants are commonly obtained from the external nares.

Bronchoalveolar lavage (BAL)

Indications: Collection of fluid for microbiology and cytology from the lower airways in cases of suspected bronchopulmonary disease (e.g. bacterial pneumonia).

Procedure:

1. The rabbit should be anaesthetized and intubated using a sterile cuffed endotracheal (ET) tube.
2. 100% oxygen should be provided prior to and following the procedure.
3. Place the rabbit in lateral recumbency. In cases with suspected unilateral lung disease the affected lung should be downwards.
4. Place a sterile 4 Fr urinary catheter through the ET tube to emerge just beyond the caudal end of the tube.
5. Flush 1–2 ml/kg warm sterile saline down the catheter, using a sterile syringe attached to the urinary catheter, and immediately apply gentle suction to collect fluid. Approximately half of the total fluid volume used should be aspirated back (Figure 7.36).
6. Samples should be collected into sterile tubes and EDTA tubes for analysis.

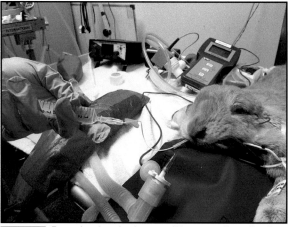

7.36 Bronchoalveolar lavage. Warm sterile saline is flushed down the catheter using a sterile syringe; approximately half the total fluid volume used should be aspirated back. See text for more details. (© Elisabetta Mancinelli)

PRACTICAL TIP

- Pre-measure the catheter alongside the ET tube prior to use to judge the length of insertion.
- Gentle elevation of the rabbit's hind end may help in sample collection, as well as gentle sideways ballottement of the thorax.
- Direct visualization is possible using bronchoscopy and this may aid sample collection.

WARNING

- The technique is relatively straightforward; however, care should be taken with severely debilitated dyspnoeic animals.
- Intubation is essential, and intermittent positive pressure ventilation (IPPV) using a ventilator to inflate the lungs is used by the authors prior to and following this procedure.

Thoracocentesis

This procedure involves the surgical puncture and drainage of the pleural space and should be carried out under ultrasonographic guidance. The technique should only be performed following appropriate diagnostic tests (thoracic radiography and ultrasonography) to confirm that the procedure is indicated. It is rarely required in rabbit medicine in the authors' experience.

Indications:

- To remove excessive accumulations of fluid (pleural effusions) or air (pneumothorax) from the pleural space to aid respiration and alleviate clinical signs of dyspnoea.
- Analysis of aspirated fluids helps aid diagnosis (culture, cytology, fluid analysis and specific gravity).

Procedure:

1. The rabbit should be placed in sternal recumbency and oxygen should be provided using a facemask.
2. The area between the 5th and 10th intercostal spaces should be clipped and surgically prepared, and the 7th intercostal space infiltrated with 1 ml of local anaesthetic.
3. Thoracocentesis is usually performed on the right side of the thorax unless diagnostic tests indicate a lesion confined to the left.
4. Insert a 21 G butterfly catheter needle or intravenous cannula with stylet carefully into the thorax at the level of the 7th intercostal space at a slight cranial angle.
5. Once the cannula is *in situ* remove the stylet.
6. Apply suction using extension tubing attached to the catheter, a three-way stopcock and a 10 ml syringe.

PRACTICAL TIP

Insert the butterfly catheter needle one-third of the way up the thorax from the ventrum in cases with pleural effusion and in the mid-thorax in cases with pneumothorax.

WARNING

Take care to avoid the blood vessels associated with the caudal border of the ribs when inserting the cannula.

Abdominocentesis

This procedure should be performed under ultrasonographic guidance, in the authors' experience, so that free peritoneal fluid can be directly visualized and sampled while minimizing the risk of iatrogenic damage to abdominal organs (in particular the large caecum and thin-walled bladder).

Indications: Diagnostic evaluation of excess free abdominal fluid (culture and sensitivity, cytology, fluid analysis). Fluid accumulations may occur associated with excessive production of peritoneal fluid (transudate, modified transudate, exudate) or leakage of intestinal contents, uterine contents, bile or urine, blood or chyle. Ascites is a relatively common finding, associated with hypoalbuminaemia and renal glomerular disease, although liver disease and intestinal disease should also be ruled out. Septic peritonitis is also often seen in rabbits, associated with gastrointestinal perforation, ruptured abdominal abscesses or uterine rupture.

Procedure:

1. The procedure can be carried out in calm, conscious animals but sedation is usually preferred to prevent sudden movements.
2. The rabbit should be restrained in dorsal recumbency and an area clipped and surgically prepared midline, caudal to the umbilicus.
3. Insert a 21–23 G butterfly catheter or intravenous catheter with stylet carefully, at a 45-degree angle to the skin, under ultrasound guidance, lateral to the midline and caudal to the umbilicus.
4. Remove the stylet and aspirate the fluid carefully into a sterile container.

PRACTICAL TIP

The bladder should be expressed prior to performing this procedure.

WARNING

- Coagulopathies should be ruled out prior to sampling, with measurement of whole blood clotting time in cases of suspected haemoabdomen.
- It is possible to puncture the bladder or intestine if ultrasonography is not used, leading to sampling of urine or intestinal contents and potential iatrogenic damage to these organs.

Diagnostic peritoneal lavage

Indications: This procedure is indicated if initial abdominocentesis is unsuccessful in retrieving a diagnostic sample.

Procedure:

1. See steps 1–3 for abdominocentesis.
2. Once the catheter has been placed, slowly instil warm saline (20 ml/kg) via the catheter, using extension tubing attached to the catheter, a three-way stopcock and a 50 ml syringe.
3. Aspirate fluid carefully for analysis.

PRACTICAL TIP
Gentle rocking of the patient to disperse the abdominal fluid may aid sampling.

WARNING
As for abdominocentesis.

Clinical techniques

Administration of medicines and fluid therapy
Routes and volumes for administration of medications are given in Figure 7.37.

Intramuscular injection

1. Identify the spine before palpating the symmetrical muscle areas within the lumbar region, approximately 2–3 cm on either side, which allows the epaxial muscles to be located (Figure 7.38a).
2. With the rabbit sitting in sternal recumbency on a non-slip surface, press the body of the rabbit against your abdomen using one arm, while securing the head of the rabbit in the crook of your elbow.
3. Use your other hand to inject into the epaxial muscles (Figure 7.38b). Always draw back the syringe before injecting, to avoid inadvertent intravenous injection.

Route	Sites	Volumes	Comments	Practical hints
Oral				
By syringe	Oral	Small volumes (0.5–3 ml) per mouthful dependent on rabbit size Supportive feeding: High-fibre 'critical care' formula: 50 ml/kg/day and 10–15 ml/kg/feed e.g. 2.5 kg rabbit has 125 ml/day, divided into 4 feeds = 31.25 ml 4x daily	Allow the rabbit to swallow between administrations. This is time-consuming and requires a good degree of patience	A hands-off approach between mouthfuls encourages the rabbit to chew and swallow
Parenteral				
Subcutaneous	Scruff of neck	Large volumes can be given (up to 50 ml in a 2.5 kg rabbit)	Usually well tolerated. Absorption rates vary but can be very slow in debilitated rabbits. With larger volumes, more than one injection site may be required	Hyaluronidase (1500 IU dissolved and injected into 1000 ml of isotonic fluids) can be added to promote absorption
Intravenous	Marginal ear vein (see Figure 7.39), lateral saphenous vein (see Figure 7.27) or cephalic vein (see Figure 7.28)	Fluid therapy: 4 ml/kg/h maintenance flow rates over 24-hour period. Dehydration deficits are added to this as a percentage of bodyweight, based on clinical signs of dehydration As a general rule assume 10% dehydration for debilitated animals; replace 50% of the fluid deficit in 12 hours and the remainder (plus maintenance and concurrent losses) in 48–72 hours. Shock fluid volumes of 100 ml/kg may be given over 60 minutes [a]. An i.v. catheter should be placed prior to drug administration	Very quick absorption rate All intravenous administrations should be given slowly and, if using a catheter, this should be flushed afterwards	As rabbits are prolific chewers, the giving set tubing should be secured away from the mouth. Alternatively, the catheter can be capped and fluids given in slow boluses via a needle and syringe at regular intervals. Elizabethan collars are rarely needed and will reduce normal eating and caecotrophy
Intraosseous	Proximal humerus, proximal tibia and proximal femur (see Figure 7.43)	As for intravenous route	Life-saving procedure to improve circulation so that intravenous catheters can then be placed to continue fluids and medications intravenously. Used for fluid therapy and administration of some intravenous drugs where rapid absorption is required in collapsed animals with poor venous access	Radiography is useful to ensure correct placement. Sedation and local anaesthesia are required

7.37 Routes and volumes for administration of medication. ([a] Paul-Murphy and Ramer, 1998) (continues) ▶

Route	Sites	Volumes	Comments	Practical hints
Parenteral				
Intramuscular	Epaxial muscles (lying either side of the vertebral column in the lumbar region; Figure 7.38), semimembranosus and semitendinosus muscles and quadriceps	Small volumes only – no more than 1 ml	The needle should be inserted at right angles to the muscle mass. Aspirate prior to injecting to ensure the needle has not entered a vessel	As this can be painful, an assistant restraining the rabbit is required to prevent sudden movements
Intraperitoneal	Paramedian or caudal to umbilicus	2.5 kg rabbit – no more than 20 ml	The rabbit should be well restrained, as there is a risk of puncturing bowel or bladder. The fluid should be warmed to reduce the risk of inducing hypothermia	Always draw back before injecting to ensure the needle has not punctured any abdominal organs
Topical				
Drops or ointment	Aural	Small volumes		The ear should be held whilst applying drops to prevent immediate shaking of medication out of the ear canal after application. Massaging the base of the ear when applying ointments improves the rabbit's tolerance of being medicated
	Dermal		Care must be taken to ensure the rabbit cannot groom the application off before it has a chance to take effect	If applying EMLA cream gloves should be worn
	Ocular	Several drops or blebs	Tenting the lower lid laterally when applying drops prevents them overflowing on to fur	Gently rolling the upper lid dorsally allows better exposure of the eye
Nebulization (see Figure 7.44)				
Inhalation	Respiratory tract	5 ml of F10 solution (1:250 dilution with water) per 15 minutes of nebulization	Extremely useful in the management of chronic respiratory disease	This is very well tolerated in rabbits

7.37 (continued) Routes and volumes for administration of medication. ([a] Paul-Murphy and Ramer, 1998)

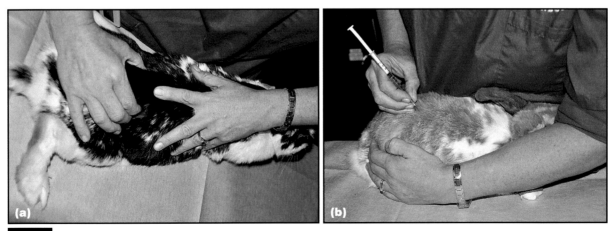

7.38 (a) Positioning and (b) restraint for intramuscular injection.

Placement of an intravenous catheter

1. Clip the fur from the back of the lateral borders of both ears and apply local anaesthetic cream (e.g. EMLA) along the line of the marginal ear vein. (With both ears clipped, if there are complications with one vein, the other ear is already prepared and ready for a second attempt at placement.)
2. Leave the rabbit for at least 15–20 minutes while the local anaesthetic takes effect and while the catheter placement materials (Figure 7.39a) are set up.
3. Use spirit to wipe the excess local anaesthetic cream off the ear and clean the skin surface.
4. Pre-flush the catheter with heparinized saline to reduce the risk of blood clotting in the catheter.
5. With an assistant raising the vein by occluding the base of the ear (Figure 7.39b), hold the ear in one hand, and hold the catheter in the other.
6. The vein is very superficial and when the bevel of the catheter is through the skin, the angle of the catheter should be almost parallel to the ear (Figure 7.39c).
7. Once in the vein, advance the stylet and catheter approximately 0.5 cm before advancing only the catheter further (Figure 7.39d). Flashback of blood is not always seen in rabbits owing to the small vessel size. Holding a finger under the ear prevents the ear from bending while the catheter is advanced.

8. Once the catheter is completely in the vein, the stylet is removed and a bung fastened to the catheter (Figure 7.39e). A T-port can be used, if preferred, in larger rabbits or in those requiring regular fluid therapy. However, T-ports can be bulky and there is potential for the rabbit to chew the attachment.
9. Use tape to secure the catheter. Place two pieces of micropore tape, one below and one above the catheter (Figure 7.39f). Leave this to hang until the ear support is added.
10. Place a folded or rolled-up swab inside the external ear canal to support the catheter and maintain the natural shape of the ear (Figure 7.39g). The tape is then secured around this. Take care not to kink the pinna and catheter in large-eared rabbit breeds.
11. A piece of silk tape can be used for further security, taking care not to tape over the bung (Figure 7.39h).
12. Flush the catheter to double-check correct positioning and patency. The fluid can often be seen running through the vessels of the ear or can be palpated entering the vessel at the level of the catheter.
13. The catheter should then be secured further with a single layer of a soft bandage (Figure 7.39i), followed by a layer of cohesive bandage (Figure 7.39j).

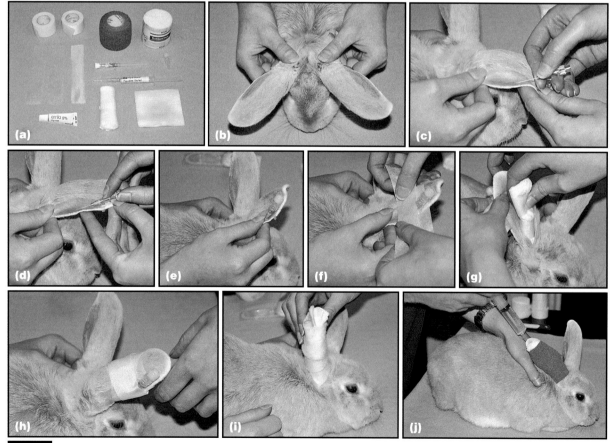

7.39 Placement of an intravenous catheter; see text for details.

Fluid therapy: Rabbits are highly tolerant of intravenous fluids (Figure 7.40). However, repeated use of the marginal ear vein for venepuncture or injection of irritant substances can lead to necrosis (Figure 7.41) or fibrosis of the vein.

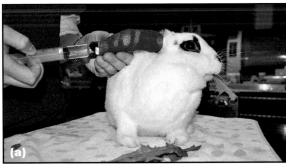

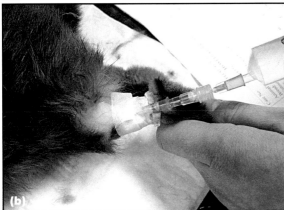

7.40 **(a)** Intravenous fluid therapy via an ear vein. **(b)** A rabbit receiving a bolus of fluids to the lateral saphenous vein, with the hind foot being held.

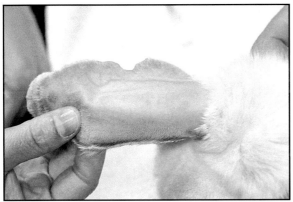

7.41 Necrosis of the marginal ear vein following long-term intravenous fluid therapy.

Intraosseous catheterization

Indications:

- Administration of fluids and/or medications in animals with shock or dehydration when peripheral blood vessels are not easily accessible.
- May also be used in juvenile animals or dwarf breeds where venous access may be difficult owing to vessel size.

Anatomical sites: The trochanteric fossa of the proximal femur, just medial to the greater trochanter and parallel to the long axis of the femur, is the site preferred by the authors. Although the proximal tibia is technically an easier site to use, needle placement involves entering the stifle joint capsule and there is therefore the potential for more complications. It is also possible to use the proximal tibia or proximal humerus in the rabbit.

Procedure:

1. The site is clipped and surgically prepared. Put on sterile gloves and place a sterile drape over the patient.
2. Infiltrate lidocaine 2% into the skin, muscle and periosteum.
3. Provide premedication with an opiate analgesic, e.g. buprenorphine at 0.03–0.05 mg/kg i.v. or s.c.
4. Make a small incision in the skin with a scalpel over the site of needle placement (if necessary).
5. Use a 1.5 inch (4 cm) spinal needle, intraosseous needle or 18–22 G 1 inch (2.5 cm) hypodermic needle with sterile surgical wire utilized as a stylet. Stabilize the bone to be penetrated with one hand and insert the needle along the long axis of the bone with a steady downward pressure (Figure 7.42). Penetration of the medullary cavity is confirmed by a sudden release of pressure and lack of resistance.

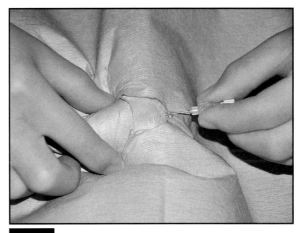

7.42 Intraosseous catheterization.

6. Remove the stylet and flush with heparinized saline. There should be no resistance to flushing and no swelling of surrounding soft tissues if the catheter is correctly placed.
7. Administer fluids or medication as required by slow continuous infusion rather than a rapid bolus (Figure 7.43b).
8. Attach a T-port or catheter bung and apply a light dressing to keep the catheter in place. Alternatively, butterfly tape can be applied to the hub and sutured to the surrounding skin to secure the catheter.
9. The catheter should be flushed after each use and three times daily if not regularly used.

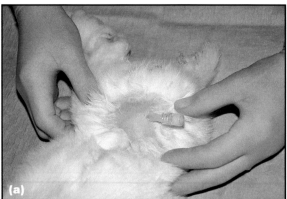

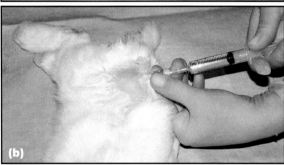

7.43 **(a)** Intraosseous catheter in place in the proximal femur. **(b)** Administration of fluids or medication by slow continuous infusion through an intraosseous catheter.

PRACTICAL TIP
- General anaesthesia or heavy sedation is required in animals that are not unconscious, because this procedure is painful.
- Radiography may be used to confirm correct placement in the medullary cavity.
- The leg may be bandaged to restrict limb mobility and reduce the risk of the catheter dislodging.

WARNING
- Do not use in fractured or poorly mineralized bones.
- Care should be taken to maintain the sterility of the catheter if remaining *in situ* over time.
- Do not leave catheter in place for longer than 72 hours, as there is an increased risk of site contamination after this time.

Nebulization
This may be performed in the clinic or by the owner in the home environment. An oxygen chamber, incubator (Figure 7.44) or covered cage/carrier box can be used (see also Chapter 11). Rabbits are very tolerant of this mode of medication.

Assisted feeding

Oral

1. Fill a 50 ml wide-nozzled dosing syringe with high-fibre 'critical care' formula (10–15 ml/kg per feed).

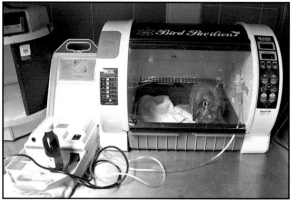

7.44 Rabbit in an incubator adapted for nebulization treatment.

2. Restrain the patient appropriately in sternal recumbency.
3. Gently insert the nozzle lateral to the incisors and advance it 2–4 cm into the mouth (dependent on rabbit size).
4. Ensure the patient's head remains in a straight (dorsoventral) position while small volumes of food are administered (Figure 7.45).
5. Remove the syringe from the oral cavity between mouthfuls to encourage chewing and swallowing.

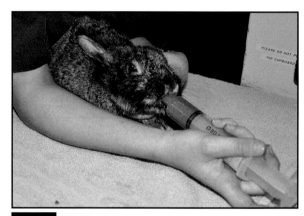

7.45 Critical care syringe-feeding.

Nasogastric intubation
Rabbits tolerate nasogastric tubes well.

Indications:

- For the administration of nutritional support, fluid therapy and medications to critically ill rabbits.
- Nasogastric intubation is indicated when a rabbit will not take syringe feeds by mouth, for example stressed and fractious rabbits, rabbits with oral pain (e.g. following dental surgery, partial mandibulectomy), rabbits with facial nerve paralysis or swallowing disorders.

Procedure:

1. Pre-measure a 5–8 Fr catheter or paediatric feeding tube from the external nares to the last rib.

2. Place topical local anaesthetic gel or a few drops of ocular local anaesthetic into the nasal opening a few minutes prior to tube placement. This is usually resented by the rabbit.
3. Apply a sterile lubricant to the catheter tip.
4. Elevate the rabbit's head and insert the tube into the ventral nasal meatus, aiming ventrally and medially. The head should be flexed as the tube passes down the proximal oesophagus.
5. Attach the tube to the fur on the head and along the bridge of the nose using tape wings, and place an Elizabethan collar if necessary (Figure 7.46).

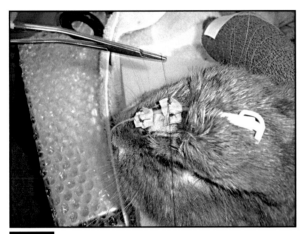

7.46   Nasogastric tube in place. (© Joanna Hedley)

PRACTICAL TIP
Correct tube placement should always be confirmed by a lateral radiograph because rabbits do not cough if the tube is placed in the trachea.

WARNING
Care should be taken if using this technique in rabbits with respiratory disease, as the tube partially occludes the nares; this may cause further dyspnoea, since rabbits are obligate nasal breathers.

Orogastric intubation

Indications:

• Single dosing of medications or fluids when the rabbit will not take syringe feeds by mouth or where nasogastric intubation is not possible.
• Decompression of gastric tympany in cases with gaseous distension or liquid stomach contents.

Procedure:

1. Sedation or general anaesthesia is required for this technique except in rabbits in a state of extreme collapse, or in very calm individuals.
2. Pre-measure and mark an 18–22 Fr round-tipped rubber catheter or feeding tube from the incisors to the last rib (Figure 7.47).

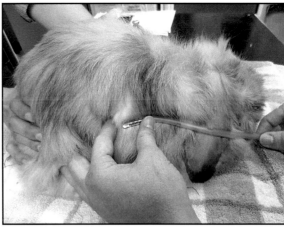

7.47   Pre-measurement of an orogastric tube prior to placement.

3. The rabbit should be held in sternal recumbency with the head supported.
4. A mouth gag should be applied to prevent the rabbit from chewing through the tube.
5. Flex the neck and pass the lubricated tube though the mouth and down the oesophagus into the stomach.

PRACTICAL TIP
Metal mouth gags (such as those used for dentistry) should only be used in anaesthetized rabbits. For conscious rabbits a mouth gag can be fashioned using a small bandage roll, otoscope cone or plastic syringe.

WARNING
Correct placement can be determined by auscultation over the stomach for gurgling noises while injecting 5–10 ml of air via the tube. If accidentally introduced into the trachea condensation will appear in the tube. A cough reflex is rarely heard, and therefore absence of a cough does not confirm placement in the oesophagus.

Nasolacrimal cannulation

Indications

• Irrigation of the nasolacrimal duct to remove debris causing a blockage or purulent material in cases with infection.
• Deposition of topical treatments directly *in situ* along the nasolacrimal duct.
• Instillation of contrast material into the duct for dacryocystography.

Procedure

1. Most rabbits tolerate this procedure while conscious, following prior topical application of local anaesthetic drops.
2. Pull the lower eyelid gently in a ventral direction. Rabbits have a single slit-shaped punctum

located on the medial aspect of the lower eyelid in the conjunctiva (see Figure 7.11).

3. Introduce a 20–27 G lacrimal cannula or intravenous cannula with stylet removed a few millimetres into the duct, directed ventromedially (Figure 7.48).
4. Flush the duct with sterile saline to confirm patency.
5. Topical medications and contrast material may be instilled into the duct.
6. If the duct is patent there should be little resistance to flushing. In cases occurring secondary to dental disease it is usually difficult to achieve full patency.

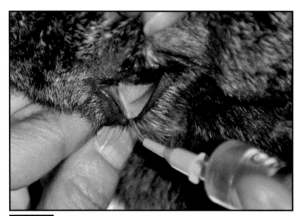

7.48 Nasolacrimal cannulation.

PRACTICAL TIP

The punctum is often dilated and easily located in chronic dacryocystitis. If not immediately obvious, gentle warm saline flushing of the area usually helps locate the punctum.

WARNING

If the globe starts to bulge while the duct is being flushed the procedure should be stopped immediately. This may occur if the duct is ruptured or the cannula is not in the punctum and fluid is being instilled into the retrobulbar space.

References and further reading

Benson KG and Paul-Murphy J (1999) Clinical pathology of the domestic rabbit, acquisition and interpretation of samples. *Veterinary Clinics of North America: Exotic Animal Practice* **2**(3), 539–551

Brown S (1997) Clinical techniques in rabbits. *Seminars in Avian and Exotic Pet Medicine* **6**(2), 86–95

Brown S (1998) General therapeutic regime for anorexia. In: *Small Mammals' Specialist Session. BSAVA Congress Proceedings*, p.32

Chitty, J (2007) Clinical techniques: the subarachnoid space: its clinical relevance in rabbits. *Journal of Exotic Pet Medicine* **16**(3), 179–182

Deeb BJ (2004) Respiratory disease and pasteurellosis. In: *Ferrets, Rabbits and Rodents: Clinical Medicine and Surgery, 2nd edn*, ed. KE Quesenberry and JW Carpenter, pp.172–182. WB Saunders, Philadelphia

Fisher PG (2010) Standards of care in the 21st century: The rabbit. *Journal of Exotic Pet Medicine* **19**(1), 22–35

Paul-Murphy J and Ramer JC (1998) Urgent care of the pet rabbit. *Veterinary Clinics of North America: Exotic Animal Practice* **1**(1), 127–152

Saunders R and Rees Davies R (2005) *Notes on Rabbit Internal Medicine*. Blackwell Publishing, Oxford

Whittington JK and Bennett RA (2011) Clinical technique: myelography in rabbits. *Journal of Exotic Pet Medicine* **20**(3), 217–221

Williams BH (2000) Disorders of rabbit and ferret bone marrow. In: *Laboratory Medicine: Avian and Exotic Pets*, ed. AM Fudge, pp.276–284. WB Saunders, Philadelphia

Online resource

Washington State University College of Veterinary Medicine: Small animal diagnostics and therapeutic techniques (www.vetmed. wsu.edu)

Rabbit History Form

Patient name:.. Case number:.................. Date: ....

Signalment

Age:.................................... Sex: .... Neutered:.......................... Bred from:..................................

Breed: .... Coat colour: ....

Ownership

BIOP (been in owner's possession): .... Acquired from:..

Previous rabbits owned: ....

Does the rabbit have animal company? (If yes, what species, sex and how many?):...

....

Housing

Housing type and size:..

Indoors/outdoors:..

....

Access to wildlife (if yes, what species?):..

Bedding:...

Litter tray trained?:...

Frequency cleaned out: ....

Diet

Food (volume and frequency given):...

....

Access to grass:...

Appetite:... Water source: ....

Treats/supplements given:...

Health and fitness

Vaccination status: ....

Behaviour: ....

Handling (how frequently?):...

Exercise: ....

Previous health problems: ....

Current medications:...

An example of a rabbit history form.

8

General nursing care and hospital management

Wendy Bament and Gidona Goodman

Appropriate nursing care for rabbits greatly aids their treatment and recovery from illness and surgery. Assessment of pain and demeanour can be difficult, and certain drugs widely used in veterinary practice are contraindicated in rabbits. This chapter lists equipment and drugs that are useful when treating rabbits. Important rabbit-specific considerations are discussed, ranging from information acquired at the time of consultation to anatomical factors affecting the nursing care of rabbits. The major components of supportive care are discussed, including nutritional support, fluid therapy, analgesia and prokinetics, with added detail on oxygen therapy, nebulization and wound management. The chapter concludes with a list of common rabbit emergencies. See also Chapter 6 for further advice on making a practice 'rabbit-friendly'.

The rabbit ward and cage

When designing a rabbit ward it is important to consider the behaviour and welfare needs of rabbits. The main driving factor is the predisposition of rabbits to become easily stressed, particularly when hospitalized.

General ward considerations

- A separate housing area should be provided, away from other hospitalized patients that could be considered predators (particularly dogs, cats, ferrets and birds of prey).
- Human and animal traffic should be kept to a minimum, as should noise (e.g. staff should avoid talking loudly).
- Rabbit cages should not be placed facing each other, so as to minimize territorial or aggressive reactions (Figure 8.1).
- Where possible rabbits should be treated before patients of predator species, to avoid rabbits detecting scents that would cause stress. Use of protective clothing or designated staff can also help.
- Staff must be aware of correct handling techniques because rabbits are predisposed to spinal and hindlimb injury (see Chapter 7 for correct handling techniques).
- The ward flooring should, where possible, be easy to scrub and disinfect, such as vinyl-type

material rather than tiling, because rabbit urine can eventually erode through concrete-based substrates (Figure 8.1).
- There should be a stable ample-sized examination table in the ward, ideally used only for small mammals (Figure 8.1).
- The environmental temperature should be maintained between 18 and 21°C as rabbits are prone to heat stress.
- Ward lights that have a dimmer switch can be useful for a rabbit ward. Lights should be switched off at night, between 9 pm and 8 am where possible.
- An emergency box (housing an accessible collection of equipment and drugs required in an emergency) can be justified in a rabbit ward, especially if the ward is located far away from the anaesthetic and theatre stations. For further discussion see Chapter 10 and Thompson and Bament (2012).
- It is useful to have a specific location where labelled animal belongings are safely stored until collection is advisable, to avoid any embarrassments.
- Separate storage areas (cupboards and fridges) are advisable for keeping rabbit food away from that used for carnivores such as dogs, cats, ferrets, snakes or birds of prey.

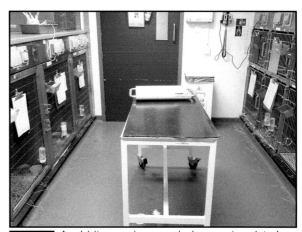

8.1 A rabbit-conscious ward where no 'predator' species (e.g. cats, dogs, ferrets) are hospitalized. Enclosures are side by side with enough space between cage fronts so as not to instigate territorial disputes. Note the large examination table, wall-mounted otoscope/auroscope and easy-to-clean flooring.

Waste and hygiene

Maintaining excellent standards of hygiene between patients is a paramount concern, particularly for nurses. Effectively, every surface a rabbit touches in the veterinary hospital must be disinfected; this is particularly important with mesh or wire cages owing to the increased surface area and opportunity for disease transmission. Some examples of suitable high-level wide-spectrum disinfectants for use in rabbit (animal) wards are shown in Figure 8.2, and some are available 'unscented', which could reduce any risk of irritation to sensitive mucous membranes or stress from an unfamiliar smell. Alcohol-based sanitizing hand gels can also be employed and dispensers placed next to doors to encourage maintenance of hygiene.

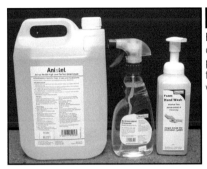

8.2

Examples of disinfectant products suitable for use in a rabbit ward.

It is suggested that *Encephalitozoon cuniculi*, which is transmitted via spores in urine, is present in more than 50% of pet rabbits, and the veterinary hospital runs the risk of being a significant contributor to disease transfer (Keeble and Shaw, 2006). Myxomatosis is a viral infection commonly seen in wild rabbits, mainly during the summer months in the UK, but domestic rabbits are also susceptible to this disease and care is required in minimizing its spread by vector transmission, e.g. fleas and mosquitos. Classic 'barrier nursing' should not be necessary between pet rabbits, but placing infected rabbits in a different room from those unaffected may help to prevent the disease spreading.

Another rabbit-specific issue regarding hygiene is their predisposition to pass thick alkaline calcium-rich urine which, if not cleaned away daily, can leave permanent crusting and cause damage to enclosures and fittings. White vinegar is excellent for removing this stain, although owing to its strong odour it should be used when no rabbits are around, to avoid causing any stress.

Zoonoses and other human safety concerns

The main risks to human health are from rabbit bites and scratches and zoonotic pathogens such as ectoparasites (e.g. fleas), *Pasteurella multocida*, *Campylobacter* spp. and *E. cuniculi*. Allergic reactions to hay or sensitivity to rabbit fur can also occur. Most people will know if they are sensitive to hay and rabbit fur and precautions should be taken, such as wearing a mask when grooming or cleaning and pre-emptive antihistamine. If staff have adverse reactions to rabbit bites/saliva, such incidents should be logged and the required first aid treatment performed.

E. cuniculi infection has been reported in humans, particularly in immunosuppressed individuals, and it is advised to maintain high levels of hygiene and wear disposable examination gloves when cleaning out cages.

Other more immediate risks from handling rabbits are bites and scratches; any wounds should be washed immediately with antibacterial handwash.

Rabbit hospital cage set-up

When planning an appropriate cage design for rabbits, both general welfare requirements and individual preferences should be considered. Therefore, it is important to gather as much information from the rabbit's owner as possible at the time of admission regarding diet (including favourite treats), toys, drinking water vessel (bowl or bottle), companions, bedding type and even grooming requirements. Another consideration that could help prepare staff is to find out from the owner the general demeanour or character of the rabbit, e.g. if they are confident or skittish, and whether they bite (see Chapter 5).

General cage considerations

A typical rabbit hospital cage is shown in Figure 8.3.

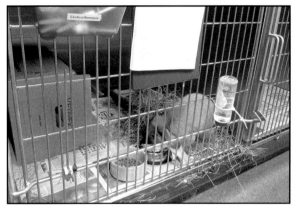

8.3 A typical rabbit hospital cage containing an appropriately sized hide box, a bundle of hay 1–2 times the size of the rabbit, a litter tray, and food and water provision.

- **Dimensions:** Cages should allow the rabbit to be able to stand up on its hindlegs and hop once or twice in succession; suggested cage dimensions are 100 cm × 80 cm × 80 cm. Despite the timid nature of rabbits, it is advisable to house them in wire-fronted enclosures in order to promote ventilation inside the cage and to enable observation of the patient without disturbing them. However, it is important to ensure that a 'hide' area is available. See also Chapter 2.
- **Hay:** Giving rabbits plenty of good quality (low dust-producing) timothy-rich hay every day is an absolute essential and, as a rough guide, a portion of hay should be about the size of the rabbit. Keeping it in a bunch rather than spreading it out will help keep it fresh and provide some enrichment by allowing the rabbit to pick through and move it around. Some rabbits like to use hay as bedding so they must be given enough to allow for bedding and feed.

- **Drinking water:** Information should be acquired from the owner as to whether the rabbit is used to drinking from a bottle or a bowl, because rabbits can reduce their water intake if not provided with the familiar vessel. If in doubt, both should be provided and drinking behaviour recorded. Recent studies have demonstrated that, when given a choice, rabbits prefer to drink from bowls rather than sipper bottles, and bowls allow a bigger intake of water in a shorter time-span (Tschudin *et al.*, 2010).
- **Newspaper:** Mainly used for flooring, but great care should be taken if the rabbit has a tendency to shred, chew and eat paper or cardboard as this can lead to gut problems or cause a tracheal obstruction (author's personal experience). If more bedding is required then extra hay is advised to allow natural digging behaviour and patient preference in bedding shape and positioning.
- **Hide or secure area:** This can be as simple as a cardboard box or placing a towel over one half of the cage door, but it is vital to incorporate this for rabbit patients to give them the choice of either investigating their outer surroundings by coming to the front of the cage or hiding and reducing stress levels in a secure area (Figure 8.3). Boxes can be particularly useful because rabbits instinctively prefer to feel the sides as they would if they were in a burrow, and if the box is relatively sturdy then more confident rabbits will enjoy jumping on top of it, which may also make them feel more secure.
- **Pellets or muesli:** Ideally owners should be encouraged to feed their rabbits complete pellets rather than selective or muesli-type mixes (see Chapter 3), but it is important not to deviate from the established diet of an individual rabbit as it can cause complications with the intestinal tract. Also, when tempting sick or recovering animals it is important to offer familiar and/or palatable food items. However, it can be considered positive to offer a small amount of pellets to test whether the rabbit will eat them. This would allow staff to advise owners on providing a more appropriate diet by gradually weaning their rabbits on to complete pellets.
- **Litter tray:** The provision of a litter tray can improve cage hygiene and daily waste assessment. Normal wood cat litter or hay can be used inside a shallow cat litter tray, and most rabbits are easily trained to use these by placing their fresh faeces inside the tray. Rabbits previously unfamiliar with litter trays show a tendency to adopt their use (author's experience), which provides another opportunity to help the owner improve hutch husbandry management and rabbit welfare.
- **Companions and familiar items:** It is important to take advantage, where possible and not contraindicated, of providing familiar items such as toys (Figure 8.4), hides or bonded companion rabbits (Figure 8.5). The decision to admit companion rabbits to accompany inpatients needs to be carefully assessed according to space available, stability of relationship between rabbits and appropriateness for the condition or procedure for the patient. Companions can be particularly useful in the recovery phase, encouraging patients to eat and exercise, but care must be taken as the stressful new environment, or discomfort, can initiate agonistic behaviours. Companion rabbits should ideally be given their own designated cage while assessing the patient's faecal output, eating or drinking measurements. The companion's cage should be fitted out with the items discussed above, but with plenty of enrichment to prevent a healthy rabbit becoming stressed and a patient itself. Companion animals admitted with a patient are still under the care of the practice.
- **Floor padding:** Cages can be fitted with highly durable rubber padding, although prolonged periods on this can lead to it being badly chewed, with possible ingestion and gut or tracheal obstruction. Use could be considered in rabbits with diseases such as severe pododermatitis.

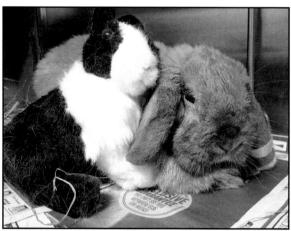

8.4 Toys may be used as 'companions' for rabbit patients, and should be considered when setting up the cage furniture.

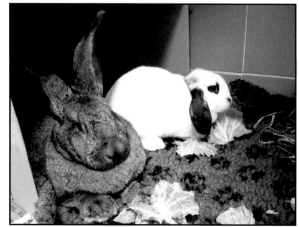

8.5 Bonded companion rabbits can be an important part of the treatment plan for hospitalized rabbits. Interactions and social time should be carefully monitored when the rabbits have experienced any time apart. Note the soft blanket, which is often given to giant breeds experiencing skeletal discomfort and pododermatitis.

Specific cage set-ups

Rabbits experiencing certain conditions or those that are physically compromised will inevitably require specific considerations for cage set-ups, and it is advisable to plan and prepare these cages before the rabbit is removed from its travel carrier. Figure 8.6 describes the commonly encountered conditions of pet rabbits and the hospitalization considerations each scenario requires.

Condition	Main concerns affecting husbandry planning	Diet	Bedding	Extra considerations
Dental disease or oral pain	Discomfort when eating, or reduced ability to eat	Softened food, e.g. moistened pellets, grated and shredded vegetables (Figure 8.7). Supportive feeding, e.g. critical care formulas	Normal (newspaper)	Where incisors have been removed it may be beneficial to offer dry food and strips of green vegetables
Recovery from anaesthesia	Inability to regulate temperature, retain upright position or acquire nutrition voluntarily	Supportive feeding, e.g. critical care formulas	Warm comfortable bedding, e.g. towels initially until coordinated movements observed and then deep hay	Remove cage furnishings and water bowls until fully recovered. Incubator can be set up with food and water for cold, slow to recover patients
Gut stasis or bloat	Abdominal discomfort	Hay and supportive feeding	Normal or deeper layer of hay for support	Minimize handling and noise in the ward
Shocked patient (after trauma)	Reduced body temperature Inability to retain upright position Sensitivity to external environment	Tempting foods	Warm comfortable bedding, e.g. towels initially until coordinated movements observed and then deep hay	Oxygen therapy Heat support: incubator (Figure 8.8), microwaveable cherry-stone heat packs Minimize handling and noise in the ward
Respiratory compromise	Discomfort of the respiratory tract Easily panicked	Tempting foods	Normal (newspaper)	Oxygen therapy Minimize handling and noise in the ward
Urinary disease (including scald)	Discomfort of urinary tract and urinary scalds to the skin Reduced body temperature if wet with urine Secondary infection due to ulcers and scalding	Tempting foods. Diets formulated for urinary disease	Absorbent and deep bedding such as Vetbed and incontinence pads, to draw urine away from the rabbit	Incontinence pads can be used plastic side up if requiring a free-catch urine sample (Figure 8.9), or an empty litter tray can work for rabbits used to using one
Ocular disease	Eye discomfort. Panic due to impaired vision (Figure 8.10)	Tempting foods	Normal (newspaper). Minimalistic furniture if surgical procedure is imminent, to reduce risk of further ocular trauma. Otherwise deep hay to promote eating and sense of security, if some degree of blindness is present	Minimal furniture or obstacles, maintained in the same locations. Place towel in front of cage to reduce light/shadow movements. Care when approaching the rabbit to pick it up
Vestibular disease	Inner ear discomfort or irritation. Panic if loss of balance	Tempting foods. Easy to eat and not likely to cause soiling of the fur	Normal (newspaper). Rolled towels padding the corners can help avoid the rabbit getting stuck in a corner (Figure 8.11)	Minimize handling, light and noise in the ward
Limb fractures	Limb discomfort	Normal or tempting foods	Normal or padded (newspaper and deep fabric blankets). Rolled towels padding the corners can help avoid the rabbit getting stuck in a corner	No boxes or raised furniture such as litter trays to avoid the rabbit jumping up and causing further trauma

8.6 Considerations for setting up cages for specific rabbit patients. Any sick rabbit is likely to show a degree of anorexia. 'Supportive feeding' refers to critical care formulas. Specific nursing support is discussed in the text. (continues) ▶

Condition	Main concerns affecting husbandry planning	Diet	Bedding	Extra considerations
Hindlimb paresis	Limb discomfort	Normal or tempting foods	Absorbent and deep bedding (e.g. Vetbed) and incontinence pads, to draw urine away from the rabbit (Figure 8.12)	No litter tray
Ectoparasite infestation, e.g. flystrike	Irritated skin	Normal or tempting foods	Normal (newspaper)	Care when handling other patients or housing near to another patient
Severe pododermatitis	Foot discomfort during locomotion or sitting position	Normal or tempting foods	Well padded, non-abrasive flooring, which may need to be placed underneath a layer of newspaper	

8.6 (continued) Considerations for setting up cages for specific rabbit patients. Any sick rabbit is likely to show a degree of anorexia. 'Supportive feeding' refers to critical care formulas. Specific nursing support is discussed in the text.

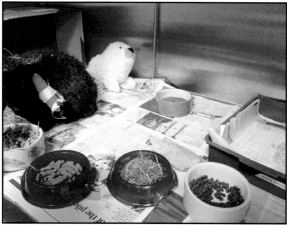

8.7 A cage set up for a patient with dental disease or oral pain, showing the provision of easy-to-eat food items (shredded and grated vegetables, softened and hard pellets and wet critical care formula). A favourite toy and the patient's own bowls are also included.

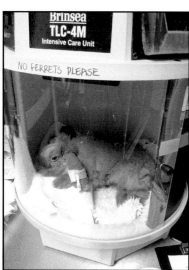

8.8 Rabbit patients can be maintained and monitored in an incubator during recovery from sedation/anaesthesia or if collapsed. Care is necessary with the use of heating devices (hot water bottles or heat packs) and with some synthetic bedding (e.g. Vetbed, towels) when patients are more coordinated and lively, to avoid potential ingestion and foreign body or choking risks.

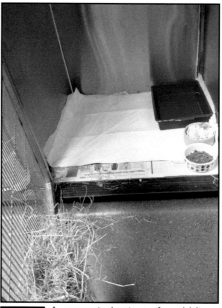

8.9 A suggested set-up of a rabbit cage if a free-catch urine sample is required. The plastic side of an incontinence pad can be used to line the cage and/or an empty litter tray for rabbits used to using them. Once the urine has been collected the cage should be re-set up appropriately.

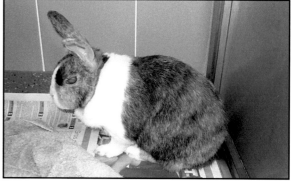

8.10 A rabbit with ocular disease and blindness just prior to anaesthesia for diagnostics and treatment. Note the rabbit's body language suggesting stress: it has backed into a corner and its ears are held forward. Prior to anaesthesia these patients should have minimalistic cage furniture.

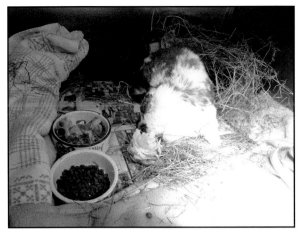

8.11 A cage set up for a rabbit with vestibular disease. Note the rolled blankets and towels in the cage corners and edges to prevent the rabbit rolling and getting stuck. Food and water must be safe and easy for the rabbit to reach.

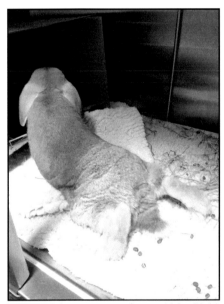

8.12 A cage set up for a rabbit with hindlimb paresis. Note the use of soft bedding to avoid the development of sores and ulcers.

Daily patient assessment

Every rabbit should be weighed when it is admitted to the ward. Bodyweight should then be recorded daily because it is a good indicator of whether the patient is eating and drinking sufficiently. The daily weight, urine and faecal output, food consumption and other clinical observations (Figure 8.13) should be recorded; an example of a patient record sheet is provided at the end of this chapter.

Daily exercise can also be beneficial to the patient. As well as the physical benefits of moving around, it encourages bowel movements. Often, rabbits that have not passed faeces overnight will pass some after exercising for a few minutes outside the confines of the cage. A patient should never be left to exercise unsupervised and all electrical wires should be out of reach, as rabbits may chew them.

Parameters to assess	Normal range or appearance	Notable observations
Animal – direct observations		
Demeanour/ behaviour	Stoical or inquisitive	Relaxed, lying stretched out *versus* stressed such as kennel guarding, teeth grinding, thumping feet or grunting
Respiratory rate	30–60 breaths/minute	Character (regularity) and sounds (fluid crackles)
Heart rate	180–300 beats/minute	Rhythm or pulse deficits
Gut sounds	Left and right abdomen should sound like a slow creaking door with a few bubbles	Noisy wet/'sloshy', quiet or no sounds
Abdominal palpation	Soft, doughy abdomen, and possibly faecal pellet palpated	Pain score. Hardened, possible tumour, foreign body, pregnancy, bloated tympany, faecal impaction, etc.
Temperature	38.5–40°C	Outside the normal range
Weight	Dependent on breed	Relative to the breed and compared with first day of hospitalization
Cage		
Faeces	Dry pellet = final faecal pellet. Wet pellet = caecotroph pellet. Caecotrophs are usually passed within 3–8 hours of eating	Size, consistency and volume
Urine	20–350 ml/kg per day (highly variable with diet and other factors). Can appear thick and reddened in some normal rabbits due to porphyrin plant staining from their diet	Amount, consistency and colour. Urinalysis for further investigation
Food intake	Measured from a given weighed amount, e.g. 20 g pellets, or score out of 10 for vegetables. Rabbits consume 5% of their bodyweight daily in dry diet	Direct observations encouraged of eating hay and food preferences or difficulties
Water intake	50–150 ml/kg/day	Variation from normal parameters

8.13 Parameters for daily patient assessment.

If the patient is unable to groom effectively, or is recumbent, the perianal area should be checked daily for any faecal matter sticking to the coat and for any evidence of urine soaking the fur. If soiling of fur is noted, the area should be washed gently with warm water and shampoo. Care must be taken to dry the fur properly to avoid scalding, hypothermia and moist dermatitis.

Nursing clinics

Owing to the increasing popularity of rabbits as pets and with growing demand from owners to optimize their husbandry, the adoption of nursing clinics for rabbits, as seen for dogs and cats, is well justified and an important opportunity to support rabbit owners. Suggested nursing clinics include: the new rabbit owner; weight clinics; behaviour clinics; and grooming services (see also Chapter 6).

The new rabbit owner (husbandry, preventive healthcare)

When people are thinking about owning a rabbit, as with dogs and cats, it is a great opportunity for veterinary teams to inform and support new rabbit owners, either prior to purchasing or when bringing in a new rabbit. It is advisable to have clearly written handouts (see examples at end of Chapter 6) as well as the practice policies and services offered for the owner to review later at their leisure. The following topics could be discussed.

- **Pre-purchasing advice:** Identify potential physical problems encountered, advise on potential allergens and zoonoses, and recommend sources of pet rabbits (e.g. rehoming centres).
- **Diet:** Promote the importance of fibre and high quality timothy-rich hay, suitable vegetables and edible plants. For pre-owned or rehomed rabbits it may be necessary to change their diet gradually to a more suitable one.
- **Housing:** Discuss space and indoor or outdoor facilities and requirements.
- **Enrichment:** Recommend safe and natural behaviour-enhancing toys, which may be sold by the veterinary hospital. Include discussions on rabbit behaviour and encourage socialization with companions (advise at least one companion) and strategies for introductions (see also Chapters 2 and 5).
- **Vaccination:** Rabbit haemorrhagic disease (RHD) and myxomatosis vaccines are now available as a single injection (see Chapter 6).
- **Neutering:** Should be encouraged to prevent breeding and reproductive disorders such as uterine neoplasia.
- **Grooming and physical checks:** Encourage a regular grooming regime, not only to habituate the rabbit to handling but also to maintain coat condition and allow regular physical assessments. Common conditions seen in pet rabbits, such as pododermatitis, should be discussed. Basic equipment can be suggested such as grooming tools and scales for weight checks.

Weight clinics

These are usually only offered for owners of overweight rabbits and weight management plans can be custom-made for the individual rabbit and the owner's capability.

- Target weights at specific dates or 'weight diaries' can be suggested, or a pre-designed sheet can be handed out.
- An obesity/body condition scoring chart is available at: http://www.pfma.org.uk/petometer.html.

Behaviour clinics

To support rabbit owners, it is advisable to consider providing clinics that target topics such as 'naughty' behaviour, litter training and socialization (see also Chapter 5). Owners may need to be reminded of the rabbit's natural prey instincts and their general dislike of being picked up. As with most animals, it can be considered appropriate to assume that they prefer to be left to decide for themselves when they want to interact with humans, and the core theme should be about building trust. Depending on time and space available, the use of veterinary clinic facilities could be considered when helping to introduce rabbits to one another, to provide a neutral environment, a slightly stressful experience that they can bond together over, or simply to help support owners and promote keeping rabbits in social pairs or groups (see Chapters 2 and 5).

Grooming

This can be offered as a service to owners who struggle to cope with the grooming requirements of some rabbits, especially with breeds such as Angoras. Some owners will also not feel confident enough to clip nails.

Supportive and postoperative care

Supportive and postoperative care in rabbits involves the following:

- Heat therapy
- Pain management
- Fluid therapy
- Nutritional therapy
- Prokinetics
- Oxygen therapy
- Nebulization
- Wound management
- Physiotherapy and exercise
- Hand-rearing neonates (see Chapter 4).

A list of the equipment, diets and drugs that may be required is shown in Figure 8.14.

Heat therapy

Animals recovering from surgery, those who are lethargic or collapsed and young animals will be prone to hypothermia and will benefit from the provision of supplemental heating. The normal body temperature range for a rabbit is 38.5–40°C. The ideal environmental temperature for normal rabbits should be maintained at 18–21°C, and consequently hypothermic rabbits may require environmental temperatures of 25–30°C and careful patient monitoring, e.g. rectal temperature recorded every 15 minutes. The rabbit's body language and behaviour should also indicate the effect of temperature extremes in

Food/feeding
Timothy-rich meadow hay, grass, pellets and fresh vegetables (e.g. spring greens, savoy cabbage) and fruit (apple). A selection of commercially produced diets. Ceramic bowels 20 cm in diameter

Clinical examination
Otoscope, paediatric stethoscope, ophthalmoscope, electronic thermometer. Rodent cheek pouch dilator and incisor gag. Scales

Diagnostics
Needles: 27–21 G 16 mm. Urinary catheters: 3–4 Fr cat catheter or 3–4 Fr Jackson cat catheter

Medication
Adrenaline, colestyramine, cisapride, **diazepam**, **doxapram**, **naloxone**, lidocaine/prilocaine cream (e.g. EMLA cream 5%), glycopyrrolate, imidacloprid, meloxicam, metoclopramide, probiotic (e.g. Bio-lapis Protexin veterinary; Avipro Vetark)

Anaesthesia
Ayres T-pece rebreathing circuit with Jackson Rees modification, facemasks, supraglottic airway device, uncuffed ET tubes (2–4 mm), ET tubes (1–5 mm), laryngoscope with a Wisconsin blade size 0 and 1 or auroscope with long nose cone. Small animal ventilator (SAV03 for patients up to 10 kg). Capnograph, Doppler and blood pressure monitor, handheld digital pulse oximeter

Supportive care
Intravenous catheters: 26 G x 19 mm/24 G x 19 mm/22 G x 25 mm. Elizabethan collar (7.5–10 cm). Bandages, dressings. 4–8 Fr paediatric feeding tube and/or 6–8 Fr dog catheter; 4–6 Fr Portex paediatric feeding tube or 3–4 Fr cat catheter. Recovery diets: e.g. Supreme Recovery Diet; Oxbow Critical Care Diet. Catheter-tip 60 ml syringe. Room heater, hairdryer, microwaveable heat pad/cherry-stone bag. Incubator, oxygen tent for rabbits, oxygen humidifier. Nebulizer and dispensing cups

Cleaning
Disinfectant, alcohol sanitizing hand gels

Grooming
Nail clippers, grooming equipment (e.g. FURminator), shaving clippers

Cage furniture
Cat litter trays, cat litter. Incontinence pads. Rubber matting

8.14 Equipment for use in a rabbit ward. The drugs in bold should be included in a crash box.

the environment, for example if too hot the rabbit will lay stretched out and be panting, if too cold the rabbit will be huddled and hunched and inactive or slow to respond to stimuli. Therefore it is important to assess the combination of specific data from environmental and rectal temperatures and the rabbit's behavioural responses. A baseline body temperature should be established for the individual rabbit.

Provision of additional heat

- **Portable room heaters** with variable settings are useful, but if directing heat into a rabbit's cage there must be a box or hide that the rabbit can shelter in if it needs to. Portable heaters are useful for when the animal has recovered and is moving around but still has a low body temperature. Given that this method is somewhat indiscriminate, it is important to assess the behaviour of other patients in the warmer environment to avoid heat stress.
- There Is a variety of **incubators** available that are suitable for rabbits (in terms of size and safety) and it is advisable for veterinary hospitals to have one dedicated for small herbivorous mammals. Most incubators will have heat and humidity controls (required values are usually 25–30°C and 40–60% humidity), and can also be used for nebulization sessions and oxygen therapy. Incubators are particularly useful when rabbits are recovering from an anaesthetic because intensive and efficient heat therapy can be applied and tailored to the patient without affecting the rest of the ward.
- When using **heating devices** to provide direct heat to the rabbit's body it is essential to ensure that there is a layer of bedding or a towel between it and the recumbent rabbit, and to consider the time it takes for the item to lose its heat, because heat may then be drawn away from the rabbit (Figure 8.15).
  - Cherry-stone 'bean' bags (unscented) can be microwaved safely and, where indicated, washed in a washing machine and tumble-dried, and they have the added advantage of being 'mouldable' to the patient's body to optimize comfort. However, to avoid hotspots, the bag must be shaken and mixed to distribute any hot beans or stones.
  - Heat pads (e.g. Snugglesafe) are very practical, easy to clean and provide relatively long periods of heat emission. Their rigidity can be uncomfortable for some animals and it is important to ensure that adequate bedding is placed between the pad and the rabbit.

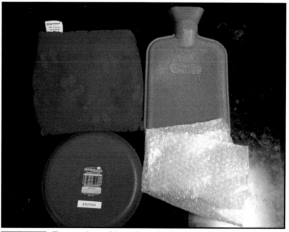

8.15 Examples of heating devices that can be used with hypothermic rabbits or patients in recovery from anaesthesia. Monitoring is essential when using these devices to prevent scalding, heat loss or potential foreign body threat when the rabbit is more active and investigating its environment.

- Electric heat mats provide heat as long as they are plugged into an electric socket, but they do not have adjustable settings and their temperature must be monitored to avoid scalds. They may also pose a risk in rabbits that recover suddenly and begin to dig and 'gnaw' at the mat.
- Hot water bottles and 'hot hands' (warm water in tied examination gloves) can be useful for instant heat provision to recumbent hypothermic rabbits, but their heat emission is usually short-lived and this will also lead to heat loss from the rabbit.

Pain management

Pain management is an integral part of supportive and postoperative care of rabbits (see also Chapter 10). It promotes healing, feeding and recovery after surgery. Pain assessment in rabbits (see also Chapters 5 and 20) can be difficult because they are a prey species and therefore alter their behaviour in the presence of a human observer, but provision of analgesia is advised even if there are no obvious signs of pain. A study on the behavioural effects of ovariohysterectomy (Leach *et al.*, 2009) demonstrated that: 'inactive' pain behaviours such as twitching, flinching, wincing and slow shuffling increased following surgery; behaviours indicative of activity, such as movement, grooming, exploring and standing, decreased; and inactivity (lying down) increased. This was more evident in the afternoon, which may be due to rabbits being naturally less active during the morning. Recently a rabbit grimace scale has been developed: the cheek or nose bulge at rest becomes progressively more pointed or flattened as the intensity of acute pain increases (Keating *et al.*, 2012). Pain may lead to a reduction of food and water intake, which in turn leads to a reduction in faecal output.

Non-steroidal anti-inflammatory drugs (NSAIDs), such as meloxicam and carprofen, and/or opioids (buprenorphine) are the analgesic agents of choice (see Chapter 10). As in other species, when using NSAIDs care should be taken if the animal is hypotensive or hypovolaemic, because of the risk of renal toxicity.

Fluid therapy

Fluid therapy involves the administration of fluids to the rabbit via the various routes summarized in Figure 8.16. This aims to support the venous circulation and optimize hydration status. Dehydration status should be determined when examining rabbits by assessing 'tenting' of the skin, sunken eyes or desiccation of the cornea and dry or tacky mucous membranes.

Rabbits that have experienced relatively long periods (>4 hours) of anorexia, more than 1 day of loose faeces or diarrhoea, or sedation and general anaesthetics will primarily require a maintenance rate of crystalloid fluids (such as compound sodium lactate or lactated Ringer's solution). Procedures and conditions that have caused significant blood loss may require colloids, either alone or mixed with crystalloids (e.g. 50:50 dilutions). The daily maintenance rate for rabbits is slightly higher than for dogs and cats: 4 ml/kg/h or 80–100 ml/kg/24h. During procedures requiring sedation or general anaesthesia it is recommended to administer 10 ml/kg/h in slow boluses every 5–15 minutes. Fluids may be provided via the oral, subcutaneous, intravenous or intraosseous routes in rabbits. Techniques and equipment for intravenous and intraosseous catheter placement are described in Chapter 7.

Fluids administered via any route should be gently warmed to body temperature; bolus syringes can be placed inside electric baby-bottle warmers to facilitate this during procedures. This will prevent discomfort when injecting and may help to prevent loss of body heat (Figure 8.17). Any warmed fluid should be tested before administration by squirting it on to the handler's skin.

Volume	Conditions indicated	Suggested equipment	Advantages	Disadvantages	Suggested fluids
Oral					
10–15 ml/kg q8h	Gut stasis, mild dehydration	Catheter-tip syringe, nasogastric feeding tube	Simple. Can be performed by one person. Non-sterile solutions used in dilute recovery formula	Slow. Variable absorption. Risk of aspirated/inhaled fluid	Lectade, soaked ground pellets, Vetark Critical Care Formula, Supreme Recovery, Oxbow Critical Care Formula, Labefer's Emeraid Nutritional Care System Herbivore
Subcutaneous injection					
Up to 100 ml total in at least two sites, depending on the size of the rabbit	Collapse, mild to moderate dehydration, gut stasis, poor venous access	Needle (23–21 G), syringe (20 ml is easier but up to 50 ml), butterfly catheter if the rabbit will tolerate it	Large volume. Simple and quick technique. Can be used in combination with intravenous routes	Slow absorption (especially if animal is significantly dehydrated). Repeated treatment can become uncomfortable and create scars. May require more than one person	Isotonic, crystalloids, hyaluronidase can be used to promote resorption: 1 vial of hyaluronidase 1500 IU in a 1 litre bag of fluids

8.16 Routes for fluid therapy in rabbits. Blood transfusion is described in the section on 'Rabbit emergencies'. (continues) ▶

Volume	Conditions indicated	Suggested equipment	Advantages	Disadvantages	Suggested fluids
Intravenous injection					
4 ml/kg/h maintenance; 10 ml/kg/h for sedated or anaesthetized patients; 100 ml/kg/h as shock dose	Collapse, moderate to severe dehydration, GI stasis, anaesthesia, oral or limb discomfort (other routes are inaccessible)	Clippers, swabs, surgical spirit, i.v. catheter (26–24 G), injection bung, T-extension set, local anaesthetic (e.g. EMLA cream), non-traumatic tape (e.g. Micropore, Durapore), bandages (e.g. Softban, Vetwrap)	Rapid rehydration, large volumes. Easy catheter placement, well tolerated, relatively non-invasive route or low disturbance for fluid administration (particularly if a T-extension adapter used)	Likely to chew through drip extension lines. Catheter placement painful unless local anaesthetic cream is used; poor technique will stress the rabbit. Requires more than one person. Placement is dependent on previous venous puncture and scarring, and adequate circulation and body temperature	Crystalloids and colloids
Intraosseous catheter (femur, tibia)					
4 ml/kg/h maintenance; 100 ml/kg/h as shock dose	Collapse, moderate to severe dehydration, severe anaemia, anaesthesia	Clippers, chlorhexidine, surgical spirit, swabs, spinal needle (20–22 G), injection bung, strong adhesive tape (zinc oxide), T-extension adaptor, bandage material	Rapid rehydration. Large volumes. Easy access if vascular collapse	Aseptic procedure. Requires general anaesthesia (sometimes local is adequate if the rabbit is collapsed) and confident placement	Crystalloids and colloids

8.16 (continued) Routes for fluid therapy in rabbits. Blood transfusion is described in the section on 'Rabbit emergencies'.

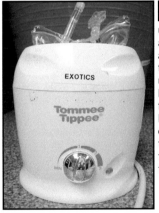

8.17 Baby-bottle warmers can be used to keep fluid boluses at body temperature to assist with fluid and heat therapy and to prevent uncomfortably cold fluids being administered. Any fluid boluses used must be checked by squirting on to the handler's skin for the ideal temperature prior to administering them to the patient.

It is widely accepted that 1% dehydration requires 10 ml/kg fluid replacement on top of any maintenance fluids administered. However, excessive fluid therapy can ensue and the following fluid administration protocol can be employed to avoid this (Girling, 2003).

Day 1: Maintenance fluids + 50% of deficit
Day 2: Maintenance fluids + 50% of deficit
Day 3: Maintenance fluids only

Nutritional therapy

Rabbits are hindgut fermenters and exhibit disturbances to their gastrointestinal tract when experiencing pain (e.g. dental disease), stress or fear (prey response) or an inappropriate or altered diet. This usually presents as anorexia, gut stasis (ileus), cessation of coprophagic behaviour, gastroenteritis, diarrhoea or bloat. As with most herbivores, rabbits must always have a high indigestible fibre content to maintain a healthy gastrointestinal tract, and their usual gut transit time is approximately 20 hours. Failure to keep up with the demands of the gastrointestinal tract will result in microflora domination and bloat, or fatal damage to the gastrointestinal mucosal lining. Currently there is a variety of nutritional care products available specifically for rabbits, and other hindgut fermenters, that are palatable and efficient at replacing nutrients, fluids and fibre content. These include Vetark Critical Care Formula, Supreme Recovery Formula and Oxbow Critical Care Formula (coarse). Some rabbit patients may prefer to lap or take these formulas voluntarily out of a bowl, which should be considered, particularly for highly strung individuals.

Syringe-feeding

See also Chapter 7. The fibrous nutritional support products (Oxbow Critical Care Formula, Lafeber's Emeraid Nutritional Care System Herbivore, and Supreme Recovery) are porridge or gruel-like with a thick consistency, and a wide-bore syringe should be used. This will ensure direct insertion into the mouth, avoiding soiling the face as seen with catheter-tip syringes. In the author's experience the following guidelines will make syringe feeding of rabbits easier:

1. The rabbit should be placed with all four legs on the table surface and its head facing away from the handler; it can be wrapped in a towel to keep it secure (the 'bunny burrito' or 'bunny roll'; Figure 8.18; see also Chapter 7).

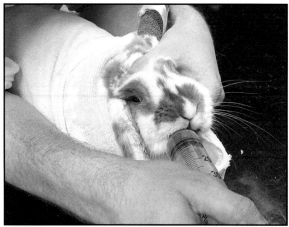

8.18   Wrapping the rabbit in a towel can be helpful for administering critical care formulas to anxious and lively patients, as it provides added support to their backs.

2. The head should be carefully but securely grasped (with a thumb on top of the head). The handler should be able to see the apex of the nose and septum of the top lip, while leaning over the rabbit providing support for its back.
3. The syringe tip can be gently passed through the rabbit's diastema, which can be found by placing the syringe tip on the incisors then gently sliding to one side.
4. A small amount (1 ml) of the formula is administered and the syringe removed immediately to facilitate mastication. It is important to ensure that the nose and side of the mouth are not touched because this is not tolerated by rabbits. More should not be administered until the first mouthful has been swallowed.
5. To encourage swallowing the rabbit can be stroked or gently repositioned, or its nose (frontal bone) scratched, as rabbits will regularly 'freeze'

and refuse to swallow. A great deal of patience and time is required in these cases.
6. Any spillages around the mouth or paws should be gently wiped clean to avoid hard crusts and dermatitis.

It is not unusual to see rabbits voluntarily eating immediately following a syringe-feeding session and therefore this should be considered as a viable method to stimulate appetite. Other techniques include simply hand-feeding rabbits with tempting foods (e.g. spring greens, dandelion leaves, banana peel, grated carrot) or bed-bathing and grooming while they are in their cages, but with consideration of the rabbit's demeanour (e.g. do not do this if they are highly stressed by human contact). Having periods of time with cage companions can relax the patient and encourage eating, but this should be done under supervision and ideally in neutral territory to avoid any aggression (unless the companion is inanimate). Probiotics, multivitamins (particularly vitamin B complex, because rabbits are coprophagic) and gut transfaunation may all be useful as supportive therapy in rabbits.

Nasogastric tube feeding
If a rabbit needs multiple feeds and is difficult to syringe feed, a nasogastric tube can be inserted. A 4–8 Fr paediatric feeding tube, or a 6–8 Fr dog catheter with extra holes cut in it, can be inserted after applying a local anaesthetic such as lidocaine spray or proxymetacaine eye drops to the nares. The technique for placing the tube is described in Chapter 7.

Prokinetics
Rabbits often present with reduced gut motility or ileus following surgery or as result of an underlying medical condition. Prokinetic drugs should be used in conjunction with high-fibre nutritional support and exercise. The drugs should not be used if gastrointestinal obstruction is suspected. Currently, four different drugs are available and they can be used in combination (Figure 8.19).

Following surgery, a single injection of metoclopramide may suffice to aid gut motility. Prolonged ileus needs to be treated more aggressively and a

Drug	Area of action within the gastrointestinal tract	Dose and route of administration	Contraindications
Ranitidine	Oesophagus, stomach, small intestine, caecum, colon	4–6 mg/kg orally/s.c. q8–24h Concentration dependent prokinetic effect in rabbits	
Metoclopramide	Oesophagus, stomach, small intestine	0.2–0.5 mg/kg orally/s.c./i.v. q4–8h	This has only been shown to be effective in adult rabbits
Domperidone	Oesophagus, stomach, small intestine	0.5 mg/kg orally q12h	
Cisapride	Oesophagus, stomach, small intestine, colon	0.5–1.0 mg/kg orally q8–24h	Combination with itraconazole, miconazole and ketoconazole is contraindicated due to fatal cardiac arrhythmias

8.19   Prokinetic drugs used in rabbit medicine.

combination of prokinetics, fluid therapy and analgesia is advised. Prokinetics are contraindicated in rabbits with an obstructive condition and corrective surgery is indicated in these cases (see *BSAVA Manual of Rabbit Surgery, Dentistry and Imaging*).

Oxygen therapy

Open-mouth breathing in rabbits indicates an emergency, because rabbits are obligate nasal breathers. The rabbit should first be stabilized by administering supplemental oxygen while attempting to establish the cause of dyspnoea.

Causes of dyspnoea in rabbits include mechanical airway obstruction by a foreign body, or upper or lower respiratory disease. Metastatic uterine adenocarcinoma of the lungs, allergies and cardiac disease can also lead to dyspnoea. By monitoring the pattern and rate of respiration and the colour of the mucous membranes and by using pulse oximetry, it is possible to assess respiratory function, oxygen saturation levels and the success of oxygen supplementation. Although the respiratory rate in undisturbed rabbits is between 30 and 60 breaths per minute, respiratory rate is almost invariably elevated owing to stress in a hospital environment. The pulse oximeter probe can be attached to the ear, tail or between the toes.

The rabbit should be placed in an oxygen-enriched environment (Figure 8.20) if handling may further compromise respiration or if one or both nasal passages are blocked. Oxygen humidifiers can also aid in improving respiration. Supplemental oxygen can also be provided directly to the patient using a face mask or intranasally via a catheter or feeding tube, provided there is no nasal or oropharyngeal obstruction.

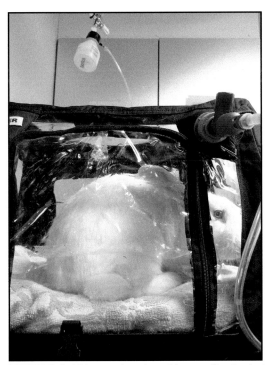

8.20 Rabbits can be placed in specifically designed 'oxygen tents' to administer accurate oxygen concentrations to patients in respiratory distress.

Nasal oxygen is administered by placing a 4–6 Fr paediatric feeding tube or a 3–4 Fr cat catheter using a similar technique to nasogastric tube placement (Figure 8.21). Local anaesthetic is first applied. The catheter or feeding tube is inserted about 1 cm into the nasal passage and secured with tape and tissue glue to the head. A flow rate no greater than 0.5–1 l/min of oxygen is recommended as at higher flow rates the pressure can detach the catheter from the connector. The advantages and disadvantages of these different approaches are given in Figure 8.22.

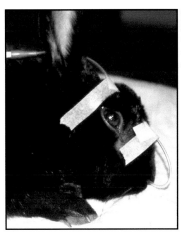

8.21 A nasal catheter is a useful method for administering supplemental oxygen.

Method	Advantages	Disadvantages
Facemask	Controlled administration of level of oxygen	Can be poorly tolerated especially in the fractious/distressed patient. Rebreathing of carbon dioxide due to size of mask and oxygen flow. If the seal is too tight around the face occlusion of the nostrils could occur (rabbits are obligate nasal breathers)
Flow-by oxygen holding pipe to nose	Less intrusive to the patient than the facemask	Difficult to monitor the exact amount of oxygen supplied to the patient
Nasal oxygen	Controlled and direct supplementation of oxygen to the patient	Not applicable with nasal obstruction, may not be tolerated by the patient
Oxygen tent (see Figure 8.20), plastic over front of cage	Allows the patient to relax within cage without being restrained	The temperature within the cage can quickly cause the patient to overheat. Opening the cage door causes the oxygen concentration to change rapidly
Incubator	Allows the patient to move around freely, temperature can be easily controlled	Cost

8.22 Methods of oxygen supplementation.

Nebulization

Nebulization is used as an adjunctive therapy for respiratory disease; it involves the aerosolization of antibiotics, decongestants or saline. An ultrasonic or compressed-air nebulizer (not an air humidifier) creating particles smaller than 5 μm should be used. The rabbit can be placed in a modified carrier or cage covered with plastic to create a confined air space and nebulized for 30 minutes 2–4 times a day as needed. Nebulization therapy bypasses the 'blood–bronchus barrier' and provides topical treatment to the airway, thus minimizing the side effects of systemic drugs and allowing topical treatment with drugs that would not reach the airway by other routes.

Nebulization with saline and systemic rehydration improves clearance of mucus. Mucolytics such as acetylcysteine and bromhexine can also be added. Others have used antimicrobial products such as F10SC (Health & Hygiene Pty) at a dilution of 1:250. Lipid-soluble antibiotics are better able to penetrate the barrier and reach adequate concentrations at the airway surface. See Chapter 11 for further details of respiratory therapy.

Exercise or coupage (percussion of the chest wall for a couple of minutes with cupped palms) following nebulization will encourage evacuation of airway mucus.

Wound management

Systemic evaluation of the patient is essential before concentrating on wound management. Underlying causes and systemic diseases should be addressed and the patient stabilized. It is important to ascertain how and when the injury occurred. Wounds can be classified based on the degree of contamination. A clean wound has been surgically created under aseptic conditions. A clean contaminated wound has minimum contamination and can be easily cleaned. A contaminated wound has gross contamination and foreign debris. An infected wound has thick viscous exudate.

Deep wounds should be filled with sterile petroleum jelly prior to clipping, to stop fur from entering the wound. The rabbit's fur should be clipped as close as possible to the skin and the wound, and the area gently and thoroughly irrigated with warm (body temperature) sterile saline (0.9% NaCl). Excessively aggressive lavage can spread contaminants and bacteria into deeper tissue. A 0.05% solution of chlorhexidine diacetate can also be used as a lavage solution. Wound debridement can be surgical, chemical (e.g. Dermisol cream, Zoetis UK Ltd), enzymatic or mechanical (e.g. adhesive bandages). Dependent on the area, size, depth and nature of the wound and the rabbit's behaviour, the wound can be treated via primary closure or left open for secondary healing. If left open, the wound should be cleaned thoroughly daily and a suitable dressing may be applied. Various products are useful in managing different types of wounds (Figure 8.23).

Bandages are made up of three layers:

- The primary or contact layer can be adhesive if the wound requires debridement, or non-adhesive. Wet-to-dry dressings should be replaced daily and are useful during initial wound

Dressing	Use and action
Hexamethyldisiloxane acrylate copolymer (spray dressing) (e.g. Opsite, Smith & Nephew)	Gently spray over surgical/closed wounds; acts as waterproof barrier. May be used for urine scald
Aloe vera cream	Helps to maintain vascular integrity and prevent ischaemia. Antibacterial properties including against *Pseudomonas*
Enzymes (e.g. trypsin, balsam of Peru, castor oil)	Enzymatic debridement, angiogenesis and improved re-epithelialization
Hydrogel dressing (e.g. Intrasite gel, Smith & Nephew)	Promotes natural debridement by loosening and absorbing slough and exudates. Used for a variety of wounds from shallow, undermined to deep wounds. Useful in pressure sores, skin ulcers, lacerations, grazes, cavity wounds and excoriated skin
Silver sulfadiazine (sterile antibacterial cream)	Useful for urine/faecal scald, pododermatitis, moist dermatitis, burns, necrotic wounds, for pressure sores and ulcers
Propylene glycol, malic acid, benzoic acid or salicylic acid (e.g. Dermisol cream and multicleanse solution, Pfizer)	Removes dead tissue and debris, encourages rapid wound healing Useful in urine/faecal scald, moist dermatitis
Low-adherent cotton absorbent dressing (e.g. Melolin, Smith & Nephew)	Useful to cover surgical wounds with the use of a sticky dressing (e.g. Hypafix). Can be used for small open wounds or surgical wounds if there is little exudate. Will need changing more frequently than other thicker dressing material
Hydrocellular polyurethane dressing (e.g. Allevyn, Smith & Nephew)	Ideal for moist wound management. Can be used with shallow granulating wounds, chronic/acute exudative wounds, pressure sores, ulcers, infected and surgical wounds. Care required in placement as fragile skin can tear easily
Exogenous collagen matrix (e.g. BioSIST, Dechra)	Acts as a matrix for wound healing

8.23 Dressings and topical treatments for rabbit wound management.

management when debridement is needed. Non-adhesive dressings retain moisture, encourage epithelialization and are applied when granulation tissue is forming. The dressing may only need to be changed every 2–4 days
- The secondary or intermediate layer is designed to absorb exudate and prevent movement of the wound and primary layer
- The outer layer is used to hold the other layers in place. Elastic adhesive tapes are often used. Body bandages are often not well tolerated; they frequently slip and tend to inhibit respiration and increase body temperature. Nich Stretch Net Sleeve (Nich Marketers Inc.), an open-weave bandage, allows greater flexibility and ventilation (Figure 8.24), whilst an absorptive pad like Allevyn (Smith and Nephew) with Intrasite gel (Smith and Nephew) can be held in place over the wound. 'Eaze-off' (Millipledge) is an adhesive bandage and tape remover that has proved useful in rabbit patients.

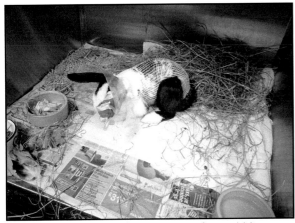

8.24 An example of a cage set up for a rabbit undergoing wound management. The rabbit is wearing body bandage and an Elizabethan collar. Note the tape used to hold the catheterized ear out of the rabbit's face, and the lack of furniture, including no litter tray to cause any obstruction to movement. Food items have been provided as large easy-to-reach pieces to facilitate feeding.

The use of Elizabethan collars may be justified to prevent rabbits from dislodging sutures or grooming wounds excessively. Rabbits can find these collars hugely frustrating, however, and caecotrophy will be interrupted, so their use should be limited. If using such collars, to account for the added awkwardness, it is advisable to do the following:

- Ensure there is plenty of hay within easy reach
- Place the water sipper bottle slightly higher
- Use large (20 cm diameter) ceramic bowls for easier access to food or water
- Tape the ear holding a catheter to the collar to prevent it dropping over the rabbit's face and subsequently getting chewed.

Urine scalding and faecal matting
Underlying causes of soiling with urine and faeces, which can lead to scalding and other complications,

are discussed in depth in Chapters 12 and 13. When managing animals with these conditions, all the matted fur should be removed by clipping as close as possible to the skin. The skin in the perineal area is extremely delicate and easily torn, and these rabbits may need to be sedated. The area should be washed gently with warm water and shampoo, and the fur and skin gently dried. Many rabbits will allow the use of a hairdryer but this depends on their temperament. Barrier cream should then be spread thickly on to the clipped areas of skin, trying to avoid the fur, as it is difficult to remove. Silver sulfadiazine cream is particularly effective, and can be followed by a layer of petroleum jelly or zinc and castor oil cream; these creams stay in contact with the skin for longer periods.

To reduce the recurrence of soiling and to prevent its occurrence in hospitalized rabbits, the animal's cage should be cleaned as soon as possible after the patient has urinated or defecated. Incontinence pads and synthetic fleece bedding can also be used to increase absorption and reduce soiling, and are particularly useful in recumbent animals. In addition to the above, to prevent flystrike, cyromazine (e.g. Rearguard) or permethrin (e.g. Xenex) can be applied topically to the rabbit.

Pododermatitis
Pododermatitis is inflammation of the plantar aspect of the fore and hind paws as a result of inadequate bedding or abrasive flooring and poor hygiene (Figure 8.25). Most pet rabbits seem to exhibit this in some form, ranging from mild parting of the hair and dry skin to painful ulcerative lesions. Every rabbit should have its feet (the plantar aspect over the caudal metatarsal and tarsal bones) checked. Treatment varies from applying a layer of a barrier cream (e.g. Sudacrem), to treatment of the area as an open wound requiring regular bandage changes and applying analgesics and antibiotics where necessary. Extra padding on the floor of the cage can be used if the rabbit will tolerate it.

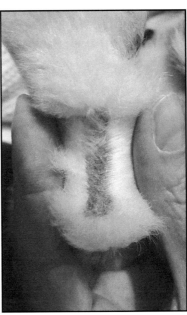

8.25
Pododermatitis. Typical presentation of linear (hocks towards toes) pododermatitis often seen on the hind feet in rabbits.

Rabbit emergencies

See Chapter 22 for approaches to common emergencies.

Blood transfusion

A blood transfusion (Figure 8.26) is generally required if the haematocrit decreases to <10–15%, but this depends on the duration of anaemia and the clinical signs. The circulating blood volume of a rabbit is 55–65 ml/kg and a loss of >20–25% results in shock. If a blood donor is unavailable, colloids or synthetic haemoglobin (e.g. Oxyglobin) at 2 ml/kg given over 10–20 minutes can be used to prevent hypovolaemic shock (Lichtenberger, 2004). A recent review in human medicine revealed that there is no evidence that colloids reduce the risk of death compared to resuscitation with crystalloids in patients with trauma, burns or following surgery. Furthermore, the use of hydroxyethyl starch might increase mortality (Perel *et al.*, 2013).

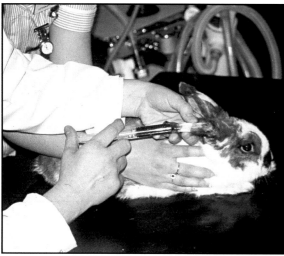

8.26 A rabbit receiving a blood transfusion via a marginal ear vein. Ideally an in-line filter should be used but direct injection can be employed in an emergency if no other suitable equipment is available.

Donors

Ideally, a donor should be a littermate or, if this is not possible, a 'house mate' to reduce the potential for disease transfer. The donor should have been vaccinated against RHD and myxomatosis in the past 12 months. The donor should weigh at least 1 kg and show no signs of clinical disease. Ideally the donor should have a normal complete blood count and biochemistry profile and be negative for antibodies to *Encephalitozoon cuniculi*.

Collection

A volume of blood equivalent to 1% of bodyweight can be safely collected from the donor. The jugular vein is the most suitable vein for collecting a large volume of blood. Citrate phosphate dextrose (CPD) adenine anticoagulant should be used, using 1 ml of anticoagulant per 9 ml of blood. Ideally, blood transfusion should take place within 4–6 hours, but blood can be kept in CPD adenine for 28–35 days. Whole blood should be stored at 4–6°C.

Transfusion

Transfusion volumes are based on quantities recommended for dogs and cats (10–20 ml/kg). A transfusion may be given via any vein. A T-connector for intravenous extension sets is connected to the intravenous cannula in the chosen vein. A disposable 18 μm blood filter (e.g. Hemo-Nate filter, Utah Medical Products Inc.) is attached to this and then to the blood-filled syringe. The syringe plunger should be depressed carefully, filling the filter with blood, slowly tilting the filter to avoid air bubbles. An initial transfusion rate of 0.25 ml/kg/h for 15 minutes is advised to detect any adverse reaction. A maximum transfusion rate of 22 ml/kg/h is recommended. Cross-matching is always recommended, because rabbits have blood groups and reactions can occur. However, initial acute transfusion reactions are rare in first-time recipients. During the transfusion, respiration and heart rate should be monitored, and the animal observed for signs of transfusion reactions. These include haemolytic and allergic reactions and hypokalaemia, resulting in clinical signs that include rigor, jaundice, renal impairment and abnormal bleeding due to intravascular coagulation.

References and further reading

Girling S (2003) *Veterinary Nursing of Exotic Species*. Blackwell Publishing, Oxford

Harcourt-Brown F (2002) *Textbook of Rabbit Medicine*. Butterworth Heinemann, Oxford

Keating SCJ, Thomas AA, Flecknell PA and Leach MC (2012) Evaluation of EMLA cream for preventing pain during tattooing of rabbits: changes in physiological, behavioural and facial expression responses. *PLoS ONE* **7**(9) [available at www.plosone.org]

Keeble E and Shaw DJ (2006) Seroprevalence of antibodies to *Encephalitozoon cuniculi* in domestic rabbits in the United Kingdom. *Veterinary Record* **158**, 539–544

Leach MC, Allweiler S, Richardson CA, Roughan JV and Narbe R (2009) Behavioural effects of ovariohysterectomy and oral administration of meloxicam in laboratory housed rabbits. *Research in Veterinary Science* **87**, 336–347

Lichtenberger M (2004) Transfusion medicine in exotic pets. *Clinical Techniques in Small Animal Practice* **19**(2), 88–95

Paul-Murphy J and Ramer JC (1998) Urgent care of the pet rabbit. *Veterinary Clinics of North America: Exotic Animal Practice* **1**(1), 127–152

Perel P, Roberts I and Ker K (2013) Colloids versus crystalloids for fluid resuscitation in critically ill patients. *Cochrane Database of Systematic Reviews*, Issue 2. Art. No. CD000567.DOI:10.1002/14651858.CD000567.pub6

Quesenberry KE and Carpenter JW (2004) *Ferrets, Rabbits and Rodents: Clinical Medicine and Surgery*. WB Saunders, St. Louis, Missouri

Thompson L and Bament W (2012) Anaesthesia and analgesia. In: *BSAVA Manual of Exotic Pet and Wildlife Nursing*, ed. M Varga *et al.*, pp.167–204. BSAVA Publications, Gloucester

Tschudin A, Clauss M, Codron A, Liesegang A and Hatt J-M (2010) Water intake in domestic rabbits (*Oryctolagus cuniculus*) from open dishes and nipple drinkers under different water and feeding regimes. *Journal of Animal Physiology and Animal Nutrition* **95**, 499–511

Tschudin A, Clauss M and Codron D (2011) Preference of rabbits for drinking from open dishes versus nipple drinkers. *Veterinary Record* **168**(7), 190–190a

RABBIT HOSPITALIZATION FORM

Animal's details	Client's details

Animal's details

Case no.:..

Name: ....

Species:..

Breed:..

Sex: Male ☐   Female ☐   Entire ☐   Neutered ☐

Age: Y ....M..................

Date:	Case clinician:
....	....
....	....
....	....

Client's details

Name: Miss/Mrs/Mr..

Address:..

....

....Postcode:........................

Primary telephone no.:..

Other contact no.: ....

Belongings description:

....

....

....

Hospitalized diet:

Food	Amount	Frequency	Own food
Pellets			
Mix			
Veg			

Admission weight:..............................kg...............

Today's weight: ....kg...............

Warnings/clinical signs..

....

....

Procedure/reason for hospitalization: Procedure date:

	Resp.rate (normal 30–60 breaths/min)	Heart rate (normal 180–300 beats/min)	Temperature (normal 38.5–40°C)	Gut sounds present		Food eaten e.g. 20 g pellets/day (Hay to be given *ad lib*)		Drinking (ml) e.g. 300 ml/day Bowl ☐ Bottle☐		Urine	Faecal pellets (Approx. no. and form)
				Left	Right	Eaten (g+?/10)	Given (g)	Drank (ml)	Given (ml)		
0900											
1200											
1400											
1600											
2100											

Medication/Procedure				0900	1200	1400	1600	1800	2100	2400
Drug/procedure		Dose mg/kg	Total dose ml							
		Freq	Route							
Drug/procedure		Dose mg/kg	Total dose ml							
		Freq	Route							
Drug/procedure		Dose mg/kg	Total dose ml							
		Freq	Route							
Drug/procedure		Dose mg/kg	Total dose ml							
		Freq	Route							
I/V catheter maintenance:		Rate: /hr	Flush							
Location: L ☐ R ☐		Freq:	Redress							

Procedures planned/instructions for the day

☐ Bloods   ☐ Urine sample

☐ Diagnostic imaging: Rads ☐   U/S ☐   C/T ☐   Endoscopy ☐

☐ GA ± surgery   ☐ Sedation   ☐ Other:...

Phone owner ☐

Charged ☐

Vet initials:

An example of a rabbit hospitalization form.

9

Clinical pathology

Petra Wesche

Age, sex, breed, husbandry conditions and circadian rhythms all affect haematological and biochemical parameters in rabbits. For example:

- Young rabbits under 12 weeks of age generally have lower red blood cell (RBC) and white blood cell (WBC) counts than adult rabbits
- The total WBC and lymphocyte counts are lowest in the late afternoon and evening, whereas heterophil and eosinophil counts tend to rise
- Urea and cholesterol levels tend to increase at the end of the day
- Caged rabbits have slightly lower packed cell volume (PCV), RBC and haemoglobin (Hb) values and lymphocyte counts than rabbits that are kept outside with plenty of exercise and natural diets.

Stress can also influence several parameters (see later). Haemolysis, often caused by excessive pressure applied at venepuncture and prolonged storage, affects several blood parameters. Anaesthesia with various anaesthetic agents may alter a variety of biochemical parameters.

Reference ranges are often based on the New Zealand White rabbit, which is the most common breed used in laboratory research, and thus interpretation of values and reference ranges must take this into consideration.

The popularity of rabbits as pet animals has led to the creation of 'wellness profiles' that can be used by veterinary surgeons and laboratories to establish individual rabbit and breed reference ranges. It is imperative always to collect a thorough clinical history and carry out a systematic physical examination. Laboratory values can only serve as a guide and have to be brought into context with the presentation and history of the patient.

Faecal and skin sampling and tests are discussed in Chapters 12 and 17.

Haematology

Blood collection

Blood may be obtained from various sites in the rabbit, including the jugular vein, cephalic vein, recurrent tarsal or lateral saphenous vein, central auricular artery and the medial saphenous artery (see Chapter 7). A maximum of 55–78 ml of blood per kilogram of bodyweight can be safely collected from well hydrated non-anaemic rabbits. Only a small volume, about 1 ml or less, is required in most cases to run a full blood profile. The laboratory should be contacted for individual instructions.

Figure 9.1 gives details of haematological parameters in the rabbit.

Parameter	Range
Erythrocytes (RBC)	5.1–7.6 x 10^{12}/l
Haematocrit/packed cell volume (PVC)	0.3–0.4 l/l
Haemoglobin (Hb)	100–150 g/l
Mean corpuscular volume (MCV)	60–69 fl
Mean corpuscular haemoglobin (MCH)	19–22 pg/cell
Mean corpuscular haemoglobin concentration	300–350 g/l
Leucocytes	5.2–12.5 x 10^9/l
Lymphocytes	30–85%
Heterophils	20–75%
Eosinophils	0–4%
Basophils	0–7%
Monocytes	0–4%
Platelets	250–650 x 10^9/l

9.1 Haematological parameters.

As rabbit blood tends to clot very quickly, the collected blood should be transferred to tubes with appropriate anticoagulant (e.g. EDTA, heparin) as soon as possible. The use of paediatric collection tubes is recommended. It is advisable to fill tubes with anticoagulant first, but care must be taken that the needle does not come into contact with the coated surface. Contamination may lead to erroneous values, especially calcium in the case of EDTA, at biochemistry. Tubes should be filled to the mark in order to avoid dilution artefacts. Gently invert the tube several times to ensure adequate mixing.

It is very important also to produce air-dried blood smears at the time of venepuncture in order to preserve the cell morphology and to avoid erroneous interpretation of ageing, transport or anticoagulant artefacts. In the event of leakage or breakage of the collection tube, or when only a very small sample can be obtained, the experienced investigator is then still able to draw a variety of conclusions from the blood smear, such as estimated general cellularity, cell counts and fractions of individual cell populations, platelet numbers, abnormal cell morphology and potential blood parasites.

RBC parameters

With an average lifespan of 57 days, which is much lower than that of the RBCs of dogs and cats, approximately 0.5% of rabbit RBCs are eliminated from the circulation on a daily basis. Consequently there is a relatively high turnover of cells showing polychromasia and anisocytosis (1–2% is considered normal; Figure 9.2). These may also be accompanied by occasional nucleated RBCs and Howell–Jolly bodies. A reticulocyte count of 2–4% in adults with a slight increase in juveniles is commonly seen with new methylene blue (NMB) staining. Regenerative anaemia will produce increased numbers of reticulocytes and polychromasia.

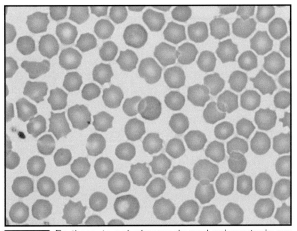

| 9.2 | Erythrocyte polychromasia and anisocytosis are a normal finding on rabbit blood smears. |

The normal haematocrit (PCV) ranges between 0.30 and 0.40 l/l, with slightly higher values in males than in females and in older compared to juvenile rabbits. Lower values may be associated with anaemia, whereas high values (>45%) are usually associated with dehydration and, occasionally, gastrointestinal stasis.

Haemoglobin concentration (Hb) should be approximately three times the number of the haematocrit and tends to range between 100 and 150 g/l. Falsely increased values may be associated with haemolysis, increased Heinz bodies or lipaemia. The mean corpuscular haemoglobin (MCH) and mean corpuscular haemoglobin concentration (MCHC) are both calculated from Hb. Normal values are 19–22 pg/cell for MCH and 300–350 g/l for MCHC.

Normal mean corpuscular volume (MCV) ranges between 60 and 69 fl. Elevations are generally associated with regenerative processes. Erythrocytes cannot store more than four haemoglobin molecules, so hyperchromasia is always an artefact due to haemolysis, increased Heinz bodies or lipaemia.

Anaemia

Regenerative anaemia is associated with increased (>2%) polychromasia, anisocytosis, nucleated RBCs and Howell–Jolly bodies. In many cases this reflects recent blood loss due to ecto- or, less often, endoparasites, trauma and haematuria, haemorrhaging uterine adenocarcinomas or endometrial aneurysms. Ingestion of potato plant leaves and stems may cause intravascular haemolysis. Eating onions, garlic and chives may lead to oxidative damage manifested by increased Heinz body formation. Owing to the introduction of lead-free paints, lead poisoning, characterized by basophilic stippling and a macrocytic hypochromic anaemia, has become a rare finding.

Non-regenerative anaemia is frequently observed in pet rabbits and is commonly associated with chronic conditions such as otitis media and dental problems, abscesses, pneumonia, mastitis, endometritis, pyometra, renal disease, pododermatitis and osteomyelitis.

Blood typing

To date, rabbit blood grouping/typing has seen extensive research with confusing results. Several conflicting nomenclatures exist and no commercial test is currently available for blood typing. In cases of severe anaemia with a PCV <10% or acute blood loss of 20–25%, a blood transfusion is advisable. Cross-matching is unnecessary for first-time recipients. Healthy blood donors can part with up to 10 ml/kg.

WBC parameters

The normal range varies between 5.2 and 12.5 × 10^9/l for adults, with mild variations with age, gender, breed and season. There is either minimal or no leukaemoid response to infection in rabbits. As mentioned above, circadian rhythms can also influence WBC values. The total WBC counts and lymphocyte counts are lowest in the late afternoon and evening, whereas heterophil and eosinophil counts tend to rise. This has to be taken into consideration when the results are interpreted.

Lymphocytes

Lymphocytes are the most frequently encountered leucocyte in rabbits and measure approximately 7–10 μm in diameter. In health they make up 30–85% of WBC. The nuclear-to-cytoplasm ratio is high, and there is a round dark-staining nucleus. The cytoplasm shows medium to occasionally intense basophilic staining properties (Figure 9.3).

Diseased rabbits often show a reduced lymphocyte count. A relative lymphopenia may also be encountered with stress. Rabbits with lymphosarcoma tend to have reduced RBCs, down to 2 × 10^{12}/l, a haematocrit of 0.10–0.25 l/l and Hb values of 35–73 g/l, whereas the total lymphocyte count often remains normal.

Heterophils

Heterophils are the equivalent of neutrophils and are the second most frequently encountered leucocyte

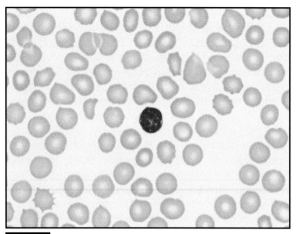

9.3 A small lymphocyte.

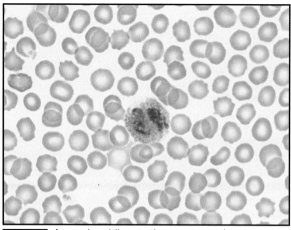

9.5 An eosinophil; note the more prominent rounded granules.

(20–75%). The nucleus is often multilobed and the cells contain mainly small, but occasionally larger, more sparsely distributed eosinophilic granules within the cytoplasm (Figure 9.4). The heterophils measure approximately 7–10 μm in diameter; they are generally smaller than eosinophils.

Rabbits may be affected by the Pelger–Huët anomaly, a rare autosomal dominant genetic condition in which the granulocytes show unsegmented or hyposegmented nuclei with a coarse, mature chromatin pattern. Dumbbell-shaped or 'pince-nez' nuclei are seen in clinically normal heterozygous rabbits. The homozygous form is generally lethal *in utero*, and few homozygous individuals are born alive. These tend to have an increased neonatal mortality rate and they often develop severe skeletal deformities including dyschondroplasia. Blood smears from homozygous rabbits show round to oval nuclei with only minimal nuclear segmentation and an extremely coarse chromatin pattern.

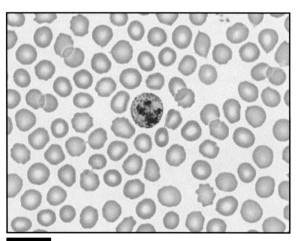

9.4 A heterophil; note the rod-shaped granules.

Eosinophils
Eosinophils comprise 0–4% of the WBC count. They measure approximately 10–15 μm in diameter. The nucleus is horseshoe-shaped or bilobed. Their cytoplasmic granules are large and stain more intensely eosinophilic with Romanowski-type stains than do those of heterophils (Figure 9.5).

Eosinophilia is encountered with chronic parasitism, especially during the tissue phase. Increases are also seen with traumatic injuries, general skin disease, and in lung, gastrointestinal or uterine disorders.

Monocytes
Monocytes comprise 0–4% of the WBC count and, at 15–18 μm in diameter, are the largest leucocytes. The nucleus is often bean-shaped but can be ovoid to lobulated (Figure 9.6). There is abundant grey to pale basophilic cytoplasm with occasional small vacuoles. Dark red granules may be observed with non-specific toxicity. Inflammatory processes or chronic infection may be associated with monocytosis.

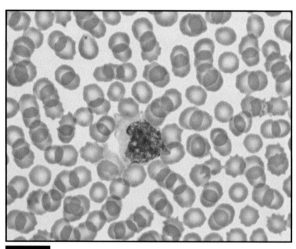

9.6 A monocyte.

Basophils
Basophils generally comprise 0–7% of the WBC count, but up to 30% may be observed in clinically healthy rabbits. At 7–11 μm in diameter they are similar in size to heterophils. The nucleus is lobulated and often obscured by metachromic purple to black granules (Figure 9.7).

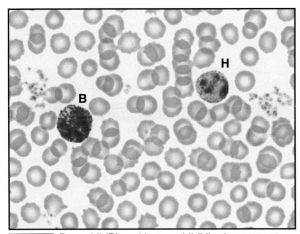

9.7 Basophil (B) and heterophil (H); also present are platelet clumps.

Platelets

Platelets are round to oval in shape and measure approximately 1–3 μm in diameter. Numbers range between 250 and 650 × 10⁹/l. The cytoplasm is usually colourless to slightly basophilic with occasional small clusters of azurophilic granules. Rabbit blood coagulates fairly quickly. Platelet clots may be due to inadequate mixing of samples leading to falsely low platelet counts read by the analyser. Large clot numbers may also lead to falsely increased leucocyte counts. It is therefore important to check the sample prior to running it through the analyser and to screen a blood smear for platelet aggregates. True thrombocythaemia may be observed with recent haemorrhage, disseminated intravascular coagulation (DIC) and acute infection.

Coagulation

Selected coagulation values are shown in Figure 9.8. These are only guidelines. Individual instruments may use different methodologies or reagents which require establishment of individual coagulation times. Newer techniques such as thromboelastometry are useful but are generally only available in diagnostic laboratories or research facilities. Rabbit haemorrhagic disease (RHD) causes DIC with increased prothrombin (PT) and activated partial thrombin (APTT) times. DIC has also been described in rabbits exposed to *Escherichia coli* endotoxins.

Parameter	Reference ranges
Activated clotting time (ACT)	4.0 ± 0.4 minutes
Activated partial thromboplastin time (APTT)	15.7–42.7 seconds
Fibrinogen	3–4 g/l
Prothrombin time (PT)	7.5 ± 0.3 seconds
Thrombin time (TT)	9.9 ± 2.1 seconds
Bleeding time	1.4 ± 0.3 to 5.4 ± 1.2 minutes

9.8 Clotting parameters.

Blood biochemistry

Blood sampling is described earlier in the chapter. Figure 9.9 gives a summary of biochemical parameters in rabbits.

Prolonged stressful conditions as well as physical restraint and haemolysis of the sample influence several biochemical parameters (Figure 9.10). Several

Parameter	Normal range
Alanine aminotransferase (ALT)	27.4–72.2 IU/l
Aspartate aminotransferase (AST)	10.0–78.0 IU/l
Creatine kinase (CK)	58.6–175.0 IU/l
Lactate dehydrogenase (LDH)	27.8–101.5 IU/l
Gamma-glutamyl transferase (GGT)	0–5 IU/l
Amylase	212–424 IU/l
Bilirubin	2.6–17.1 μmol/l
Blood urea nitrogen (BUN)	10.1–17.1 mmol/l
Total protein	49–71 g/l
Albumin	27–50 g/l
Globulin	15–33 g/l
Albumin:globulin ratio	0.7–1.89
Creatinine	74–171 μmol/l
Glucose	5.5–8.2 mmol/l
Triglycerides	1.4–1.76 mmol/l
Cholesterol	0.1–2.0 mmol/l
Calcium	2.2–3.9 mmol/l
Inorganic phosphate	1.0–2.2 mmol/l
Sodium	130–155 mmol/l
Chloride	92–120 mmol/l
Bicarbonate	16–32 mmol/l
Potassium	3.3–5.7 mmol/l

9.9 Biochemical parameters.

Increased

- Total protein (TP)
- Lactate dehydrogenase (LDH)
- Aspartate transaminase (AST)
- Creatine kinase (CK)
- Potassium (K⁺)
- Phosphate (PO₄⁻)

Decreased

- Red blood cells (RBCs)
- Haematocrit (PCV)
- Amylase

9.10 Artefacts caused by haemolysis.

parameters are also influenced by the age and sex of the rabbit and by the time of sampling, as rabbits follow a circadian rhythm.

Protein

Normal values for total protein (TP) range between 49 and 71 g/l, with an albumin-to-globulin (A:G) ratio of 0.7–1.89. Physiological variations due to age, reproductive status, pregnancy, breed and strain have been reported. Excessive compression during venepuncture may lead to falsely increased TP readings.

True hyperproteinaemia is associated with dehydration, chronic and immune-mediated disease, hypovolaemia and prolonged hyperthermia.

Hypoproteinaemia is observed with protein loss due to haemorrhage or chronic malabsorption based on poor diet or dental disease. Protein-losing nephropathies and enteropathies are uncommonly observed.

Measurement of albumin and globulin fractions aids in determining the cause further. Serum protein electrophoresis has been used as a tool to screen for and identify specific problems but requires an experienced laboratory. In general, alpha-globulins tend to increase with pyrexia and acute disease, such as bacterial infection or a developing abscess. Beta-globulins (also termed acute-phase proteins) include fibrinogen, which is only infrequently raised in inflammatory conditions in rabbits. Gamma-globulins consist predominantly of antibodies and are elevated in subacute to chronic inflammation.

Albumin

Reference values suggest a range between 27 and 50 g/l. Hyperalbuminaemia, especially when accompanied by an increased PCV, is consistent with dehydration. A low PCV with raised albumin and globulins indicates haemolysis.

Hypoalbuminaemia can be a physiological finding in pregnant does. Reduced caecotrophy also leads to primarily low albumin levels. Pathological conditions with hypoalbuminaemia but not hypoglobulinaemia include advanced liver disease, which may be related to hepatic coccidiosis or migrating tapeworm larvae.

Globulin

The normal range is 15–33 g/l. Hyperglobulinaemia indicates an inflammatory condition, ranging from acute to chronic. Further investigation of individual fractions requires more in-depth tests such as electrophoresis. A serum sample is generally preferred. Hypoglobulinaemia indicates losses, predominantly due to haemorrhage, burns or wound exudation.

Fibrinogen

Fibrinogen is lower in young rabbits (<2 g/l) than in adults (3–4 g/l) and is only infrequently increased with inflammation. Measurement requires a sample of plasma.

Enzymes

Rabbits do not have liver-specific enzymes. Thus hepatocellular damage can only be suspected from a combination of increased enzyme values and clinical signs. In advanced stages hypoalbuminaemia may be observed.

Alanine aminotransferase

Unlike in other herbivores, ALT is not liver-specific in the rabbit. It also has a very short half-life of about 5 hours. Normal values are 27.4–72.2 IU/l. Increases in ALT values are somewhat in proportion to the degree of liver necrosis present. Moreover, ALT is not affected by stress and handling, which makes the enzyme suitable as a diagnostic tool. Slight elevations in clinically healthy rabbits may be associated with resin and other solvent fumes from wood shavings and anaesthetic agents. Mycotoxins can also produce mild elevations. Hepatic coccidiosis, liver lobe torsion and advanced hepatic neoplasia produce a more pronounced increase and are usually accompanied by raised alkaline phosphatase (ALP), bilirubin and gamma-glutamyl transferase (GGT) values.

Aspartate transaminase

AST has a very short half-life of only 5 hours in the rabbit and is distributed in a variety of tissues. The normal range is reported as 10.0–78.0 IU/l. Elevated values can be seen with liver damage due to necrosis as well as muscle damage, hyperthermia, and stress at the time of handling and collection of the sample. Haemolysis also increases values.

Lactate dehydrogenase

The normal concentration of LDH is 27.8–101.5 IU/l. LDH is produced in muscle and liver and is present in most cells within the body including erythrocytes, thus rendering it a non-specific enzyme in this species. Haemolysis increases values.

Creatine kinase

CK originates primarily from the skeletal muscles and, in small amounts, from the heart and mitochondria. Normal concentration range is 58.6–175.0 IU/l. Increased values are a good indicator of muscle damage and, as CK has a short half-life, the duration of the insult can be estimated. Increased values may also be seen as a result of struggling in response to venepuncture or handling, and with haemolysis.

Gamma-glutamyl transferase

GGT concentrations between 0 and 5 IU/l are considered to be within the normal range. Activity in the circulation is low, and increased values are associated with bile stasis and possibly hepatic coccidiosis but to a lesser extent than in other animals.

Alkaline phosphatase

ALP is widely distributed within the body, with several isoenzymes present. ALP does not increase as a consequence of hepatocellular damage. Physiological elevations are seen in growing animals, and ALP also increases with bone remodelling, enteric disease and bile stasis associated with hepatic coccidiosis, liver abscesses, hepatic lipidosis or neoplasia. Extrahepatic obstruction of bile ducts due to abscesses or neoplasia may also increase ALP values. Pregnancy is frequently associated with physiologically low levels and diarrhoea may also decrease values. ALP does not rise as a consequence of normal handling, and increases most likely reflect true tissue damage.

Glutamate dehydrogenase
GDH is a mitochondrial enzyme that is present predominantly in liver, heart and kidney and to a lesser degree in skeletal muscle, brain and leucocytes. Within the liver GDH is located primarily within the centrilobular cells, thus an increase in GDH suggests centrilobular hepatic injury.

Amylase
Amylase in the rabbit is highly organ-specific with only minute concentrations in salivary gland tissue, liver and intestine. Normal values are 212–424 IU/l. Therefore an increase is almost always consistent with pancreatic injury due to duct obstruction, pan-creatitis, peritonitis or abdominal trauma. Occasionally, raised values are also observed with renal disorders when clearance of amylase is impaired or with endogenous or exogenous corticosteroids. Falsely decreased values can be observed with sample haemolysis.

Lipase
Increased lipase concentrations are non-specific and thus of little diagnostic value if used alone. A rise may indicate pancreatic damage if consistent with clinical signs and concurrently elevated amylase. Decreased values can be observed with sample haemolysis.

Triglycerides and cholesterol
Normal triglyceride concentration is 1.4–1.76 mmol/l. Levels peak after a meal and accurate measurement requires a fasted sample, which is not feasible in rabbits owing to caecotrophy. Hypertriglyceridaemia in conjunction with hypercholesterolaemia can be observed with lipid-rich diets, obesity and hepatic impairment.

Normal cholesterol concentration is 0.1–2.0 mmol/l. Hypercholesterolaemia in anorexic rabbits is seen as a poor prognostic value and suggests end-stage hepatic lipidosis. Increased values can also be seen with hepatic disease, pancreatitis, diabetes mellitus, nephritic syndrome, chronic renal failure, elevated cortisol and low thyroid hormone levels. A familial hypercholesterolaemia has been recognized in some breeds, e.g. the Watanabe rabbit. Physiologically low values of up to 30% below the reference range can be seen during pregnancy. Hypocholesterolaemia can also be linked to chronic malnutrition and liver failure.

Bile acids
Rabbit bile production is considerable. Bile acids are derived from cholesterol and are produced in a circadian rhythm in rabbits. Caecotrophy significantly hampers collection of a fasted sample. Normal levels are <40 μmol/l. Only persistently raised levels are of value in clinical practice. Significantly increased values of >100 μmol/l have been associated with hepatic coccidiosis.

Bilirubin and biliverdin
Normal values for bilirubin are reported as 2.6–17.1 μmol/l; however, only 30% of biliverdin is converted into bilirubin in rabbits, owing to their low biliverdin reductase activity. Almost all bilirubin measured in the plasma is in the conjugated form.

Hyperbilirubinaemia is predominantly due to cholestasis. In juveniles this is most often correlated with hepatic coccidiosis whereas neoplasia is the primary cause in adult rabbits. Aflatoxicosis due to ingestion of mouldy food causes hyperbilirubinaemia and is usually accompanied by elevated ALT values. RHD causes severe hepatic necrosis with concurrent elevation of all hepatocellular enzymes and subsequent jaundice in rabbits that survive the initial insult. Haemolysis subsequent to, for example, immune-mediated haemolytic anaemia also releases bilirubin.

Blood urea nitrogen
Urea is the end-product of the protein catabolism performed by the liver and is excreted via the kidneys. Normal concentration is 10.1–17.1 mmol/l. In health about 25–40% of BUN is reabsorbed via the renal tubules. Levels follow a circadian rhythm, with a peak observed during late afternoon or early evening. Values relate to diet, nutritional condition, liver function, hydration, intestinal absorption and urease activity within the caecum. Slight elevations and fluctuations are common in clinically healthy rabbits and difficult to interpret. Breed and sex variations have also been reported.

Increased values can be differentiated into pre-renal, renal and post-renal causes:

- Pre-renal elevations are predominantly associated with dehydration or water deprivation. Creatinine should also be elevated. Both values should return to normal shortly after fluid administration. Other causes include protein-rich diets, gastrointestinal haemorrhage, strenuous exercise, and decreased renal perfusion subsequent to stress-induced shock and cardiac disease
- Renal causes are observed when at least 50–70% of nephrons are impaired. Increased BUN and creatinine values suggest renal azotaemia, usually accompanied by hypokalaemia, hypercalcaemia and hyperphosphataemia, non-regenerative anaemia and isosthenuria. The most common cause of chronic renal insufficiency is attributed to *Encephalitozoon cuniculi* infection, but chronic interstitial nephritis, glomerulonephritis, pyelonephritis, nephrolithiasis, renal cysts and lymphosarcoma are important differentials
- Urine flow obstruction caused by sludgy urine, uroliths or neoplasia, as well as perforation of the urinary tract, results in post-renal azotaemia.

Decreased BUN values suggest hepatic insufficiency, a diet insufficient in proteins, loss of muscle mass due to inadequate food intake or dental disease, or administration of anabolic steroids.

Creatinine

Creatinine is produced by the muscle as an endogenous protein catabolite. The normal range is 74–171 μmol/l. Values are not reliable in samples older than 24 hours. Creatinine is not reabsorbed in the renal tubules and therefore the excretion rate is equivalent to glomerular filtration capacity, making it a more reliable indicator of renal function than urea. In health, the glomerular filtrate has the same concentration as plasma. Increased blood levels indicate decreased renal blood perfusion or dehydration and water deprivation. In the latter case rehydration should return values to normal within a short period of time. Raised values can also be seen with severe muscle damage and exposure to mycotoxins. With uroabdomen, creatinine levels in the abdominal fluid should be higher than blood plasma levels.

Glucose

Glucose metabolism in herbivores differs from that in carnivores owing to their continuous feeding behaviour and the caecal production of volatile fatty acids, which are the primary source of energy. Caecotrophy hampers collection of a fasted sample.

Only in neonates <2 weeks old do glucose values decrease after starvation. Normal values are 5.5–8.2 mmol/l.

Hyperglycaemia is frequently encountered in stressful conditions, e.g. due to transport, handling and hyperthermia. Acute intestinal obstruction causes marked elevation in glucose (mean 24.7 mmol/l), whereas gut stasis often produces only mildly elevated values (mean 8.5 mmol/l) but warrants a guarded prognosis because it may imply hepatic lipidosis. Elevations can also be observed with early mucoid enteritis and glucocorticoid therapy.

Hypoglycaemia occurs after prolonged starvation or anorexia of more than 48–96 hours and with terminal mucoid enteritis, sepsis, liver failure and other chronic diseases.

True diabetes is rare in rabbits and is barely described in the literature, with the exception of some strains of New Zealand White rabbits and some obese individuals. Both type 1 and 2 diabetes have been observed. Type 2 is more common in obese rabbits. When present, diabetes manifests itself with the typical clinical signs observed in other species and very high glucose levels. Serum fructosamine >335 mmol/l may help to confirm the diagnosis.

Electrolytes

Breed-specific differences have been reported for many electrolytes and results should be interpreted bearing this in mind.

Calcium

Normal values are 2.2–3.9 mmol/l. Calcium metabolism in rabbits differs from that in other animals because they absorb the electrolyte in proportion to the concentration of the ion in the intestine and excrete the excess via the kidneys. Parathyroid hormone (PTH) regulates blood-to-bone calcium ratios. It takes a higher concentration of blood calcium in rabbits to turn off the production of PTH than in dogs and cats. Therefore blood concentrations in adult rabbits are relatively high. Blood levels are lower than normal adult rabbit values during pregnancy and in growing individuals, where they rarely rise, independent of dietary calcium intake. As long as dietary intake is sufficiently high, vitamin D plays an insignificant role in calcium absorption. Calcium is excreted via the kidneys at a rate of between 45 and 60% in rabbits, which causes turbid to mildly sludgy urine and physiological crystalluria but may also predispose the rabbit to urolith formation. The excretion rate is far higher than in most other mammals, which limits their renal calcium excretion rate to no more than 2%. Free ionized calcium does not vary with fluctuating albumin levels and reflects more accurately the physically relevant and available blood level, but owing to sample requirements and expense total calcium, which is the sum of bound and ionized calcium, is generally measured.

Hypercalcaemia has been observed with chronic renal failure and paraneoplastic syndrome. Hypocalcaemia is rare but has been reported in connection with hypoalbuminaemia due to insufficient dietary uptake or severe liver failure, diarrhoea, hyperparathyroidism, and occasionally with late stage pregnancy and lactation.

Phosphate

The predominant role of phosphate lies in the formation of bone and teeth but it can be found within all cells of the body. The normal range is 1.0–2.2 mmol/l. It is regulated by the kidneys and thus can be an indirect indicator of kidney function. Calcium-to-phosphorus (Ca:P) ratios indicate mineral balance and these elements should be evaluated together. Hyperphosphataemia can be observed with chronic renal failure and loss of >80% of functional tubules but also with soft tissue trauma. Hypophosphataemia may be associated with insufficient dietary uptake or malabsorption and diarrhoea.

Sodium

Normal concentration is 130–155 mmol/l. Hypernatraemia is predominantly seen with dehydration or fluid loss due to diarrhoea, peritonitis, exudating wounds and burns, as well as myiasis (fly strike). Artefactual increases can be due to lipaemic samples or hyperproteinaemia. Hyponatraemia has been associated with polyuria due to acute or more frequently chronic renal failure.

Potassium

Potassium is the main regulator that maintains membrane potential and is itself regulated by several hormones. Hypoadrenocorticism has not been reported in rabbits. Low potassium concentration causes 'floppy rabbit syndrome'; such rabbits present with sensory depression and muscle weakness.

Hyperkalaemia can be observed with acute renal failure, urinary flow obstruction, severe tissue trauma, metabolic acidosis and as an artefact with haemolysis.

Hypokalaemia is seen with dietary deficiency, increased salivation, diarrhoea, alkalosis, renal failure and release of catecholamines due to stress. Furthermore, administration of diuretics and the use of pentobarbital also cause decreased levels of potassium. Artefacts that cause hypokalaemia include hyperproteinaemia and lipaemia.

Hormones

It is common practice to neuter pet rabbits in order to avoid pregnancy and deal with aggression and other behavioural issues. There are no significant hormone differences between male and female neutered rabbits. Hormonal abnormalities have been observed with incomplete gonadectomy, adrenal disease and other conditions and thus may help to identify the origin of the behaviour problem (for reference values of selected hormones see Chapter 19).

Cortisol

Intact rabbits generally have higher values than their neutered counterparts. Levels may also be elevated by any stressful situation such as transport, handling and poor husbandry.

Urinalysis

Urinary output varies widely depending on the diet and ranges between 20 and 350 ml/kg/day. Figure 9.11 lists urine parameters for the rabbit.

Description	Reference range
Glucose	Negative to trace (depending on stress levels of rabbit)
Bilirubin	Negative
Erythrocytes (RBCs)	Negative
pH	7.5–9 (average 8.2)
Protein	Negative to trace
Ketones	Negative
Leucocytes	Negative
Specific gravity (g/l)	1.003–1.036
Urinary protein:creatinine ratio (UPC)	0.11–0.40

9.11 Urinalysis values.

Collection

Urine can be obtained in a variety of ways (see also Chapter 7):

- Rabbits trained to use a litter tray will generally urinate into a clean, empty tray placed in the usual location; veterinary medical litter can be added for encouragement
- In rabbits used to handling, a free-catch sample may be attempted. The first, most contaminated, part of the urine should be freely voided before collecting the midstream sample. Urine should be collected in a clean, unused, preferably sterile container (e.g. a universal container). The sample should be tested as soon as possible. Litter tray and free-catch samples should not be used for culture owing to contamination from the urogenital tract and possibly the collection surface
- Many rabbits will also spontaneously urinate after the urinary bladder has been palpated. Manual expression of the urinary bladder is another way to collect urine and, if the first voided part is discarded, may be used for culture. Expression is contraindicated in rabbits with stranguria or haematuria and suspected urethral obstruction because the bladder may be extremely distended and thus prone to rupture. If perforation of the urinary tract is suspected, creatinine levels can be determined in the abdominal fluid and plasma. With uroabdomen, creatinine levels in the abdominal fluid should be higher than blood plasma levels. With chronic cystitis the bladder wall is generally hyperplastic
- The most appropriate way to collect a sterile urine sample is by urethral catheterization, or ideally cystocentesis. However, an overexpanded urinary bladder should be catheterized rather than sampled by cystocentesis.

Physical characteristics

Rabbit urine is naturally turbid with colour variations from white to yellow, but orange to red–brown urine may result from the presence of porphyrin pigments from consumed plant material. Clear urine may be observed from pregnant, lactating or very young rabbits.

Specific gravity is best measured with a refractometer. Dipsticks are not calibrated for the rabbit and have a large error margin.

Chemical characteristics

- Glucose readings should be negative. Stress, anorexia, hepatic lipidosis and ketosis may increase values.
- Bilirubin should be negative. Positive values may be due to haemolysis.
- A low pH has been associated with a high-protein diet or with starvation anorexia, but also pregnancy toxaemia and fever. Urine left at room temperature will become more alkaline as a result of the decomposition of urea.
- Traces of protein in urine are a normal finding in young rabbits. If the protein reading is positive in adults, the specific gravity (SG) should be taken into consideration. Abnormal findings may be associated with renal disease and renal damage but also increased muscular activity, seizures and stress. Persistent proteinuria in a urine

sample with an inactive sediment is considered pathognomonic for tubular or glomerular disease. Chronic renal failure is a common problem in rabbits.

- The urine protein:creatinine ratio (UPC) does not vary between rabbits infected with *Encephalitozoon cuniculi* and uninfected individuals. However, routine calculation of UPC in a rabbit suspected of having renal disease is considered to be advantageous in monitoring progression of the disease. The reference range for UPC in clinically healthy rabbits has been calculated as 0.11–0.40.
- Ketone readings should be negative. They may be increased with hepatic lipidosis, pregnancy toxaemia, severe dental problems or caecal impaction.

Sediment

Sediment preparations from a urine sample collected under sterile conditions should be free of epithelial cells, bacteria and casts.

Rare erythrocytes may be observed. However, more than three RBC per high power field (HPF) is considered abnormal and may suggest inflammation, infectious processes, calculi with subsequent irritation of the mucosa or neoplasia of the urinary or reproductive tract. Haematuria and haemorrhagic vaginal discharge are the most frequently encountered clinical signs of cystic endometrial hyperplasia. Haematuria and serosangineous vaginal discharge are also common clinical signs associated with uterine adenocarcinoma in rabbits. Manual expression of the bladder may cause pseudohaematuria.

Crystals, especially calcium carbonate monohydrate, anhydrous calcium carbonate and occasionally ammonium magnesium phosphate (triple phosphate, struvite) as well as rare calcium oxalate crystals, may be observed in normal rabbit urine. Casts suggest renal disease but their number does not correlate with severity, and their absence does not exclude renal pathology because casts may disintegrate with prolonged storage or vigorous mixing. The type of cast suggests the location of damage.

Cerebrospinal fluid

Rabbits should be anaesthetized for the collection of CSF. It should be collected into a sterile glass or plastic container, preferably from the atlanto-occipital joint (or through a lumbar approach) using a 22 G, 1.0–1.5 inch (2.5–4 cm) spinal needle (see Chapter 7). Immediate analysis of glucose and total and differential cell counts will provide the best results.

If examination is delayed the CSF can be diluted with rabbit serum at a ratio of 1:10 (serum:CSF) to preserve cellular morphology. The tube must be clearly marked because this diluted sample cannot be used for protein evaluation, which requires a separate undiluted aliquot.

Blood contamination can be assumed when samples are bright red. Intracranial haemorrhage due to either disease or trauma is generally associated with brown–red haemorrhage, whereas turbidity suggests pleocytosis and possibly bacterial meningitis (e.g. due to listeriosis). Increased protein concentration with lymphomonocytic pleocytosis has been reported in connection with *E. cuniculi* infection but these changes can also be seen with other viral, protozoan or immune-mediated encephalitides and with central nervous system (CNS) lymphoma.

Figure 9.12 shows CSF parameters for the rabbit.

Parameter	Reference range
White blood cells (WBCs)	0–7 cells/mm^3
Lymphocytes	40–79%
Monocytes	21–60%
Total protein (TP)	59 mg/dl
Red blood cells (RBCs)	0

9.12 Normal cerebrospinal fluid (CSF) parameters.

Bone marrow

Bone marrow examination is warranted to evaluate anaemia, leucopenia or thrombocytopenia and to examine further the presence of increased immature or abnormal cells. Samples can also be collected for bacterial culture if infection is suspected. Samples for cytology and core biopsy can be obtained from the proximal femur, proximal tibia, proximal humerus or pelvis (see Chapter 7). Samples for cytology should be collected prior to bone marrow biopsy, and an air-dried smear should be made without delay after aspiration to preserve cellular morphology. Biopsy specimens should be placed in 10% formalin immediately after collection. Samples collected in formalin should always be sent in separate packages from all other samples because fumes may leak and cause fixation artefacts. The approximate myeloid:erythroid (M:E) ratio for adult rabbits is 1:1, with about 20% of cells within the proliferation pool and 80% in the storage pool.

Figure 9.13 lists bone marrow parameters for the rabbit.

Parameter	Reference range
Myeloid:erythroid (M:E) ratio	Approximately 1:1
Proerythroblasts, myeloblasts, undifferentiated blasts and lymphocytes	6.5 ± 2.4%
Promyelocytes and myelocytes	14.5 ± 4.4%
Storage pool (late precursors and mature cells)	81.5 ± 4.8%

9.13 Bone marrow values for adult rabbits.

Serology

Serological tests are available for antibodies against a number of pathogens. Some of these are less significant when dealing with individual pet rabbits housed exclusively indoors but may be useful for breeders and sanctuaries. Adequate quarantine periods accompanied by relevant screening protocols should be observed before socializing new additions with established groups or individuals.

Encephalitozoon cuniculi

E. cuniculi is a widespread obligate intracellular microsporidian parasite with a high prevalence in clinically healthy rabbits in the UK (52%). Several species of *Encephalitozoon* including *E. cuniculi* are known to be zoonotic, especially for immunocompromised persons. Infected rabbits are positive for antibodies on serology about 3–4 weeks after infection. This is about 4 weeks earlier than histopathological changes in kidney and brain are visible or the organism (spores) can be detected in urine or faeces. Antibodies are passively transferred from infected does to their offspring and the latter may test positive for the first 4 weeks of life without being infected. Once maternal antibody levels decrease, the juveniles are susceptible to natural infection. A single positive enzyme-linked immunosorbent assay (ELISA) result on a blood sample cannot differentiate among active, early, reactivated or chronic infection because the measured IgG only demonstrates exposure. A second IgG test, performed at least 4 weeks later, should ideally show a rise in titre if true infection is present. However there is significant individual variation, and thus interpretation of equal or lower titres is challenging. Recently, testing of IgM, which is more indicative of current active infection, has become available in the UK. This test should be run concurrently with the IgG test to obtain a better insight into the infective status. A negative test result, obtained after the appropriate infection period, should be considered a true negative, even when neurological signs are present, and other differentials should be explored.

In one study, apparently clinically healthy rabbits were compared with those suspected of *E. cuniculi* infection as well as other clinically abnormal rabbits (Cray *et al.*, 2009). The latter two groups showed a higher gamma-globulin concentration that was accompanied by a decreased albumin-to-globulin ratio when measured by protein electrophoresis. A PCR test to screen urine and faeces to detect actively shedding rabbits is also available in the UK. See also Chapter 15.

Treponema paraluis cuniculi

Treponematosis, or rabbit syphilis, is a venereal disease limited to rabbits that affects both bucks and does. Transmission occurs via mating and from infected does to their offspring. The incubation period is between 3 and 6 weeks. Small vesicles, erythematous papules and ulcers that are ultimately covered with scabs form predominantly in the genital region but occasionally also around the lips and ocular region of infected animals. Inapparent infection of seropositive animals has been reported. Wet-mounted scabs can be examined under dark-field microscopy where available for the presence of spirochaetes. Several serological tests are available, with the microhaemagglutination test outperforming the rapid plasma reagin (RPR) test. Both tests are human tests which use *T. pallidum* as the antigen. Since antibody levels are slow to rise, false negatives are possible and suspect animals may have to be tested multiple times over several weeks to ensure a negative status. A single positive test result in a clinically healthy rabbit has no clinical relevance because many rabbits harbour the organism within their nasal cavities without ever becoming infected, or have previously been exposed. Rabbits <2 months old still may have maternal antibodies and positive results are difficult to interpret.

Pasteurella multocida

P. multocida is transmitted between rabbits by direct contact, aerosol and fomites. Vaginal infection of newborns has also been reported. The organism is generally harboured within the nasopharynx. Many carriers are asymptomatic. Active infection may be triggered by a variety of causes. The typical clinical presentation is a catarrhal or mucopurulent nasal exudate. Outbreaks can be acute, subacute or chronic. Serology for antibodies against *P. multocida* is useful when culture has yielded no results. However a single positive titre merely indicates exposure, and seroprevalence in clinically healthy animals is high. Molecular detection by PCR is available and offers a more sensitive method for confirming current infection.

Clostridium piliforme

C. piliforme is the causative agent of Tyzzer's disease. The prevalence in pet rabbits is unknown. Transmission occurs via ingestion of spores from the environment or the faeces of an infected animal. Zoonotic potential is generally confined to immunocompromised persons. Infection in rabbits may be clinically inapparent and immunocompetent animals may clear the infection within a few weeks. Poor husbandry, stress and immunosuppression predispose to disease. Serology has a good negative predictive value but false positives are possible. If the animal in question shows no clinical signs a false-positive result or a non-toxic strain is likely.

Cytology

Cytology is a cost-effective, relatively non-invasive procedure that generally requires only physical restraint, light sedation or local anaesthesia. Samples can be examined in house by the trained clinician or nurse/technician for a quick first impression or even confirmation of clinical suspicion. It is often possible to classify the lesion and fluids as inflammatory (Figure 9.14) or neoplastic, and to differentiate round cell from mesenchymal

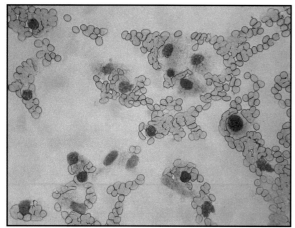

9.14 Fine-needle aspirate from a case of steatitis in the dewlap of a rabbit. There are abundant erythrocytes, with a few macrophages and a few heterophils. As there is no fat on this smear, a diagnosis of steatitis would not be possible from it alone, only chronic active inflammation. (May–Grünwald Giemsa; original magnification X400) © Chris Knott.

or epithelial lesions. Further investigation regarding malignancy, completeness of excision and possible metastasis generally requires histopathology. In addition to blood, bone marrow, CSF and urine, material for cytology can be obtained by sampling organs and lesions (Figures 9.15 and 9.16), aspirating synovial fluid and effusions in the thoracic and abdominal cavities and performing bronchoalveolar washes. See Chapter 18 for additional information on neoplastic diseases.

Sampling techniques

Sampling requires cleaning of the lesion. Surgical preparation is only required when bacteriology is needed. Aspiration requires a small needle (22 G

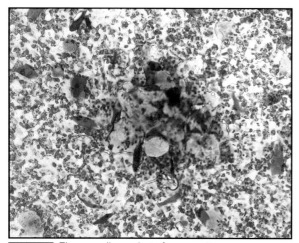

9.15 Fine-needle aspirate from a cutaneous mass. Apart from erythrocytes (probably contamination during sampling) it consists largely of keratin squames (nucleated and non-nucleated) and clumps of keratinous debris. This is typical of a keratinizing cystic lesion such as an epidermal cyst, infundibular keratinizing acanthoma, or one of the various benign skin adnexal tumours such as trichofolliculoma, trichoepithelioma or pilomatrixoma. (May–Grünwald Giemsa; original magnification X200) © Chris Knott.

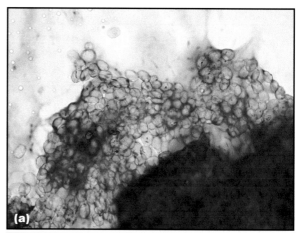

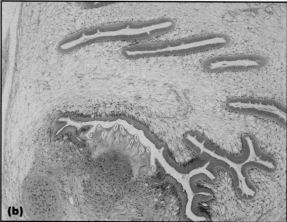

9.16 **(a)** Fine-needle aspirate from a subcutaneous cystic swelling. There are abundant moderately cohesive cells, which look at first sight somewhat like adipocytes from a lipoma, but they are smaller. These are very suggestive of mesenchymal stellate cells from the larval cestode in a coenurus cyst (probably *Taenia serialis*). (May–Grünwald Giemsa; original magnification X200) **(b)** Histology of the lesion, which was removed a few days after aspiration, shows multiple larval cestodes within the coenurus. Note the hooklets on the protoscolex and the abundant parenchymal stellate cells. (H&E; original magnification X100) © Chris Knott.

or slightly smaller), a 2 ml syringe and several clean slides, preferably with a frosted edge, as well as a pencil.

1. If the lesion is a mass it should be firmly fixed with one hand while the other hand approaches with the unattached needle. Most cutaneous lesions and organs exfoliate fairly well and aspiration is not required.
2. The needle should be advanced using the 'woodpecker' technique, whereby it is shifted in a backwards and forwards motion while repositioning the needle in different directions and depths of the tissue. Many neoplastic lesions as well as abscesses have a necrotic centre, so sampling along the margins is often more rewarding.
3. Once the needle has been withdrawn, it is attached to a syringe with the plunger drawn back to the 1 or 2 ml mark.
4. The sample material is then expressed with a little pressure on to a clean slide.

Fluids must be aspirated with the syringe attached.

Once the material is positioned on the slide, it is spread carefully according to its consistency. Cells are often very fragile and too much pressure will cause cell lysis and streaming, which renders many samples non-diagnostic. Liquid droplets should be spread like a blood smear, whereas more mucoid material can be spread with the slide-over-slide technique or the 'starfish' technique. Multiple sampling attempts and the preparation of several air-dried slides ensure a better diagnostic value. Never heat-fix slides for cytology.

When samples are collected for histopathology, impression smears can be made after blotting the tissue on paper to remove excess blood. Smears should be air-dried and never heat-fixed.

Clearly mark slides with the patient's name, species and location of lesion. Be as specific as possible. Number multiple lesions with a code that is reflected on the clinical record and submission form. When submitting slides to the laboratory use appropriate containers.

WARNING

Under no circumstances should formalin containers be sent together with blood or cytology samples in the same package. Fumes may leak, even though the container appears to be locked, especially during warm weather or where packages are stored in a heated environment. Formalin fumes may create artefacts that render haematology and cytology samples non-diagnostic.

Inflammatory lesions

Abscesses

Abscesses are frequently encountered in rabbits and often form subsequent to oral trauma or dental root problems (see *BSAVA Manual of Rabbit Surgery, Dentistry and Imaging*). They are often accompanied by a suppurative nasal discharge that is similar in appearance to that observed with chronic rhinitis due to pasteurellosis or treponematosis.

Another common location for abscesses is the abdominal cavity, where they are presumed to form within mesenteric lymph nodes following bacterial invasion from the intestinal tract. The most common isolates from these intra-abdominal abscesses are *Pasteurella multocida*, *Escherichia coli* and *Staphylococcus* spp.

Cutaneous abscesses are generally well encapsulated and can often easily be removed by surgical excision.

Cytologically, abscesses present with numerous heterophils and macrophages admixed with lower numbers of plasma cells and lymphocytes. The background frequently contains blood, necrotic amorphous and cellular debris and mineral fragments, as well as extra- and intracellular bacteria. Staphylococcal infections are often accompanied by eosinophilic debris arranged in a homogeneous, club-like structure.

Cutaneous treponematosis

Also commonly known as 'rabbit syphilis', this venereal disease causes vesicles and erythematous lesions that are later covered by scabs and crusts (see Chapter 17). The lesions are predominantly located around the genitalia, oral mucous membranes and ocular region. Cytology reveals epidermal hyperplasia accompanied by variable hyperkeratosis or parakeratosis with moderate inflammation. The corkscrew-like bacteria (spirochaetes) are located between the epithelial cells of deeper regions. They can be demonstrated with dark-field microscopy or silver staining. However, a biopsy or serological tests are generally required for confirmation (see above).

Bronchoalveolar lavage

Normal BAL fluid contains predominantly macrophages and to a lesser extent small mononuclear cells and mucus.

Round cell lesions

Lymphoma

Lymphomas are the most commonly observed neoplasm in young rabbits but are also frequently found in adults. Distribution is generally multicentric. Affected tissues often include skin, lymph nodes, eyes and oral cavity. The majority of lymphomas are high-grade variants with significant anisocytosis. The cells have dark intensely basophilic cytoplasm, large nuclei and multiple nucleoli, a high nuclear:cytoplasmic ratio and increased mitotic figures. Final grading and differentiation requires histopathology.

Thymoma

Apart from metastatic neoplasia and lymphoma, thymomas are the most common intrathoracic tumours observed in rabbits. Ultrasound-guided fine-needle aspiration is an accurate diagnostic tool. They are usually benign but their space-occupying nature can impinge on the lung capacity. On cytology mainly small and occasionally larger more pleomorphic lymphoid cells are intermixed with reticuloendothelial cells. Thymomas are also occasionally associated with paraneoplastic syndromes such as hypercalcaemia and dermatopathies.

Mesenchymal cell lesions

Nodular dermal fibrosis

The lesions are predominantly found in the skin along the back and flanks. They often appear as small, barely visible and palpable nodules within the dermis possibly due to developmental hamartomas or subsequent to previous traumatic insults. The nodules generally exfoliate poorly and may require aspiration. Cytology often reveals only scant fibrocytes and blood but occasionally also broad bands of dermal collagen delineated by low numbers of well differentiated mesenchymal cells can be observed that may be accompanied by mild epithelial hyperplasia. Inflammation or adnexal hyperplasia is only infrequently reported in connection with this lesion.

Soft tissue sarcoma

These tumours appear to be common neoplastic lesions of the skin and underlying muscle in middle-aged rabbits. The cells are often not well differentiated and it remains a challenge to diagnose their true origin. Fibrosarcomas, rhabdomyosarcomas, leiomyosarcomas and histiocytic sarcomas are the most frequently reported sarcomas. Typically they are highly invasive yet metastasis is found to be rare and slow. Complete excision is often difficult and once surgical intervention has been attempted local recurrence often appears to be more aggressive than the original tumour. Sarcomas commonly exfoliate poorly and in these cases aspiration rather than just using the woodpecker technique is advised. It is advisable to quick-stain a slide to check that adequate cellularity is present before releasing the patient. Tumours often show a high cellular pleomorphism ranging from round to spindle-shaped cells with variable anisokaryosis and nucleoli, as well as bi- and multinucleated cells. Histology is generally required for a final diagnosis.

Lipoma

Lipomas are reported in rabbits on a regular basis and are commonly found along the trunk. Cells often exfoliate poorly and may also wash off during the staining process, leaving only individual cells or small clusters of well differentiated adipocytes (Figure 9.17). When submitting samples to the

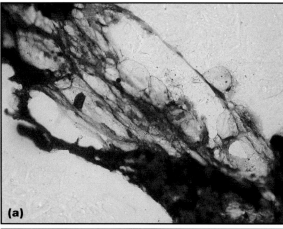

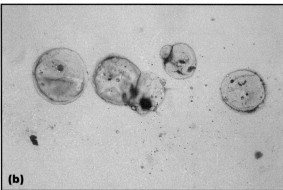

9.17 **(a)** The typical appearance of a fine-needle aspirate from a lipoma, showing a sheet of ruptured and collapsed adipocytes. **(b)** This aspirate contains a few intact adipocytes. (May–Grünwald Giemsa; original magnification X400) © Chris Knott.

laboratory it is advisable to mark relevant slides as 'fatty'. Clinical presentation of the mass and the history may help to differentiate between subcutaneous fat and a diagnosis of lipoma.

Epithelial cell lesions

Polyps

Polyps are found involving the rectum, vulva or penile shaft. They are fairly common in rabbits. A viral origin has been proposed based on similarity with viral-induced lesions in other mammals. Cytology reveals well differentiated but often hyperplastic squamous epithelium with hyperkeratosis, accompanied by occasional parabasal cells and inflammation within fibrous components. Secondary bacterial infections are commonly reported. Erosions and crusts suggest self-trauma due to pruritus or other irritation.

Basal cell tumour

These typically occur as solitary benign masses on the trunk and leg. Complete excision is generally curative but rare invasive forms with metastatic potential occur. Basal cell tumours exfoliate well. Cells are round to oval with scant basophilic cytoplasm and small round dark nuclei with minimal anisokaryosis. Occasionally the cells contain small amounts of melanin pigment.

Trichoepithelioma

In essence these tumours are basal cell tumours with variable squamous or follicular differentiation. The distribution and clinical behaviour of the two types of neoplasm is alike, but on the cut surface trichoepitheliomas often have a laminated core of keratin or a cystic appearance. The majority of these tumours are benign, but with irritation or rupture they may cause a foreign body reaction. The cytological appearance closely resembles that of basal cell tumours with additional keratinous debris and/or squamous cells.

Squamous papilloma

Lesions primarily involve the face and shoulder region and are caused by papillomaviruses. The Shope papillomavirus, which causes only benign disease in wild rabbits, shows a high transformation rate to squamous cell carcinoma in domestic rabbits. Oral papillomatosis of domestic rabbits is induced by oral papillomavirus but the lesions generally regress with time. Cytological features comprise marked epithelial papilliform hyperplasia with a prominent granulosa cell layer and occasional koilocytes embedded within the granular layer. With this particular lesion impression smears are often more rewarding than aspiration. Squamous cells predominate in the preparation, admixed with occasional parabasal cells and infrequent atypical cells, which show some anisokaryosis.

Squamous cell carcinoma

Common locations include the skin of the ears, face and feet. SCC is fairly commonly observed and often invasive, with the potential for metastasis.

Concurrent heterophilic inflammation is a common feature that can disguise the neoplastic component, especially in cytological preparations. Multiple samples taken from different angles and depths may help to elucidate the tumour type.

Mammary gland tumours

Tumours and cysts of the mammary gland are occasionally observed, with the majority of these being diagnosed as adenocarcinomas. Concurrent uterine adenocarcinomas are common. Frequently these tumours are cystic or inflamed with a highly variable cytological appearance. Epithelial cells may be admixed with proteinaceous fluid, resembling matrix, blood and/or mixed inflammatory cells. These features are challenging even for the experienced investigator.

Uterine adenocarcinoma

Uterine carcinomas are the most frequently observed intra-abdominal neoplasm of intact female rabbits. They usually present with abdominal distension and a palpable mass. Cytology frequently reveals significant hyperplasia and dysplasia that may also be observed with endometrial hyperplasia and adenomyosis. Thus diagnosis should be approached conservatively and a final decision should be made by an experienced specialist.

Testicular tumours

Testicular tumours are occasionally seen in rabbits. The most commonly reported appears to be the benign interstitial or Leydig cell tumour with sheets of large polygonal cells and moderate to large amounts of pale basophilic occasionally foamy cytoplasm. Nuclei are generally small and ovoid and contain a single small nucleolus. On rare occasions Sertoli cell tumours and testicular teratomas have been described.

References and further reading

Benson KG and Paul-Murphy J (1999) Clinical pathology of the domestic rabbit: acquisition and interpretation of samples. *Veterinary Clinics of North America: Exotic Animal Practice* **2**, 539–551

Cohen C (1962) Blood groups in rabbits. *Annals of the New York Academy of Sciences* **97**, 26–36

Cray C, Arcia G, Schneider R, *et al.* (2009) Evaluation of the usefulness of an ELISA and protein electrophoresis in the diagnosis of *Encephalitozoon cuniculi* infection in rabbits. *Journal of the American Veterinary Medical Association* **70**(4), 478–482

Fecteau KA, Deeb BJ, Rickel JM, *et al.* (2007) Diagnostic endocrinology: Blood steroid concentrations in neutered male and female rabbits. *Journal of Exotic Pet Medicine* **16**, 256–259

Garner MM (2007) Cytologic diagnosis of diseases of rabbits, guinea pigs and rodents. *Veterinary Clinics of North America: Exotic Animal Practice* **10**, 25–49

Harcourt-Brown F (2002) *Textbook of Rabbit Medicine*. Butterworth-Heinemann, Oxford

Harkness JE (1987) Rabbit husbandry and medicine. *Veterinary Clinics of North America: Small Animal Practice* **17**, 1019–1044

Hawkins MG, Vernau W, Drazenovich TL, *et al.* (2008) Results of cytologic and microbiologic analysis of bronchoalveolar lavage fluid in New Zealand White rabbits. *Journal of the American Veterinary Medical Association* **69**(5), 572–578

Keeble E and Shaw DJ (2006) Seroprevalence of antibodies to *Encephalitozoon cuniculi* in domestic rabbits in the United Kingdom. *Veterinary Record* **158**, 539–544

Kunzel F and Hittmair KM (2012) Thymomas in rabbits: Clinical evaluation, diagnosis and treatment. *Journal of the American Animal Hospital Association* **48**(2), 97–104

Manning PJ, Ringler DH and Newcomer CE (1994) *The Biology of the Laboratory Rabbit, 2nd edn.* Academic Press Limited, London

Melillo A (2007) Rabbit clinical pathology. *Journal of Exotic Pet Medicine* **16**, 135–145

Mitchell M and Tully TN (2009) Rabbits. In: *Manual of Exotic Pet Practice*, ed. M Mitchell and TN Tully, Chapter 14, pp.375–405. Saunders Elsevier, St. Louis

Paré JA and Paul-Murphy J (2004) Disorders of the reproductive and urinary systems. In: *Ferrets, Rabbits and Rodents: Clinical Medicine and Surgery, 2nd edn*, ed. KE Quesenberry and JW Carpenter JW, pp.183–193. Elsevier Saunders, St. Louis

Putwain S (2008) Clinical pathology updates: haematology and biochemistry of the rabbit. *UK Vet* **13**(6), 75–77

Quesenberry KE and Carpenter JW (2012) *Ferrets, Rabbits and Rodents: Clinical Medicine and Surgery, 3rd edn*. Elsevier Saunders, St. Louis

Richardson VCG (2000) The urinary system. In: *Rabbits: Health, Husbandry and Diseases*, ed. VGC Richardson, pp.64–72. Wiley-Blackwell Science Ltd, Oxford

Ritter JM, von Bomhard W, Wise AG, Maes RK and Kuipel M (2012) Cutaneous lymphomas in European pet rabbits (*Oryctolagus cuniculus*). *Veterinary Pathology* **49**(5), 846–851

Saunders RA and Davies RR (2005) Common laboratory abnormalities. In: *Notes on Rabbit Internal Medicine*, pp.69–88. Blackwell Publishing Ltd., Oxford

Siller-Matula JM and Plasenzotti R (2008) Interspecies differences in coagulation profiles. *Thrombosis and Haemostasis* **100**(3), 397–404

Vaissaire J, Brochet MF, Labadie JP, *et al.* (1979) Interest of serum protein electrophoresis in rabbit pathology. *Annals of Zootechnology* **28**, 142

von Bomhard W, Goldschmidt MH, Schofer FS, *et al.* (2007) Cutaneous neoplasms in pet rabbits: A retrospective study. *Veterinary Pathology* **44**(5), 579–588

Weisbroth SH, Flatt RE and Kraus AL (1974) Anatomy, physiology, and biochemistry of the rabbit. In: *The Biology of the Laboratory Rabbit*, pp.549–572. Academic Press, New York

10

Analgesia, sedation and anaesthesia

Kevin Eatwell

Most practices will have some experience of anaesthetizing rabbits. However, a 2006 study found that 1.39% of rabbits anaesthetized in general veterinary practice in the UK died under general anaesthesia, with most of these deaths due to cardiorespiratory problems. This compared to an anaesthetic death rate of 0.17% in dogs and 0.00167% in humans (Brodbelt, 2006).

Rabbit owners expect a high level of veterinary care, but many owners are reluctant to take advantage of referral and it therefore falls upon general practitioners to take a number of measures to minimize mortality and morbidity. This chapter will cover a number of useful critical care techniques and recent advances in rabbit analgesia, sedation and anaesthesia to assist the veterinary surgeon in minimizing the risks, allowing an increasing array of clinical procedures to be performed. It is important to provide some pre-sedation or anaesthetic advice to owners on how to transport their rabbit and how to improve the quality of the rabbit's hospital stay. This is possible in cases where an elective procedure is being performed but may not be possible where an emergency procedure has to be performed. See Chapter 6 for further details.

Anaesthesia and analgesia related to surgery and dentistry are discussed in detail in the *BSAVA Manual of Rabbit Surgery, Dentistry and Imaging.*

Analgesia

Rabbits are a prey species and therefore hide illness well. It can be difficult to evaluate pain in the rabbit, although some of the possible signs are noted in Figure 10.1 and a number of pain-scoring techniques are being developed.

Remote observation, via a window or closed circuit television for example, helps greatly to identify underlying pain because any preservation responses are reduced. As signs are limited it is often considered best practice to offer analgesia routinely to rabbits, at the same level provided for similar procedures in dogs or cats. If there is any doubt as to the level of pain in a rabbit, analgesia should be provided. Although, typically, analgesia is geared towards pain induced by veterinary interventions, it should also feature prominently in the treatment of both acute and chronic disease processes, where the level of pain is likely to be underestimated by the owner and the veterinary surgeon.

- Immobility
- Abnormal posture such as belly pressing
- Guarding behaviour
- Reduced food consumption
- Reduced water consumption
- Increased aggression
- Tooth grinding
- Hiding
- Increased respiratory rate
- Increased heart rate
- Reduced grooming
- Altered facial expression
- Restlessness

10.1 Signs of pain in rabbits.

Rabbits should be kept away from natural predator species to reduce anxiety and encourage normal activity and feeding (see Chapter 6). Placing a rabbit close to potential predators will increase anxiety and reduce feed intake; this in itself will reduce gastrointestinal motility, leading to intestinal gas build-up and pain. Immobilizing or covering traumatized areas may also assist in stabilizing wounds and will reduce the level of pain generated by ongoing trauma. This does, however, have to be balanced against the additional stress of having a dressing placed.

There are essentially five drug classes that can be used to provide analgesia in rabbits. Pre-emptive analgesia should be given wherever possible, because it reduces central nervous system 'wind-up' (which causes prolonged and exaggerated central responses to pain) and results in smoother anaesthesia and recovery. It is often best to combine agents to provide multimodal analgesia. There are few data confirming the level of analgesia provided by the agents used in rabbits, and regimes and doses that have been commonly used in other species are often utilized.

Local anaesthesia

Local anaesthetic agents
Local anaesthetics such as lidocaine and bupivacaine are underutilized in companion animal practice. These agents block pain transmission from the painful focus and are most usefully applied to block an area prior to a procedure being performed (Figure 10.2). They can be applied topically, by infiltration of the tissue, or administered by injection

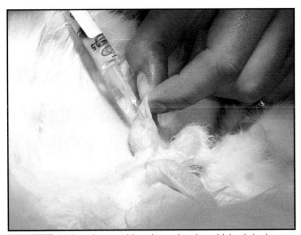

10.2 Lidocaine and bupivacaine local block being applied to the spermatic cord prior to surgical castration of a rabbit.

directly into a joint, regionally as a nerve block, or intrathecally by epidural or subarachnoid injection. Local anaesthesia can be used as an adjunct to general anaesthesia to reduce the amount of anaesthetic that is used. It may also reduce postoperative analgesic requirements.

Lidocaine has a rapid onset of action but a limited time of action (2–3 hours), whereas bupivacaine takes longer to block an area but does have a longer duration of action (2–6 hours). These agents can be used for specific blocks or as a line block over the anticipated area of a surgical incision. Toxicity is a concern: typically 4 mg/kg is the maximum dose of lidocaine administered and 2 mg/kg the maximum dose of bupivacaine. Generally doses of 1 mg/kg of each agent are combined in the same syringe and administered as required.

It is common to anaesthetize the skin over the site of intravenous catheter placement. The most commonly used agent is an emulsified mixture of local anaesthetics (e.g. EMLA 5% cream) which contains both lidocaine and prilocaine. The area is shaved and the cream is applied to the area in a thick layer (but not rubbed in). The cream is covered with an occlusive dressing (such as cling film). Full-thickness analgesia is achieved 45–60 minutes later. Other options include 4% lidocaine cream. For intraosseous needle placement, analgesia is required as far as the periosteum. In this case the area is clipped and surgically prepared. A syringe containing both lidocaine and bupivacaine can be used to inject down to the periosteal membrane.

For nasogastric tube placement local anaesthetic agents are applied intranasally. Agents typically used include lidocaine jelly (e.g. Xylocaine) or those intended for topical anaesthesia of the glottis (e.g. Intubeaze oromucosal spray). The tube can be placed 3 minutes after application of the agent. Further details of catheter and tube placement are found in other chapters in this Manual.

Local nerve blocks

Nerve blocks are most commonly used for dental procedures. There is considerable variation in skull dimensions among rabbit breeds. The infraorbital nerve block and the mental nerve block can be used to provide local anaesthesia for incisor removal and also to block the surrounding soft tissue. Other cranial nerve blocks can be performed, such as those of the mandibular nerve, maxillary nerve or palatine nerve, but these are hard to accomplish owing to limited oral access and the small size of rabbits. See *BSAVA Manual of Rabbit Surgery, Dentistry and Imaging* for more details.

Epidural anaesthesia

Epidurally administered agents can be used for the management of surgical cases (see *BSAVA Manual of Rabbit Surgery, Dentistry and Imaging*) and for rabbits with postoperative or chronic pain. This is achieved with lower doses compared with systemic therapy and may achieve a greater level of analgesia. The location and duration of analgesia produced will depend on the volume and agent used (Dollo *et al.*, 2004). Local anaesthetics are the drugs most commonly used for epidural analgesia, but opioid agonists, alpha-2 agonists and ketamine have also been used.

The spinal cord in rabbits continues until the sacral vertebrae, with the endpoint showing individual variation. The epidural and intervertebral spaces are small, and the cranially directed dorsal spinous processes that overlie the intervertebral spaces make the technique more challenging than in larger mammals.

Rabbits are placed in a prone position with the spine flexed. The area over the lumbar spine is shaved and surgically prepared. Local anaesthetic can be injected subcutaneously over the desired intervertebral space. Generally a 25 G needle is used for epidural anaesthesia, and this is inserted in the midline between the dorsal spinous processes. Cerebrospinal fluid is seen when the needle is in the subarachnoid space. When the needle is in the epidural space, there is no fluid and a drop of flush easily enters the space.

Lidocaine 2% can be administered at a rate of 0.4 ml/kg. Analgesia develops within 5–15 minutes and lasts from 60–90 minutes. Bupivacaine can provide 4.5–6 hours of surgical analgesia.

If opioid agonists are used, sensory loss occurs and hindlimb function is retained. When local anaesthetic agents are used, either alone or with opioids, motor and sensory losses are produced, often causing hindlimb paralysis. Caution is advised when administering high concentrations of local anaesthetics because toxicity has been reported (Malinovsky *et al.*, 2002; Yamashita *et al.*, 2003). Epidural anaesthesia is contraindicated in rabbits with endotoxaemia, meningitis and coagulation abnormalities.

Analgesic agents

Ketamine

When used in very low doses, ketamine acts to block *N*-methyl-D-aspartate (NMDA) receptors in the dorsal horn of the spinal cord. The NMDA receptor is involved in the transmission of painful (nociceptive) impulses from the peripheral to the central nervous system (CNS). Blocking this receptor prevents 'wind-up' of the CNS. Microdoses of ketamine do not cause dissociative anaesthetic effects, but do induce blockade of the NMDA receptor.

Ketamine is often used as part of a standard anaesthetic regime in rabbits and the NMDA antagonism and analgesic effects should be borne in mind. It can be provided as a premedicant, but some clinicians use ketamine intravenously to facilitate intubation. It is commonly used in human medicine for its analgesic properties at a low dose, and is often given as a continuous rate infusion.

Alpha-2 agonists

Alpha-2 agonists are often used in anaesthetic regimes in rabbits, but they also provide some analgesia. There are dense concentrations of alpha-2 receptors in the dorsal horn of the spinal cord and the analgesic benefits of microdoses of medetomidine or dexmedetomidine can be significant. Alpha-2 agonists contribute to analgesia in a variety of conditions, including those involving pain of musculoskeletal, visceral and neuropathic origin. When these agents are used as an adjunct to provide analgesia, the doses used are much smaller than those used for sedation or anaesthesia.

Opioids

Opioids are used commonly in companion animal medicine. It is important to consider any planned anaesthetic regime and ensure that there is no antagonism between the opioids utilized. Opioids provide sedation along with pain relief and they may be used as part of premedication prior to anaesthetic induction, or in combination with other agents to provide general anaesthesia/sedative cocktails. Two main drugs are readily used in clinical practice:

- Butorphanol is a partial agonist and antagonist at the mu opioid receptor, and a kappa agonist. It provides analgesia for only 2 hours. Doses of 0.1–0.5 mg/kg are often used (Flecknell, 2000)
- Buprenorphine is a partial mu agonist with a bell-shaped response curve. It provides analgesia over a 6–8-hour period. Doses of 0.01–0.1 mg/kg have been recommended (Flecknell, 2000), although doses up to 0.05 mg/kg are typically used in practice.

The use of pure mu agonist opioids is to be preferred for more severe pain. Morphine at a dose of 2–5 mg/kg can be given every 4 hours (Flecknell, 2000). Fentanyl is often used in combination with fluanisone (Hypnorm). Fentanyl/fluanisone provides analgesia for up to 3 hours and is given via the subcutaneous or intramuscular route (Flecknell et al., 1989). This combination often forms part of a sedative or anaesthetic regime.

Mixed agonists or antagonists such as buprenorphine or butorphanol can be used after pure mu opioids to reduce unwanted side effects or to provide follow-on analgesia. Low doses of butorphanol are often used to reduce side effects of pure mu opioids (such as respiratory depression, dysphoria, hyperalgesia) without reducing analgesia, and in some circumstances may actually have synergistic analgesic effects. This may be due to preferential binding to the excitatory mu receptors (Briggs et al., 1998; Smith et al., 1999). There is some evidence to support the use of very low doses of butorphanol concurrently with pure mu opioids, and doses up to 0.1 mg/kg have been suggested (Briggs et al., 1998; Smith et al., 1999).

Painful procedures or conditions will require the use of shorter-acting pure mu opioids throughout the day, but typically buprenorphine is preferred overnight because of its longer duration of action. It is important that painful procedures are completed early in the day so that the level of analgesia can be evaluated and titrated based on need. If oral opioids are required, buprenorphine can be given by this route at 10 times the parenteral dose. Tramadol at a dose of 10 mg/kg once a day can be used for longer-term opioid analgesia.

Non-steroidal anti-inflammatory drugs

NSAIDs can be used as routine for any surgical procedure or for longer-term analgesia, provided the animal is well hydrated. They can be given orally or parenterally. Meloxicam has been evaluated, and parenteral doses up to 1 mg/kg daily may be required to reduce pain (Leach et al., 2009). This agent does have the advantage of an oral preparation which is palatable and is useful for owners to administer at home, both in the short and the long term.

Figures 10.3 and 10.4 summarize the analgesic drugs available for use in rabbits.

Agent	Dose	Route	Indications	Contraindications
Ketamine	Up to 10 mg/kg	i.v., i.o., i.m., s.c.	Used as part of a sedative cocktail	
Medetomidine	Up to 0.05 mg/kg	i.v., i.o., i.m., s.c.		Can cause cardiorespiratory depression so care needed in sick rabbits
Dexmedetomidine	Up to 0.025 mg/kg	i.v., i.o., i.m., s.c.		Can cause cardiorespiratory depression so care needed in sick rabbits

10.3 Analgesic agents for rabbits. i.o.=intraosseous. (continues) ▶

Agent	Dose	Route	Indications	Contraindications
Butorphanol	0.1–0.5 mg/kg 6 times daily	i.v., i.o., i.m., s.c. Oral dose is 10 times parenteral dose	Mild pain after surgery. Used for partial reversal of pure mu opioids	
Buprenorphine	0.01–0.05 mg/kg 2–4 times daily	i.v., i.o., i.m., s.c. Oral dose is 10 times parenteral dose	Moderate pain and useful opioid due to duration of action. Used for partial reversal of pure mu opioids	
Morphine	2–5 mg/kg 6 times daily	i.v., i.o., i.m., s.c.	Severe pain in the perioperative period	
Fentanyl	0.005 mg/kg	i.v.	Can be used at this dose per hour for a continuous rate infusion	
Fentanyl (in combination with fluanisone)	0.1575 mg/kg	i.m., s.c.	Useful as a preoperative sedative for painful procedures	
Tramadol	10 mg/kg once daily		Useful for longer-term medication at home	
Meloxicam	0.6 mg/kg 2 times daily	i.v., i.o., i.m., s.c., oral	Any painful condition	Ensure well hydrated
Carprofen	2–4 mg/kg once daily	i.v., i.o., i.m., s.c., oral	Any painful condition	Ensure well hydrated
Ketoprofen	1–3 mg/kg 1–2 times daily	i.v., i.o., i.m., s.c., oral	Any painful condition	Ensure well hydrated

10.3 (continued) Analgesic agents for rabbits. i.o.=intraosseous.

Condition/patient type	Drug	Dose
Acute mild to moderate pain, e.g. postoperative or wound	Meloxicam	0.3 mg/kg q24h s.c., orally
	+ Buprenorphine	0.03–0.05 mg/kg q8h s.c., i.v., orally
	or Tramadol	5 mg/kg q8h s.c., i.v., orally
Acute severe pain, e.g. fracture, burn	Fentanyl	25 μg per rabbit transdermal patch or fentanyl in combination with fluanisone (as Hypnorm, VetaPharma) 0.05–0.1 ml/kg s.c., i.m.
	or Morphine	0.5–2 mg/kg s.c., i.m.
	+ Meloxicam	0.6–1 mg/kg s.c., orally
Critically ill, e.g. liver disease [a], renal disease, gastrointestinal stasis	Fentanyl [a]	25 μg per rabbit transdermal patch or fentanyl in combination with fluanisone (as Hypnorm, VetaPharma) 0.05–0.1 ml/kg s.c., i.m. if mild sedation and muscle relaxation required
	or Morphine [a]	0.5–2 mg/kg s.c., i.m.
	or Buprenorphine [a]	0.03–0.05 mg/kg q8h s.c., i.v., orally
Dyspnoea (see Chapter 11)	Meloxicam	0.3–1 mg/kg s.c., orally
Chronic pain, e.g. dental disease, orthopaedic cases	Meloxicam	0.3–1 mg/kg q12h then reduce to lowest effective dose
Geriatric (see Chapter 20)	Buprenorphine	0.03 mg/kg q8h i.v., s.c., orally
	or Tramadol	5–15 mg/kg q12h s.c., i.v., orally
	and/or Meloxicam	0.3–1 mg/kg q12h then reduce to lowest effective dose

10.4 Suggested analgesic drugs for specific patient types. i.o.=intraosseous. [a] A change in the dose or dosing interval may be required.

Sedation in rabbits

Sedation of rabbits can be performed for minor procedures, such as radiography, ultrasonography or computed tomography (CT) examination. However it is still important to provide supportive care measures, particularly thermal support, fluid support and oxygenation, during the period of sedation. Ocular lubricants should be used routinely for sedated and anaesthetized rabbits because their blink reflex will be diminished and there may be a reduction in tear production (Ghaffari *et al.*, 2009).

Routine anaesthetic monitoring should also be undertaken. There are a number of agents that can be used to sedate rabbits but the decision on which agents to use and at what dose depends on the clinical condition of the rabbit and the procedures to be undertaken.

Generally, subcutaneous administration of injectable agents is sufficient and leads to maximum effect within 10–15 minutes. With intramuscular injections the absorption rate and time to onset of action tend to be more consistent, though the administration causes more discomfort than the subcutaneous route. Sedative agents are used to provide analgesia, reduce anxiety and provide some muscle relaxation and sedation. Combining agents can help because the side effects of each are minimized and all will provide some analgesia (preemptive multimodal analgesia).

Sedative agents

Alpha-2 adrenergic agonists
Alpha-2 agonists, such as medetomidine, are commonly used in sedative cocktails for rabbits. In medetomidine there is a mixture of the *levo* and *dex* isomers. It is the *dex* isomer that is active, providing consistent dose-dependent effects. In contrast, levomedetomidine is agonistic at lower doses but can be antagonistic at higher doses, leading to variable effects. Dexmedetomidine is shorter acting than medetomidine and its analgesia lasts longer than its sedative effects (it is the other way around with medetomidine). The cardiovascular effects of these two agents are identical: they cause initial vasodilation followed by marked vasoconstriction. Both the heart rate and respiratory rate are depressed.

Dissociative anaesthetics
Ketamine alone has minimal sedative effects in rabbits but is commonly used in combination with other agents. The main benefits of ketamine are the minimal effects on cardiovascular parameters, reduction in the dose of other agents and additional analgesia. Tiletamine is longer acting and is available in combination with zolazepam.

Benzodiazepines
Diazepam and midazolam are used commonly in rabbits by a variety of routes. They cause muscle relaxation, sedation and amnesia. Their cardiovascular effects are minimal but they do not provide analgesia. Diazepam should not be mixed with other agents but midazolam can be. Midazolam is shorter acting than diazepam and water-soluble, and is preferable. Zolazepam is potent and long acting and is available in combination with tiletamine, though this combination may lead to nephrotoxicity in rabbits (Hedenqvist and Hellebrekers, 2003). Benzodiazepines can increase recovery times and the use of benzodiazepine reversal agents such as flumazenil should be considered.

Neuroleptics
Fluanisone (a butyrophenone) is commonly used for sedative protocols in rabbits, primarily because it is combined with fentanyl in a commercially available product authorized in the UK. It does prolong recovery, having a duration of action of 4 hours. Therefore, if fentanyl/fluanisone sedation is considered, the rabbit will usually need to be kept in overnight. Other protocols, or modification of the standard doses used for fentanyl/fluanisone (by adding in a third agent), may be used to speed recovery. This combination is often reserved for use when follow-on procedures may lead to significant pain. As an example, fentanyl and fluanisone can be used to sedate a rabbit for radiography followed by intravenous induction for dental abscess surgery. Fluanisone causes some hypotension due to vasodilation.

Opioids
These are often used as a standard component of sedation protocols. Many disease processes and their treatments are painful. It is important to select the correct opioid on the basis of its duration of action and the level of analgesia it will provide, as outlined earlier in this chapter. Typical opioids used include butorphanol and buprenorphine, although fentanyl is commonly used in combination with fluanisone.

Rabbit sedation protocols
Medetomidine or dexmedetomidine is often combined with ketamine and an opioid, such as butorphanol or buprenorphine, to sedate rabbits, given via the intramuscular or subcutaneous route. Xylazine has been used in a number of protocols and is still a frequently used large animal sedative but is not in common use in companion animal practice, having been superseded by medetomidine, and will not be discussed further. A combination of medetomidine and ketamine is the most commonly used protocol in rabbits, and the level of sedation may be deepened with isoflurane or sevoflurane administered by mask (Brodbelt, 2006). However, among the adverse drug reactions in rabbits most commonly reported to the Veterinary Medicines Directorate in the UK are those due to medetomidine or dexmedetomidine. The effects reported are dyspnoea, tachypnoea, apnoea, bradycardia, cardiac arrest and death in some cases (Diesel, 2011). However, the use of medetomidine or dexmedetomidine did not appear to increase the risk of anaesthetic death over other agents in a survey undertaken in the UK (Brodbelt, 2006).

A secure airway and an intravenous catheter are important to allow remedial action to be taken when any sedatives are administered to rabbits. Many clinicians use very regimented sedation and anaesthetic protocols and lack the confidence to explore other regimes. However, if significant problems occur (e.g. with medetomidine or dexmedetomidine), being confident with other regimes is important because critical patients do need a different approach. There is merit in using low doses of these agents intravenously; this can provide additional analgesia with the benefit of being reversible, thus speeding recovery and reducing the doses of other agents (e.g. ketamine) that cannot be reversed. This is discussed in more detail under rabbit anaesthesia protocols. Should the clinician wish to avoid the use of alpha-2 agonists altogether another protocol can be considered, using a benzodiazepine, ketamine and an opioid.

Fentanyl with fluanisone can be used to provide sedation. This combination is authorized in the UK, and as such should be the first-choice agent. There are some advantages to consider. First, some peripheral vasodilation occurs (as opposed to vasoconstriction produced by the alpha-2 agonists) which facilitates venepuncture and catheter placement. The heart rate and respiratory rate are also kept at a more acceptable level. The presence of pink mucous membranes is reassuring prior to anaesthesia. In addition, pulse oximetry is more reliable because peripheral perfusion is better. However, respiratory depression is still a concern with fentanyl/fluanisone, and the use of doxapram (at 5 mg/kg) has been suggested as a routine agent with this combination. It has been shown to reverse the respiratory depressant effects, without increasing rabbit activity, for the first 45 minutes after administration (Flecknell *et al.*, 1989). Thus the use of doxapram should be considered where respiratory depression is of concern when using fentanyl/fluanisone.

Alfaxalone has recently become available in the UK and has been used alone as an intramuscular agent or after the administration of medetomidine or xylazine. In the latter regime medetomidine was given subcutaneously and alfaxalone was given intramuscularly (Marsh *et al.*, 2009).

Routes used for the administration of sedative protocols include subcutaneous (between the scapulae), intramuscular (into the epaxial muscles), intraperitoneal (in the caudal quadrant on the right side) and intravenous (marginal ear vein). Intraperitoneal routes have fallen out of favour given the ease of intravenous access in rabbits, allowing doses to be titrated more accurately.

Doses of sedative agents used in rabbits are shown in Figure 10.5.

Reversal of sedative protocols

Medetomidine and dexmedetomidine can be reversed using atipamezole. For medetomidine 5 times the medetomidine dose is used and for dexmedetomidine 2.5 times the dose is used. This can be administered subcutaneously or intramuscularly. Intravenous use has been performed in an emergency situation but may cause excitation. Reversal of these agents reverses any analgesia provided and so is best avoided if significant pain is present. If a low dose of medetomidine was used, or the sedation was longer than 45 minutes in duration, reversal may be unnecessary because it will have minimal effect on recovery time. Atipamezole has a shorter duration of action than medetomidine and re-sedation is possible if it is used shortly after

Option	Drug	Dose	Route	Notes on use
1 [a]	Medetomidine or Dexmedetomidine	0.1–0.5 mg/kg or 0.05 mg/kg	s.c., i.m.	Young and healthy patients that need a quick recovery
	Ketamine	10–35 mg/kg		
	Buprenorphine or Butorphanol	0.03 mg/kg or 0.1–0.5 mg/kg		
2	Diazepam	1–5 mg/kg	s.c., i.m.	Non-painful procedures
	Ketamine	20–40 mg/kg		
3	Midazolam	0.25–0.5 mg/kg	s.c., i.m.	Painful procedures in debilitated rabbits
	Buprenorphine	0.03–0.05 mg/kg		
4	Fentanyl	0.0315–0.1575 mg/kg	s.c., i.m.	Painful procedures requiring a pure mu opioid
	Fluanisone	1–5 mg/kg		
5	Alfaxalone	5–10 mg/kg	i.m.	
6 [b]	Medetomidine	0.25 mg/kg	s.c., i.m.	
	Alfaxalone	5 mg/kg		

10.5 Dosages of sedative drugs. [a] Nevalainen *et al.* (1989); Hedenqvist *et al.* (2001); Difilippo *et al.* (2004); Orr *et al.* (2005); [b] Marsh *et al.* (2009).

administration of the medetomidine or used intravenously in an emergency. Thus, delaying its use or providing a subcutaneous dose as well may be required. If ketamine has been used in combination with medetomidine, administration of atipamezole should be delayed for 45–60 minutes because ketamine alone causes tremors and muscular rigidity (Harcourt-Brown, 2002).

Reversal of fentanyl can be achieved using a number of mixed agonist/antagonist agents such as butorphanol (0.1–0.5 mg/kg) or buprenorphine (0.01–0.05 mg/kg). Naloxone should be available to reverse any opioids completely in the event of an emergency. This will reverse any analgesia and is usually reserved for an inadvertent overdose or where complications have occurred.

A benzodiazepine reversal agent such as flumazenil can be used to reverse diazepam or midazolam where these have been used.

Pre-anaesthetic considerations

Nitrous oxide
Nitrous oxide has been used in rabbits in a number of experimental situations and has also been used clinically but in general is not recommended for use in rabbits because it only reduces the required concentration of volatile agents by a small percentage (0.25–0.5%). It may also diffuse into gas-filled intestines (Hedenqvist and Hellebrekers, 2003). It can be used at a concentration of up to 60% of the inhaled gas with oxygen to carry volatile anaesthetics for the induction and maintenance of anaesthesia. At induction it accelerates the uptake of volatile anaesthetics and speeds induction. During maintenance it reduces the inspired concentration of volatile anaesthetic required, lowering the adverse effects of the latter. Recovery is more rapid because less volatile anaesthetic has been administered over a given time.

Continuous rate infusion
CRI (sometimes referred to as constant rate infusion, although technically the rate can be altered at any point during the infusion) is an excellent method for delivering analgesia because it eliminates the peak and trough effects of intermittent dosing. Opioids (such as morphine, fentanyl, butorphanol), ketamine, dexmedetomidine and lidocaine are commonly used as CRIs in human medicine and similar methods have been applied in rabbits. This technique is likely to be more widely used in the future.

One of the limiting factors is the availability in clinical practice of syringe drivers capable of delivering reliable low volume infusions. However, syringe drivers are becoming increasingly available, and a change in the UK legislation that will come into force in the near future will mean that many units delivering fluids in mm/h will become redundant in human medicine. This may lead to second-hand units becoming available for veterinary use at a low cost (Figure 10.6).

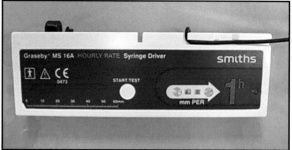

10.6 Syringe driver calibrated in mm/h capable of delivering fluid rates between 0.2 and 16.5 ml per hour, ideal for setting up continuous rate infusions.

These units can be used to provide maintenance fluid therapy during anaesthesia, during sedation, postoperatively or in the critically ill rabbit. However many clinicians prefer to use intermittent bolus administration of fluids in conscious animals owing to the risk of a rabbit chewing the intravenous line (Figure 10.7).

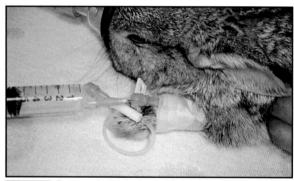

10.7 Bolus administration of fluids into the cephalic vein of a rabbit.

CRI is commonly employed in rabbits by the author, most typically with dexmedetomidine and ketamine, and the low doses have minimal cardiovascular effects. The regime used mirrors that used in human patients. Generally a loading dose is followed by a standard infusion rate. Ketamine and dexmedetomidine are generally used by CRI in any procedure where significant pain is anticipated (generally if more pain is expected than would be generated by a routine ovariohysterectomy). However, in human medicine, CRI is considered for use in all cases and may reduce dependence on opioids, particularly pure mu opioids which may induce hyperalgesia or dysphoria. Therefore, the use of low doses of ketamine + dexmedetomidine, or dexmedetomidine alone, with or without analgesics such as morphine, fentanyl or butorphanol, and administered as a CRI, should be considered for all surgical cases in rabbits.

Typically the higher end of CRI doses used in other small animal species are applied in rabbits (Figures 10.8 and 10.9). The infusion rate can be altered according to patient need, particularly if a Y-port is used to facilitate additional fluid therapy as required. It is important to realize that CRI is used to augment other analgesics and not to replace them.

Agent	Intravenous loading dose	Intravenous maintenance dose
Ketamine	0.25–0.5 mg/kg	0.02–0.2 mg/kg/h
Morphine	0.5 mg/kg	0.1–0.4 mg/kg/h
Fentanyl	0.005 mg/kg	0.005 mg/kg/h
Butorphanol	0.2–0.4 mg/kg	0.1–0.2 mg/kg/h
Dexmedetomidine	0.005 mg/kg	0.001 mg/kg/h
Medetomidine	0.01 mg/kg	0.002 mg/kg/h

10.8 CRI rates used in dogs and cats. The higher end of the dose range is recommended for rabbits as they have a higher metabolic rate.

Adding a ketamine CRI to a standard rate of fluid therapy for a 2 kg rabbit undergoing surgery

Fluid requirement is 10 ml/kg/h; 2 x 10 ml = 20 ml is required per hour.
Ketamine requirement is 0.2 mg/kg/h. Concentration is 100 mg/ml.
0.2 x 2/100 = 0.004 ml is required per hour. This is added to 20 ml of fluid therapy and the syringe driver set to deliver 20 ml/h.

10.9 Calculating a ketamine constant rate infusion.

Clinical examination and hospitalization

Rabbits undergoing anaesthesia are often assumed to be healthy or to have only localized disease, but the rabbit may well be in a worse physical state than anticipated and it is worth reviewing the American Society of Anesthesiologists (ASA) physical status classification system, which was developed in 1963:

1. A normal healthy patient.
2. A patient with mild systemic disease.
3. A patient with severe systemic disease.
4. A patient with severe systemic disease that is a constant threat to life.
5. A moribund patient that is not expected to survive without the operation.

It is important to evaluate where each patient fits on this scale and many rabbits assumed to be healthy may in fact have a higher grade. Rabbits identified as grades 1–2 have been reported as having a 0.73% chance of an anaesthetic death; those of grades 3–5 have a 7.37% chance of anaesthetic-related death (Brodbelt, 2006). Most rabbits undergoing anaesthesia are, in reality, of grades 2–4.

A full clinical examination, including obtaining an accurate weight (on scales weighing to the nearest 5 g is ideal), is important because rabbits are a prey species and hide disease well (see Chapter 7). Subtle signs of illness may be missed by their owners. The examination may pick up subtle illness or behavioural changes that may lead to other treatment or diagnostic procedures being required.

Clinical examination also allows for baseline parameters to be obtained for the individual. This is important because the reference ranges for physiological parameters in rabbits are quite broad

and this acts as a point of reference for the rest of the procedure. These should be clearly marked on the anaesthetic sheet as the pre-anaesthetic parameters that should be maintained during and after anaesthesia. It is important to realize, however, that stress and anxiety will influence these parameters. The respiration rate should be taken by observation at a distance and the heart rate can often be obtained by gently opposing a stethoscope to the side of the patient without physical restraint. Once the rabbit has been fully evaluated it should be transferred to a quiet warm hospital cage.

Critical care techniques

Elective procedures may require minimal supportive care before anaesthesia, because the rabbits are clinically healthy. However, sick rabbits will benefit from a period of supportive care prior to anaesthesia; supportive fluid therapy, nutritional support, thermal support and analgesia are all important (see Chapter 8). In mild cases supportive care may be instigated at the point of anaesthesia to minimize stress on the patient. Rabbit sedation and anaesthesia will create some side effects and possible complications, depending on which agents are used, and it is important to provide adequate supportive care to reduce these effects during the sedation or anaesthetic period and after the procedure. A sedated rabbit still requires the same level of supportive care provided to an anaesthetized rabbit, and requires full attention and diligence.

Fluid therapy

Fluid therapy is important. It may be impossible to quantify deficits, so many patients are assumed to be dehydrated and a standard rate of fluid therapy provided. Rabbits have a high metabolic rate and their daily fluid requirement is 100 ml/kg/day. The route of administration depends on the severity of illness. During anaesthesia 6 ml/kg/h is used for normovolaemic rabbits undergoing diagnostic procedures. However, 10 ml/kg/h is used for those rabbits undergoing surgery, particularly if the body cavity is being opened and there is an increased risk of haemorrhage and evaporative losses. A variety of routes can be used.

Generally, fluids such as lactated Ringer's solution or normal saline (0.9%) are given via the subcutaneous route. Injectable solutions containing glucose can also be given, but it is important to realize that the concentration of sugars in the fluid does not provide any real nutritional support and is a potential risk factor for abscess formation.

Intraperitoneal fluids can be given and are less painful and more rapidly absorbed than fluids given by the subcutaneous route. However, they do cause dilution of the peritoneal fluid, hinder inflammatory responses in the abdominal cavity (for example those fighting bacterial contamination) and can reduce effective clotting. They also lead to increased pressure on the diaphragm and may cause some respiratory compromise if given to excess. There is also a risk of organ perforation during administration, with subsequent peritonitis.

An intravenous catheter can be placed for routine fluid therapy in rabbits and this is the preferred route in all animals. The additional benefits of intravenous access are not to be underestimated.

In severely dehydrated or collapsed animals intraosseous fluids can be given, although this is usually reserved for those cases where intravenous access was not possible or in an emergency situation. See Chapter 7 for further details on techniques of administration.

Fluids should be warmed to body temperature prior to administration; infant bottle warmers can be used to provide a low-cost method. These can be positioned in the wards and in induction areas. The choice and rate of fluid therapy depends on the nature of the presenting complaint, the physical examination of the rabbit and the results of any preoperative blood sampling.

Feeding prior to anaesthesia

Rabbits undergoing routine procedures do not usually require assisted feeding prior to anaesthesia, but will benefit from familiar food sources being offered. Debilitated rabbits will benefit from supportive nutrition prior to anaesthesia yet should still be offered easy access to familiar foods. Nasogastric tubes can be placed via the ventral nasal meatus for supportive nutrition. However, these are of a small gauge (typically 4 Fr) and do not allow for the coarser fibrous foods to be given.

If assisted feeding is being performed (prior to anaesthesia) this has to be taken into account when planning anaesthesia because it is important to ensure that there is a clear oropharynx. When rabbits have been allowed to feed, it is unusual for a rabbit to have food at the back of the pharynx during intubation. However assisted feeding should be stopped 30 minutes before premedication. Once rabbits have been given premedication, all food should be removed so that they do not become sedated with an oropharynx full of food.

Thermal support

Maintaining normothermia is important for all rabbits, but those that are ill, sedated or anaesthetized present an increased challenge. All sedative or anaesthetic agents will induce a degree of hypothermia and thermal support must be instigated at the time of premedication or sedation. Sick animals may well require thermal support throughout their stay at the veterinary clinic.

Patient size is also an important factor to consider. Rabbits have a large surface area-to-volume ratio and hypothermia is a risk; however, rabbits have poor thermal tolerance, and hyperthermia and hypothermia can both develop quickly. If the measures used are highly effective at controlling hypothermia, then hyperthermia is also a risk during anaesthesia and surgery. Avoiding hypothermia starts with the identification of normothermia for each patient on that day, and therefore it is essential to record baseline parameters.

Sick rabbits, and patients during and after anaesthesia, will be unable to regulate their temperature (for example, shivering thermogenesis is lost under anaesthesia) and provision of a heat source is important. In many cases focal heat is contraindicated because the patient may be unable to move away from or towards a heat source. Providing an even heat source over the entire cage is important and monitoring rectal temperature is vital to ensure that normothermia is maintained (Figure 10.10).

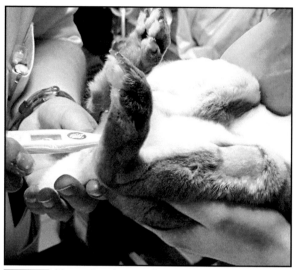

10.10 Measuring the rectal temperature provides an essential benchmark when controlling hypothermia.

There are two main methods of reducing the risk of hypothermia:

- Heat loss during anaesthesia should first be controlled by increasing insulation:
  - The procedure room or operating theatre should be kept warm by turning off the air-conditioning
  - Heat mats (either electric or circulating hot water) can be used, and towels placed to prevent heat loss by conduction through the theatre table
  - Wrapping part of the animal in aluminium foil or bubble wrap can help to reduce heat loss; bubble wrap is especially useful for radiography
  - Aseptic skin preparation for minor procedures, such as intraosseous needle placement or biopsy of a mass, will involve clipping fur and using disinfectants, which may cool the patient; excessive skin preparation should be avoided. Warming scrubbing fluids in an infant bottle warmer can help to reduce chilling (Figure 10.11)
  - Clear sterile plastic drapes allow a clear view of the patient but also act to retain more heat than the standard cloth drapes
  - Theatre lights used to facilitate the procedure will also help to keep the animal warm
- Active heating of the patient should be performed. Methods of providing heat are summarized in Figure 10.12.

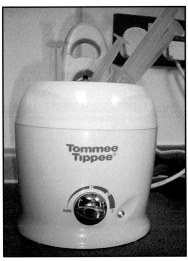

10.11 An infant bottle warmer is an inexpensive way of keeping parenteral fluids and scrub solutions warm.

Increase insulation and decrease heat loss
• Wrap extremities in bubble wrap
• Warm scrubbing fluid prior to use in infant bottle warmer and avoid or reduce alcohol
• Portex thermovent
• Minimize spirit use
• Space blanket
• Wrap the animal in a towel
• Wrap extremities in aluminium foil
• Reduce surgical time
• Minimize clipping area
• Use plastic drapes instead of cloth or paper drapes
• Switch off air conditioning

Provide a continuous heat source
• Warm parenteral fluids in infant bottle warmer
• Theatre lighting used as a radiant heat source (avoid desiccation)
• Raise room temperature
• Electric heat mats [a]
• Bair hugger
• Water recirculating heat mats
• Hairdryer
• Heat lamps [a]
• Hot Dog
• Heated theatre table [a]
• Incubators (after premedication and in recovery)

Heat sources that may cool if not monitored or reheated
• Hot hands (gloves with warm water) [a]
• Warm parenteral fluids in the microwave or hot water
• Microwaveable bean bag or plastic disc [a]
• Hot water bottle [a]

10.12 Options available for maintaining normothermia. Above all, monitor the rectal temperature continuously. [a] Care must be taken to prevent burns at the site of contact with the heating device.

Arterial blood gas analysis

Arterial blood gas analysis should be considered a part of the routine evaluation of rabbits. It has been shown to be superior to capnography and pulse oximetry in the evaluation of acid–base or electrolyte disturbances, ventilation and oxygenation of the patient in a variety of species including rabbits (Eatwell *et al.*, 2013). Capnography and pulse oximetry are used as non-invasive methods to give near real-time results, but lack the accuracy of arterial blood gas analysis. Arterial blood gas analysis is simple to perform in the rabbit (Figure 10.13).

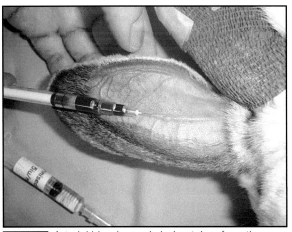

10.13 Arterial blood sample being taken from the medial ear artery.

Arterial blood gas analysis is best used to evaluate the status of the patient over time. Samples are usually taken every 30 minutes to allow for processing and for remedial action to be taken, and to evaluate its beneficial effects. The main limiting factor is not failure to take the sample, nor the cost or time involved in running a near-patient test, but the initial outlay on a patient-side blood analyser.

A variety of parameters can be measured but typically include: pH, PCO_2, PO_2, SO_2, sodium, potassium, chloride, ionized calcium (iCal), glucose, haematocrit and haemoglobin (Hb). From these the bicarbonate (HCO_3^-), total carbon dioxide content (TCO_2) and base excess are typically calculated automatically. The dead-space fraction, anion gap and arterial alveolar gradient can be calculated manually.

There are a number of techniques employed to assist in the interpretation of blood gas analysis and the necessary remedial action to be taken (Foxhall, 2008).

Preparation

Preparation is the key to any anaesthetic procedure. As rabbits are higher-risk patients, minimizing the length of any anaesthetic procedure is important and identifying all items likely to be needed and preparing these in advance is important. Preparing all the emergency drugs is also important, including complete reversals for any agents used. As an alternative, simple dosing charts can be created and kept in a 'crash' box nearby (Figure 10.14). Note that 80% of rabbits have atropinases, limiting the beneficial effects of atropine, and so glycopyrrolate is to be preferred. Where possible, emergency agents should be administered intravenously. If a catheter has not been placed, the intraosseous route may be preferable if the clinician is experienced in the placement of intraosseous catheters.

Agent	Indications	Dose
Lidocaine	Ventricular fibrillation	1–2 mg/kg
Propranolol	Tachyarrhythmias	0.1 mg/kg
Atropine	Bradyarrhythmias	≤3 mg/kg
Glycopyrrolate	Bradyarrhythmias	0.1 mg/kg
Doxapram	Hypoventilation	2–10 mg/kg
Adrenaline	Asystole	0.1 ml/kg of 1 in 10,000 (asystole)
Vasopressin	Hypotension	0.8 IU/kg

10.14   Emergency drug dosages for rabbits.

Antibiotic therapy

Pre-emptive antibiotic therapy may be indicated if significant infection is suspected or a contaminated procedure is going to be performed. If bacterial culture and sensitivity testing is not possible presumptive therapy for likely pathogens is required.

Respiration under anaesthesia

Ventilation is depressed under sedation and anaesthesia, and appropriate monitoring is discussed later in this chapter. However, elevation of the thorax or laying the patient in ventral recumbency can facilitate ventilation of an anaesthetized patient (Figure 10.15). Supplemental oxygen should be given wherever possible to sedated (Figure 10.16) and anaesthetized patients because this elevates PO_2.

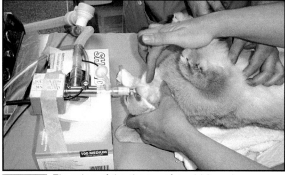

10.15   Elevation of the thorax of a rabbit under anaesthesia. Chest elevation is important to aid respiration.

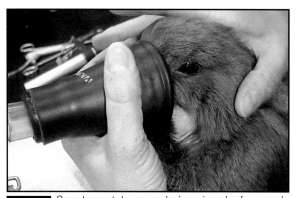

10.16   Supplemental oxygen being given by facemask to a sedated rabbit.

Anaesthesia

The level of experience in anaesthetizing rabbits varies among individual veterinary surgeons, although there may be a practice protocol in place which is typically used. However the effectiveness of this protocol and its safety may be less than ideal. Anaesthesia may be planned well in advance (in the case of an elective procedure) or may be more urgent owing to an emergency presentation; nonetheless, it is a rare occasion where adequate preparation for the procedure cannot be undertaken.

Formulating anaesthetic techniques that work consistently is important. There are a number of factors that put rabbits at a potentially higher anaesthetic risk. Rabbits are a prey species, are prone to stress and have a very good preservation response. As a result they mask disease well. Despite this, anaesthesia of a sick patient may well be preferred over physical restraint or sedation, particularly given the incidence of underlying respiratory pathology. Rabbits are near obligate nasal breathers and open-mouth breathing is a poor prognostic indicator. Nasal and sinus disease is common, leading to respiratory compromise. Rabbits may also suffer from lower respiratory tract disease and cardiac disease.

Premedication of rabbits is often performed and can help with muscle relaxation, analgesia and sedation of the patient (providing all three aspects of the anaesthetic triad). Premedicants can cause hypothermia, however, in addition to cardiovascular and respiratory depression, and so supportive care measures should be implemented at the point of premedication.

Waiting until the patient is in theatre prior to dealing with thermal support is a mistake, and patients can quickly become markedly hypothermic. Suitable premedicants include a variety of different agents such as alpha-2 agonists, ketamine, benzodiazepines, neuroleptics, opioids and acepromazine. Anticholinergics can be used as premedicants; however glycopyrrolate has to be used because a large percentage of rabbits possess atropinases. The exact choice depends on whether sedation alone or full anaesthesia is required; many sedative protocols will be deepened by the addition of inhaled anaesthetic gas. In addition, the choice of opioid depends on the level of analgesia required intra- and post-operatively. Caution is required because the use of butorphanol or buprenorphine preoperatively for moderately painful conditions will preclude the use of pure mu opioids as premedicants when corrective surgery is performed, which may elevate the level of pain suffered in the immediate postoperative period.

Food should be removed once premedication has occurred, to avoid any food being left in the oropharynx. Rabbits are usually placed in a basket, kept in a quiet darkened room and covered with a towel (Figure 10.17). The time is noted and the patient is evaluated regularly. Premedicated rabbits should be moved to a heated room to counteract any hypothermia and this avoids patients that are in the ward being subjected to higher temperatures.

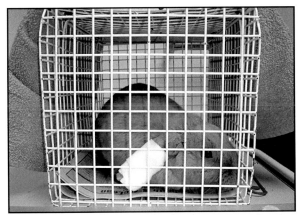

10.17 A rabbit in a cage that has been covered and placed in a quiet room after premedication. Sedated rabbits should be kept under close observation.

Ideally, premedication is used to provide sedation, analgesia and muscle relaxation. This is followed by intravenous induction and securing an airway to provide oxygen and gaseous anaesthetic. Parenteral anaesthetic induction is typically preferred over gaseous induction. Intravenous administration allows lower doses to be used, reduces the lag time so they can be dosed to effect (as opposed to intramuscular or intraperitoneal use where a set dose is given), and if intravenous induction is achieved immediate intubation is possible.

Gaseous anaesthetic agents used commonly in rabbits include isoflurane and sevoflurane. Halothane was used historically, but will not be discussed further because isoflurane has now replaced this agent. Sevoflurane has a very low solubility in blood and, therefore, induction and recovery are more rapid than with isoflurane. Mask induction with agents such as isoflurane and sevoflurane has been shown to cause marked breath holding (for up to 3 minutes) and anxiety, leading to prolonged induction times. As a result sevoflurane, despite its lower lipid solubility compared with isoflurane, does not lead to faster induction in rabbits (Flecknell *et al.*, 1999). Should mask induction be performed, there is a benefit in preoxygenation of the rabbit for a few breaths first, prior to adding in the anaesthetic gas. One human study showed a marked improvement in oxygenation after four deep breaths in 100% oxygen immediately prior to induction; 1–2 minutes is therefore excessive and increases anxiety (Fleureaux *et al.*, 1995). The circuit should be flushed because there may be residual anaesthetic in the circuit or machine. Wrapping the rabbit in a towel is usually required (Figure 10.18). However, mask induction is stressful for any rabbit and vocalization (screaming) may occur; this method should therefore be avoided in a fully conscious rabbit.

Breath holding is still evident with mask induction even after premedication or sedation, although the level of physical restraint required to enable mask induction may be less, and so some premedication is advised as a minimum (Flecknell *et al.*, 1999). Restraint must be secure because even if mild sedation is utilized the noxious stimuli from the gaseous agent can still lead to struggling.

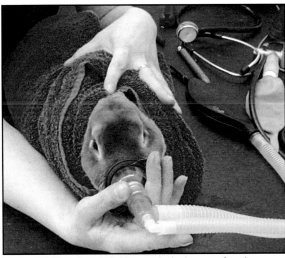

10.18 Towel restraint is needed when performing mask induction with inhalant agents.

In one study, slowly increasing the percentage of anaesthetic gas (every 30 seconds) during induction did not reduce induction time, nor did it reduce breath holding, anxiety or struggling, although this is a popular technique. The rabbits held their breath for 30–180 seconds while the lower levels of anaesthetic gas were being administered and started breathing once high concentrations were applied (Flecknell *et al.*, 1999). If this technique is to be employed then a potential solution may be to apply a low concentration for the first 3 minutes of induction, prior to incrementally increasing the concentration. Mask induction with isoflurane is usually performed at 5% and sevoflurane at 8% (owing to its higher minimum alveolar concentration). Chamber induction leads to similar anxiety: rabbits will lift their heads to the top of the chamber to avoid the agent, with subsequent struggling and breath holding once they are forced to inhale the anaesthetic gas.

Facemasks should be tight fitting with a membrane over the rabbit's face. Clear masks allow the rabbit to be visualized during induction. There are facemasks marketed that allow for some scavenging of waste gases (either active or passive) to reduce environmental contamination.

In general, T-pieces are suitable for rabbits because they have little resistance and low dead space. The addition of a reservoir bag enables positive pressure ventilation to be performed. Dead space can be minimized by using low dead space connectors. The gas flow rate used is typically 3 times the minute volume (tidal volume, 4–6 ml per breath per kg, multiplied by the respiratory rate, 30–60 breaths per minute) of the rabbit. Small patients can require very low flow rates, but the flowmeter on many anaesthetic machines is not accurate below 1 l/min, so this should be used as a minimum setting for all patients. Scavenging is an important part of an anaesthetic system, removing inhalant agents safely to reduce exposure of personnel. This may be performed by connection of the waste gases to an active scavenging system, or to activated charcoal for adsorption.

Mask or chamber induction can be used alone, after any of the premedicants or sedative protocols listed, or avoided by using intravenous induction. The latter is to be preferred in most cases.

Rabbit anaesthesia protocols

Most of the anaesthetic agents used in premedication have already been discussed under rabbit sedation. Acepromazine (a phenothiazine) is not commonly used in rabbits as a premedicant, but doses of 0.1–1 mg/kg can be used. No analgesia is provided, there is a long duration of action, it can lead to variable levels of sedation and hypotension occurs due to peripheral vasodilation. Acepromazine will, however, reduce the doses of other agents required.

Respiratory secretions do not appear to be a problem in this species and if anticholinergics are used they may increase viscosity, increasing the risk of obstruction further (Bateman *et al.*, 2005). Glycopyrrolate is used in rabbits because they possess atropinases.

Induction agents used in rabbits include propofol (an alkyl phenol) which enhances gamma-aminobutyric acid (GABA) function. Perivascular administration is not irritant, induction is rapid and propofol is rapidly metabolized, leading to quick recovery. Side effects include a moderate fall in systolic blood pressure, a small reduction in cardiac output and significant respiratory depression. The respiratory depression may result in a reduced respiratory rate or reduced tidal volume and oxygen should be supplemented. The cardiorespiratory depression is dose dependent and slow administration will avoid apnoea, which is common in rabbits. Analgesia is minimal.

Alfaxalone (a steroidal anaesthetic) appears to be a safe and effective intravenous induction agent in rabbits. Inductions are smooth and peripheral perfusion is maintained. Catheterization is easy and intravenous injection does not appear to cause any discomfort. Recovery is usually smooth. Alfaxalone is not reversible (Grint *et al.*, 2008). Intramuscular or subcutaneous use is also possible but can lead to a variable effect, and typically twice the intravenous dose is used.

Dosages and protocols for anaesthetic agents used in rabbits are summarized in Figures 10.19 and 10.20.

Reversal of agents used for rabbit anaesthesia will speed recovery. However, selection and use of the correct reversal agents is important. Analgesia and the duration of action of the agents used should be taken into consideration when reversing anaesthesia in a rabbit.

Pure mu opioid agonists can be reversed using naloxone, which reverses all analgesia, and this is typically only used in an emergency situation. Buprenorphine is commonly used as a reversal agent as it provides a quick recovery and offers improved and extended analgesia over butorphanol (Flecknell *et al.*, 1989). However, some clinicians prefer butorphanol and believe it to lead to quicker recovery (despite published reports to the contrary).

Option	Drug	Dose	Route	Use
1	Medetomidine or Dexmedetomidine	0.05 mg/kg or 0.025 mg/kg	i.v. induction to effect	Young and healthy patients that need a quick recovery
	Ketamine	5 mg/kg		
	Buprenorphine or Butorphanol	0.03 mg/kg or 0.1 mg/kg		
2 [a]	Diazepam Midazolam	1–5 mg/kg 1 mg/kg	i.v. induction to effect	Non-painful procedures
	Ketamine	10–40 mg/kg		
3	Midazolam	0.25–0.5 mg/kg	Premedication i.m., s.c.	Painful procedures in debilitated rabbits
	Buprenorphine	0.03–0.05 mg/kg		
	Ketamine	7–10 mg/kg diluted to 1 ml in 0.9% saline	i.v. induction to effect	
4 [b]	Fentanyl	0.0315–0.1575 mg/kg	Premedication i.m., s.c.	Markedly painful procedures requiring a pure mu opioid
	Fluanisone	1–5 mg/kg		
	Midazolam or Diazepam or Propofol or Alfaxalone	0.2–2 mg/kg or 2 mg/kg or 1–6 mg/kg or 1–2 mg/kg	i.v. induction to effect	
5 [c]	Buprenorphine	0.03 mg/kg	Premedication i.m., s.c.	Moderately painful procedures requiring a partial mu opioid
	Alfaxalone	2–3 mg/kg	i.v. induction to effect	
6 [d]	Propofol	10 mg/kg	i.v. induction to effect	

10.19 Rabbit anaesthetic dosages. [a] Gil *et al.* (2004); Mader (2004); [b] Flecknell and Mitchell (1984); Harcourt-Brown (2002); Heard (2004); Martinez *et al.* (2009); [c] Grint *et al.* (2008); [d] Leach *et al.* (2009); Allweiler *et al.* (2010).

Condition/patient type	Pre-anaesthetic medication	Induction	Special considerations
Planned anaesthesia of a young and healthy rabbit	Fentanyl/fluanisone 0.1–0.3 ml/ kg s.c., i.m.	Midazolam i.v. to effect (mean dose 0.7 mg/kg)	
	or no pre-anaesthetic medication	*or* Ketamine 15 mg/kg and medetomidine 0.25 mg/kg i.m., s.c.	Buprenorphine 0.03 mg/kg i.v./s.c./i.m. could be given pre-anaesthetic if a painful procedure is planned
Chronic dental disease and in poor body condition	Fentanyl/fluanisone 0.1 m/kg s.c., i.m.	Midazolam i.v. to effect (mean dose 0.7 mg/kg)	Fluid therapy is essential from pre-anaesthetic through to post anaesthetic and eating and drinking. Employ multimodal analgesia. Provide nutritional support pre- and post-anaesthetic
Respiratory disease	Buprenorphine 0.03 mg/kg i.v. or butorphanol 0.3 mg/kg i.v. and midazolam i.v. to effect (mean dose 0.7 mg/kg)	Ketamine i.v. to effect (mean dose 10 mg/kg). Dilute in 5 ml of saline to ensure slow IV injection to effect can be achieved	• Preoxygenate by mask • Assess the rabbit's ability to oxygenate and ventilate before anaesthesia using capnography and pulse oximetry. If the S_pO_2 levels are <90% on room air and the $ETCO_2$ levels >45 mmHg, anaesthesia should be postponed if possible for stabilization and treatment, e.g. antibiosis • Intubate the trachea so that IPPV is possible if necessary • Maintain with inhalation agents delivered in 100% oxygen • Do not use nitrous oxide • Supplement oxygen and monitor S_pO_2 during recovery from anaesthesia
Emergency anaesthesia of critically ill rabbit	Fentanyl/fluanisone 0.05–0.1 ml/kg s.c., i.m.	Midazolam i.v. to effect (mean dose 0.7 mg/kg) or Chamber induction with sevoflurane and maintain on sevoflurane or isoflurane	Aggressive fluid therapy may be required pre-anaesthetic and continued until the rabbit is stabilized, recovered and eating and drinking
Geriatric	Midazolam or Fentanyl/ fluanisone 0.05–0.1 ml/kg s.c., i.m.	Chamber induction with sevoflurane and maintain on sevoflurane, or isoflurane and maintain on sevoflurane or isoflurane	Fluid therapy is essential from pre-anaesthetic through to post anaesthetic and eating and drinking. Employ multimodal analgesia

10.20 Suggested anaesthetic doses for specific cases.

In these cases buprenorphine may be administered 2 hours later, when the effects of the butorphanol have waned. In cases where severe postoperative pain is likely the fentanyl should not be reversed but analgesia continued with morphine (generally 3–4 hours after the original fentanyl dose).

Propofol, alfaxalone, benzodiazepine antagonists and/or dexmedetomidine have all been used intravenously in combination with fentanyl/fluanisone intramuscularly in order to speed recovery by reducing the dose of the benzodiazepine induction agent. To date only the beneficial effects of propofol use after fentanyl/fluanisone have been reported in the peer-reviewed literature (Martinez *et al.*, 2009). Propofol can still lead to cyanosis and is avoided by some clinicians, and long-term use under anaesthesia has been linked to anaesthetic deaths (Aeschbacher and Webb, 1993). As yet no peer-reviewed data have been reported on alfaxalone use after fentanyl/fluanisone.

Sarmazenil (a benzodiazepine antagonist) has been used extensively by this author, with low doses given intravenously or applied to the buccal mucosa (0.05 mg/kg) to speed recovery. This drug has now been removed from the market, but these findings suggest that other benzodiazepine antagonists, such as flumazenil, may have a significant role in rabbit anaesthesia.

Dexmedetomidine (or medetomidine) can be administered after premedication (possibly at a lower dose) prior to intravenous induction to effect, with a lower dose of an induction agent. Doses used in this fashion may be as low as 0.005–0.02 mg/kg depending on which agent is used. Equally, ketamine could be provided at a low dose to reduce the dose of induction agent further. In either of these cases the dose used could simply be used as the loading dose for a CRI of the agent.

Total intravenous anaesthesia has not been investigated widely in rabbits. Agents commonly used in other species include propofol and alfaxalone (Waelbers *et al.*, 2009). These agents are commonly used incrementally to top up short-term anaesthesia when dental examinations are being performed, with no apparent clinical problems. However no CRI doses have been evaluated in rabbits.

Intubation

One study has reported that only 29% of rabbits are intubated in practice in the UK (Brodbelt, 2006). Rabbit intubation can be a tricky procedure and it takes time to master. However, facemask anaesthesia has been shown to create clinically significant hypoxaemia and hypercapnia and is best avoided (Bateman *et al.*, 2005). Significant tracheal trauma, haemorrhage and oedema can occur with poor intubation technique and respiratory arrest is a potential complication of protracted failed attempts at intubation (Grint *et al.*, 2006; Phaneuf *et al.*, 2006). If a rabbit is going to be maintained on a facemask there is little point in performing an intravenous induction. However agents such as propofol, midazolam and alfaxalone can be diluted in saline to reduce the risk of inadvertent overdose and used to top up an anaesthetic when intubation may not be warranted. Dilutions of up to 1:9 can be used. Many dental procedures are performed without intubation (although it is easy to perform a dental procedure around an endotracheal tube).

All rabbits should be intubated where possible. Techniques such as nasal intubation have been described but should ideally be abandoned once tracheal intubation is mastered (DeValle, 2009). Direct visualization of the larynx is best because this reduces the risk of tracheal trauma and allows evaluation of the oropharynx for food material or foreign bodies. Generally 2–4 mm endotracheal tubes are utilized. Tracheal trauma is a real risk and repeated attempts to intubate can lead to tracheal and glottal oedema and necrosis. This becomes evident usually within a few days post anaesthesia.

Caution and practice are required. Rabbits have a long narrow mouth with a large fleshy tongue and a small gape. This restricted oral access means that intubation is a challenge and makes it difficult to see the larynx. Rabbits are also obligate nasal breathers and therefore the soft palate will have to be disengaged from the epiglottis prior to intubation. There are laryngoscopes specifically marketed for rabbits (such as the Flecknell or Wisconsin blade 0 or 1). A long otoscope cone is used as an alternative by many clinicians. If metal, the otoscope cone can be autoclaved between patients. Perfect restraint is needed although solo intubation is possible with practice. Most rabbits will give a cough response upon intubation; many will be quite light by the time they are intubated and some tooth grinding is to be expected. A set time (e.g. 5 minutes) or number of attempts at intubation (e.g. three) before giving up and resorting to mask induction to reduce the risk of tracheal trauma, cyanosis and death is a sensible protocol. Preoxygenation before and between attempts is vital.

Visual intubation

The rabbit can be positioned in dorsal or ventral recumbency. The head must be held in line with the rest of the body, with the tongue gently extended and held with atraumatic dressing forceps or digital pressure. The head is then hyperextended to pass the tube over the back of the tongue. The front end of the rabbit may also be elevated off the end of the table. The otoscope cone can then be inserted on the other side through the diastema. There are two vascular plexuses, either side of the soft palate, which can be visualized easily. Some clinicians use an introducer which is placed via the otoscope into the glottis. The epiglottis can be seen as a V-shaped silhouette behind the soft palate. Flipping the soft palate up with the endotracheal tube or introducer will lead to breathing sounds being heard up the otoscope and the glottis can be directly visualized. Local anaesthetic (lidocaine) spray can be applied and trickled down the otoscope on to the glottis (Figure 10.21). The otoscope can be removed and the rabbit oxygenated whilst this takes effect.

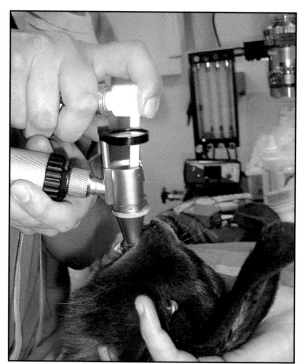

10.21 An otoscope has been used to visualize the glottis, and lidocaine spray is being applied to the glottis.

Cyanosis is common after the soft palate has been displaced, so speed is important, as is oxygenation of the rabbit between attempts. The otoscope or laryngoscope is then removed and a pre-measured endotracheal tube is passed over the introducer into the glottis (Figure 10.22). Suitable introducers can include urinary catheters (usually 6 Fr) with the luer lock cut off. Other clinicians simply pass an endotracheal tube (with the connector removed) without an introducer. A fairly straight endotracheal tube 2–4mm in diameter will be required. A slight twist of the tube encourages it to

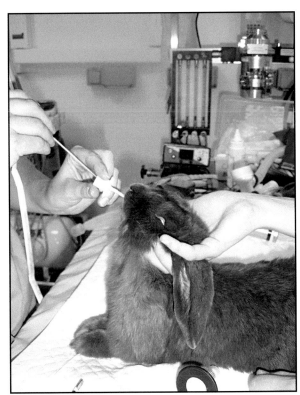

10.22 The endotracheal tube is introduced into the glottis.

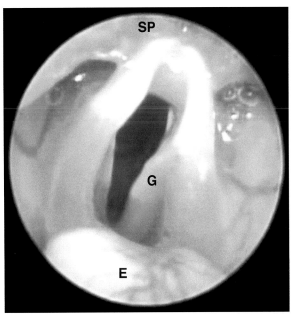

10.23 Endoscopic view of the glottis (G), epiglottis (E) and soft palate (SP).

fall into place. The dead space can be increased with this technique because a slightly longer tube is required and there is an increased risk of bronchial intubation. Some rabbits may be quite light and the otoscope cone can be used as a mouth gag. A few breaths of inhalant usually allow the rabbit to deepen sufficiently to remove the otoscope cone. Once this is performed the endotracheal tube can be secured in place. Intubation rapidly reverses any cyanosis, and capnography can be used to confirm correct placement. Condensation can also be visualized in the endotracheal tube or on a glass slide.

Bronchial intubation is a possible complication and the tube length must be measured accurately. The maximum length is from the point of the lips back to rib number four. Using an otoscope cone necessitates use of a longer tube. The tube must be secured to the head using surgical tape or a bandage.

Endoscopic intubation can also be performed: essentially the endotracheal tube is passed over the endoscope and proximal tracheoscopy is performed with the endotracheal tube then slid off the endoscope. A similar technique involves the endoscope being used to visualize the oropharynx, allowing accurate endotracheal tube placement (Figure 10.23).

Blind intubation

Blind intubation is also commonly performed and can work well if the veterinary surgeon is skilled in this procedure. Listening to breathing noises, rather than gurgling or swallowing noises, guides the clinician while placing the tube. It is important to measure the length of tube that needs to be inserted to reach the level of the larynx from the lips.

However visualization is not possible and foreign bodies may be present, or trauma may occur. It is also difficult to ensure that local anaesthesia has been applied to the larynx. If this technique is attempted it is best to use an otoscope to ensure that the oropharynx is clear and that the lidocaine spray has actually been applied to the glottis.

Once the rabbit is intubated the tube is taped in place (suturing is also an option for facial surgery). A small filter can be attached to reduce respiratory fluid loss and the rabbit is then connected to the anaesthetic circuit.

Laryngeal masks or devices

Alternatives to intubation include a human laryngeal mask or a supraglottic airway device (e.g. V-gel, Docs Innovent) which engages over the glottis (Bateman *et al.*, 2005; Crotaz, 2010; Figure 10.24). The V-gel provides a secure airway, minimizes the risk of tracheal or glottic trauma and is easy to apply.

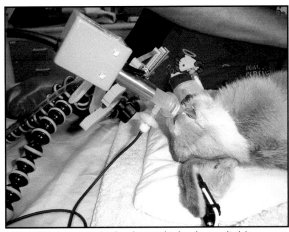

10.24 A supraglottic airway device is a suitable alternative to endotracheal intubation.

Capnography can be used to confirm placement. However tongue compression can be a problem, with some swelling and cyanosis possible, and as it is a blind technique, checking for a clear oropharynx is common sense prior to use. It is impossible to predict whether supraglottic airway devices will replace endotracheal intubation, but they certainly provide a superior alternative to facemask anaesthesia and provide arterial blood gas analysis results that show no statistically significant differences from those of intubated rabbits (Cruz *et al.*, 2000).

Maintenance of anaesthesia

Once the airway is secure the rabbit can be maintained on oxygen with or without the addition of nitrous oxide. The inhaled anaesthetic agent is usually either isoflurane or sevoflurane. Generally, the minimum alveolar concentration (MAC) required is consistent across species and usually 1.5–2 times the MAC is required to maintain anaesthesia. For isoflurane (MAC 2.05% in the rabbit) a 3% setting on the vaporizer is sufficient. For sevoflurane 4–5% may be required. It is important to titrate the level of anaesthesia required based on any premedicants or analgesics used, which will reduce the percentage required. The level of stimulation the patient receives will also influence the concentration required. Keeping the percentage of inhalant as low as possible, based on patient need, reduces patient morbidity and any side effects, as opposed to setting the vaporizer to a particular value and leaving it there.

Any anaesthetic reduces cardiovascular output and ventilation. Mechanical ventilation can be used to ensure sufficient oxygenation of tissues and facilitate carbon dioxide removal. Intermittent positive pressure ventilation (IPPV) is indicated for all rabbits that have been intubated where pulse oximetry and capnography indicate respiratory compromise. Oxygenation is increased and end-tidal carbon dioxide decreased by ventilation. Capnography and pulse oximetry can be used to monitor the effectiveness of mechanical ventilation.

Whilst IPPV can be performed by a veterinary nurse, this may not be practical. In order to achieve effective ventilation the nurse should be focused solely on this task for the duration of anaesthesia; otherwise there is increased risk of ventilation–perfusion mismatching as the pressure, volume and frequency of ventilation are altered markedly. Low-cost pressure cycling systems can be used which measure the pressure at the end of the endotracheal tube (Figure 10.25). They can replace a T-piece and can be set for IPPV or normal ventilation. This system allows IPPV to be instigated and stopped at any point during the procedure, depending on the requirements of the patient. This is of particular importance during thoracic surgery or for laparoscopic procedures. These units measure pressure at the end of the endotracheal tube and allow a unidirectional flow of gas until a particular pressure is reached, which then opens a valve. Expiration is achieved by the patient's natural recoil, and after a time lag (set by the operator) a valve shuts, causing the animal's lungs to fill with oxygen (inspiration)

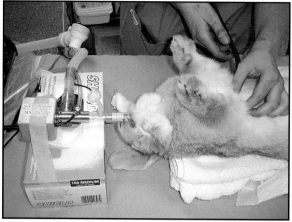

10.25 Mechanical positive pressure ventilators can be used to improve oxygenation and ventilation under anaesthesia.

until the set pressure is reached again. This is a simple system to use and the pressure setting is gauged by observing the animal's chest movements, which should equate to those expected in a conscious rabbit. It is best to start at lower pressures, observe the chest movements of the patient and increase pressure slowly to achieve normal chest movements. Increasing pressure increases lung volume (based on lung compliance). The frequency should also be set to the normal anticipated respiratory rate (typically 30–60 breaths per minute). Volume-limited units deliver a set volume, and both types have potential problems. If the pressure increases pressure-limited units will not inflate the animal's lungs, and if there is a leak they may never inflate them sufficiently. Volume-limited units deliver the set volume whatever the pressure, and if there is a leak and the gas escapes the patient will not be ventilated. It is important to monitor the effectiveness of a mechanical ventilation system at all times.

When used appropriately, IPPV facilitates and stabilizes anaesthesia, and ensures delivery of the inhalational agent to the lungs, oxygenation of the lungs and removal of carbon dioxide from the alveoli.

Monitoring rabbits during anaesthesia

Monitoring patients under anaesthesia is important and is typically performed by a veterinary nurse. However, particularly if IPPV is employed, the clinical parameters used to monitor anaesthesia can be limited in rabbits and monitoring devices can help to reduce both morbidity and mortality under anaesthesia.

The reflexes and parameters typically monitored to evaluate the plane of anaesthesia include the following.

Toe pinch/withdrawal reflex and ear pinch

These are commonly performed but are not reliable as an indicator of anaesthetic depth in all cases. For a surgical plane of anaesthesia the ear pinch and hindlimb toe pinch reflexes should be absent and the forelimb toe pinch reflex barely present. Loss of the forelimb toe pinch reflex can indicate a dangerous depth of anaesthesia.

Heart and respiratory rate and rhythm

All anaesthetic agents depress cardiorespiratory function and continuous monitoring of the heart and respiratory rates is important. A stethoscope or an oesophageal stethoscope can be utilized in rabbits and the results obtained used to check the functioning of monitoring devices (Figure 10.26). Peripheral pulses, mucous membrane colour, tackiness and refill time can also help to evaluate perfusion. The central auricular artery is easy to find in rabbits.

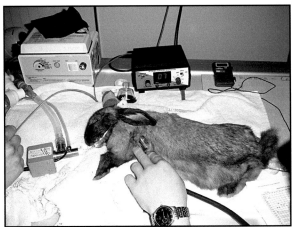

10.26   The use of a stethoscope to monitor heart rate and respiratory rate during anaesthesia. Standard monitoring techniques should be routinely performed and compared with those provided by monitoring devices.

Eye position and palpebral reflex

The palpebral reflex may not be lost until the rabbit is very deeply anaesthetized, and patients anaesthetized with ketamine can have unpredictable results, with the reflex being lost early on.

Voluntary movement and response to surgery

Ideally these should be pre-empted and the plane altered accordingly to the level of surgical stimulation.

Temperature

The rectal or oesophageal temperature must be monitored throughout anaesthesia and recorded. Supportive care measures to maintain core temperature were discussed earlier in this chapter.

Pulse oximetry

Pulse oximetry measures the oxygenation of the patient by using the oxygen saturation of the haemoglobin molecules (S_pO_2). This correlates well with the arterial oxygen (P_aO_2) levels. The machines are based on the human oxygen–haemoglobin dissociation curve, and normal values should be 96% or more. Caution is advised if alpha-2 agonists are utilized because poor peripheral perfusion can lead to improper functioning of the unit, as can skin pigmentation when it is placed on the ear. Probes can be difficult to attach to the ear in some of the smaller rabbits, but they can be attached to the tongue (Figure 10.27) or inserted in the rectum, thus avoiding any issues with pigmentation. Pulse

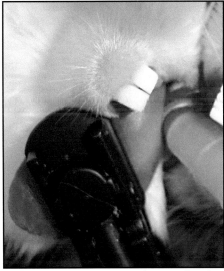

10.27   Pulse oximetry probes can be placed on the tongue.

oximetry does not provide information on blood flow or oxygenation of the rabbit's tissues (which is the important objective). Many machines are manufactured for human use and are unable to detect heart rates over 250 beats per minute. There are machines on the market that can record rates up to 350 beats per minute; this can still be exceeded by rabbits but is unusual in the clinical setting. Pulse oximetry does not give information about the effective ventilation of the patient. The machines are also quite insensitive because patients are being given 100% oxygen and there has to be significant respiratory compromise before the S_pO_2 drops below 93%. Monitoring the trend can be more useful. For these reasons pulse oximetry has fallen out of favour with some anaesthetists.

Capnography

This measures effective ventilation of the patient. Ventilatory failure is the most common cause of morbidity and mortality under anaesthesia. Capnography is highly sensitive and reacts far more quickly than pulse oximetry in an emergency situation. Capnography measures the end-tidal CO_2 ($ETCO_2$) level. It depends on the rapid exchange of gases between the lungs and the circulation and $ETCO_2$ correlates well with P_aCO_2 in anaesthetized rabbits. This is a real-time monitoring system and is highly sensitive. Hand-held units are available that detect CO_2 in the air flow in the anaesthetic circuit. Most units available are side-stream monitors that continuously remove a small portion of air for analysis. This can be a problem in small patients where there are low flow rates and creates a small delay as it takes a little time for the air to reach the unit. In-circuit analysers would be better in these circumstances, but they are more expensive and side-stream sampling has not caused an obvious problem clinically when ventilating small patients.

A capnograph can be used on anaesthetized or conscious patients (to help in the clinical assessment of hypercapnia for example, because mucous membrane colour is unreliable), and all species have similar $ETCO_2$ values. The display is simple to use and interpret. Side-stream units are most commonly used (as opposed to mainstream units which are more costly), but it is important to ensure that these have a low flow rate to avoid interrupting the gas flow for small patients. Small adapters can be utilized to minimize dead space (Figure 10.28). Respiratory rates up to 120 breaths per minute can be recorded. A capnograph also displays a real-time waveform of the level of CO_2 in the gas flow, allowing the clinician to evaluate underlying pathology, the respiratory rate and the $ETCO_2$.

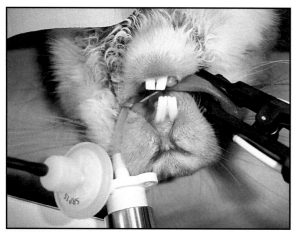

10.28 A small dead space connector can be fixed on to the endotracheal tube and used for capnography.

The normal capnograph display consists of a number of phases:

- **Phase I:** Expiration of air from the dead space. This air has not been in contact with alveolar air and should not contain a high level of CO_2
- **Phase II:** Expiration of air from the dead space and air in contact with respiratory surfaces. Increasing CO_2 levels occur until there is expiration only of air in contact with the respiratory membranes
- **Phase III:** Expiration of air in contact with respiratory membranes. The plateau is the $ETCO_2$
- **Phase 0:** Inspiration, with zero CO_2. The level of CO_2 is low in inspired air.

Evaluation of the waveform involves the frequency, rhythm, height, baseline and overall shape. The tracings can be used to verify intubation (CO_2 from expiration can be detected), rebreathing (elevated baseline), hypoventilation (ascending plateau), hyperventilation (descending plateau), $ETCO_2$ (height), airway obstruction (no CO_2 can be detected), leakage of gas from the system (varying plateau and $ETCO_2$), and a fall in cardiac output will reduce overall height as a result of decreased gaseous exchange. The $ETCO_2$ should be 4.5–5.9% (34–45 mmHg) in most cases. Artificial ventilation should be tailored to maintain these levels. If ventilation is not being performed routinely, interpretation of

the capnograph is important so that manual positive pressure ventilation can be used if needed. Should ventilatory problems continue then doxapram can be used to reverse the depressant effects of opioids, in particular fentanyl.

Capnography requires a secure airway and this can limit its usefulness if the rabbit is not intubated. Adequate oxygenation does not equal adequate ventilation, and adequate ventilation does not equate to adequate oxygenation. However, failure to provide adequate ventilation is far more likely than inadequate oxygenation. There is a lot to be said for using both oximetry and capnography where possible.

Doppler ultrasonography

Doppler devices have become increasingly available in clinical practice for monitoring blood pressure in other species. They are easy to use and allow an audible continuous readout of the heart rate and blood flow. The rhythm and rate can be assessed. The probes can be taped in place over a peripheral vessel. Flat probes are best for these purposes, although a pen-style probe can be used for intermittent evaluation. The heart rate can be calculated or the anaesthetist can concentrate on the rhythm and pick up subtle changes in rate in real time. The second advantage of these units is for indirect blood pressure monitoring (Figure 10.29). All anaesthetic agents will create some hypotension during anaesthesia (as a result of reduced baroreceptor reflex and vasodilation). Measuring blood pressure will allow fluid therapy to be titrated, particularly if colloids are used. Usually systolic pressure in the anaesthetized rabbit ranges between 92 and 135 mmHg (lower than in dogs and cats). The foreleg is typically used but the hindlimb can also be used, allowing the best access for the anaesthetist and surgeon. The cuff is placed high up on the limb with the Doppler probe below. The cuff width should be 40% of the limb circumference for optimal results.

The probe is placed on the caudal aspect of the midline of the foot behind the carpus or tarsus, which can be shaved and/or have a copious amount of lubricating jelly applied. The pulse can be palpated

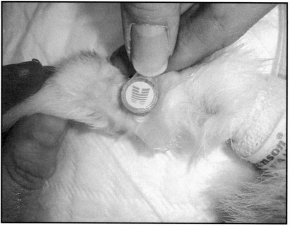

10.29 Blood pressure monitoring can provide useful information and allow anaesthetic depth and fluid therapy to be titrated to the requirements of the rabbit.

or the Doppler used to locate the artery. Once the artery is identified, surgical tape can be used to secure the Doppler probe in place. The cuff is placed higher up the limb, over the antebrachium or tibia. Blood flow is confirmed again and the Doppler probe adjusted if required. The cuff is inflated until sounds are lost. The cuff is then slowly deflated until the systolic flow is audible again. This is repeated three times and the average systolic blood pressure reading is taken. In the anaesthetized rabbit the Doppler technique has been shown to underestimate systolic blood pressure by an average of 5 mmHg (±9 mmHg) and to overestimate mean blood pressure by an average of 10 mmHg (±8 mmHg) (Harvey and Murison, 2010).

Electrocardiography

This is more time-consuming and it is difficult to obtain consistent readings. Use of electrical items (such as radiosurgery) can lead to electrical interference and therefore electrocardiography is less commonly used as an anaesthetic monitoring tool. However, specific patients, based on their presentation, may well require electrocardiography recording as part of a safe anaesthetic regime.

- The red cable (white in the USA) attaches to the right foreleg.
- The yellow cable (black in the USA) attaches to the left foreleg.
- The green cable (red in the USA) attaches to the left hindleg.
- The black cable (green in the USA) is the earth cable and attaches to the right hindleg.

Filed-down crocodile clips can be used to reduce trauma. The development of smaller oesophageal electrocardiography probes (such as those made by Vetronic services) has greatly simplified the use as a monitoring tool and the popularity is likely to increase.

Complications arising from anaesthesia

Respiratory compromise is the most important complication that can occur with anaesthesia (Brodbelt, 2006) and can largely be prevented by securing the airway and using capnography and mechanical ventilation. Arterial blood gas analysis can also be useful in detecting longer-term abnormalities. If the airway is not secure, placement of a supraglottic airway device is a very quick method that allows oxygenation and mechanical ventilation in a crash situation. If oxygen is not immediately available then an Ambu bag or a resuscitator can be used to deliver room air as an alternative. However, increasing the inspired oxygen level has a marked effect on arterial oxygenation and should be performed as quickly as possible.

Cardiovascular complications typically result from anaesthetic overdose, and having an intravenous line and reversal agents on standby is important for rapid correction of a dropping heart rate. The use of Doppler ultrasonography allows any reduction in heart rate to be identified immediately, and a reduction in blood pressure can also be detected. Fluid therapy, including colloids, can be used to maintain blood pressure. Emergency drugs (see Figure 10.14) and aggressive (but not excessive) fluid therapy can be administered in critical situations while cardiac compression is instigated.

Cardiorespiratory resuscitation techniques

Respiratory arrest: If the rabbit's trachea is intubated, it is necessary first to check that the tube is patent and has not become dislodged or blocked with secretions or debris. After patency has been confirmed, IPPV can be applied (at 20–30 breaths per minute) using 100% oxygen and an appropriate breathing system until spontaneous ventilation returns.

If the rabbit's trachea is not intubated, the head and neck should be extended, the tongue pulled forward, oxygen supplied using a tightly fitting facemask, or a laryngeal mask or device, and IPPV started. A supraglottic airway device can be inserted as an alternative. Capnography can be used to identify carbon dioxide in exhaled air.

The volatile agent should be turned off and specific antagonists for any components of the anaesthetic protocol administered (e.g. atipamezole to reverse alpha-2 adrenergic agonists, naloxone to reverse opioids, and flumazenil to reverse benzodiazepines; Figure 10.30).

Agent	Dose
Atipamezole	Give 5 times the medetomidine dose or 2.5 times the dexmedetomidine dose (the same volume for many available products)
Naloxone	10–100 µg/kg
Flumazenil	0.025 mg/kg

10.30 Reversal agents used in rabbits.

Doxapram (10 mg/kg i.v. or sublingual) is a central respiratory stimulant that may increase the rate and depth of breathing, but also increases oxygen demand so should be used with caution.

Cardiac arrest: The steps described above should be carried out, and cardiac compressions started at approximately 100 compressions per minute. The anaesthetist's thumb and forefinger should compress the chest directly over the heart at a regular rhythm. If an ECG is available the heart rhythm should be monitored and emergency drugs (see Figure 10.14) can be administered as appropriate.

Recovery from anaesthesia

The postoperative period is a period of high risk and accounts for 64% of perioperative rabbit deaths (Brodbelt, 2006). Once gaseous agents have been turned off, continued respiratory support is indicated because respiratory compromise is common during recovery. Rabbits are generally left on oxygen until extubated, and ventilation may be required. Further oxygenation can then be provided via a facemask (Figure 10.31) and supplemental oxygen provided in the recovery cage if indicated. Reversal agents should be administered at the completion of the procedure, but this has to be balanced with the analgesic effects of agents such as the alpha-2 agonists or opioids, which may be beneficial in the immediate postoperative period. If low doses have been used reversal may not hasten the return to mobility and feeding.

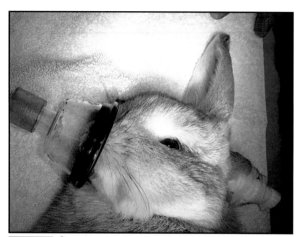

10.31 Supplemental oxygen is important during recovery. Oxygen can be given by facemask after removal of the endotracheal tube.

Monitoring of the rectal temperature, pulse and respiration should be continued, every 5 minutes or more frequently as needed. Most rabbits benefit from an ambient temperature of 26–30°C in the recovery period and therefore they are best held in incubators. Rabbits need to be transferred to lower temperatures once they are mobile, and then require further observation to ensure that normothermia is maintained once thermal support is removed. A potential solution to this is to reduce the temperature of the incubator gradually while continuing to monitor the rabbit's rectal temperature. Continuous recording devices (Figure 10.32) are helpful because the temperature can be recorded

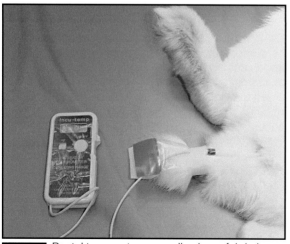

10.32 Rectal temperature recording is useful during recovery. Digital temperature recording devices provide a continuous readout of rectal temperature.

remotely with minimal disturbance of the patient and loss of heat from the incubator, for example. Higher relative humidities can also benefit recovering patients and reduce the risk of dehydration.

Jaw tone and movement are indications that recovery is imminent and the endotracheal tube can be removed. In many cases the tube stimulates the patient and once it has been removed many patients will tolerate further oxygen by mask. The return of shivering thermogenesis is also an indication of recovery. Once the rabbit stops tolerating oxygen by facemask it can be moved to a warm recovery cage for further close observation.

It is important to plan the recovery and have a warmed recovery cage prepared. This may be an incubator, propagator or a cage in a warmed room. It is important to continue to monitor respiration, heart rate and rectal temperature throughout the recovery period. All measures used to maintain normothermia during anaesthesia should be maintained during the initial phase of recovery. It can be more difficult to apply many of the techniques, but continuous monitoring is possible alongside the use of towels, blankets and heat mats (caution is advised because these can be damaged by nails or teeth), as both hypothermia and hyperthermia are possible. Once moved into the brooder or cage, the rabbit is still at risk of hypothermia, but this risk decreases as the rabbit's ability to regulate its own temperature returns. At this point, close observation is still required but a gradual reduction in thermal support is indicated. Rectal temperature monitoring should be provided throughout this period. It is important to ensure that a rabbit is capable of maintaining its rectal temperature without thermal support before being transported to the usual hospital cage. Rectal temperature will require further monitoring.

Food and water should be provided once the rabbit is coordinated; some rabbits will get wet if bowls of water are provided, and this can chill the patient. It is important to provide hide boxes, towels, blankets and nesting material where appropriate to allow recovering rabbits to hide. The ward temperature may be elevated slightly in the initial period or maintained overnight. Digital fan heaters are available with a thermostat, which can be used to keep a ward at an even overnight temperature. Feeding, drinking and faecal and urine outputs should be monitored post anaesthesia. Fluid therapy and analgesia will need to be continued during this period. Nutritional support is important. On recovery from anaesthesia, support of any problems detected in the pre-anaesthetic examination should be continued. Assessment and support is continued until the rabbit is eating well and passing normal faecal pellets. Assisted feeding with high-fibre diets also stimulates gastrointestinal motility.

A period of hospitalization may be indicated, depending on the condition of the animal. Further antibiotics and analgesics may also be required. Keeping rabbits in overnight will allow provision of further analgesia and monitoring of faecal output. Assisted feeding can also be instigated.

It is important to advise the owner on homecare at the discharge appointment. The rabbit must be mobile and eating and drinking before discharge. Minimizing stress and pain and providing palatable foods help to promote this. Monitoring faecal and urinary output is vital. Occasionally there will be small, dry firm pellets produced initially but defecation should quickly return to normal.

References and further reading

Aeschbacher G and Webb AI (1993) Propofol in rabbits. 2. Long term anaesthesia. *Laboratory Animal Science* **43**, 365–373

Allweiler S, Leach MC and Flecknell PA (2010) The use of propofol and sevoflurane for surgical anaesthesia in New Zealand White rabbits. *Laboratory Animals* **44**, 113–117

Bateman L, Ludders JW and Gleed RD (2005) Comparison between facemask and laryngeal mask airway in rabbits during isoflurane anesthesia. *Veterinary Anaesthesia and Analgesia* **32**, 280–288

Briggs SL, Sneed K and Sawyer DC (1998) Antinociceptive effects of oxymorphone-butorphanol-acepromazine combination in cats. *Veterinary Surgery* **27**, 466–472

Brodbelt DC (2006) *The Confidential Enquiry into Perioperative Small Animal Fatalities*. PhD thesis, Royal Veterinary College

Crotaz IR (2010) Initial feasibility investigation of the v-gel airway: an anatomically designed supraglottic airway device for use in companion animal veterinary anaesthesia. *Veterinary Anaesthesia and Analgesia* **37**, 579–580

Cruz M, Sacci T, Luna S, Braz J and Cassu R (2000) Use of a laryngeal mask for airway maintenance during inhalation anaesthesia in rabbits. *Veterinary Anaesthesia and Analgesia* **27**, 112–116

DeValle JMS (2009) Successful management of rabbit anaesthesia through the use of nasotracheal intubation. *Journal of the American Association for Laboratory Animal Science* **48**(3), 166–170

Diesel G (2011) Review of adverse events following off-label use of medicines. *Veterinary Record* **168**, 205–207

Difilippo SM, Norberg PJ, Suson UD, et al. (2004) A comparison of xylazine and medetomidine in an anaesthetic combination in New Zealand white rabbit. *Contemporary Topics in Laboratory Animal Science* **43**, 32–34

Dollo G, Malinovsky JM, Péron A, et al. (2004) Prolongation of epidural bupivacaine effects with hyaluronic acid in rabbits. *International Journal of Pharmacology* **272**, 109–119

Eatwell K, Mancinelli E, Hedley J, et al. (2013) Use of arterial blood gas analysis as a superior method for evaluating respiratory function in pet rabbits (*Oryctolagus cuniculus*). *Veterinary Record* **173**(7), 166

Flecknell PA (2000) Anaesthesia. In: *Manual of Rabbit Medicine and Surgery*, ed. PA Flecknell, pp.103–116. BSAVA Publications, Gloucester

Flecknell PA, Liles JH and Wootton R (1989) Reversal of fentanyl/fluanisone neuroleptanalgesia in the rabbit using mixed agonist/antagonist opioids. *Laboratory Animals* **23**, 147–155

Flecknell PA and Mitchell M (1984) Midazolam and fentanyl-fluanisone: assessment of anaesthetic effects in laboratory rodents and rabbits. *Laboratory Animals* **18**, 147–160

Flecknell PA, Roughan JV and Hedenqvist P (1999) Induction of anaesthesia with sevoflurane and isoflurane in the rabbit. *Laboratory Animals* **33**, 41–46

Fleureaux O, Estbe JP, Blery C, Douet N and Mallenant Y (1995) Effects of preoxygenation methods on the course of PaO₂ and PaCO₂ in anaesthetic post induction apnea. *Cahiers de Anaesthésiologie* **43**(4), 367–370

Foxhall F (2008) The parameters. In: *Arterial Blood Gas Analysis: An easy learning guide*, ed. F Foxall, pp.1–12. M&K Publishing, Cumbria

Ghaffari MS, Moghaddassi AP and Bokaie S (2009) Effects of intramuscular acepromazine and diazepam on tear production in rabbits. *Veterinary Record* **164**, 147–148

Gil AG, Silvan G, Illera M, et al. (2004) The effects of anaesthesia on the clinical chemistry of New Zealand white rabbits. *Contemporary Topics in Laboratory Animal Science* **43**, 25–29

Grint NJ, Sayers IR, Cecchi R, Harley R and Day MJ (2006) Postanaesthetic tracheal strictures in three rabbits. *Laboratory Animals* **40**, 301–308

Grint NJ, Smith HE and Senior JM (2008) Clinical evaluation of alfaxalone in cyclodextrin for the induction of anaesthesia in rabbits. *Veterinary Record* **163**, 395–396

Harcourt-Brown F (2002) Anaesthesia and analgesia. In: *Textbook of Rabbit Medicine*, ed. F Harcourt-Brown, pp.121–139. Butterworth-Heinemann, Oxford

Harvey L and Murison P (2010) Comparison of direct and Doppler arterial blood pressure measurements in rabbits during isoflurane anaesthesia. Abstract presented at *Spring AVA Conference, Cambridge, UK, 30–31 March 2010*

Heard JD (2004) Anesthesia, analgesia and sedation of small mammals. In: *Ferrets, Rabbits and Rodents: Clinical Medicine and Surgery*, ed. KE Quensenberry and JW Carpenter, pp.356–369. Saunders, St Louis

Hedenqvist P and Hellebrekers LJ (2003) Laboratory animal analgesia, anesthesia, and euthanasia. In: *Handbook of Laboratory Animal Science*, 2nd edn, No. 1, ed. J Hau and GL Van Hoosier, pp.413–455. CRC Press, Boca Raton, FL

Hedenqvist P, Roughan JV, Orr HE, et al. (2001) Assessment of ketamine/medetomidine anaesthesia in the New Zealand White rabbit. *Veterinary Anaesthesia and Analgesia* **28**, 18–25

Leach MC, Allweiler S, Richardson C, et al. (2009) Behavioural effects of ovariohysterectomy and oral administration of meloxicam in laboratory housed rabbits. *Research in Veterinary Science* **87**, 336–347

Mader D (2004) Rabbits: Basic approach to veterinary care. In: *Ferrets, Rabbits and Rodents: Clinical Medicine and Surgery*, ed. KE Quensenberry and JW Carpenter, pp.147–154. Saunders, St Louis

Malinovsky JM, Charles F, Baudrimont M, et al. (2002) Intrathecal ropivacaine in rabbits: pharmacodynamic and neurotoxicologic study. *Anesthesiology* **97**(2), 429–435

Marsh MK, McLeod SR, Hansen A and Maloney SK (2009) Induction of anaesthesia in wild rabbits using a new alfaxalone formulation. *Veterinary Record* **164**, 122–123

Martinez MA, Murison PJ and Love E (2009) Induction of anaesthesia with either midazolam or propofol in rabbits premedicated with fentanyl/fluanisone. *Veterinary Record* **164**, 803–806

Nevalainen T, Phyhala L, Voipio HM, et al. (1989) Evaluation of anaesthetic potency of medetomidine-ketamine combination in rats, guinea-pigs and rabbits. *Acta Veterinaria Scandinavica* **85**(Suppl), 139–143

Orr HE, Roughan JV and Flecknell PA (2005) Assessment of ketamine and medetomidine in the domestic rabbit. *Veterinary Anaesthesia and Analgesia* **32**, 271–279

Phaneuf LR, Barker S, Groleau MA and Turner PV (2006) Tracheal injury after endotracheal intubation and anaesthesia in rabbits. *Journal of the American Association for Laboratory Animal Sciences* **45**, 67–72

Smith MA, Barrett AC and Picker MJ (1999) Antinociceptive effects of opioids following acute and chronic administration of butorphanol: influence of stimulus intensity and relative efficacy at the mu receptor. *Psychopharmacology* **143**, 261–269

Uilenreef JJ, Murrell JC, McKusick BC and Hellebrekers LJ (2008) Dexmedetomidine continuous rate infusion during isoflurane anaesthesia in canine surgical patients. *Veterinary Anaesthesia and Analgesia* **35**, 1–12

Waelbers T, Vermoere P and Polis I (2009) Total intravenous anaesthesia in dogs. *Vlaams Diergeneeskundig Tijdschrift* **78**(3), 160–169

Yamashita A, Mishiya M, Satoshi M, et al. (2003) A comparison of the neurotoxic effects on the spinal cord of tetracaine, lidocaine, bupivacaine, and ropivacaine administered intrathecally in rabbits. *Anesthesia and Analgesia* **97**, 512–519

11

Respiratory disease

Joanna Hedley

Respiratory problems are one of the most common reasons for which pet rabbits are presented to a veterinary practice. Unlike dogs and cats, rabbits have the disadvantage of being almost obligate nasal breathers owing to the anatomical positioning of their epiglottis over the soft palate. This effectively separates the oral cavity from the respiratory system. Consequently, upper respiratory tract disease may result in significant respiratory compromise that should not be underestimated.

Pasteurella multocida is the most common infectious agent involved but many other causes exist, so a full diagnostic work-up should always be carried out. Underlying factors such as inadequate ventilation, overcrowding or concurrent disease may contribute significantly to the progression of respiratory problems and should always be considered.

Clinical investigation

Clinical examination
On clinical examination it is important to attempt to determine whether respiratory disease is affecting the upper or lower respiratory tract (or both) because this will affect further diagnostics and treatment.

Observation
Initially the patient should be evaluated in its carrier to assess the respiratory rate and pattern before handling. The normal respiratory rate in a calm rabbit is 30–60 breaths per minute. However, many individuals will be tachypnoeic owing to the stress of transport and being in an unfamiliar environment. Despite this, a normal rabbit should show minimal abdominal effort and no respiratory noises should be heard from a distance. An asynchronous breathing pattern (when the thorax and abdomen contract at different times) may be observed in cases of pleural disease and requires further investigation. After observation from a distance, a full clinical examination may be performed.

Very dyspnoeic animals (Figure 11.1) may benefit from being supplemented with oxygen prior to examination, but most cases will tolerate at least a brief assessment before a decision is made regarding investigations and treatment.

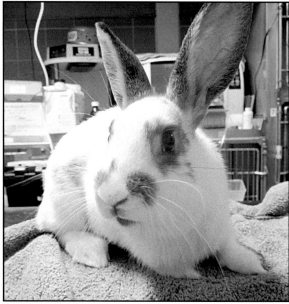

11.1 Rabbit mouth-breathing as a result of a tracheal stricture. Open-mouth breathing or cyanosis is always a poor prognostic indicator and these cases should be treated with extreme care, supplemented with oxygen, and handling should be minimized until the patient is more stable.

Upper respiratory tract disease
Rabbits with upper respiratory tract disease often present with nasal discharge, snuffling and sneezing. Some animals may be anorexic and they can be markedly dyspnoeic if the upper airways are becoming obstructed. Nasal discharge is not always noticed by owners if the rabbit is grooming it away, but matted fur on the medial forelimbs and paws usually indicates that discharge has been present. Both nares should be checked for patency; if in any doubt, a clear glass slide recently wetted with alcohol may be placed beneath the nares. Fogging of the slide indicates that the associated nasal canal is patent. The head should be examined for symmetry and the margins of the nasal cavity and sinuses palpated thoroughly.

A full oral examination should also be performed (see *BSAVA Manual of Rabbit Surgery, Dentistry and Imaging*) because dental disease is often associated with upper respiratory problems. Ocular discharge may be observed associated with conjunctivitis and dacryocystitis, and pressure over the lacrimal sac at the medial canthus of the eye may result in a discharge from the nasolacrimal punctum. In these cases the nasolacrimal ducts should be flushed to ensure their patency (Figure 11.2); copious discharge may be expelled. Neurological signs such as a head tilt or circling may also be observed if infection has ascended via the Eustachian tube to affect the middle and inner ear.

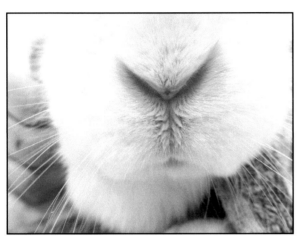

11.2 Fluorescein dye may be instilled into the eyes in dacryocystitis. If nasolacrimal ducts are patent, the dye should be visible at both nares.

Lower respiratory tract disease

Rabbits with lower respiratory tract disease usually present with dyspnoea, and respiratory noises such as wheezing may be heard. Coughing is possible but does not commonly occur. Such rabbits may be lethargic, and have a reduced appetite and associated weight loss.

Unfortunately disease is often subclinical or only associated with subtle signs until fairly advanced. Exercise tolerance can be difficult for owners to assess but activity levels may be reduced. Rabbits that have been sitting still for longer periods often have moderate to severe bilateral hock pododermatitis, and detection of these lesions should lead the clinician to question the rabbit's activity levels, especially if lesions have not previously been present.

Auscultation

The whole thorax and trachea should be thoroughly auscultated. Paediatric stethoscopes can be particularly useful for auscultation of a rabbit's small lung fields. Inspiration and expiration are normally fairly quiet in a calm rabbit, although some stressed individuals may grunt on examination. Adventitious lung sounds may include crackles (rales) or wheezes. Crackles are usually inspiratory and occur as a result of the re-opening of airways that have closed during expiration. Wheezes may be inspiratory or expiratory but are usually higher pitched sounds that occur because of the passage of air through narrowed bronchi. Upper respiratory noise may be referred to the thorax, thus making it difficult to assess lung sounds fully, especially in a stressed tachypnoeic patient. However, these noises often diminish if the rabbit is allowed time to calm

down and for its respiratory rate to slow to normal levels, allowing better evaluation of the lower respiratory system. Patchy loss of sounds may indicate lung consolidation or an underlying mass. The chests of larger rabbits may also be percussed, which can be useful in identification of areas of consolidation. Finally, the heart should be thoroughly auscultated in order to rule out cardiovascular abnormalities, which may present with similar clinical signs.

Radiography

Radiography is usually the first step in diagnosis of a respiratory condition. Regardless of whether the disease appears to be affecting the upper or lower respiratory tract, multiple skull and thoracic views should be taken in order to confirm the extent of disease. Sedation or general anaesthesia is generally required for adequate positioning. However, in collapsed dyspnoeic patients in which general anaesthesia carries a higher risk, conscious radiographs may be preferred initially and more detailed views taken once the patient is stabilized. Mild sedation with midazolam and butorphanol may be used to reduce stress and allow positioning to obtain more diagnostic films.

Skull radiographs should include lateral, dorsoventral, left and right oblique and rostrocaudal views in order to assess the nasal cavity, sinuses, dental arcades and tympanic bullae. Changes may be subtle but any asymmetry, increased opacity or areas of bone lysis may indicate underlying disease.

Thoracic radiographs should include both lateral and dorsoventral views. Interpretation of thoracic radiographs, especially the cranial lung lobes, may be challenging owing to the small size of the thoracic cavity. Ideally the forelimbs should be extended cranially, the rabbit intubated and the film taken on inspiration. An increased bronchial, interstitial, alveolar or mixed pattern may indicate pneumonia, but radiographic changes may not be present in early stages of the disease process. Increased radio-pacity of the cranial lung lobe, displacement of the heart caudally and elevation of the trachea may indicate a cranial thoracic mass such as a thymoma. The heart should be evaluated and measured to rule out potential cardiac disease (see Chapter 14).

Ultrasonography

Ultrasonography is of limited use in most cases of respiratory disease but may be helpful in the investigation of a suspected thoracic mass such as a thymoma. In these cases, aspirates may be obtained under ultrasound guidance to confirm diagnosis.

Computed tomography and magnetic resonance imaging

Computed tomography (CT) is an extremely useful tool in the diagnosis of respiratory disease. Sedation or a short general anaesthetic is usually required but excellent images of the skull and thoracic cavity can be obtained. It is the imaging modality of choice for detection and full evaluation of rhinitis, sinusitis (Figure 11.3), dental disease, otitis media and pulmonary disease. However, availability in practice may

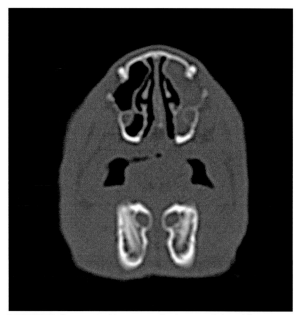

11.3 Computed tomography is a useful tool for detecting sinusitis. The left sinuses of this rabbit were found on surgical exploration to be filled with purulent material.

be limited and, although costs are reducing, CT is still more expensive than radiography.

Magnetic resonance imaging (MRI) is more useful for soft tissue imaging, such as further evaluation of a thoracic mass. However it is more expensive, often less easily available than CT and usually requires a longer period of general anaesthesia so is not yet commonly used in practice.

Endoscopy

Endoscopy is extremely useful in the diagnosis of respiratory disease and is usually more readily available in practice than CT or MRI. For upper respiratory disease, rhinoscopy may be performed. This is a relatively easy technique in rabbits >2 kg and to a limited extent in smaller individuals. Rabbits should be anaesthetized and intubated for this procedure, but even at a surgical plane of anaesthesia a certain amount of sneezing may be expected in those individuals with rhinitis. The use of a 1.9 mm rigid endoscope with sheath is recommended. The endoscope may be advanced from the nares caudally along the ventral and middle nasal meatus to assess the nasal cavity and sinus openings (Figure 11.4). Biopsy samples of the nasal mucosa can be taken for histopathology and culture. A small amount of haemorrhage may be expected, especially with diseased tissue, but should not be significant if the endoscope is used gently. Care should be taken, however, to avoid damaging the nasal turbinates, which may bleed profusely if traumatized.

The nasal cavity may also be flushed under endoscopic guidance to aid removal of any excess mucus or debris. Flushing should only be performed in an intubated patient; the oral cavity should be packed with gauze and the rabbit positioned at an angle to allow fluid to drain out of the mouth, in

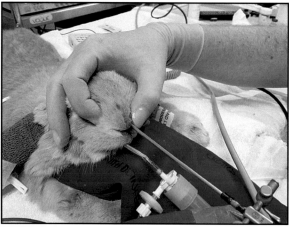

11.4 A rigid endoscope can be used to investigate upper respiratory tract disease.

order to avoid aspiration. Both nasal canals should ideally be evaluated but if significant haemorrhage or swelling is encountered on one side the clinician may opt not to evaluate the other side at the same time, in order not to compromise respiration. Retrograde flexible endoscopy may also be used to evaluate the caudal nasopharynx, especially in cases with a suspected foreign body. It can, however, be a more challenging procedure owing to the anatomy of the elongated soft palate, and often requires practice.

For lower respiratory disease, tracheoscopy may be performed. Rabbits should be anaesthetized and either rigid or flexible endoscopy may be used, as in cats and dogs.

Haematology and biochemistry

It is useful to check haematology and biochemistry in any sick rabbit. Haematological abnormalities may be revealed in cases with respiratory disease, though parameters are often within normal limits.

Bacterial diseases

Pasteurellosis

Pasteurella multocida is a Gram-negative bacterium and the most common cause of respiratory disease in rabbits (Rougier *et al.*, 2006). However various other infectious agents may also be isolated and are thought to play a significant role in respiratory disease. It is therefore important not to assume automatically that pasteurellosis is the problem in every rabbit with respiratory signs.

P. multocida appears to be a commensal bacterium of the respiratory tract in most if not all pet rabbits, and prevalence increases with age. However, not all infected rabbits will develop respiratory disease. Some will have no clinical signs, others develop a low-grade chronic infection and some develop acute disease. Various strains of *P. multocida* exist, with a few types causing septicaemia and death within 24 hours, often with no respiratory signs. Factors determining the course of the disease include the strain and virulence of the bacterium, and the host immune response. Any potential stressor, such as moving to a new home, heat stress, overcrowding, a change in social structure or concurrent disease will potentially predispose to clinical pasteurellosis. Chronically poor standards of hygiene with inadequate ventilation and elevated environmental ammonia levels will also predispose to disease. Alternatively, treatment with corticosteroids will cause immunosuppression and may result in pasteurellosis.

Transmission is generally via direct contact with nasal secretions, aerosols or fomites, or vertical. Aerosol transmission from an infected rabbit to others in adjacent cages usually requires a prolonged period of contact. Alternatively, inoculation via wounds or the oral, conjunctival or vaginal routes may occur.

Clinical signs of upper and lower respiratory tract disease may be seen in addition to associated middle/inner ear disease in some cases. Abscesses are common and occasionally neurological signs may also be seen as a consequence of abscesses affecting the brain. Reproductive problems such as mastitis and metritis may also be seen in breeding animals.

Other bacterial agents causing respiratory disease

Bordetella bronchiseptica is another Gram-negative bacterium and the second most common isolate from rabbits with upper respiratory disease (Rougier *et al.*, 2006). Usually a commensal of the upper respiratory tract, *Bordetella* rarely causes a problem itself but has been shown to predispose to the development of pasteurellosis. It is generally found more commonly as rabbits age. It can also cause disease in other species such as guinea pigs. Other common isolates from cases of upper respiratory tract disease include *Pseudomonas* spp. and *Staphylococcus aureus*. *Moraxella catarrhalis* and *Mycoplasma* spp. have also been detected.

Lower respiratory tract disease often involves the same bacteria, but *Escherichia coli*, *Chlamydophila*, *Mycobacterium*, *Pneumocystis oryctolagi* and cilia-associated respiratory (CAR) bacillus (different from the rat variant) have also been isolated. Usually mixed bacterial infections are detected on culture.

Diagnosis of bacterial respiratory infections

For suspected upper respiratory tract infections, a deep nasal swab is required for culture. The swab should be moistened with sterile saline and ideally be inserted about 2–3 cm into the ventral meatus (Figure 11.5). Sedation is normally required for this and sampling often stimulates a bout of intense sneezing. Unfortunately false-negative results are common, and more superficial samples or a culture of nasal discharge are usually contaminated by environmental bacteria. Alternatively, culture of a nasolacrimal duct flush may be performed but again false-negative results are common. Endoscopically obtained biopsy samples of the nasal mucosa submitted for culture are a preferred alternative

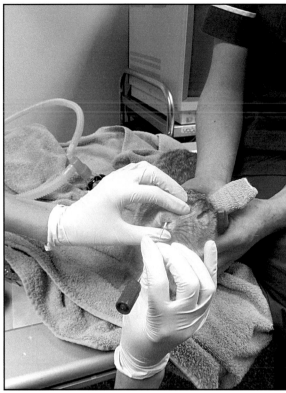

11.5 Deep nasal swabs may be taken under sedation.

wherever possible and are more likely to give an accurate representation of any pathogens present.

For suspected lower respiratory tract infections a tracheal wash or bronchoalveolar lavage (BAL) may be performed via the lumen of a sterile endotracheal tube. The catheter size will depend on the diameter of the endotracheal tube but usually 1–2 ml of sterile saline is introduced (depending on patient size) and then aspirated. A sample may be submitted for culture and cytology. Alternatively, mucus or pus from the end of the endotracheal tube may be cultured but the chances of contamination are higher with this technique.

Definitive diagnosis of pasteurellosis or other respiratory infections ideally requires isolation of the pathogen and demonstration of associated pathology (on biopsy specimens or post-mortem examination). In practice this may be difficult to prove in a live animal, so diagnosis is usually based on culture of the bacteria in association with typical respiratory signs. Serology for *Pasteurella* is possible but not widely available; paired samples (3–4 weeks apart) are needed to demonstrate rising antibody titres. Unfortunately false negatives are common in immunosuppressed individuals, and false positives can occur owing to cross-reactions with other bacteria. Polymerase chain reaction (PCR) testing for *Pasteurella* and *Bordetella* may be more useful in future but is not widely available at present.

On post-mortem examination, rhinitis with turbinate atrophy, sinusitis, otitis, well demarcated red–grey foci in the lungs consistent with bronchopneumonia, pulmonary abscesses and pericarditis may be observed (Figure 11.6).

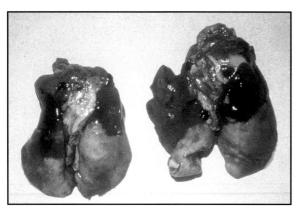

11.6 Rabbit lungs affected by *Pasteurella multocida* infection, showing cranial lobe consolidation.

General treatment of bacterial respiratory infections

Severe dyspnoea, open-mouth breathing or cyanosis should be treated as an emergency. The patient should be placed in a quiet, dark environment to reduce stress and should be supplemented with oxygen. Handling should be minimized for at least an initial 30 minutes unless absolutely necessary. Oxygen for longer-term therapy should be humidified and <40%. Mild sedation with midazolam may be necessary for particularly stressed patients, but generally the frequency of treatments should be minimized.

General treatment of respiratory disease usually involves antibiotic therapy for a minimum of 14 days in an attempt to eliminate the bacteria. In cases of pasteurellosis, infection and clinical signs are often only suppressed, with disease recurring at any time of stress. Chronic or severe infections may need treatment for up to 3 months, so owner compliance is important. Antibiotic choice should ideally be based on culture and sensitivity, and bactericidal drugs are preferred for treatment of severe disease such as pneumonia. Choice of antibiotic may also be guided by in-house Gram stains. In cases where empirical therapy is required (or while awaiting culture results) it is worth considering that mild cases appear to respond well to potentiated sulphonamides; however, these are not as effective in the treatment of established purulent infection.

Ideally fluoroquinolones should not be used as first-line antibiotics in mild infections unless indicated by culture and sensitivity. Enrofloxacin has been shown to be effective in the majority of cases although may not totally eliminate the disease. Marbofloxacin has been shown to be equally effective *in vitro* and also to be slightly more effective against most other commonly isolated bacteria so may be considered as an alternative (Rougier *et al.*, 2006). Most strains of *Pasteurella* also appear sensitive to ciprofloxacin, parenteral penicillin, tetracycline, gentamicin and chloramphenicol. However, the effect on gut flora of some of these antibiotics (such as gentamicin) should be considered, as systemic use may not be appropriate. Tilmicosin is also authorized as an in-feed medication for rabbits and has been reported to be effective at treating pasteurellosis. It is authorized to be used for up to 7 days but can cause a fatal adverse reaction in rabbits, so the injectable version is not generally used in practice.

Nebulization (Figure 11.7) is commonly used as a method of topical treatment alongside systemic antibiotics for both upper and lower respiratory tract disease. A nebulizer should be chosen that is capable of producing particles <0.5 μm. A wide range of drugs may be nebulized, including antibiotics, mucolytics, bronchodilators, and also F10 disinfectant (Figure 11.8). Ideally, antibiotics should be chosen that can penetrate the lipid barrier within the respiratory system to reach an adequate concentration at the airway surface. These include fluoroquinolones, tetra-cycline, azithromycin and metronidazole. However, even nebulization with saline alone may be useful to rehydrate the natural mucociliary escalator and enable the rabbit's natural defences to remove bacteria from the lungs. Recommendations for nebulization vary but generally 2 or 3 times daily for a period of 15 minutes is sufficient for most drugs. Mucolytics and bronchodilators may also be administered either parenterally or orally if indicated.

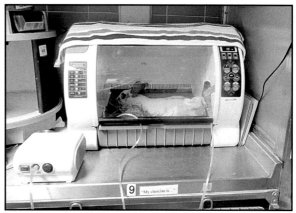

11.7 A rabbit undergoing nebulization therapy in an incubator.

Drug	Dose
Acetylcysteine	200 mg in 9 ml sterile water
Amikacin	50 mg in 10 ml saline
Aminophylline	25 mg in 9 ml saline
Amphotericin B	100 mg in 15 ml saline
Doxycycline	200 mg in 15 ml saline
Enrofloxacin	100 mg in 10 ml saline
Erythromycin	200 mg in 10 ml saline
F10	1:250 dilution in sterile water
Gentamicin	50 mg in 10 ml saline
Piperacillin	100 mg in 10 ml saline
Tylosin	100 mg in 10 ml saline

11.8 Suggested drug dosages for nebulization.

Supportive care is vital, especially for the inappetent rabbit, and includes offering tempting foods, syringe feeding if necessary and fluid therapy. The use of non-steroidal anti-inflammatory drugs (NSAIDs) should also be considered, especially as these patients are often in considerable discomfort. Grooming may have been neglected in chronic cases and will help to improve the rabbit's general comfort, especially where ocular and nasal discharges have built up. For rabbits with pneumonia, regular coupage and gentle exercise may also aid in expulsion of respiratory secretions.

While medical treatment is usually the preferred option in the majority of cases, some rabbits with chronic rhinitis and associated sinusitis may require surgical intervention (see *BSAVA Manual of Rabbit Surgery, Dentistry and Imaging*). Rhinotomy or rhinostomy procedures may be performed to debride and flush affected tissue and an indwelling catheter may be left in place for at least a week to allow continued topical therapy.

Treatment of associated disease should always be considered. This may include topical treatment for conjunctivitis, regular flushing of the nasolacrimal ducts, and treatment of otitis media, dental disease or abscesses (see *BSAVA Manual of Rabbit Surgery, Dentistry and Imaging*).

Control of bacterial respiratory infections

Pasteurellosis is a ubiquitous problem in pet rabbits but the development of disease can be reduced by good standards of husbandry and minimizing stress. Enclosures should be spacious, well ventilated and cleaned out regularly to reduce ammonia levels. New individuals should be quarantined and observed carefully for respiratory signs before introduction to established pet rabbits.

The use of corticosteroids should be avoided wherever possible. Vaccinations have been successfully trialled in laboratory rabbits but are not currently authorized in the UK. However nowadays laboratory rabbits are usually *Pasteurella*-free as a result of selective breeding.

> **WARNING**
> Very occasionally, pasteurellosis may be a zoonotic risk to humans and young, old or immunosuppressed individuals in particular should be warned of this. Susceptible individuals may suffer from skin infections, pneumonia, arthritis, meningitis and septicaemia.

Viral diseases

Myxomatosis

Myxomatosis is a viral disease spread by biting insects such as fleas and mosquitoes and is usually fatal (see Chapter 17). Common signs include swelling around the eyes and genitals but upper respiratory signs may also be seen. Diagnosis is usually based on clinical signs and although supportive

treatment may be given, euthanasia should be considered owing to the poor prognosis. Prevention by regular vaccination is strongly advised and a new vaccine was introduced in Europe in 2012. This has marked benefits over the previous vaccine, being administered by subcutaneous injection (instead of partly intradermal as required for the previous vaccine), with immunity lasting 1 year, and being combined with rabbit haemorrhagic disease vaccination (Spibey *et al.*, 2012). Good flea control is still recommended, especially in the summer months.

Rabbit haemorrhagic disease

Rabbit haemorrhagic disease (RHD) is a rapidly fatal disease caused by a calicivirus (closely related to the agent of European brown hare syndrome). Rabbits <2 months of age appear resistant to the disease but may become long-term carriers (Ferreira *et al.*, 2004). Older animals are normally found dead. There are often no ante-mortem signs but sometimes dyspnoea and haemorrhagic discharges from the nares and anus may be observed. Diagnosis is therefore generally on post-mortem examination. Haemorrhages in the lungs, liver and other visceral organs may be seen. Treatment is unsuccessful and therefore euthanasia is advised. A possible interaction between myxomatosis and RHD has been suggested (Marchandeau *et al.*, 2004).

As mentioned above, a new vaccine was introduced in 2012. This is authorized for use in rabbits >5 weeks of age with immunity lasting 1 year and appears very effective. There was, however, a new variant of RHD detected in France in 2010 and it is not yet known whether the new vaccine will be effective against this variant (Le Gall-Reculé *et al.*, 2011).

Herpesvirus

Herpesvirus is a rare cause of respiratory disease but should be considered in group situations. One outbreak was reported in a rabbitry in Alaska, caused by leporid herpesvirus-4 (Jin *et al.*, 2008). Rabbits presented with dyspnoea, conjunctivitis, periocular swelling, anorexia, weakness, ulcerative dermatitis and abortion. Many died or were euthanased due to the severity of disease. Further disease outbreaks have been reported in Canada in both pet and commercial rabbits (Brash *et al.*, 2010). Herpesvirus has not yet been reported in pet rabbits in the UK.

Neoplasia

Carcinoma and adenocarcinoma of the turbinates should be considered where bone destruction with or without proliferation is visible radiographically. In the lower respiratory tract the only primary neoplasia reported is pulmonary carcinoma. However, lymphosarcoma may affect the lungs and mediastinal lymph nodes. This is mainly seen in young rabbits and can also involve other visceral organs including the liver, spleen and kidneys.

The lungs are one of the most common sites for metastases, and in entire female rabbits these are usually secondary to uterine adenocarcinoma.

Prognosis is poor, so any rabbit with suspected uterine pathology should be radiographed to detect pulmonary metastases at an early stage. However, any tumour could potentially metastasize to the lungs. Once clinical signs of dyspnoea are noted euthanasia is advised as treatment is unsuccessful.

Hypertrophic osteopathy has been described in one rabbit secondary to metastatic uterine adenocarcinoma, with a large thoracic mass affecting the lungs (DeSanto, 1997). Although the condition is uncommon, thoracic radiographs should be considered for lame rabbits undergoing radiography.

Further details on neoplastic conditions are given in Chapter 18.

Thymoma

The thymus is particularly large in rabbits and persists into adulthood. Both benign neoplasms (thymomas) and malignant neoplasms such as thymic lymphomas have been reported, and affected individuals may present with respiratory signs. The aetiology of thymic neoplasia has not been established in any species, although a genetic basis for thymoma was identified in one report of three rabbits. In these cases thymoma was also associated with immunodeficiency and haemolytic anaemia.

Most commonly, a gradual onset of dyspnoea and exercise intolerance may be noted as the thymus slowly increases in size, restricting space in the thoracic cavity. Alternatively, the patient may present in acute respiratory distress with tachypnoea, dyspnoea and open-mouth breathing. Bilateral exophthalmos, and head, neck and forelimb oedema may also be seen as a result of impaired venous return to the heart (Wagner et al., 2005). Both eyes can usually be retropulsed normally and without pain, but exophthalmos may be induced by ventroflexion. One case of exfoliative dermatitis thought to be associated with a thymoma has also been reported (Florizoone, 2005).

Thoracic radiographs are the most useful diagnostic aid. A rounded soft tissue opacity is generally visible cranial to the heart. The trachea is often displaced dorsally and the lungs displaced caudally. Sometimes a pleural effusion is also present (Pilny and Reavill, 2008), and CT may provide more detailed information. Abdominal imaging should also be performed (both radiography and ultrasonography) to look for metastases.

Bone marrow cytology may be useful if metastatic disease is suspected. An ultrasound-guided fine-needle aspirate of the mass (see Chapter 18) will help to differentiate between thymoma and thymic lymphoma but histopathology of the mass is usually necessary to diagnose thymic neoplasia definitively. Thymomas are composed of a mix of well differentiated (usually small) mature lymphocytes and epithelial cells. Thymic lymphomas are usually composed of large lymphoblasts.

Surgical excision is currently the treatment of choice, via a median sternotomy for optimum visualization (see *BSAVA Manual of Rabbit Surgery, Dentistry and Imaging*), although an approach via a left lateral thoracotomy has also been reported. Intensive postoperative care, including a thoracotomy tube and excellent analgesia, is required. Radiotherapy may be useful if the neoplasm appears invasive or as follow-up treatment after surgery (Sanchez-Migallone et al., 2006). However, the proximity of the thymus to the heart and lungs will limit the radiation dose, and will predispose to side effects such as fibrosis and pneumonitis.

Other diseases of the respiratory system

Respiratory irritation

There are many potential respiratory irritants in a pet rabbit's environment, including smoke, dust, household chemicals, wood shaving vapours and elevated ammonia levels from inadequate cleaning. Cigarette smoke has been shown to cause severe lung changes in laboratory rabbits, including congestion, thrombosis and haemorrhage within the lungs, emphysema and alveolar destruction (Fidan et al., 2006).

Allergic rhinitis and bronchitis

Allergic respiratory disease has not been proven to exist in pet rabbits, but does appear to be a problem in practice. Rabbits may present acutely or following chronic exposure. Acute cases may appear severely dyspnoeic but will usually self-resolve once the rabbit has been removed from the source. Owners should be advised to place the rabbit in a well ventilated room or ideally outside if not too hot or cold. If severe dyspnoea is still present by the time of presentation, rabbits may be given supplementary oxygen as described above, and the administration of bronchodilators especially by nebulization may be useful. Antihistamines have been used but their efficacy is uncertain. They may be more appropriate for use in chronic cases alongside improvements in hygiene, ventilation and removal of any potential irritant. Saline nebulization may also be useful.

Identifying the exact cause is not always easy. The substrate and hay should be changed (ideally for dust-free varieties), the use of any aerosols around the rabbit should be minimized and animals should never be exposed to smoke. Owners should be asked to keep a daily record in an attempt to identify the pattern of disease, and to determine whether it is seasonal or coincides with any changes in the environment or routine.

Foreign bodies

Foreign bodies are often seen in rabbits as a consequence of their curious nature. Small pieces of rubber, towel or other inappropriate material may become lodged in the pharynx, causing dyspnoea or gagging. Alternatively, strands of hay and grass seeds may become lodged in the nasal cavity causing irritation and serving as a nidus for infection.

Sneezing and snuffling are often observed alongside nasal discharge, which may be unilateral. Identification of a foreign body usually involves general anaesthesia to allow endoscopy to be performed. Forceps may be used to grasp the foreign body under endoscopic guidance and gently remove it. Antibiotic cover and NSAIDs will generally need to be provided owing to the resulting soft tissue trauma.

Aspiration pneumonia is possible but uncommon. However, care should always be taken when administering oral medications or syringe feeding to give the rabbit time to swallow.

Trauma

Trauma to the respiratory system is uncommon but should be considered. Facial trauma such as a bite from another animal may introduce infection to the upper respiratory system and may disrupt airflow. Thoracic trauma causing conditions such as diaphragmatic hernias or pneumothorax may occur but appears to be rare in pet rabbits.

Tracheal stricture has been reported following intubation. Possible causes include movement of the endotracheal tube against the tracheal mucosa if not secured appropriately, or a reaction to disinfectants that have not been thoroughly rinsed off the tube. Clinical signs of dyspnoea are usually seen 2–3 weeks following anaesthesia and prognosis is poor (Grint *et al.*, 2006).

Congenital abnormalities

Congenital abnormalities are rare but may be seen in younger patients. Incomplete tracheal rings have been reported in one case, resulting in tracheal collapse. So far there has been no successful treatment reported.

Other differential diagnoses

Cardiovascular disease should always be ruled out in a dyspnoeic rabbit. Other non-respiratory problems should also be considered such as gastric dilation, which may cause increased pressure on the thoracic cavity and also result in dyspnoea.

References and further reading

Brash ML, Nagy É, Pei Y, *et al.* (2010) Acute hemorrhagic and necrotizing pneumonia, splenitis, and dermatitis in a pet rabbit caused by a novel herpesvirus (leporid herpesvirus-4). *Canadian Veterinary Journal* 51(12), 1383–1386
Broome RL and Brooks DL (1991) Efficacy of enrofloxacin in the treatment of respiratory pasteurellosis in rabbits. *Laboratory Animal Science* 41, 572–576
Campagnolo ER, Ernst MJ, Berninger ML, *et al.* (2003) Outbreak of rabbit hemorrhagic disease in domestic lagomorphs. *Journal of the American Veterinary Medical Association* 223(8), 1151–1155
Clippinger TL, Bennett RA, Alleman AR, *et al.* (1998) Removal of a thymoma via median sternotomy in a rabbit with recurrent appendicular neurofibrosarcoma. *Journal of the American Veterinary Medical Association* 213, 1140–1143
Cundiff DD, Besch-Williford CL, Hook RR, *et al.* (1994) Characterisation of cilia-associated respiratory bacillus isolates from rats and rabbits. *Laboratory Animal Science* 44, 305–312
Deeb BJ, DiGiacomo RF, Bernard BL and Silbernagel SM (1990) *Pasteurella multocida* and *Bordetella bronchiseptica* infections in rabbits. *Journal of Clinical Microbiology* 28, 70–75
Dei-Cas E, Chabe M, Moukhlis R, *et al.* (2006) *Pneumocystis oryctolagi* sp. *nov*, an uncultured fungus causing pneumonia in rabbits at weaning: review of current knowledge and description

of a new taxon on genotypic, phylogenetic and phenotypic bases. *FEMS Microbiology Review* 30, 853–871
DeSanto J (1997) Hypertrophic osteopathy associated with an intrathoracic neoplasm in a rabbit. *Journal of the American Veterinary Medical Association* 210, 1322–1323
DiGiacomo RF (1989) Atrophic rhinitis in New Zealand White rabbits infected with *Pasteurella multocida*. *American Journal of Veterinary Research* 50, 1460–1465
DiGiacomo RF, Garlinghouse LE and Van Hoosier GL (1983) Natural history of infection with *Pasteurella multocida*. *Journal of the American Veterinary Medical Association* 183, 1172–1175
DiGiacomo RF, Jones CDR and Wathes CM (1987) Transmission of *Pasteurella multocida* in rabbits. *Laboratory Animal Science* 37, 621–623
Dugal F, Belanger M and Jacques M (1992) Enhanced adherence of *Pasteurella multocida* to porcine tracheal rings preinfected with *Bordetella bronchiseptica*. *Canadian Journal of Veterinary Research* 56, 260–264
Ferreira PG, Costa-e-Silva A, Monteiro E, *et al.* (2004) Transient decrease in blood heterophils and sustained liver damage caused by calicivirus infection of young rabbits that are naturally resistant to rabbit haemorrhagic disease. *Research in Veterinary Science* 76(1), 83–94
Fidan F, Unlu M, Sezer M, *et al.* (2006) Acute effects of environmental tobacco smoke and dried dung smoke on lung histopathology in rabbits. *Pathology* 38, 53–57
Florizoone K (2005) Thymoma-associated exfoliative dermatitis in a rabbit. *Veterinary Dermatology* 16(4), 281–284
Grint NJ, Sayers IR, Cecchi R, *et al.* (2006) Postanaesthetic tracheal strictures in three rabbits. *Laboratory Animals* 40(3), 301–308
Jin L, Valentine BA, Baker RJ, *et al.* (2008) An outbreak of fatal herpesvirus infection in domestic rabbits in Alaska. *Veterinary Pathology* 45, 369–374
Le Gall-Reculé G, Zwingelstein F, Boucher S, *et al.* (2011) Detection of a new variant of rabbit haemorrhagic disease virus in France. *Veterinary Record* 168(5), 137–138
Mahler M, Stunkel S, Ziegowski C and Kunstyr I (1995) Inefficacy of enrofloxacin in the elimination of *Pasteurella multocida* in rabbits. *Laboratory Animals* 29(2), 192–199
Marchandeau S, Bertagnoli S, Peralta B, *et al.* (2004) Possible interaction between myxomatosis and calicivirosis related to rabbit haemorrhagic disease affecting the European rabbit. *Veterinary Record* 155(19), 589–592
Marlier D, Mainil J, Linde A, *et al.* (2000) Infectious agents associated with rabbit pneumonia: isolation of amyxomatous myxoma virus strains. *Veterinary Journal* 159, 171–178
McKay SG, Morck DW, Merrill JK, *et al.* (1996) Use of tilmicosin for treatment of pasteurellosis in rabbits. *American Journal of Veterinary Research* 57, 1180–1184
Peshev R and Chrostova L (2003) The efficacy of a bivalent vaccine against pasteurellosis and rabbit haemorrhagic disease virus. *Veterinary Research Communications* 27, 433–444
Pilny A and Reavill D (2008) Chylothorax and thymic lymphoma in a pet rabbit (*Oryctolagus cuniculus*). *Journal of Exotic Pet Medicine* 17(4), 295–299
Roels S, Wattiau P, Fretin D, *et al.* (2007) Isolation of *Morganella morganii* from a domestic rabbit with bronchopneumonia. *Veterinary Record* 161(15), 530–531
Rougier S, Galland D, Boucher S, *et al.* (2006) Epidemiology and susceptibility of pathogenic bacteria responsible for upper respiratory tract infections in pet rabbits. *Veterinary Microbiology* 115, 192–198
Sanchez-Migallon DG, Mayer J, Gould J, *et al.* (2006) Radiation therapy for the treatment of thymoma in rabbits (*Oryctolagus cuniculus*). *Journal of Exotic Pet Medicine* 15(2), 138–144
Spibey N, McCabe VJ, Greenwood NM, *et al.* (2012) Novel bivalent vectored vaccine for control of myxomatosis and rabbit haemorrhagic disease. *Veterinary Record* 170(12), 309
Suckow MA (2000) Immunisation of rabbits against *Pasteurella multocida* using a commercial swine vaccine. *Laboratory Animals* 34(4), 403–408
Suckow MA, Haab RW, Miloscio LJ, *et al.* (2008) Field trial of a *Pasteurella multocida* extract vaccine in rabbits. *Journal of the American Association of Laboratory Animal Science* 47(1), 18–21
Suckow MA, Martin BJ, Bowersock TL and Douglas FA (1996) Derivation of *Pasteurella multocida*-free rabbit litters by enrofloxacin treatment. *Veterinary Microbiology* 51(1–2), 161–168
Vernau KM, Grahn BH, Clarke-Scott HA and Sullivan N (1995) Thymoma in a geriatric rabbit with hypercalcaemia and periodic exophthalmos. *Journal of the American Veterinary Medical Association* 206, 820–822
Villa A, Gracia E, Fernandez A, *et al.* (2001) Detection of mycoplasmas in the lungs of rabbits with respiratory disease. *Veterinary Record* 148, 788–789
Wagner F, Beinecke A, Fehr M, *et al.* (2005) Recurrent bilateral exophthalmos associated with metastatic thymic carcinoma in a pet rabbit. *Journal of Small Animal Practice* 6(8), 369–370

12

Digestive system disease

Frances Harcourt-Brown

Many diseases affect the digestive system of rabbits. There can be a complex interrelationship between them, so an exact diagnosis is often difficult. Clinical examination, clinical pathology, imaging techniques and, in some cases, surgery or post-mortem examination may be the only way to make a diagnosis. This chapter describes the features of the common digestive system diseases that affect rabbits kept as pets rather than those that are reared in intensive conditions for meat or fur production, or for laboratory purposes. Knowledge of the digestive physiology and the anatomy of the gastrointestinal tract is helpful (Figure 12.1).

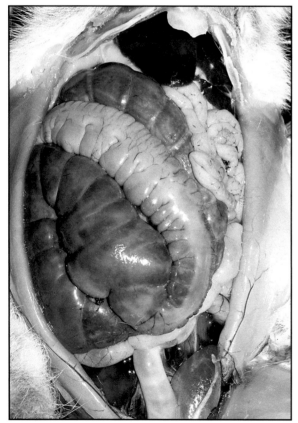

12.1 Normal appearance of the caecum and proximal colon. Abdominal contents of a juvenile male wild rabbit that was killed by a car, showing the size of the caecum and proximal colon, which were full of ingesta. The rabbit was killed in the morning and had just filled its digestive tract with food. The size of the caecum gives an idea of the amount of caecotrophs that are expelled and consumed each day.

Signs of digestive disease

The signs of digestive disease and their clinical significance are summarized in Figure 12.2.

Anorexia

Anorexia is a sign of many diseases in rabbits, such as dental disease, upper respiratory tract infections or urinary tract problems. In any anorexic rabbit, it is always important to perform a full clinical examination, including examination of the oral cavity. Radiography is often necessary (Harcourt-Brown, 2013; Lennox, 2013). Other imaging techniques, such as ultrasound examination to assess gut motility, can be useful alongside blood glucose levels and other biochemical parameters. Anorexia is associated with slow gut motility, although it can be difficult to determine whether the anorexia is due to the primary disease or a secondary effect of the associated stress-induced reduction in gut motility. Once gut motility is reduced, food and fluids do not move through the digestive tract, the stomach does not empty and anorexia is the result.

Abnormal appearance and amount of faeces

Gross examination
The amount, size and texture of faeces and/or caecotrophs that are produced are an important part of the clinical history. Some owners will bring faecal samples with them (Figure 12.3). Other owners are not always able to provide this information, especially if their rabbit is housed with others. Hospitalization can be helpful to observe faecal output. A description of the types of faeces that may be produced and the significance of any abnormalities is given in Figures 12.4 and 12.5.

Microscopic examination
Microscopic examination of faeces can yield additional information (Figure 12.6). Plain and stained (Gram's stain) faecal smears will show the presence and amount of fibre particles and microorganisms. Flotation techniques can be used to detect parasites. A quick and easy technique is to mix a small amount of faecal material with saturated salt solution prior to spinning the mixture in a centrifuge. After removing the tube containing the mixture from the centrifuge, it

Disease	Demeanour	Appetite	Faecal output	Gastric dilation	Gas in caecum	Blood glucose	Other features
Oesophageal obstruction: complete	Distressed; choking and regurgitating	Not eating	Normal at outset	No	In late stages	Normal to slightly elevated (stress response)	
Oesophageal obstruction: partial	Quiet						Radiographically, there may be gas in stomach and throughout gastrointestinal tract due to aerophagia
Megaoesophagus	Normal	Normal or reduced appetite	Normal or reduced	No	No	Normal to slightly elevated (stress response)	May periodically regurgitate liquid stained with food
Gastrointestinal hypomotility: early	Quiet and less responsive	May pick at food	Reduced; small hard faeces	No	May be small amounts	May be low, normal or slightly elevated	Always a secondary condition; stress response; may be due to moving foreign body or other source of pain such as dental disease
Gastrointestinal hypomotility: late (>48 hours)		Complete anorexia	None		Yes	Normal to slightly elevated (stress response) (<15 mmol/l)	
Hepatic lipidosis	Quiet; cold; often ataxic	Complete anorexia	None	No	Yes	Variable; often high	Blood results often bizarre with evidence of organ failure; lipaemia, ketosis, acidosis common
Gastric ulceration: not perforated	Quiet	Anorexic	Reduced	No	Maybe in late stages of gastrointestinal hypomotility	Normal to slightly elevated (stress response) (<15 mmol/l)	Difficult to diagnose during life
Gastric ulceration: perforated	Unresponsive; cold; often ataxic					Often elevated	Anterior abdominal pain
Liver lobe torsion	Quiet; cold; may be ataxic depending on severity of torsion	Sudden-onset anorexia	May pass normal faeces at outset	Not at outset. Many develop after 24–72h due to paralytic ileus	No	Normal or elevated depending on degree of torsion. Increases in terminal stages due to paralytic ileus	Anaemia is a feature; enlarged liver lobe may be palpable as hard mass in cranial abdomen on right side just behind ribs
Small intestinal obstruction: complete	Unresponsive	Sudden-onset anorexia	May pass normal faeces at outset	Yes	No	Marked elevation (usually >20 mmol/l)	Sudden onset; rabbit often hiding in strange places; dilated stomach often palpable during clinical examination
Small intestinal obstruction: moving	Quiet demeanour; may improve if foreign body passes through ileocolic valve	Sudden-onset anorexia but may start eating if foreign body passes through		Yes	Yes if foreign body passes through ileocolic valve	Elevated (>15 mmol/l)	
Paralytic ileus	Unresponsive	Complete anorexia	No	Yes	Yes	Marked elevation (usually >20 mmol/l)	Follows major abdominal surgery or crisis
Enterotoxaemia	Unresponsive	Complete anorexia	Diarrhoea; may be haemorrhagic	No	Usually	Marked elevation (usually >20 mmol/l)	Often sudden onset
Heavy metal toxicity	Quiet	Reduced appetite	No	No	May be small amounts	May be low, normal or slightly elevated	Often see radiodense flakes in digesta on abdominal radiographs; blood changes in advanced cases

12.2   Clinical features of some digestive diseases of rabbits. (continues)

Disease	Demeanour	Appetite	Faecal output	Gastric dilation	Gas in caecum	Blood glucose	Other features
Pancreatitis	Quiet; unresponsive	Anorexic	Reduced or absent	No	Not in early stages	Variable	Abdominal pain may or may not be present; difficult disease to diagnose without exploratory surgery
Infectious enteritis	Quiet	Variable	Diarrhoea	No	Often	Variable	Severity of signs varies with pathogen; usually young recently purchased rabbits
Coccidiosis	Variable	Variable	Diarrhoea; may be haemorrhagic and liquid or soft and pasty	No	Maybe	Normal to slightly elevated (stress response)	Coccidial oocysts easily identified in faeces
Mucoid enteropathy	Responsive at outset; progressively quieter until cold and unresponsive	May eat at outset but progressive loss of appetite	May be liquid faeces in mucus, just mucus or no faeces at all	Yes in later stages	Gas may be seen around impacted caecal contents	Variable depending on stage of disease and degree of pain	Usually young recently purchased rabbits
Megacolon	Normal; may be intermittent periods of unresponsiveness	Often very hungry but may have periods of anorexia	Voluminous quantities of loose 'cow pat' faeces or soft faeces that vary in size; some can be very large; may have periods of reduced faecal output	No	May be periods of caecal tympany or caecal impaction	Variable depending on stage of disease and degree of pain	Usually older rabbits, often with spotted markings; faecal output varies but is never normal; microscopically, faeces are a mixture of hard faeces (long strands of fibre) and caecotrophs (range of microorganisms
Intestinal anomalies, e.g. adhesions, diverticulosis	Variable; may be unresponsive during periods of intermittent colic	Variable; may be anorexic during periods of intermittent colic	Often normal	Variable; may be dilated during periods of intermittent colic	No	Variable depending on stage of disease and degree of pain	Intermittent abdominal pain; exploratory surgery is needed to make the diagnosis
Caecal impaction	Quiet	Variable; often reduced	Reduced or absent	No	May be gas surrounding impacted caecal contents	Slight to moderate elevation (<15 mmol/l)	Palpable impacted caecum; may be linked with dehydration, e.g. due to chronic renal failure; or mucoid enteropathy or megacolon
Uneaten caecotrophs: soft liquid caecotrophs	Normal	Good	Hard faeces plus caecotrophs; soft caecotrophs that often stick to fur	No	No	Normal to slightly elevated (stress response from handling)	Rabbit is well in itself and passing hard faeces; often due to dietary change or insufficient dietary fibre
Uneaten caecotrophs: firm caecotrophs			Hard faeces plus caecotrophs; firm bunches of mucus-coated caecotrophs that may be seen in the bedding				Rabbit is well in itself and passing hard faeces; often linked with obesity and excessive amounts of concentrated foods; can be due to flexibility problems (e.g. spondylosis, kyphosis or lordosis) that affect the rabbit's ability to reach the anus
Yersiniosis	Quiet	Reduced appetite or complete anorexia	Reduced	No	No	Variable depending on stage of disease and degree of pain	Difficult disease to diagnose without exploratory surgery

12.2 (continued) Clinical features of some digestive diseases of rabbits.

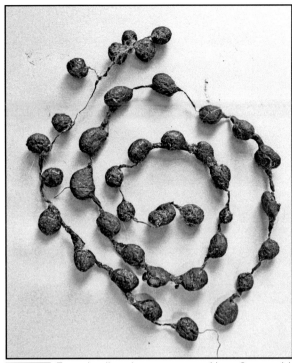

12.3 Faecal pellets that were passed by a 3-year-old Lionhead neutered female. Rabbits ingest a lot of fur, especially during moulting. The fur passes through the digestive tract and is compressed into hard faecal pellets, which may be joined by long strands of hair in long-haired breeds.

Type of faeces	Gross appearance
Normal caecotrophs	
Normal hard faeces	
Soft caecotrophs	

12.4 Gross appearance of faeces.

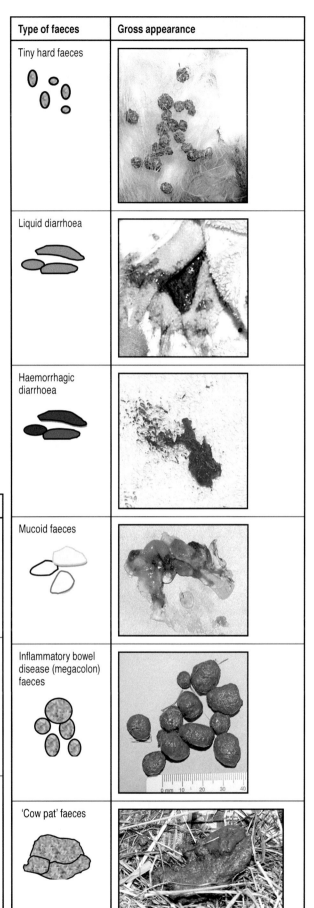

Type of faeces	Gross appearance
Tiny hard faeces	
Liquid diarrhoea	
Haemorrhagic diarrhoea	
Mucoid faeces	
Inflammatory bowel disease (megacolon) faeces	
'Cow pat' faeces	

Appetite	Hard faeces	Appearance of faeces	Caecotrophs	Conclusion	Reason
Good	Copious quantities of normal sized faeces (approx 100 per day)		Not seen (consumed)	Normal	
Not eating	Normal sized faeces		Not seen (consumed)	Gastrointestinal function was normal; disease was sudden onset	Peracute disease, e.g. intestinal obstruction, liver lobe torsion
Good	Copious quantities of normal sized faeces		Seen as bunches of soft but formed, strong smelling faeces in bedding or under tail	Rabbit is not eating caecotrophs but caecotrophs are normal	Obesity; excessive amounts of concentrates; vertebral abnormalities; incisor problems, etc. (see text)
Not eating	Absent		Seen as formed or pasty soft, strong smelling faeces in bedding or under tail	Rabbit is not eating caecotrophs because its appetite is reduced; rabbit does not have complete gut stasis	Any condition that reduces food intake (dental disease, stress, etc.); after period of gut stasis, soft caecotrophs are a sign that the rabbit is starting to recover
Good	Small faecal pellets		Seen as unformed pasty or liquid faeces in bedding or under tail	Mild disruption of caecal microflora or insufficient fibre to provide firm consistency to caecotrophs; not same as enterotoxaemia	Novel foods; stress; disruption of daily routine; insufficient dietary fibre (self-limiting if dietary fibre is increased)
Good	Small faecal pellets		Not seen (consumed)	Insufficient long particles of indigestible dietary fibre passing through gastrointestinal tract	Often seen in rabbits with chronic dental problems; can't or won't eat fibrous foods, especially hay
Poor or not eating anything	Small faecal pellets or reduced amounts (<50 per day)		Not seen (not produced)	Food is slowly passing through the digestive tract	Early stages of gut stasis; potentially fatal if left untreated
Not eating	Absent		Not seen (not produced)	Food is not passing through digestive tract at all	Late stages of gut stasis; gut motility reduced by pain and/or stress; treatment is essential
Good (may be ravenous)	Copious quantities of huge irregular faeces		Not seen (consumed)	Colon is not functioning correctly; ingesta is not compressed into small pellets	Megacolon syndrome
Good or reduced (often weight loss, despite ravenous appetite)	Voluminous softish faeces ('cow pat' faeces)		Absent (no separation of hard and soft faeces)	Colon is not functioning properly; it is not separating particles into large and small particles so caecum cannot function normally either	Megacolon syndrome in adults; coccidiosis in young rabbits
Reduced or not eating	Liquid		Absent (no separation of hard and soft faeces)	Complete disruption of intestinal function	Enteritis; much more common in young rabbits; potentially fatal
Not eating	Liquid and haemorrhagic		Absent (no separation of hard and soft faeces)	Complete disruption of intestinal function plus signs of severe inflammation	Often fatal; enterotoxaemia or severe coccidiosis in young rabbits
Reduced appetite or not eating	Absent or mixed with mucus, or just mucus		Absent (not produced)	Abnormal colonic function with stimulation of mucus production	Mucoid enteropathy; can occur with other hypomotility disorders, e.g. megacolon syndrome

12.5 Significance of faecal output.

Finding	Appearance	Significance
Large fibre particles	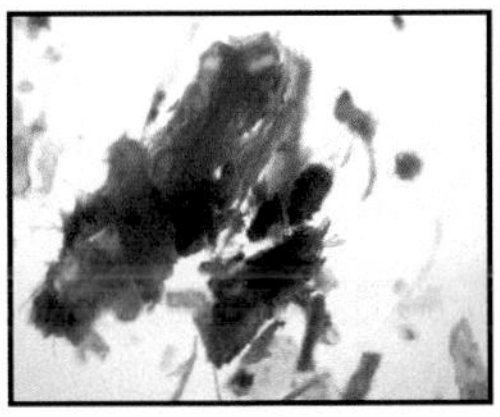	Normal feature of hard faecal pellets, which may contain hair, fibre and little else
A range of microorganisms and no fibre particles	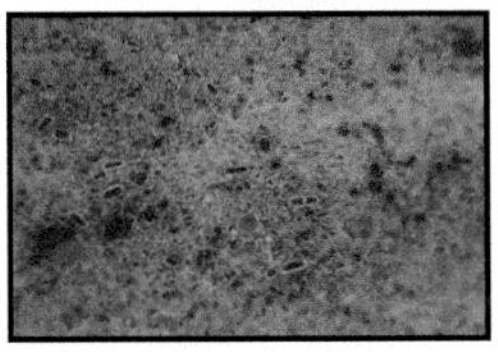	Normal appearance of caecotrophs
A mixture of large fibre particles and microorganisms	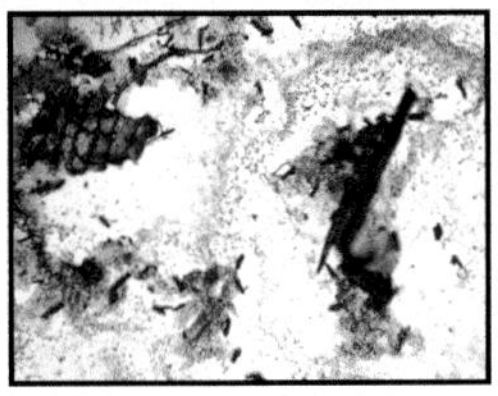	Mixture of hard faeces and caecotrophs; failure of hindgut to separate ingesta; occurs in cases of enteritis, coccidiosis or megacolon; in cases of enteritis, pathogenic bacteria, such as *Clostridium spiroforme*, may be identified by clinical pathologist
Coccidial oocysts	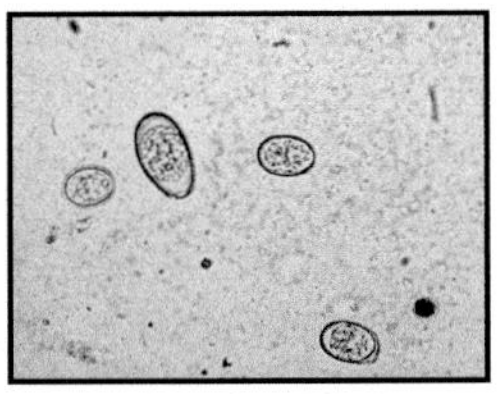	Large numbers may be seen in cases of coccidiosis; there are seven different species that affect rabbits, differentiated by size and shape of oocysts; mixed infections usually occur; *Eimeria stiedae* oocysts have an operculum
Yeasts, *Saccharomyces* (*Cyniclomyces*) *guttulatus* (red arrow) with coccidial oocyst as a comparison (black arrow)	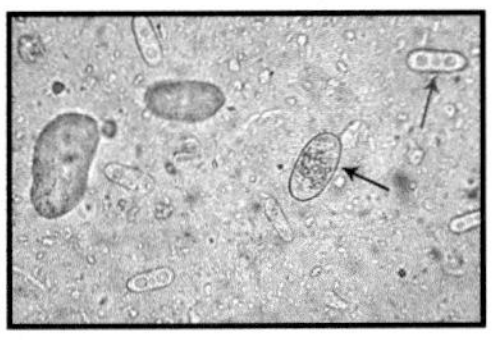	*S. guttulatus* is not pathogenic; small numbers are a normal feature of caecotrophs and are sometimes seen in hard faecal pellets; large numbers are often present in faeces of abnormal consistency, e.g. soft caecotrophs or diarrhoea
Passalurus ambiguus eggs	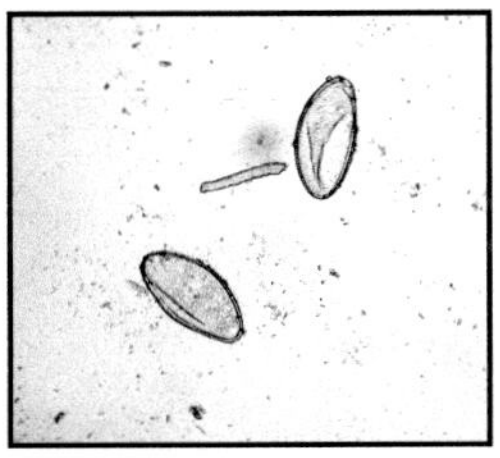	*Passalurus ambiguus* is a small oxyurid that is found in the caecum and colon. Adult worms may be visible in the faeces. The worm is non-pathogenic
Nematode egg (e.g. *Obeliscoides cuniculi*) NB. This picture shows coccidial oocysts for comparison	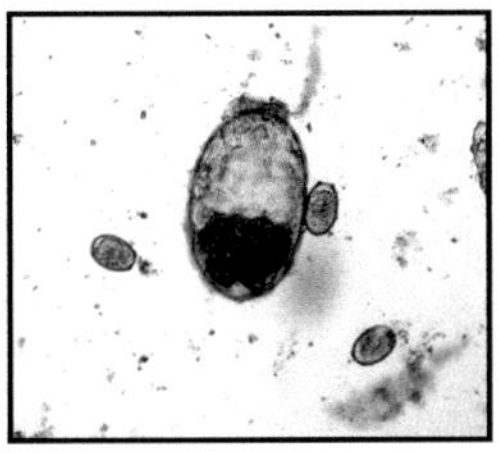	Many nematode species affect wild rabbits and this faeces sample is from a wild rabbit. In pet rabbits, food that has been contaminated by faeces from wild rabbits may be a source of nematodes
Cittotaenia ctenoides eggs	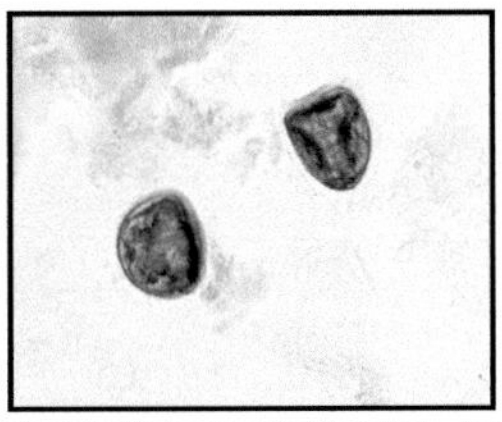	*Cittotaenia ctenoides* is a tapeworm that is rare in pet rabbits. Segments may be seen on gross examination of the faeces. Free-living mites act as intermediate hosts. The infestation may be introduced by eating wild plants. Heavy infestation may cause clinical signs

12.6 Microscopic examination of faeces. Please note that magnification varies in the images.

can be held upright in a container and saturated salt solution added to the tube to form a meniscus. A coverslip can be placed over the meniscus and left for 20–30 minutes before removing it from the tube and placing it on a microscope slide for examination. Although this method does not give a quantitative result, it is a simple way of finding parasites.

Abdominal pain

Unlike other species, rabbits with serious abdominal diseases do not exhibit overt signs of pain and tend to hide away from view when they are seriously ill. Rabbits cannot vomit or sweat and their normal heart rate is 150–300 beats per minute; this is hard to count accurately and a high rate can be normal. A history of sudden-onset anorexia and hiding, perhaps with some signs of abdominal discomfort such as 'flopping down' or 'pressing its stomach to the ground' needs to be taken seriously and investigated. Loud tooth grinding is another sign of abdominal pain. If these signs are overlooked, the presence of a serious, but potentially treatable, abdominal disease may be left until the rabbit becomes obviously shocked, hypothermic, ataxic or moribund.

Any pain detected during abdominal palpation is significant. Palpation should be performed carefully and gently because tympanitic viscera can rupture or localized abscesses can burst. Peritonitis can cause flinching. Localized signs of pain may be detected in damaged organs such as a liver with a twisted lobe or a hydronephrotic kidney.

Accumulation of gas, fluid or food

Many digestive diseases result in the accumulation of gas, fluid or food in parts of the digestive tract.

Distended, dilated parts of the gastrointestinal tract may be palpable or visible. Gastric or caecal tympany will cause abdominal distension, and gastric dilation is usually obvious during abdominal palpation when the stomach can be palpated as a balloon-like structure behind the ribs on the left side of the abdomen. Intestinal gas acts as an excellent contrast medium and the shape and distribution of gas shadows on abdominal radiographs can be informative or even diagnostic (Harcourt-Brown, 2013; Lennox, 2013). Impacted stomach or caecal contents may be visible.

Abnormalities in haematology and biochemistry

Digestive disease may be reflected in haematological and biochemical changes. A full profile can be helpful in assessing the status of the animal and the involvement of other organs, e.g. acute renal failure or hepatic lipidosis (see Chapter 9). In some cases, financial or equipment constraints may limit the number of diagnostic tests and a small, in-house profile that is cheap and easy to perform on a few drops of blood can be a useful compromise. Blood glucose, haematocrit (packed cell volume; PCV), total protein and visual examination of the serum can be performed using a glucometer, centrifuge and spectrometer. These parameters help in the differential diagnosis and prognosis of many digestive disorders.

Blood glucose measurement can be extremely helpful in rabbits (Figure 12.7). It can aid differential diagnosis between surgical and medical cases and be a prognostic indicator. In a study by Harcourt-Brown and Harcourt-Brown (2012), which

Blood glucose concentration (mmol/l)	Significance	Possible reasons	Comments
<2	Severely hypoglycaemic	Insulinoma; paraneoplastic syndrome; artifact; metabolic disease; pancreatitis	Further investigations and repeat blood samples are necessary
2–4.1	Moderately hypoglycaemic	Lack of food	Often a feature of early gastrointestinal hypomotility and insufficient uptake of glucose and its precursors from the gut
4.2–8.2	Within reference range		Reassuring
8.3–12	Within normal range for pet rabbits that have been transported to unfamiliar surroundings	Mild stress	Reassuring but indicative that the rabbit is stressed; if other signs (anorexia, abdominal pain, suspected gastric dilation) are present then resampling is indicated
12.1–15	Slightly hyperglycaemic	Stress	Probably stress-induced but could be start of serious disease; resample unless clinical signs resolve rapidly
15.1–20	Significantly hyperglycaemic	Stress; pain	Possibly but not definitely surgical; resample after 30–60 minutes; take radiographs
20.1–25	Severely hyperglycaemic	Severe pain; deranged glucose metabolism	Serious disease is present; needs a diagnosis and surgery is likely; exploratory laparotomy is indicated, unless gas can be seen in the caecum indicating that an intestinal foreign body has passed through; monitoring and supportive care are essential
>25	Critically hyperglycaemic or diabetic	Severe pain; deranged glucose metabolism	If rabbit is ill, its condition is probably surgical or terminal; other findings from clinical examination and radiography need to be examined as well; if the rabbit is eating well, the possibility of diabetes needs to be investigated

12.7 Interpretation of blood glucose results.

involved the analysis of over 900 samples for blood glucose levels in pet rabbits, severe hyperglycaemia (>20 mmol/l) was associated with conditions with a poor prognosis. Rabbits with confirmed intestinal obstruction had a mean blood glucose of 24.7 mmol/l (n = 18). This was significantly higher than the level in rabbits with confirmed gut stasis, which had a mean value of 8.5 mmol/l (n = 51). However, blood glucose is a dynamic parameter that can rise and fall rapidly so any blood sample is only a snapshot and repeated sampling may be necessary to detect trends. There is a short time lag between the onset of clinical disease and the rise in blood glucose. Similarly, blood glucose levels may take 15–20 minutes to fall if the source of pain is resolved. The most common scenario for this is when an intestinal foreign body moves through the ileocolic valve to release the gas and fluid that has built up in the stomach and small intestine into the hindgut (see Chapter 14 in the *BSAVA Manual of Rabbit Surgery, Dentistry and Imaging*).

Assessment of the PCV can indicate anaemia or dehydration if this is looked at alongside the total protein. Acute anaemia may be seen in association with liver lobe torsion. Visual examination of the serum can show jaundice or lipaemia. Lipaemia is a sign of hepatic lipidosis.

Digestive diseases

There are many ways in which digestive diseases can be classified. They may be divided with reference to the regions of the intestinal tract that are affected or the causes of disease (e.g. viral, bacterial, parasitic). Each system has its drawbacks because of the interrelationships among stress, pathogens, diet and gut motility. For this reason, the common diseases that affect the digestive tract will be described individually.

Dental disease

Dental problems are often encountered in pet rabbits and may be due to congenital prognathic defects, jaw or tooth fractures, tumours or, most commonly, part of a progressive syndrome that is acquired and due to an incorrect diet. Dental disease is covered in detail in the *BSAVA Manual of Rabbit Surgery, Dentistry and Imaging*.

Regurgitation and oesophageal disease

Oesophageal obstruction

Occasionally, oesophageal obstruction can occur in rabbits that consume an item of food that lodges in the oesophagus. If the obstruction is complete, the syndrome is manifested by a sudden inability to swallow, loud pharyngeal noise and regurgitation of saliva, which may be stained with food (Figure 12.8). If the obstruction is partial, the rabbit may not show many signs other than inappetence and aerophagia, which may be seen on radiographs (Figure 12.9). Examination under anaesthetic and passage of a stomach tube may dislodge the obstruction. Endoscopic examination of the mouth, pharynx and oesophagus is useful

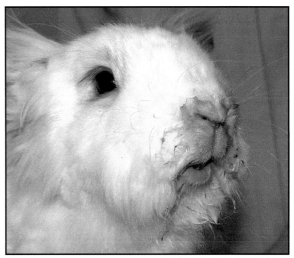

12.8 This 4-year-old neutered female rabbit suddenly stopped eating and started to make choking noises as she was eating nuggets. Green fluid came out of her nose and mouth. She was dyspnoeic. Anaesthesia was induced with intravenous propofol and maintained by continuous infusion while a tube was passed down her oesophagus into her stomach. Some resistance was felt and the respiratory noise and fluid regurgitation stopped. Subsequent endoscopic examination of the oesophagus showed no obstruction or abnormality apart from green liquid. The rabbit recovered uneventfully. A presumed diagnosis of oesophageal obstruction by nuggets of food was made. The rabbit was known to eat greedily.

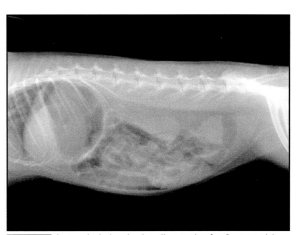

12.9 Lateral abdominal radiograph of a 3-year-old neutered male Dwarf Lop that had chewed a cushion. One end of a piece of the kapok stuffing had caught around a curved elongated tooth and the remaining section, which was 4 cm long, was lodged in the oesophagus. The rabbit was not eating but was bright and active. The radiograph shows that there is little or no food in the gastrointestinal tract, but it is filled with air instead. The stomach is not enlarged. It is contained within the costal arch and does not meet the ventral abdominal floor. The rabbit recovered after the piece of kapok was removed.

Oesophageal reflux

Nasogastric tubes carry a risk of causing gastric reflux as they allow a portal of entry for stomach acid to leak into the oesophagus through the cardiac sphincter. Iatrogenic complications such as inhalation pneumonia, gastric reflux, oesophagitis and stricture can occur with the use of nasogastric or naso-oesophageal tubes (Powers, 2006).

Myasthenia gravis

A presumptive diagnosis of myasthenia gravis has been made by the author in some rabbits with chronic regurgitation but no evidence of physical obstruction of the oesophagus. One case was a rabbit that died suddenly following thymoma removal. Post-mortem examination showed a dilated oesophagus filled with caecotrophs. Some caecotrophs had obstructed the larynx.

Diseases of the stomach

Gastric ulceration

Gastric ulcers are a common post-mortem finding in rabbits, especially in those that have been anorexic prior to death. The majority of the ulcers are seen in the fundic area of the stomach. There are no specific clinical signs associated with gastric ulceration and they often occur in rabbits that are already inappetent or in pain from other causes. The possibility of gastric ulceration is always a consideration when treating anorexic rabbits. Perforation and death can occur (Figure 12.10). It is not known whether non-steroidal anti-inflammatory drugs (NSAIDs) contribute to gastric ulceration in rabbits (as in other species), but it has been shown in rabbits that ranitidine is effective in decreasing gastric acid and pepsin secretion (Redfern *et al.*, 1991). Ranitidine also stimulates gastric motility. It is a safe and useful adjunct to the treatment of anorexic rabbits.

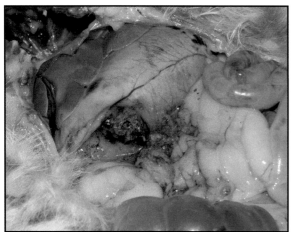

12.10 Immediate post-mortem appearance of a rabbit that had not eaten for 2–3 days, with presumed gut stasis. There was a perforated gastric ulcer with food in the abdominal cavity, a fatty liver but no other obvious abnormality. The referring practitioner had prescribed a high dose (1.5 mg/kg) of meloxicam in the preceding days and it is not known whether this was a contributory factor to the gastric ulceration.

Gastric dilation

Gastric dilation in rabbits is usually due to small intestinal obstruction (Harcourt-Brown, 2007), although it can be a feature of paralytic ileus and the late stages of mucoid enteropathy. The condition is readily detectable on abdominal palpation and by radiography (Figure 12.11). Rabbits cannot vomit or eructate and saliva is produced continuously. Normal stomach contents often include caecotrophs that contain gas-producing organisms so they can rapidly ferment and produce gas. If the exit from the stomach is blocked by obstruction of the small intestine, gas and liquid rapidly accumulate in the stomach and small intestine, proximal to the site of the obstruction. Distension of the stomach and intestine is often rapid and painful and some owners report seeing a sudden change in their rabbit's demeanour, from an active greedy individual to one that is immobile and unresponsive. The enlarged stomach impairs circulation and quickly becomes inflamed. Ulceration, necrosis, perforation and peritonitis can occur at the site of the obstruction or in the tympanitic stomach (Figure 12.12). Dehydration and electrolyte imbalances develop as fluid and electrolytes are

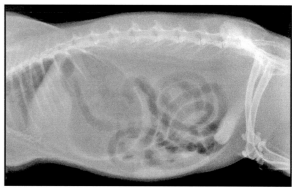

12.11 This 4-year-old male neutered Angora rabbit presented unresponsive 3 hours after the sudden onset of anorexia. A dilated stomach was palpated in the cranial abdomen and a blood sample showed a high blood glucose level (19.6 mmol/l). The radiograph shows a dilated stomach filled with fluid and dilated gas-filled sections of small intestine. The stomach is in contact with the ventral abdominal floor. The hyperglycaemia and clinical signs are typical of an obstruction of the small intestine.

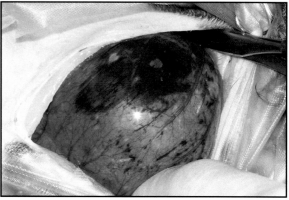

12.12 Appearance of the stomach of a rabbit with severe gastric dilation and tympany. The mucosa is inflamed and haemorrhagic.

sequestered into different compartments. Acute renal failure can be a further complication of gastric dilation. The endstage of this syndrome is either: recovery because the obstruction is surgically removed or moved through the ileocolic junction; or death from gastric or intestinal rupture, shock or acute renal failure. Death can occur within 8 hours of onset of acute anorexia. (Surgical treatment of intestinal obstruction is described in the *BSAVA Manual of Rabbit Surgery, Dentistry and Imaging.*)

Gastrointestinal hypomotility

If gut motility is reduced by stress or pain, slow gastric emptying results in dehydration and impaction of the stomach contents and, because hair is ingested during grooming, the impacted stomach contents often contain large amounts of hair. At one time, it was believed that the balls of impacted hair caused anorexia by obstructing the pylorus, so surgical removal of hairballs was the recommended treatment. Nowadays, it is recognized that gastric hairball formation is a secondary problem and that treatment of the underlying cause along with provision of food, fluids and prokinetic therapy is indicated rather than gastrotomy. In cases of gut stasis, the stomach can often be palpated as a small doughy hard structure. Impaction of the stomach with a ball of ingesta, often surrounded by a halo of gas, is a characteristic radiographic sign of gastrointestinal hypomotility (Figure 12.13).

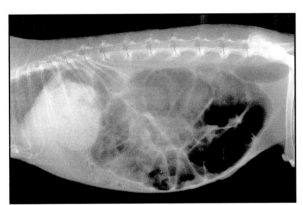

12.13 Radiographic appearance of the stomach in a rabbit with gastric impaction and caecal tympany due to advanced gut stasis. The stomach is small and contracted and contains a ball of ingesta surrounded by a halo of gas. There is a considerable amount of gas in the ileocaecocolic complex. The rabbit died and hepatic lipidosis was confirmed during post-mortem examination. A dental spur was the inciting cause.

In addition to delayed emptying of the stomach, there is also slow intestinal motility, and the food in the intestines can ferment to produce gas. Small pockets of gas may be seen throughout the small intestine and in the ileocaecocolic complex as well as in the stomach. In the later stages of gut stasis the amount of ileocaecocolic gas can be large, so caecal tympany occurs and the rabbit might appear bloated. By this stage, the rabbit will be completely anorexic and depressed. It will be in pain and other problems, such as gastric ulceration, can develop. The rabbit might start to chew paper, wood or bedding in a frantic manner. There may be audible tooth grinding, especially if the caecum is tympanitic.

Development of hepatic lipidosis

Once gut motility is reduced and food does not move through the digestive tract, there is a reduction in the absorption of fluid and nutrients from the foregut and a reduction in the supply of fluids and nutrients to the caecal microflora in the hindgut. Absorption of carbohydrates from the small intestine is reduced and volatile fatty acid synthesis and absorption from the caecum decrease. As a result, the rabbit goes into a negative energy balance, which stimulates the mobilization of free fatty acids from adipose tissue. These are transported to the liver to be metabolized as an energy source using beta-oxidation, which causes ketone body production and metabolic acidosis. The free fatty acids infiltrate the liver and cause fatty degeneration (Figure 12.14). The fatty liver is fragile and easily ruptures, which can cause abdominal haemorrhage. Free fatty acids accumulate in the kidneys as well as the liver, so the rabbit may die from ketoacidosis, abdominal haemorrhage, liver failure, kidney failure, shock or a combination of any of these conditions.

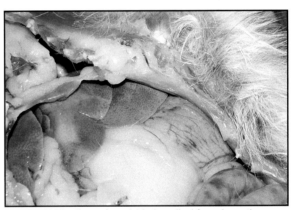

12.14 The liver of a rabbit that died from hepatic lipidosis. The rabbit had undergone coronal reduction 3 days previously after a molar spur was detected. The rabbit did not start to eat after discharge so the owners sought a second opinion. The rabbit died despite treatment, and post-mortem examination confirmed the presence of a pale, fatty, friable liver.

The clinical signs of hepatic lipidosis are total anorexia and no faecal output. The rabbit is often ataxic and hypothermic and has not eaten or defecated for several days, although the owners may not have noticed. Blood results may reflect liver and kidney failure. Lipaemia is usually present, often in conjunction with hyperglycaemia. Urine samples show a low pH and ketones. There are no pathognomonic radiographic signs of hepatic lipidosis, although ultrasonography can be useful to detect fatty infiltration of the liver.

Hepatic lipidosis occurs more readily in rabbits that already have fatty infiltration of the liver (obese rabbits) or those with a high energy demand (pregnancy and lactation).

Small intestinal obstruction

Intestinal obstruction is a common emergency in rabbits and a cause of collapse, shock and sudden death. The most common cause of intestinal obstruction in rabbits is a small solid impacted pellet, which is similar in appearance to a large hard faecal pellet but is composed of tightly matted hair instead of indigestible plant material. Obstruction by these pellets is more common during moulting and in long-haired rabbits, but also occurs in short-coated breeds, including Rex, and in captive wild rabbits. The most plausible explanation for their presence is that they are the pellets formed by compression of ingested hair (see Figure 12.3) that are ingested again once they have passed out of the anus. Rabbits are known to eat hard faecal pellets as well as caecotrophs (Ebino *et al.*, 1993) and owners often report that they have seen their rabbits doing this. Rabbits may also eat the faeces of a larger, hairier companion. This is not a problem if the pellet is small enough to pass through the digestive tract but if the rabbit consumes a large pellet of compressed hair then it can obstruct the intestine.

Complete obstruction of the small intestine

Causes of complete intestinal obstruction are ingested foreign bodies (e.g. pellets of compressed fur, locust bean seeds, dried sweetcorn, carpet fibre), strangulations or tumours. Obstruction of the small intestine results in pain, shock, gastric dilation and eventual tympany. The section of small intestine proximal to the site of the obstruction becomes dilated with gas and fluid (Figure 12.15).

This can often be seen on abdominal radiographs. Exploratory surgery is diagnostic and always indicated for the rabbit with sudden, complete anorexia, gastric dilation and no evidence of gas in the caecum. The surgical technique is described in the *BSAVA Manual of Rabbit Surgery, Dentistry and Imaging.*

Partial obstruction of the small intestine

Partial obstruction of the small intestine may be caused by strictures, adhesions, tumours or other conditions that occasionally occur in rabbits, some of which are obscure (Figures 12.16 and 12.17). Strictures or adhesions may be the result of previous episodes of inflammation in the gastrointestinal tract, or from previous surgery. Affected rabbits experience repeated bouts of abdominal pain and anorexia, which often resolve spontaneously or with analgesics and other medication. Gastric dilation may or may not be present during these episodes, or it may not be evident to the owner. Although radiography, ultrasonography, laparoscopy or computed tomography (CT) and magnetic resonance imaging (MRI) may indicate that an abnormality is present, exploratory surgery is the best way of making the diagnosis.

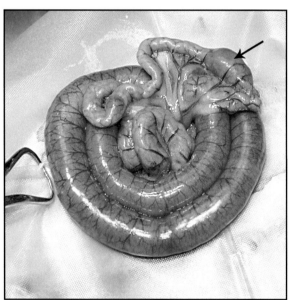

12.15 Intestinal foreign body in a section of small intestine that was exteriorized during surgery. The foreign body was obstructing the lumen. The section of intestine that is proximal to the obstruction is distended with gas and fluid in contrast to the distal section. In this case, the foreign body was successfully milked through the small intestine and through the ileocolic valve, which released the gas and fluid into the hindgut. The rabbit recovered.

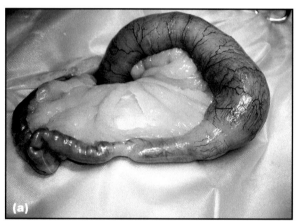

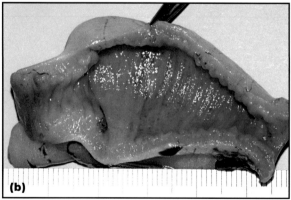

12.16 Intestinal hypertrophy. **(a)** A section of small intestine from a rabbit that was suffering from intermittent bouts of anorexia and colic that were becoming more frequent and severe. Exploratory surgery was performed when gastric dilation developed. A section of hypertrophied mucosa **(b)** was causing a partial obstruction. Histopathology confirmed that it was not neoplastic. The author has seen several similar cases but the aetiology is unknown.

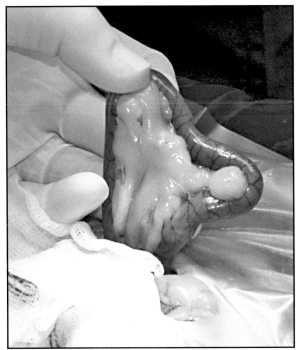

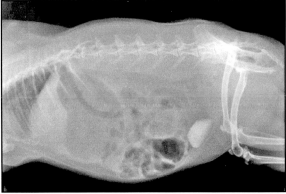

12.18 Radiograph of the rabbit in Figure 12.11, taken 1 hour later. The rabbit had been given fentanyl/fluanisone (0.2 ml/kg) in the interim. The radiograph shows that the stomach is still dilated but less so than in Figure 12.11, and the intestinal gas has moved into the ileocaecocolic complex. This was interpreted as a good prognostic sign, indicating that the obstruction had moved into the hindgut. The blood glucose had fallen to 14.6 mmol/l. The rabbit started to eat 1 hour later.

12.17 A section of the small intestine of a 2-year-old male neutered rabbit that showed signs of intermittent colic, gastric distension and anorexia. Part of the intestine followed an anomalous path, forming a U-bend that could obstruct the flow of ingesta. The anomaly was discovered during exploratory laparotomy and was corrected by carefully sectioning a narrow part of the mesentery within the U-bend and repairing it so the intestine followed a straight path. The rabbit recovered from surgery and survived for at least 3 years without signs of colic.

Moving foreign bodies

The most common moving foreign body is a medium-sized pellet of compressed hair (Harcourt-Brown, 2007), which is suspected to obstruct the small intestine periodically, causing pain but eventually moving through to the hindgut. When the foreign body passes through the ileocolic valve, all the gas and fluid that has built up in the stomach and small intestine is suddenly released into the colon and the caecum (Figure 12.18). These rabbits often make a spontaneous recovery unless they are shocked by the pain and stress of the gastric dilation.

In the cases that recover, no post-mortem examination or exploratory surgery is performed so no foreign body is seen and intestinal obstruction is not confirmed. These cases are often misdiagnosed as gut stasis, and recovery may be attributed to the variety of home remedies that are given to rabbits with 'stasis', which include pineapple juice, exercise, massaging the abdomen and simethicone. Some of these remedies are contraindicated. Massaging the abdomen of a rabbit with gastric tympany could cause the organ to rupture. Simethicone is used to treat frothy bloat in ruminants and human babies, by breaking up the bubbles of gas so they can be expelled from the stomach by eructation. Rabbits do not develop frothy bloat and cannot eructate, so simethicone is not indicated, although it will do no harm. Treatment with prokinetics, analgesia and fluid therapy may be beneficial to a rabbit with a moving foreign body as reduced gut motility will be a complicating factor due to the pain of an intestinal obstruction. However, there is a risk of inducing rupture of a tympanic stomach or small intestine by administering prokinetic therapy. Judgment should be based on clinical signs, radiography and blood tests, including glucose measurement.

Differentiating between anorexia due to a moving foreign body and anorexia due to gut stasis can be difficult, but differentiation is important because complete obstruction of the small intestine is inevitably fatal, unless the obstruction is removed. Prompt surgery for these cases can be very rewarding (Harcourt-Brown, 2013). The pellet is easily located and can be milked through the small intestine and pushed through the ileocolic valve. Knowing whether the foreign body would have gone through on its own is always difficult. Figure 12.19 summarizes the most useful diagnostic features that differentiate gut stasis from intestinal obstruction.

Diarrhoea

Enteric disease is a common reason for pet rabbits to be presented for veterinary treatment. Diarrhoea due to enteritis is a subject that is widely covered in the literature about rabbits because it is a condition that is important to breeders. Enteric disease is a major cause of death in breeding colonies and accounts for 10–12% of the mortality in intensively farmed rabbits in France (Dewrée *et al.*, 2007). In pet rabbits, there is sometimes confusion about what is and what is not diarrhoea. A brief explanation of the normal digestive physiology of rabbits is often required for rabbit owners to understand the difference between caecotrophs and diarrhoea.

Feature	Intestinal obstruction	Moving foreign body	Gut stasis
Speed of onset	Rapid: owner often says rabbit was 'fine' a few hours before	Rapid	Slow: owners often can't say when signs began
Demeanour of rabbit at outset	Depressed, immobile, may hide in corners, may show signs of colic	Variable	Progressively quieter; becomes more depressed when anorexia has been present for 2–3 days (unless another condition is making rabbit ill)
Palpation of stomach	Large, balloon-like structure behind ribs on left-hand side	Dilated stomach is often palpable	Stomach is not palpable or can be felt as small, hard mass
Abdominal radiology	Gastric dilation; may or may not be distended loops of intestine (depending on site of obstruction); no gas in ileocaecocolic complex	Gastric dilation; distended loops of intestine usually visible, unless they are filled with fluid; large amount of gas in ileocaecocolic complex once foreign body passes through	Small stomach with or without impacted contents and halo of gas, depending on stage of gut stasis; gas in caecum is common; may be large amounts of caecal gas in later stages
Blood glucose	High >20 mmol/l	Raised 15–25 mmol/l	Low, normal or slightly raised (>15 mmol/l); low or within normal range in early stages

12.19 A summary of the differences between gut stasis, a moving foreign body and complete intestinal obstruction. (Reproduced from the *BSAVA Manual of Rabbit Surgery, Dentistry and Imaging*)

In order to ascertain whether a rabbit truly does have diarrhoea, visual and possibly microscopic examination of any material that is passed may be necessary (see Figures 12.4, 12.5 and 12.6).

Uneaten caecotrophs

Uneaten caecotrophs are often mistaken for diarrhoea because the owner sees a large amount of soft material that looks and smells like faeces. The amount and nature of dietary fibre is important for the ingestion and consistency of caecotrophs (see Chapter 3). Rabbits that eat diets that contain large amounts of indigestible fibre are more likely to eat their caecotrophs and are less likely to be overweight. The caecotrophs also tend to be firmer.

Although it has not been proven, sugars and starches are sometimes cited as a cause of soft caecotrophs and the syndrome is sometimes called 'caecal dysbiosis' or 'caecal diarrhoea'. The consistency of normal caecotrophs may be variable. Laboratory studies have shown that dietary starch has no influence on the chemical composition of caecal contents or on the production or composition of soft and hard faeces (Carabaño *et al.*, 1988).

Ingestion of caecotrophs is triggered by stimulation of rectal mechanoreceptors and the odour of the caecotrophs. When food is scarce, all the caecotrophs are consumed. When plenty of food is available, the protein and fibre contents of the ration influence the amount of caecotrophs consumed. Increased levels of fibre increase caecotrophy whereas high protein levels reduce it.

Although uneaten caecotrophs do not directly represent a life-threatening condition, the implications for the welfare of the rabbit are far reaching. The condition is unpleasant for the owners and difficult to manage. Owners may be deterred by the presence of the faecal mass and the constant smell. The inconvenience of constantly bathing and cleaning their rabbit's perineum can result in owners abandoning their pet. Uneaten caecotrophs lead to skin infections and attract flies so affected rabbits are high-risk candidates for myiasis.

There are many reasons why rabbits do not eat their caecotrophs (Figure 12.20). Identifying the cause of uneaten caecotrophs is very important if the condition is to be treated successfully. Dietary modification is usually necessary and can be very successful if owners can be motivated to change the rabbit's feeding habits. Clipping off the soiled fur and treating any underlying skin infection is also important.

Loss of appetite for caecotrophs
• Too much commercial concentrated rabbit food • Insufficient dietary fibre • Loss of appetite in general, i.e. ill for another reason • Taints from certain food items or new foods that the rabbit does not like • Stress, e.g. from transport
Inability to reach anus to ingest caecotrophs
• Obesity • Spondylitis • Spinal deformities such as kyphosis, lordosis, scoliosis • Arthritic joints • Restricted space • Matted fur over the anus (fluffy rabbits or those that can't groom effectively because they have incisor problems) • Folds of skin over the anus • Balance problems, e.g. rabbits with a head tilt • Hindlimb weakness
Pain or discomfort on ingestion of caecotrophs
• Dental disease, e.g. molar spurs, incisor abnormalities • Sore perineal skin, e.g. from urine scalding or secondary dermatitis under mats of fur contaminated with caecotrophs and/or urine • Infected perineal skin folds • Respiratory disease making it difficult for the rabbit to breathe while its head is bent round
Loss of awareness that caecotrophs are emerging from the anus
• Problems with sense of smell, e.g. rhinitis • Neurological problems, e.g. fractured or dislocated vertebrae, encephalitozoonosis

12.20 Some reasons why rabbits fail to ingest their caecotrophs.

True diarrhoea

True diarrhoea occurs when no hard faecal pellets are passed and copious amounts of soft or liquid faeces are passed with little or no voluntary control. The rabbit may show signs of systemic illness, such as abdominal pain or dehydration. In this situation, diarrhoea is usually due to intestinal inflammation in response to exposure to a pathogen or due to the non-inflammatory syndrome of mucoid enteropathy (see later).

Enteric disease

Enteric disease is a major cause of losses in rabbits reared for meat production. Many terms are used to describe enteric disease in rabbits, including enteritis, enterotoxaemia, mucoid enteritis, mucoid enteropathy, dysbiosis, colibacillosis, enteropathy, enteritis complex and dysentery. This list is not exhaustive and there is overlap between the conditions. In pet rabbits, enteric disease is rare and is usually seen in newly acquired juvenile rabbits that have been purchased from a breeder or pet shop. These cases can be difficult because the rabbit may have only been in its new home for 2–3 weeks and the owners may have gone to some expense to buy hutches, pens and food and the family are already attached to their new pet. It can be hard to make an exact diagnosis (Figure 12.21). The rabbit often appears depressed and has abnormal faeces. Treatment is difficult because success depends on the pathogens involved, which can be hard to establish in the practice situation. The approach and treatment for any form of enteric disease is non-specific (Figure 12.22).

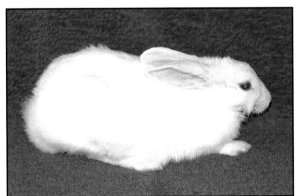

12.21 Typical appearance of a juvenile rabbit that could have been suffering from any one (or a combination) of the range of digestive disorders that can affect young rabbits. He was thin but there was abdominal distension. His coat was staring and he was inappetent. He was passing loose faeces which contained coccidial oocysts. The radiograph and subsequent post-mortem examination showed typical signs of mucoid enteropathy.

Infectious enteritis

The first sign of infectious enteritis may be weight loss and loose pasty faeces with no formed hard faecal pellets, or it may be a collapsed rabbit with

- Perform a clinical examination, paying attention to demeanour, body score, hydration status, abdominal pain or other abnormalities. A blood sample may be helpful.
- Examine the faeces macroscopically and microscopically to make sure the diarrhoea is not due to uneaten caecotrophs and to look for coccidial oocysts.
- Give fluids (either Hartmann's solution intravenously or an oral rehydration fluid such as Lectade).
- Make sure body temperature is maintained.
- Treat with opioids. These may slow gut motility and also provide analgesia for any abdominal pain.
- Give a spasmolytic if diarrhoea is severe and associated with abdominal pain, which is evident from loud tooth grinding, e.g. metamizole/butylscopolamine (Buscopan) 0.1 ml/kg s.c. or loperamide 0.1 mg/kg orally q8–24h.
- Give antibiotics. Oral metronidazole (20 mg/kg q12h) is the antibiotic of choice.
- Give colestyramine (0.5 g/kg q8–12h). Colestyramine is an ion exchange resin that binds to enterotoxins and reduces the risk of death from enterotoxaemia.
- Treat with coccidiocidal medication if coccidial oocysts are present. Toltrazuril 3 mg/kg (daily for 2 days, miss 5 days and give for another 2 days) is recommended.
- Ensure a source of palatable fibre is available. Fresh grass and/ or good quality hay are ideal. For recovery to take place the caecum needs to be repopulated with a healthy microflora, which requires the correct substrate (i.e. fibre).
- Syringe-feed the rabbit if it is not eating. Use a recovery or critical care diet.
- Consider the use of probiotics.

12.22 An approach to rabbits with true diarrhoea.

watery diarrhoea. Adult pet rabbits seldom suffer from enteritis because they are not exposed to many pathogens and the predisposing factors are reduced or absent. They may also have some immunity. In young rabbits, there are many infections that can cause enteritis and the condition is often multifactorial. Several pathogens may be involved (Figure 12.23). Providing dietary fibre has a protective effect and minimizes losses from enteric conditions.

Bacteria
• *Escherichia coli* (several strains of varying pathogenicity) • *Clostridium spiroforme* • *Clostridium difficile* • *Clostridium piliforme* (Tyzzer's disease) • *Clostridium perfringens* • *Klebsiella pneumoniae* • *Klebsiella oxytoca* • *Lawsonia intracellularis* • *Pseudomonas aeruginosa* • *Salmonella* spp.

Viruses
• Rotavirus • Coronavirus

Parasites
• Coccidia • *Cryptosporidium parvum*

12.23 Infections that can cause enteritis in rabbits.

Young rabbits are very susceptible to enteritis for a number of reasons.

- They are exposed to a number of pathogens when the caecal microflora is not yet established and they have no immunity.
- Pathogenic strains of *Escherichia coli*, *Clostridium* spp. or viruses may be present in the environment of newly weaned rabbits. Several animals sharing a small space increases faecal contamination and the risk of cross-infection.
- Coccidiosis is highly infectious and is present in most breeding establishments.
- The stomach pH of suckling rabbits is approximately 5–6.5 whereas adult rabbits have a stomach pH of 1–2, except during digestion of caecotrophs when the pH rises. This high pH of suckling rabbits not only permits healthy bacteria to pass through the digestive tract and colonize the hindgut, but also permits the passage of pathogens.
- Weaning is a stressful period for rabbits.
- After weaning, rabbits are often stressed by change of housing and diet, transport and mixing with different individuals. Intercurrent disease such as pasteurellosis can be present and is itself stressful.

Specific treatment of enteritis depends on the pathogen that is involved and on effective supportive care. Oral rehydration, spasmolytics and antibiotics can be successful (Banerjee *et al.*, 1987) especially if the causative organism can be isolated so any antibiotic sensitivity is known. Non-specific treatment is described in Figure 12.22. The role of probiotics in the prevention and treatment of infectious enteritis is unclear. Although the faecal enterococci have been characterized, the fate of introduced probiotics *in vivo* has not been established (Linaje *et al.*, 2004).

Coccidiosis

Coccidiosis is one of the most common enteric infections of rabbits. As many as 16 species of *Eimeria* have been described in the rabbit including *E. intestinalis*, *E. flavescens*, *E. magna*, *E. irresidua* and *E. piriformis*. All but one of the species are found in the small intestine, caecum or colon and cause intestinal coccidiosis. The exception is *E. stiedae*, which inhabits the epithelial cells of the bile ducts and causes hepatic coccidiosis. There is no cross immunity among the different *Eimeria* species, and mixed infections can occur. *E. magna* and *E. irresidua* are the two most pathogenic coccidial species that affect the intestine of rabbits, and coccidia are often found in conjunction with other pathogenic agents such as *Escherichia coli*. It is not always clear how important the role of intestinal coccidiosis is during an outbreak of enteritis. Experimentally, the introduction of a pathogenic species into a susceptible population can prove fatal, especially in young rabbits around the time of weaning. Concurrent infection with other pathogens is common.

Rabbits that are naturally exposed to infection may or may not show clinical signs depending on the species of coccidia, the rabbit's stress levels, diet and exposure to other pathogens. Recovered rabbits are immune to infection so the disease is extremely rare in adult pets. Clinical signs of coccidiosis vary in severity from weight loss, abdominal distension and mild pasty diarrhoea to anorexia, depression and diarrhoea that can be haemorrhagic.

Infection is introduced by oral ingestion of sporulated oocysts. There are two asexual stages during the life cycle and oocysts appear in the faeces 7–8 days after infection. Various preparations are available to prevent and treat coccidiosis, but in pet rabbits toltrazuril (2.5–5 mg/kg) appears to be the treatment of choice (Redrobe *et al.*, 2010), although oocyst numbers will increase if only a single dose is given. If medication is repeated so it is given during schizogony or gamogony (2 days of treatment, repeated after 5 days), clinical signs and oocyst output are rapidly reduced and immunity against re-infection develops (Peeters and Geeroms, 1986). Diclazuril is an alternative treatment (Vanparis *et al.*, 1989).

Coccidia are highly prolific organisms, and one viable oocyst can yield thousands more in the host. Oocysts are extremely resistant to changes in the environment and can survive for several years. They are not destroyed by most commonly used disinfectants and can resist high temperatures for short periods of time (Varga, 1982). Cleaning of the pens with mild disinfectants may be ineffectual in completely removing oocysts (Wilkinson *et al.*, 2001) and oocysts cannot be eliminated from outdoor runs, so the parasite is likely to be present in the environment of most or all breeding establishments, pet shops, rescue centres and multi-rabbit households. Good hygiene is important, especially for young susceptible rabbits, because the environmental burden is greater in intensive damp, dirty conditions. Coccidial oocysts are susceptible to desiccation, so the use of a blowtorch to 'flame' hutches is a simple method of killing oocysts, or a 10% solution of ammonia is effective. Soil may need to be removed and replaced in outdoor enclosures. Wild rabbits can be a source of infection by contaminating pasture or plants that are picked for pet rabbits, although long grass picked by hand is less likely to be contaminated than short grass grazed by large numbers of wild rabbits.

Enterotoxaemia

In rabbits, enterotoxaemia is usually caused by *Clostridium* spp. or *Escherichia coli*, which are capable of producing powerful enterotoxins. *Clostridium spiroforme* is the major pathogen in rabbit enterotoxaemia, although *C. difficile* and *C. perfringens* may also be involved. Nearly all rabbit isolates of *C. spiroforme* are toxigenic, although this is not the case in other species. These pathogens can reside in the gut without causing disease but, under certain conditions, they proliferate, produce enterotoxins and cause enteritis. This is most likely to occur in rabbits kept in intensive conditions where they are crowded into small spaces and the pathogen is prevalent in the environment. They may also be stressed and exposed to intercurrent infections and disease. In pet rabbits, enterotoxaemia is usually encountered in the newly acquired juvenile but also occurs sporadically in adults, sometimes after periods of stress or administration of certain antibiotics. In many cases there is no obvious precipitating factor.

In colonies of breeding rabbits, recently weaned animals are most susceptible to enterotoxaemia, especially if they are fed on a low-fibre high-carbohydrate diet, and for this reason it has been postulated (but not proven) that high-carbohydrate diets cause enterotoxaemia by allowing unabsorbed carbohydrate to reach the hindgut, which provides a source of glucose to the caecal microflora. Substantial amounts of glucose are required by *C. spiroforme* for toxin production, so providing the correct substrate might enhance toxin production (Cheeke, 1987). Undigested starches could also provide the correct substrate for *E. coli* and clostridia to proliferate. This 'carbohydrate overload' theory is supported by studies that show that young rabbits do not digest and absorb starch in the small intestine as efficiently as adults. However, in adult rabbits, over 99% of ingested starch is hydrolysed and absorbed in the small intestine, so the carbohydrate overload theory does not apply to adults (De Blas and Gidenne, 1998). This explains why so many pet rabbits can exist for years, albeit unhealthily, on high-carbohydrate cereal mixes and sugary treats without dying from enterotoxaemia.

Enterotoxaemia is manifested by diarrhoea, collapse or sudden death. It is an acute disease, although it is sometimes preceded by a short period of anorexia. Death is due to toxaemia, dehydration and electrolyte loss. Peracute cases can be found dead with no prior evidence of disease. Others are found moribund, often with liquid tarry brown diarrhoea. Treatment is described in Figure 12.22.

The diagnosis of enterotoxaemia is usually made during post-mortem examination, which has to be performed promptly to differentiate the changes caused by enterotoxaemia from normal autolysis of the gut. The rabbit is often in good bodily condition. There may or may not be liquid faeces oozing from the anus and staining the perineum and hindlegs. On opening the abdomen, inflammation and hyperaemia of the caecum may be seen, which may extend to the small intestine or proximal colon. Haemorrhages on the serosal surface of the caecum are characteristic of enterotoxaemia. These haemorrhages may look as though they have been applied with a paint brush (Figure 12.24) and may extend to the mucosal surface of the caecum, which can be ulcerated. The submucosa can be thickened and oedematous. The caecal contents are very liquid and may contain gas.

Sometimes, enterotoxaemia can be confirmed by detection of spiral- or comma-shaped organisms (*C. spiroforme*) on Gram-stained caecal smears, but usually in the practice setting confirmation of the diagnosis and identification of the

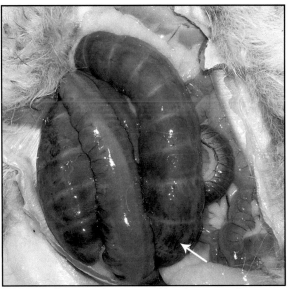

12.24 Caecum of a 4-year-old male neutered Netherland Dwarf that died after developing acute haemorrhagic diarrhoea. The liquid haemorrhagic caecal contents can be seen through the caecal wall. Parts of the serosal surface of the caecum look as if they have been brushed with red paint (arrow). This is typical of enterotoxaemia.

causative pathogen is difficult or impossible. Anaerobic culture for 24–48 hours on blood agar is required to grow the organism and specialized techniques are required to identify the toxin. If a diagnosis is important, anaerobic conditions can be preserved by tying off a section of the caecum and/or intestine at each end before it is removed and submitted to the laboratory. Alternatively, a swab of intestinal contents can be immediately plunged to the bottom of the transport medium where conditions remain anaerobic.

Antibiotic-associated diarrhoea
Antibiotic choice is important in rabbits but can be difficult because of the potential to kill bacteria selectively in the digestive tract. The caecal microflora is composed of a wide range of aerobic and anaerobic bacteria, and disruption of the balance of microorganisms can allow pathogenic species to proliferate and cause disease. Although it is counterintuitive, many of the pathogenic bacteria that induce antibiotic-associated diarrhoea are susceptible to the antibiotics that cause it. This is because the spores are resistant, so the intestinal tract can be recolonized by pathogenic bacteria after the antibiotic has disrupted the normal microflora. As a result of the recolonization, diarrhoea may develop some time after the antibiotic has been withdrawn (Bartlett, 1992).

The consequence of antibiotic administration to rabbits is not completely predictable. In the majority of cases no adverse effects are seen after administration of antibiotics, even those that are known to have the potential to cause enterotoxaemia. In other cases, transient mild diarrhoea may occur after administration of a 'safe' antibiotic. It can be hard to establish the exact sequence of events. Not all rabbits have pathogenic bacteria in their gut and the choice of antibiotic and route of administration are important factors in the development of antibiotic-associated diarrhoea and enterotoxaemia. Oral administration carries a greater risk than parenteral administration. A guide to antibiotic use is given in Figure 12.25. Rabbits with milder cases of antibiotic-associated diarrhoea can survive if the antibiotic is discontinued, although it may take some time for a healthy caecal microflora to be re-established; treatment is described in Figure 12.22.

Safe orally and parenterally
• Enrofloxacin • Marbofloxacin • Trimethoprim/sulphonamide • Metronidazole • Oxytetracycline • Doxycycline • Chloramphenicol
Safe orally but not parenterally
• Gentamicin (potentially nephrotoxic if given parenterally)
Safe parenterally but NOT orally
• Penicillin • Cephalosporins • Streptomycin • Ampicillin • Amoxicillin
Safe topically (and therefore orally)
• Fusidic acid • Gentamicin • Chloramphenicol • Chlortetracycline • Ciprofloxacin
Not safe by any route
• Lincomycin • Clindamycin • Erythromycin

12.25 A guide to antibiotic use based on current knowledge and anecdotal information. Few antibiotics are authorized for use in rabbits and the responsibility for the use of unauthorized products lies with the prescribing veterinary surgeon. 'Unsafe' antibiotics have the potential to cause antibiotic-associated diarrhoea, which may be fatal.

Mucoid enteropathy

Mucoid enteropathy is a specific non-inflammatory enteric condition of rabbits that is poorly understood. It appears to be the result of hypomotility in the caecum and colon. Like enteritis, the condition is usually seen in juvenile rabbits and in breeding does. It is rare in adult pet rabbits and, as with enteritis, a high-fibre diet appears to have some protective effect. Alterations in the caecal microflora and volatile fatty acid production are seen in association with mucoid enteropathy although it is not clear whether this is a primary or secondary event. Mucoid enteropathy is characterized by caecal impaction and the presence of large amounts of mucus in the colon.

The clinical signs of mucoid enteropathy develop gradually. In the initial stages the rabbit is often eating, before it develops abdominal distension, depression and a crouched stance. A feature of the disease is tooth grinding, presumably due to abdominal pain. There is a disruption of normal faecal production. Hard faecal pellets are not produced. Diarrhoea may be present in the early stages but in the later stages large amounts of mucus, either on its own or mixed with faecal material, are excreted. As the disease progresses, faecal production may cease completely and appetite is reduced to the point of complete anorexia.

A solid impacted caecum may be palpable and seen radiographically. Gas shadows may be seen in the caecum and small intestine. In the terminal stages, there is gastric distension with large amounts of fluid and/or gas in the stomach. At post-mortem examination, inflammatory changes are minimal and the caecum is often impacted with dried contents and gas. The colon is distended with gelatinous mucus. The stomach and small intestine may also be distended with fluid and gas. In the terminal stages, the rabbit may die from a number of secondary causes associated with gut dysfunction, such as malnutrition, gastric dilation, inhalation pneumonia, secondary bacterial infections or abdominal catastrophes associated with the disease.

The aetiopathogenesis of mucoid enteropathy is far from clear. It is not known what roles diet, stress, pathogens or caecal microflora play. Some cases appear to be infectious and associated with neurogenic dysfunction. There may be different causes in individual outbreaks.

Dysautonomia

Some outbreaks of mucoid enteropathy show signs that are similar to dysautonomic disease in horses and cats, i.e. mydriasis, dry mucous membranes, reduced tear production, bradycardia (<100 bpm), urine retention and intestinal impaction. A syndrome of caecal impaction in conjunction with pulmonary oedema, mydriasis, dry mucous membranes, reduced tear production, bradycardia and urine retention has been described in rabbits (Van der Hage and Dorrestein, 1996; Whitwell and Needham, 1996). Dysphagia and inhalation pneumonia are often seen as terminal events; affected rabbits have problems swallowing and may have uneaten food in the mouth and pharynx. The diagnosis of dysautonomia was confirmed by finding neural degeneration in the coeliac and mesenteric ganglia. No viruses, infectious agents, aflatoxins or other causative agents were discovered on food analysis or on extensive examination of the liver and intestinal contents of affected animals. A neurotoxin (e.g. from *Clostridium botulinum*) is a possible explanation for the condition.

Epizootic rabbit enteropathy

In 1996, in France, a severe digestive disease appeared in fattening domestic rabbits. The condition was named 'epizootic rabbit enteropathy'. It is highly contagious with 30–40% mortality and 100%

morbidity (Liçois *et al.*, 2005). Despite extensive research, the aetiological agent has not yet been identified, but it has been shown that the disease can be transmitted via intestinal contents from affected rabbits to those that are specific pathogen-free. Common clinical signs are anorexia and mild watery diarrhoea with considerable distension of the abdomen.

On post-mortem examination, gastric and intestinal distension without gross evidence of acute or chronic enteric lesions is seen. The caecal contents may be watery or impacted and mucus may be present in the colon. Histopathology shows cellular infiltration of the lamina propria and submucosa of various parts of the intestine with polymorpho-nuclear leucocytes, lymphocytes, macrophages and occasional plasma cells, and these cells are observed near Auerbach's plexus (Dewrée *et al.*, 2007). This myenteric plexus is in the muscular layers of the proximal colon and contains many autonomic fibres (Snipes *et al.*, 1982). Although epizootic rabbit enteropathy has great significance in farmed rabbits, it is unlikely to be encountered in the individual pet.

Other conditions associated with altered gastrointestinal motility

Although gut stasis is a non-specific response to pain and stress in rabbits, there are some conditions that change the motility of all or part of the gastrointestinal tract and affect digestion.

Paralytic ileus
Paralytic ileus is an uncommon condition that affects seriously ill rabbits. It follows major abdominal crises such as liver lobe torsion. There is complete loss of gastrointestinal motility, which results in dilation and tympany of the stomach, intestines and ileocaecocolic complex (Harcourt-Brown, 2013). Paralytic ileus is also a problem in humans, horses and other species, in which it often follows serious abdominal surgery. An imbalance between sympathetic and parasympathetic activity, plus endotoxaemia, has been postulated as a cause in horses (Koenig and Cote, 2006).

Caecal impaction and caecolith formation
In the adult pet rabbit, caecal impaction occurs sporadically. As with gastric stasis, there is often a history of a stressful situation. Dehydration may play a part in the aetiopathogenesis and it can be associated with chronic renal failure.

Caecal impaction can also occur after feeding products that are rich in small particles that cannot be degraded by the caecal microflora. Bulk laxatives such as methylcellulose or psyllium are examples, especially as they absorb water. Ground-up lignified material can have a similar effect. Small particles, such as chalk, barium or clay cat litter, can also become impacted as they are moved into the caecum during mixing and separation of ingesta in the proximal colon.

The onset of caecal impaction can be insidious. In the initial stages, the rabbit may not look particularly unwell, but is inappetent and loses weight. The condition may be mistaken for dental disease as the rabbit may pick at food, eat a little and then drop it uneaten. Affected rabbits adopt a hunched stance. Faecal output is reduced or absent. There is often mucus production. The impacted organ can usually be palpated as a hard sausage-shaped structure in the ventral abdomen that can be seen on abdominal radiographs (Figure 12.26). On post-mortem examination, the caecal contents are solid and dry. Occasionally, a large lump of hard dry caecal contents can move into the colon and cause an obstruction. Caecal dilation may be the result.

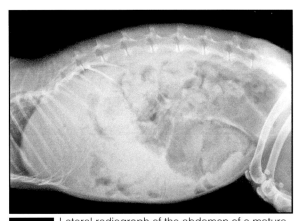

12.26 Lateral radiograph of the abdomen of a mature neutered female spotted rabbit that was thin with a distended abdomen. Large pieces of impacted ingesta surrounded by gas can be seen in the caecum. The rabbit was eating a little but not passing faecal pellets. Blood urea and calcium were raised. The rabbit was euthanased and samples sent for histopathology. Chronic interstitial granulomatous inflammatory lesions consistent with encephalitozoonosis were found in the kidney. It is not known why the caecal impaction occurred. It could have been part of a megacolon syndrome, or linked with chronic dehydration and kidney disease, or due to another disorder. Kyphosis affecting the thoracic vertebrae was believed to be an incidental finding.

Caecal impaction is difficult to treat. Surgery is unlikely to be successful. Medical treatment is directed at providing nutrition, relieving pain, promoting gastrointestinal motility, softening the caecal contents and promoting caecal evacuation. Fluid therapy by all routes (intravenous, subcutaneous and oral) is indicated. Liquid paraffin (mineral oil) and/or lactulose may help to lubricate and soften the caecal contents. Foods that are reputed to cause 'diarrhoea', such as lettuce or fruit, may tempt an inappetent rabbit to eat and provide additional fluid in addition to stimulating intestinal motility. As in all gastroenteric conditions in rabbits, good quality hay or fresh grass must be constantly available as a source of indigestible fibre. Motility stimulants such as domperidone, ranitidine, cisapride and metoclopramide can be useful.

Analgesics are indicated although, theoretically, interference with prostaglandin production by NSAIDs could have an inhibitory effect on the fusus coli, as prostaglandins stimulate caecal motility (Pairet *et al.*, 1986). Opioids such as buprenorphine or tramadol (0.5 mg/kg s.c. or i.v. q8–12h) may be preferable.

Heavy metal poisoning

The common heavy metals (lead, mercury, silver, zinc, copper, arsenic and iron) are all potential toxins. Lead poisoning in particular is a known cause of anorexia and other clinical signs in rabbits. Information about other metal poisoning is sparse but rabbits that are allowed free access to the house, garden or garage are at risk of toxicity because of their propensity to chew hard objects. Sources of lead include old paint, pipes, linoleum, golf balls and some plumbing materials. Lead shot and air gun pellets are other possible sources.

As in other species, heavy metal poisoning can be acute or chronic. Inappetence, anorexia and slow gut motility are the most commonly described clinical signs. Radiographically, radiodense flakes may be seen throughout the gastrointestinal tract and in the faeces (Figure 12.27) and in these cases

treatment with motility agents is recommended in addition to a chelating agent, such as sodium calcium edetate or penicillamine, to facilitate excretion of the lead and other heavy metals from the gut. An advantage of the rabbit's digestive physiology is the rapid elimination of large particles. Once flakes of lead paint or particles of metal pass out of the stomach, they should be rapidly passed out in the hard faeces rather than moved into the caecum and retained in the body for longer periods. Small particles of toxic material pose a greater risk if they pass into the caecum because they will be re-ingested. Slow gut motility also poses a problem if toxic material is in the stomach because it can be retained within the stomach contents. Gastrotomy and surgical removal may be necessary.

Chronic diarrhoea syndrome (megacolon)

Some pet rabbits suffer from a syndrome of chronic or intermittent diarrhoea. It is most common in mature rabbits, usually over 3 years old, and rabbits with spotted markings (e.g. English) are more prone to the condition (Figure 12.28). A genetic predisposition has been described in the literature (Bödeker *et al.*, 1995). This syndrome is sometimes described as 'megacolon' or 'cow pat faeces' because the colon and caecum can be very large and distended and the faeces may be voluminous and pasty (see Figure 12.4). Alternatively, the faeces may be soft but variable in size with some very large

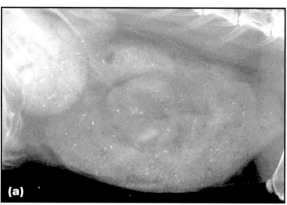

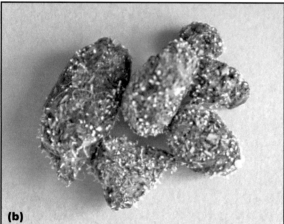

12.27 Heavy metal poisoning. **(a)** Lateral view of the abdomen of a 6-year-old neutered female rabbit that lived in an old house and had chewed the skirting boards. The rabbit was referred for specialist treatment because of anorexia that had not responded to prokinetic, analgesic and intravenous fluid therapy. Speckles of radiodense material can be seen throughout the digestive tract. **(b)** White flakes appeared in the faeces once the rabbit started to defecate after syringe-feeding and treatment with penicillamine and prokinetics. This is a good example of the benefits of taking abdominal radiographs of anorexic rabbits.

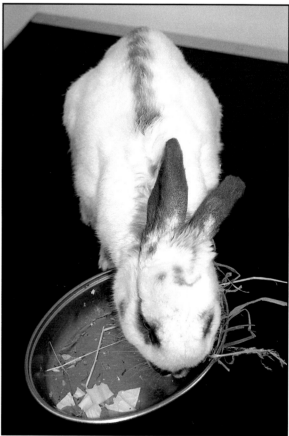

12.28 This rescue rabbit shows many typical signs of megacolon syndrome. He is a spotted breed, thin with a distended abdomen and ravenously hungry.

(marble sized) pellets passing through. In some cases the faeces vary between 'cow pat' faeces and large soft pellets. No normal faeces or caecotrophs are seen and the pellets that are passed are a mixture of the two. They are soft but contain long strands of undigested fibre. The course of the disease is slow (months or years), and affected rabbits lose weight and develop a pendulous abdomen. They may eat ravenously between bouts of anorexia and caecal tympany. Large faecal pellets, large amounts of food in the caecum, or caecal gas and tympany may be evident on abdominal radiographs (Figure 12.29) during these episodes.

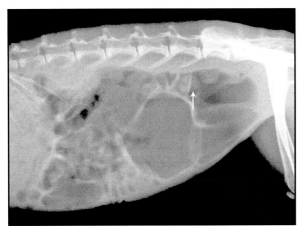

12.29 Lateral view of the abdomen of a 5-year-old English Spot neutered male showing some of the typical signs of megacolon syndrome. The caecum is dilated and filled with gas (the radiograph was taken during an intermittent bout of anorexia) and there are some very large faecal pellets in the rectum (arrow).

Blood samples often show anaemia, hypoproteinaemia and hypoglobulinaemia. A Gram stain of a faecal smear shows a range of microorganisms in the same sample as long fibre particles, suggesting that the colon is not separating the large and small particles. Histopathological examination shows lymphocytic/plasmacytic inflammation.

The condition is incurable, but manageable if the bouts of diarrhoea or caecal tympany are controlled. Dietary modification and an exclusion diet hold out the best hope. Many cases develop diarrhoea as soon as they eat any commercial rabbit foods and treats. Fruit, vegetables or human foods are often not tolerated but each case is different. The author has seen one rabbit that could only tolerate grass-based food, i.e. hay and nuggets, and would develop problems if any other food, even herbs or leafy green vegetables, was introduced into the diet. This case contrasted with another rabbit that did not tolerate any grass-based food, and could only eat fruit, vegetables and alfalfa without developing diarrhoea or impactions.

Motility stimulants such as domperidone and ranitidine can help to control the condition. They may be given continually or only during episodes of diarrhoea. Opioid analgesics may help during periods of tympany. There are pros and cons of treatment with NSAIDs as they could inhibit caecal

motility but, in most instances, the benefits outweigh the potential problems. Each case needs to be judged on its own merit and reassessed regularly. In the author's experience, prednisolone can be helpful in recalcitrant cases.

Miscellaneous digestive diseases

Yersiniosis

Pseudotuberculosis, caused by the bacterium *Yersinia pseudotuberculosis*, is a common infection in rodents, especially guinea pigs. It is also occasionally encountered in pet rabbits, in which it can cause non-specific anorexia, gut stasis and weight loss. Lesions of pseudotuberculosis include large areas of caseous necrosis in the mesenteric lymph nodes, liver, spleen and gut-associated lymphoid tissue (Figure 12.30). Yersiniosis is probably contracted from food, such as hay, that has been

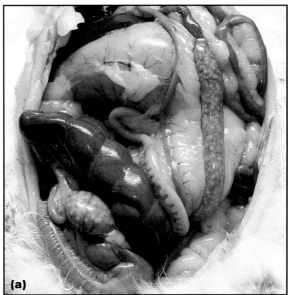

(a)

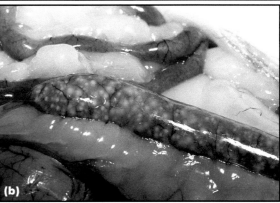

(b)

12.30 Post-mortem appearance of the sacculus rotundus **(a)** and appendix **(b)** of a rabbit with *Yersinia pseudotuberculosis* infection. Both organs have a pale spotted appearance. The clinical signs were non-specific: the rabbit was anorexic and losing weight despite a range of treatments including enrofloxacin. Blood sample results showed lymphopenia, mild anaemia and slightly raised alkaline phosphatase. An abdominal mass was thought to be present, so exploratory laparotomy was performed. The mass proved to be the sacculus rotundus.

contaminated by mice and rats. The disease is difficult to diagnose during life and is usually discovered during exploratory laparotomy or post-mortem examination. Theoretically, the infection should be responsive to antibiotic therapy but the diagnosis is often not made until it is too late for treatment.

Neoplasia

Neoplasia affecting any part of the gastrointestinal tract can occur spontaneously and a variety of tumours has been described (Shibuya *et al.*, 1999). Lymphoma appears to be the most common. Clinical signs depend on the site of the tumour but weight loss, anorexia, gastric dilation and palpable abdominal masses are all possible signs. The diagnosis is usually made during exploratory laparotomy (Figure 12.31) or post-mortem examination. See also Chapter 18.

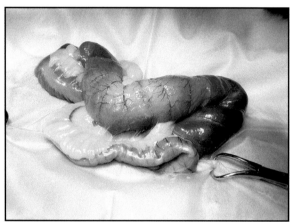

12.31 Caecum of a rabbit with multicentric lymphoma. The kidneys were also affected. The tumour was discovered during exploratory surgery for chronic inappetence, weight loss and the suspicion of an abdominal mass.

Diverticulitis

Diverticulitis occurs when infection develops in evaginations of the colonic mucosa and submucosa through weaknesses in the muscle layers. Ingesta collects in the pouches (diverticula), which may cause further distension and enlargement. Perforation of the mucosa and abscess formation can occur. Although this condition has not been reported as a naturally occurring disease in rabbits, the author has encountered four cases. All were diagnosed during exploratory surgery or at post-mortem examination. All the rabbits had a history of intermittent anorexia and colic. In three of the four cases, painful palpable masses were detected during abdominal palpation. A section of colon from one of the cases is shown in Figure 12.32.

Helminth infection

Parasitic enteritis is rarely a cause of clinical signs, although intestinal obstruction due to large numbers of tapeworms or tapeworm cysts is described in some textbooks (Harcourt-Brown, 2002). In general, the rabbit is the secondary host for tapeworms, e.g. *Taenia pisiformis*, *T. serialis* and *Echinococcus*

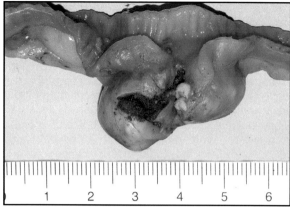

12.32 Section of the distal colon of a rabbit with intermittent bouts of colic and anorexia. Palpable masses were present in the abdomen. On exploratory laparotomy, these masses proved to be evaginations of the intestinal mucosa containing ingesta. Two of these had formed abscesses, one of which is shown. The rabbit was euthanased.

granulosus, but the rabbit can be a primary host for some tapeworms (*Cittotaenia* spp.; Figure 12.33a) that have free-living mites as the intermediate host. Occasionally tapeworm segments are seen in the faeces of rabbits (Figure 12.33b) and can be distinguished from the more common worm (*Passalurus ambiguus*) that is encountered in pets.

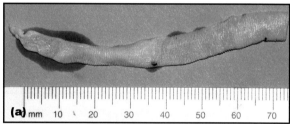

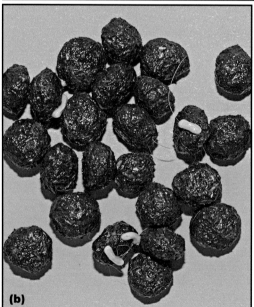

12.33 **(a)** Part of a *Cittotaenia* tapeworm that was passed out after the rabbit had been treated with praziquantel (20 mg in 0.5 ml spot-on solution) because segments had been seen in the faeces.
(b) Several *Cittotaenia* species can affect rabbits, but the condition is rare in pets. Eggs are shown in Figure 12.6.

P. ambiguus is an oxyurid that is found in the caecum and large intestine. The adult worms measure 5–10 mm and no acquired resistance appears to develop (Boag, 1985). Although the worm is usually described as non-pathogenic, heavy infestations in young rabbits may cause perianal pruritus and may be part of the enteritis complex. The small, thread-like worm is seen in both the hard faeces (Figure 12.34) and caecotrophs. The life cycle is direct, so *P. ambiguus* is susceptible to most anthelmintics, e.g. fenbendazole (10–20 mg/kg, repeated in 10–14 days; Reusch, 2005).

There are other helminth parasites that principally affect wild rabbits and are rarely seen in the domestic pet, although their eggs may be found in the faeces. Examples include *Graphidium strigosum*, *Trichostrongylus retortaeformis* and *Obeliscoides cuniculi* (Allan *et al.*, 1999).

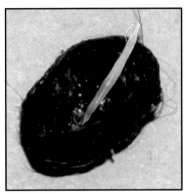

12.34
A *Passalurus ambiguus* pinworm in a hard faecal pellet from an adult pet rabbit. Eggs are shown in Figure 12.6.

Liver lobe torsion

Liver lobe torsion is a condition in rabbits that is increasingly recognized and may have been under-diagnosed in the past (Saunders *et al.*, 2009). The right caudal liver lobe, which overlies the right kidney, is most commonly affected, although torsion of other lobes can occur. The condition often occurs spontaneously in otherwise healthy rabbits. The outcome is variable, presumably depending on the size and site of the liver lobe and the degree of torsion. Affected rabbits may be presented dead or dying, or they may present with a transient period of anorexia from which they recover. If surgical removal of the affected liver lobe is not performed promptly, death may occur after 2–3 days from endotoxic shock or paralytic ileus; or the rabbit may recover as the affected lobe degenerates and atrophies. Degenerate tissue in the area of the liver is sometimes present as an incidental finding on post-mortem examination. Rabbits with life-threatening torsion of a liver lobe are presented with sudden-onset severe anorexia and lethargy. The twisted, congested liver lobe may be palpable as a painful mass in the right cranial abdomen. Gas distension of parts of the gastrointestinal tract may or may not be evident on abdominal palpation. Anaemia, which may be severe, and raised liver enzymes are often present. Blood in the peritoneal cavity may be present.

Abdominal radiography is seldom diagnostic although it rules out other differential diagnoses. Suspicion may be raised by a homogeneous area in the cranial abdomen or the presence of fluid separating the liver lobes. Ultrasound examination is useful to confirm the diagnosis of liver lobe torsion (Redrobe, 2013). An enlarged structure with mixed echogenicity is seen attached to the liver, and dilated thrombosed blood vessels may be detected within that structure. Free fluid within the abdominal cavity may be detected ultrasonographically and a small sample may be collected for examination. The fluid may be a modified transudate, exudate, or haemorrhagic effusion. The presence of a neoplastic or septic effusion may alter prognosis and treatment decisions (Stanke *et al.*, 2011).

Prompt exploratory laparotomy is indicated for any rabbit showing signs of liver lobe torsion (see Saunders, 2013). Although recovery without surgery is possible, surgery to remove the twisted lobe is the safest option. Successful lobectomy has been reported in rabbits, and the surgery is straightforward (see *BSAVA Manual of Rabbit Surgery, Dentistry and Imaging*). Early surgical intervention is recommended because the course of the disease can be rapid and paralytic ileus develops easily, presumably due to endotoxaemia related to the ischaemic tissue.

Pancreatitis

Pancreatitis occurs in rabbits as an apparently spontaneous disease. Obesity appears to be a predisposing factor but is not a universal feature. The diagnosis is usually made at post-mortem examination or during exploratory laparotomy by visual examination of the pancreas, and confirmed by histopathology. Clinical signs are non-specific, with anorexia, anterior abdominal pain and occasional tooth grinding. Fat necrosis occurs in the local mesentery with marked local peritonitis. Peritoneal effusion may be present, which may be detected with ultrasonography. Blood sample results may or may not be helpful (see Chapter 9). Treatment is problematic because withholding food is not an option for rabbits and gut stasis is a serious complication of this disease. The author has known a single case to survive after the diagnosis was made during exploratory laparotomy because the rabbit had shown signs of abdominal pain for 1 week. During this period the pain was controlled with opioids and the rabbit was treated with ranitidine, domperidone and syringe-feeding.

Anorectal papilloma

Anorectal papillomas occur at the junction between the anal and rectal mucosa in some rabbits (Figure 12.35). The aetiology is unclear but the rabbits are often overweight. Chronic inflammation and bleeding of the exposed mucosa is a common complication. The papillomas can be removed surgically (see *BSAVA Manual of Rabbit Surgery, Dentistry and Imaging*) but recurrence is common.

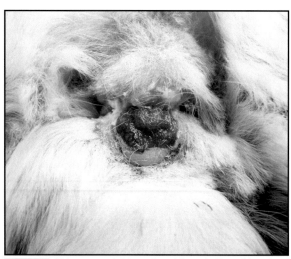

12.35 This overweight neutered female Dwarf Lop had a bleeding mass protruding from the anus. The mass was surgically removed.

References and further reading

Allan JC, Craig PS, Sherington J, *et al.* (1999) Helminth parasites of the wild rabbit *Oryctolagus cuniculus* near Malham Tarn, Yorkshire, UK. *Journal of Helminthology.* **73**, 289–294

Banerjee AK, Angulo AF, Dhasmana KM, *et al.* (1987) Acute diarrhoeal disease in the rabbit: bacteriological diagnosis and efficacy of oral rehydration in combination with loperamide hydrochloride. *Laboratory Animals* **21**, 314–317

Bartlett JM (1992) Antibiotic-associated diarrhea. *Clinical Infectious Diseases* **15**, 573–581

Berezina TP and Ovsiannikov VI (2005) Mechanisms of inhibition of the contractile activity in the ileo-caecal zone in rabbits under psychogenic stress. *Rossiiskii fiziologicheskii zhurnal imeni IM Sechenova* **91**, 893–202

Boag B (1985) The incidence of helminth parasites from the wild rabbit *Orcytolagus cuniculus* (L.) in Eastern Scotland. *Journal of Helminthology* **59**, 61–69

Bödeker D, Türck O, Lovén E, Wiebernett D and Wegner W (1995) Pathological and functional aspects of the megacolon-syndrome of homozygous spotted rabbits. *Journal of the American Veterinary Medical Association* **42**, 549–559

Carabaño R, Fraga MJ, Santoma G and de Blas J (1988) Effect of diet on composition of cecal contents and on excretion and composition of soft and hard feces of rabbits. *Journal of Animal Science* **66**, 901–910

Cheeke PR (1987) *Rabbit Feeding and Nutrition.* Academic Press, Orlando

De Blas E and Gidenne T (1998) Digestion of starch and sugars. In: *The Nutrition of the Rabbit*, ed. C de Blas and J Wiseman, pp.17–38. CABI Publishing, Wallingford

Dewrée R, Meulemans L, Lassance C, *et al.* (2007) Experimentally induced epizootic rabbit enteropathy: Clinical, histopathological, ultrastructural, bacteriological and haematological findings. *World Rabbit Science* **15**, 91–102

Ebino KY, Shutoh Y and Takahashi KW (1993) Coprophagy in rabbits: autoingestion of hard faeces. *Jikken Dobutsu* **42**, 611–613

Harcourt-Brown FM (2002) *Textbook of Rabbit Medicine.* Butterworth Heinemann, Oxford

Harcourt-Brown FM (2007) Gastric dilation and intestinal obstruction in 76 rabbits. *Veterinary Record* **161**, 409–414

Harcourt-Brown FM (2013) Gastric dilation and intestinal obstruction. In: *BSAVA Manual of Rabbit Surgery, Dentistry and Imaging*, ed. F Harcourt-Brown and J Chitty, pp.172–189. BSAVA Publications, Gloucester

Harcourt-Brown FM and Baker SJ (2001) Parathyroid hormone, haematological and biochemical parameters in relation to dental disease and husbandry in pet rabbits. *Journal of Small Animal Practice* **42**, 130–136

Harcourt-Brown FM and Harcourt-Brown SF (2012) Clinical value of blood glucose measurement in pet rabbits. *Veterinary Record* **170**, 674; Epub 2012 Jun 1

Koenig J and Cote N (2006) Equine gastrointestinal motility – ileus and pharmacological modification. *Canadian Veterinary Journal* **47**, 551–559

Lennox A (2013) Radiographic interpretation of the abdomen. In: *BSAVA Manual of Rabbit Surgery, Dentistry and Imaging*, ed. F Harcourt-Brown and J Chitty, pp.84–93. BSAVA Publications, Gloucester

Liçois D, Wyers M and Coudert P (2005) Epizootic rabbit enteropathy: experimental transmission and clinical characterization. *Veterinary Research* **36**, 601–613

Linaje R, Coloma MD, Perez-Martinez G and Zuniga M (2004) Characterisation of faecal enterococci from rabbits for the selection of probiotic strains. *Journal of Applied Microbiology* **96**, 761–771

Pairet M, Bouyssou T and Ruckesbuch Y (1986) Colonic formation of soft feces in rabbits: a role for endogenous prostaglandins. *American Journal of Physiology* **250**, G302–G308

Peeters JE and Geeroms R (1986) Efficacy of toltrazuril against intestinal and hepatic coccidiosis in rabbits. *Veterinary Parasitology* **1**, 21–35

Powers LV (2006) Techniques for drug delivery in small mammals. *Journal of Exotic Pet Medicine* **15**, 201–209

Redfern JS, Lin HJ, McArthur KE, Prince MD and Feldman M (1991) Gastric acid and pepsin secretion in conscious rabbits. *American Journal of Physiology* **261**, G295–G304

Redrobe S (2013) Ultrasonograohy. In: *BSAVA Manual of Rabbit Surgery, Dentistry and Imaging*, ed. F Harcourt-Brown and J Chitty, pp.94–106. BSAVA Publications, Gloucester

Redrobe SP, Gakos G, Saunders R, Martin S and Morgan ER (2010) Comparison of toltrazuril and sulphadimethoxine in the treatment of intestinal coccidiosis in pet rabbits. *Veterinary Record* **167**, 287–290

Reusch B (2005) Rabbit gastroenterology. *Veterinary Clinics of North America: Exotic Animal Practice* **8**, 351–375

Saunders R (2013) Exploratory laparotomy. In: *BSAVA Manual of Rabbit Surgery, Dentistry and Imaging*, ed. F Harcourt-Brown and J Chitty, pp.157–171. BSAVA Publications, Gloucester

Saunders R, Redrobe S, Barr F, *et al.* (2009) Liver lobe torsion in rabbits. *Journal of Small Animal Practice* **50**, 562

Shibuya K, Tajima M, Kanai K, *et al.* (1999) Spontaneous lymphoma in a Japanese White rabbit. *Journal of Veterinary Medical Science* **61**, 1327–1329

Snipes RL, Clauss W, Weber A and Hörnicke H (1982) Structural and functional differences in various divisions of the rabbit colon. *Cell and Tissue Research* **225**, 331–346

Stanke NJ, Graham JE, Orcutt CJ, *et al.* (2011) Successful outcome of hepatectomy as treatment for liver lobe torsion in four domestic rabbits. *Journal of the American Veterinary Medical Association* **238**, 1176–1183

Van der Hage MH and Dorrestein GM (1996) Caecal impaction in the rabbit: Relationships with dysautonomia. *Proceedings of the 6th World Rabbit Congress* **3**, 77–80

Vanparis O, Desplenter L and Marsboom R (1989) Efficacy of diclazuril in the control of intestinal coccidiosis in rabbits. *Veterinary Parasitology* **34**, 185–190

Varga I (1982) Large-scale management systems and parasite populations: Coccidia in rabbits. *Veterinary Parasitology* **11**, 69–84

Whitwell K and Needham J (1996) Mucoid enteropathy in UK rabbits: dysautonomia confirmed. *Veterinary Record* **139**, 323–324

Wilkinson MJ, Bell S, McGoldrick J and Williams AE (2001) Unexpected deaths in young New Zealand White rabbits (*Oryctolagus cuniculus*). *American Association for Laboratory Animal Science* **40**, 49–51

13

Urogenital system and reproductive disease

Elisabetta Mancinelli and Brigitte Lord

Rabbits are frequently presented to the veterinary surgeon with signs of urogenital disease. The aim of this chapter is to demonstrate how urogenital disease in rabbits can be investigated and managed by using the same approach as that used in other small animals. Relevant species differences, normal reference values and considerations will also be discussed.

Urinary system

Physiology

Rabbits excrete alkaline urine. The average volume of urine produced is 130 ml/kg/day (range 20–350 ml/kg/day, depending on diet). The kidneys of the rabbit are unipapillate, i.e. one papilla and calyx enter the ureter directly; most other mammals have multipapillate kidneys. Also, unlike most mammals, total blood calcium levels in rabbits reflect dietary intake. Dietary calcium is readily absorbed from the intestines and this absorption does not depend on activated vitamin D. As a result, both ionized and total calcium serum concentrations are higher than those in other species (ionized calcium 1.6–1.82 mmol/l, total calcium 2.17–4.59 mmol/l). The rabbit is absolutely dependent on the kidney for calcium osmoregulation. The renal fractional excretion of calcium in the rabbit is 45–60%, compared with <2% in mammals that regulate calcium uptake from the gut and eliminate excess calcium in the faeces. The excreted calcium precipitates in the alkaline urine to form calcium complex crystals, giving the urine a thick and creamy appearance (Figure 13.1).

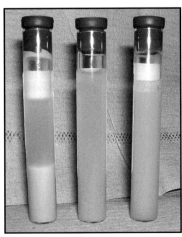

13.1 Normal rabbit urine sediment can be seen in these three urine samples. Note the variation in appearance of this sediment on visual inspection.

Urine pigments, or urochromes, give rabbit urine a yellow, brown or red colour. Some of these pigments are a result of the breakdown of endogenous compounds (e.g. bile pigments, porphyrins, flavins). The food ingested can also lead to urine coloration, either through the direct excretion of specific plant pigments (e.g. red beets) or by affecting how bile pigments and their urinary derivatives are metabolized (cabbage, cauliflower, broccoli) (Vella and Donnelly, 2012).

Kidney disease and failure

Causes of kidney disease and failure are listed in Figure 13.2. Renal insufficiency is often subclinical. Clinical signs similar to those in other mammals are seen with acute and chronic renal failure in the rabbit.

Acute kidney injury

Clinical signs and diagnosis: Non-specific signs of acute kidney injury include anorexia, lethargy, depression, dehydration, gastrointestinal ileus and stasis, and bruxism (due to pain). Urine production may be normal initially and progress to oliguria. Azotaemia with concurrent isosthenuria or hyposthenuria is diagnostic. Historical evidence of exposure to nephrotoxins (e.g. therapeutics, including aminoglycosides and sulphonamides, lead batteries) will aid diagnosis and target treatment. Prerenal azotaemia and an inability to concentrate urine (e.g. severe hypercalcaemia, overzealous furosemide use) may mimic acute kidney injury, but fluid therapy resolves the azotaemia. Hypercalcaemia causes constriction of the afferent glomerular arteriole which decreases the glomerular filtration rate. This is a functional problem and is reversible. Chronic hypercalcaemia may result in nephrocalcinosis and structural renal damage. Urine concentration is impaired as hypercalcaemia interferes with the effect of antidiuretic hormone (ADH) on the collecting duct. Animals that become oliguric will also develop hyperkalaemia and a metabolic acidosis. On physical examination, uraemic breath may be noted and enlarged swollen kidneys may be palpable, which may be confirmed by ultrasonography and radiography.

Treatment and prognosis: Acute kidney injury is potentially reversible if diagnosed quickly and treated aggressively. All potentially nephrotoxic drugs should

Category	Condition/cause	Clinical signs
Hereditary or congenital	**Polycystic kidney syndrome:** Described in rabbits, with multiple small cysts of glomerular and/or tubular origin, interstitial fibrosis of cortex and/or medulla and basement membrane alterations in the Bowman's capsule. Thought to be an inherited condition; several similarities to polycystic kidney disease seen in humans, dogs and Persian cats (Maurer *et al.*, 2004)	Most rabbits show signs of CRF by 2–3 years of age
	Renal cysts: Of tubular origin and due to an autosomal recessive mutation. Although they affect the normal structure of the renal cortex, no effect on renal function is seen, but they may be detected on ultrasonography	Subclinical
	Renal agenesis: Congenital absence of one kidney is an autosomal recessive trait seen with high incidence in Havana rabbits. The condition affects both sexes, but in the males the ipsilateral testis is also often absent	Usually subclinical
Metabolic	**Hypercalcaemia:** Leads to metastatic mineralization of soft tissues, especially affecting the kidney. Rabbits are predisposed to hypercalcaemic effects on their urinary system because this is their main route for calcium excretion. Causes of hypercalcaemia in rabbits include: renal failure (secondary hyperparathyroidism); nutritional hyperparathyroidism; paraneoplastic syndrome (lymphoma, thymoma); hypervitaminosis D (rodenticides, plants, excessive supplementation)	Initially subclinical. Progressive mineralization of kidney causes nephron damage and CRF. Uroliths can cause transient or permanent urinary outflow obstruction. Hydronephrosis, hydroureter and renomegaly may be seen
Inflammatory/ infectious	***Encephalitozoon cuniculi:*** Causes granulomatous interstitial nephritis and is a common cause of kidney disease in pet rabbits	Subclinical disease and CRF seen. Other signs depend on location of lesion (see Chapter 15)
	***Pasteurella multocida* and *Staphylococcus* spp.:** Most common bacterial causes of pyelonephritis. Glomerulonephritis, nephritis and pyelitis have also been diagnosed in rabbits	CRF
	Amyloidosis: Causes glomerulonephropathy. Usually associated with a chronic inflammatory focus (e.g. pyometritis, chronic nephrolithiasis), but spontaneous cases have been reported	CRF
	Renal fibrosis: Destruction of nephrons and dystrophic calcification of the kidney. This has been seen relatively frequently, in rabbits >2 years of age	CRF
	Focal interstitial fibrosis: May be associated with *E. cuniculi* or leptospirosis. Various serotypes of *Leptospira* have been found in wild rabbits and hares in the UK, central Europe and in the USA and Canada. No cases of zoonotic disease have been reported	Subclinical
Neoplasia	**Benign embryonal nephroma:** The third most common tumour in rabbits. Has been found in all ages of rabbit, unilateral or bilateral tumours, typically 1–2 cm in size; one case of a 6 cm tumour has been reported	Most cases subclinical, although signs due to polycythaemia, presenting as congested mucous membranes, may be seen
	Nephroblastoma: Uncommon, benign tumour	Asymptomatic
	Renal carcinoma and adenocarcinoma: Infrequently seen in rabbits of 1–6 years of age, commonly bilateral	Asymptomatic or CRF
	Lymphoma: The second most common tumour of rabbits, and the most common tumour of young rabbits, although has been seen in rabbits up to 9.5 years of age. Multiple organs often involved, including the kidney. Duration of illness can be from 1 week to 10 months	Anorexia, lethargy, peripheral lymphadenopathy, weakness, bilateral blepharitis, diarrhoea, alopecia
	Metastatic: e.g. squamous cell carcinoma	CRF. Signs dependent on site of primary tumour
Toxic	**Antimicrobials:** Several are potentially nephrotoxic in rabbits, including aminoglycosides (especially gentamicin) and sulphonamides. The risk of toxicity is greatly increased if renal perfusion is decreased	AKI
	Other potential nephrotoxins: Free-range or house rabbits may be exposed to lead, ethylene glycol, pesticides, herbicides and solvents	AKI

13.2 Causes of renal disease and chronic renal failure. AKI, acute kidney injury; CRF, chronic renal failure. (continues) ▶

Category	Condition/cause	Clinical signs
Vascular	**Systemic hypotension:** Secondary to dehydration, shock, sepsis, deep anaesthesia; causes decreased renal perfusion which, if uncorrected, rapidly leads to AKI with decreased glomerular filtration rate	AKI
	Renal hypertension. Caused by continued activation of the renin–angiotensin–aldosterone system (RAAS). Angiotensin II stimulates vasoconstriction and increased sodium and water retention, resulting in systemic hypertension and progressive impairment of renal blood flow leading to renal insufficiency. RAAS is stimulated by decreased renal perfusion (e.g. hypotension, hypovolaemia, heart failure, renal vasoconstriction), decreased sodium delivery to the distal macula densa (e.g. reduced glomerular filtration rate and nephron damage) and catecholamines	AKI or CRF
	Renal infarction	AKI or CRF

13.2 (continued) Causes of renal disease and chronic renal failure. AKI, acute kidney injury; CRF, chronic renal failure.

be discontinued and ingested toxins treated appropriately. Aggressive fluid therapy is essential to replace fluid deficits, correct electrolyte imbalances and reduce azotaemia. The aim is to 'buy time' for the nephrons to repair and hypertrophy; however if there are insufficient functional nephrons remaining the prognosis is grave. Supportive therapy of gastrointestinal ileus and gastric ulceration is recommended. The prognosis is dependent on the severity of the azotaemia and response to therapy. Tubular regeneration can occur within 3 days and is a good prognostic sign which may be seen as an improving response to treatment. The long-term prognosis is usually fair to good, provided the rabbit survives the initial period of decompensation, but a full recovery may take several months.

Prevention of gentamicin nephrotoxicity by concurrent vitamin B6 supplementation has been reported. Nine rabbits received 10 mg vitamin B6 per animal while on 40 mg/kg gentamicin, both injected intramuscularly once daily for 5 days. Acute tubular necrosis was found on histopathology in the control animals, which received only gentamicin, but these lesions were not seen in the treated group (Enriquez *et al.*, 1992). Verapamil, a calcium channel blocker used to reduce postsurgical adhesion formation in rabbits, has been shown to provide functional protection of the proximal tubules, with significantly increased creatinine clearance in acute renal ischaemia in rabbits (Alvarez *et al.*, 1994; Kim *et al.*, 1998). Verapamil may therefore be clinically beneficial in early acute kidney injury. The rabbits in the treatment group received an intravenous infusion of verapamil for 30 minutes prior to initiation of renal artery clamping. Their results suggest that the beneficial effects of verapamil may be attributed to effects other than vasodilation.

Chronic renal failure

Clinical signs: Unlike acute renal failure, chronic renal failure develops over weeks to years. Clinical signs are often mild for the magnitude of the azotaemia. A history of weight loss, polydipsia/polyuria,

poor body condition, occasionally haematuria (due to renal infarction) and non-regenerative anaemia may be noted. On clinical examination the kidneys may feel small and irregular. Lower urinary tract signs (e.g. dysuria, stranguria) often develop secondary to hypercalciuria. Intermittent anorexia and gastrointestinal ileus is a common feature in rabbits, and is most likely due to intermittent pain caused by secondary urolith formation with hypercalciuria.

Systemic hypertension is a common feature of renal failure due to the renin–angiotensin–aldosterone system. Indirect Doppler blood pressure measurement, using the same technique as for cats, is well tolerated by most rabbits. A summary of some published reference ranges for rabbits gives: mean arterial blood pressure 80–91 mmHg; systolic blood pressure 92.7–135 mmHg; and diastolic blood pressure 64–75 mmHg (Carroll *et al.*, 1996; Van Den Buuse and Malpas, 1997).

Diagnosis:

Biochemistry: Serum biochemistry often reveals hypercalcaemia and significantly elevated creatinine. Serum phosphate and potassium levels may also be elevated in severe cases. Urea may or may not be elevated. In many mammals urea is commonly used to assess renal function but in rabbits it follows a circadian rhythm and largely depends on the protein intake and nutritional status of the animal. Furthermore, rabbits have a reduced capacity to concentrate urea, and intestinal absorption, activity of the caecal flora, liver function, gastrointestinal haemorrhage, stress and hydration status can also influence blood urea levels (Jenkins, 2008). Creatinine is freely filtered through the glomerulus and excreted at a constant rate (Melillo, 2007). It is considered a more reliable indicator of kidney function than the blood urea level because it does not show the same variability due to extrarenal factors. Traditional clinical pathology indicators of nephrotoxicity, such as blood urea nitrogen, serum creatinine and urinalysis parameters, including total protein, albumin, electrolytes and sediment examination, are considered relatively insensitive and non-specific indicators of modest renal dysfunction because changes in these biomarkers tend to occur after extensive damage has been sustained by the kidneys (Mader, 1997; Ferguson *et al.*, 2008). At least 65% to 75% of the nephrons need to be damaged before a significant increase in serum creatinine is observed and changes in routine urine analysis can be detected. Routine urinalysis (Figure 13.3) and bacterial culture are recommended. Measurement of urine production can be used to adjust fluid therapy and will also facilitate assessment of endogenous creatinine clearance, providing a more accurate estimate of glomerular filtration rate (GFR) than does serum creatinine alone. Urine measurement requires an indwelling catheter and closed collection system. The creatinine clearance rate for the rabbit is 2.2–4.2 ml/min/kg (Weisbroth *et al.*, 1974). Haematuria and proteinuria may be associated with urolithiasis.

Characteristic	Normal values
Colour	Pale cream: high calcium precipitate. Yellow/orange. Brown/red: pigments from metabolic breakdown of endogenous compounds (e.g. urochromes) or ingested plant pigments
pH	8.2
Specific gravity	1.003–1.036 (1.115 average)
Urine protein to creatinine ratio (UPC)	0.11–0.4 [a]
Crystals	Large amounts of calcium carbonate monohydrate, anhydrous calcium carbonate and calcium oxalate, and ammonium magnesium phosphate (struvite) may be seen
Leucocytes and erythrocytes	Occasionally seen, <5 RBCs/hpf
Protein	Trace, albumin occasionally seen in young rabbits
Glucose	Trace
Ketones and occult blood	Absent
Casts, epithelial cells and bacteria	Absent

13.3 Urinalysis. [a] Reusch *et al.* (2009).

In renal disease, proteinuria seems to occur earlier than biochemical changes, although protein levels need to be evaluated along with urine specific gravity and sediment because healthy young rabbits may normally have a small amount of albumin in the urine and adult rabbits may have trace proteinuria (Kraus *et al.*, 1984). Measuring urinary protein and creatinine (UPC ratio of 0.11–0.40 is reported to be normal in rabbits) may be a more useful test in clinical practice, especially in association with urine specific gravity, to quantify the proteinuria (Reusch

et al., 2009). Persistent proteinuria, in urine with no signs of infection or inflammation on cytology, is an indication of renal tubular or glomerular disease and can be used as a marker of the severity of renal disease, to monitor disease progression and as an important prognostic factor. If protein loss is severe, oedema and ascites often occur.

Many toxicological studies have suggested that the anatomical integrity of the kidney may be reflected by the output of urinary enzymes. Gamma-glutamyl transferase (GGT) is one of the numerous renal tubular enzymes that are excreted in the urine of many mammal species (Bush, 1991). GGT exhibits its highest activity in the straight proximal renal tubule (Melillo, 2007); therefore validation of a non-invasive screening test for detection of this urinary enzyme, as a possible indication of early renal damage in rabbits, could be extremely useful. One author (EM) has completed a preliminary study to establish the reference ranges for GGT and the GGT index (GGT to creatinine ratio) in fresh urine from healthy domestic rabbits (Mancinelli *et al.*, 2012). These values were found to be 2.7–96.5 IU/l and 0.043–1.034, respectively.

Serology: Chronic renal disease may be caused by *Encephalitozoon cuniculi* infection (Figure 13.4). Serological testing for antibodies to this parasite is not useful in the short term for diagnosis, but elevated titres or rising titres with paired samples can be suggestive of current infection (see also Chapter 9). Classically a 4-fold rise in antibody titre is taken to indicate active infection with an organism (Addie and Ramsey, 2001). This rise may not be seen when the rabbit is immunosuppressed or the titre is already maximal at first presentation. Care must be taken with interpreting the results because 52% of healthy pet rabbits have been found to be seropositive in the UK (Keeble and Shaw, 2005; see Chapter 15). Simultaneous testing of IgM, which is more indicative of a current active infection, in combination with IgG testing is now widely available and gives a better indication of the infective status

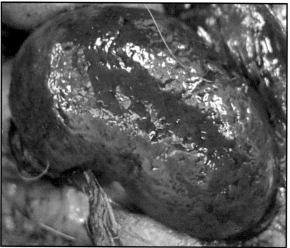

13.4 A kidney from a rabbit with encephalitozoonosis. Typical lesions appear as focal, irregular, depressed areas.

of the affected rabbit. The presence of IgM antibodies is indicative of an active infection and a requirement to institute antimicrosporidial therapy.

Imaging: Radiographic findings in rabbits with chronic renal failure include mineralization of soft tissues, including renal vessels and the aorta, and osteosclerosis. Discrete uroliths and renomegaly due to hydronephrosis may also be present. The presence of radiodense crystal sediment in the bladder is a normal radiographic finding in rabbits. Intravenous pyelograms or excretory urography can also be used to evaluate the shape, size, position and internal structure of the kidneys, ureters and bladder, to rule out the presence of masses and calculi or to identify other obstructive patterns. Ultrasonography usually shows diffuse hyperechoic renal cortices with loss of the normal corticomedullary junction, due to fibrous scar tissue. Hypoechoic regions may be seen with renal infarction and haemorrhage. Ultrasound-guided fine-needle aspiration (FNA) or laparoscopic renal biopsy can be used to diagnose renal tumours, but a clotting profile should be obtained before this is undertaken. Published values for rabbits include: activated clotting time 4.3 ± 0.6 minutes; activated partial thromboplastin time 15.7–42.7 seconds; prothrombin time 7.5 ± 0.3 seconds; bleeding time 1.9 ± 0.8 to 5.4 ± 1.2 minutes (McLaughlin and Fish, 1994).

Treatment and prognosis: All nephrotoxic drugs should be discontinued. Although chronic renal failure is usually irreversible, the severity of the clinical signs can be reduced with appropriate management. Treatment should be aimed at the underlying cause where identified, otherwise general supportive treatment is indicated.

Supportive treatment: Management of problems caused by polyuria, which may be present in some cases, is discussed later (see also Chapter 17). Fluid balance and loss of the water-soluble vitamins B and C must also be addressed. Prophylactic treatment for gastric ulceration may be advisable, because gastritis is a common sequel to uraemia in other mammals, and stress-induced ulceration, as a consequence of the stress of disease, may occur in rabbits (Hinton, 1980).

If anaemia is present, erythropoietin alpha (50–150 IU/kg i.m. or s.c. q48h) or anabolic steroids (nandrolone 2 mg/kg s.c.) may be administered; if the anaemia is severe (packed cell volume (PCV) <18%) blood transfusions may be required. Since systemic hypertension may exacerbate renal failure, treatment with angiotensin converting enzyme (ACE) inhibitors or calcium channel blockers should be considered. Treatment with benazepril, an ACE inhibitor, has been shown in a preliminary study to decrease proteinuria and reduce azotaemia, indicating improved renal function, in rabbits. Further work is being carried out to establish safe dosages, because evidence suggests that rabbits may be highly sensitive to the hypotensive effects of benazepril (Girling, 2003). Currently, a dose of <0.1 mg/kg orally once daily is recommended. Regular monitoring of blood pressure, serum creatinine, urea and electrolytes is strongly recommended if ACE inhibitors are administered. In some cases GFR is dependent on hypertension, and treatment with ACE inhibitors can be associated with an increase in azotaemia; this and hypotension, or hyperkalaemia, are all indications to stop or reduce ACE inhibitor treatment.

Rabbits with proteinuria may benefit from antiplatelet therapy. A low dose of aspirin (8 mg/kg q24h) has been shown to inhibit platelet aggregation and thrombus formation and to reduce kidney infarctions substantially in rabbits; these effects were not seen at higher doses of aspirin (e.g. 12 mg/kg). There is increasing evidence that platelets and their thromboxanes are integrally involved in the pathogenesis of glomerulonephritis. Antiplatelet treatment has been shown to decrease proteinuria, fibrin deposition and glomerular damage and preserve the GFR in rabbits with experimental glomerulonephritis (Erlich *et al.*, 1997).

Dietary manipulation is the cornerstone of chronic renal failure management in cats and dogs; however, physiological differences, in particular those related to calcium homeostasis, make such therapy complex in rabbits. Development of secondary hyperparathyroidism as a complication of chronic renal failure in rabbits is very dependent on the mineral content of the diet. Rabbits fed on a normal diet of approximately 1.2% calcium and 0.6% phosphorus have been shown to develop hypercalcaemia, hypophosphataemia and low parathyroid hormone levels in the course of chronic renal failure, therefore suggesting that rabbits are resistant to renal secondary hyperparathyroidism (Bas *et al.*, 2004). However, hyperparathyroidism can develop if uraemic rabbits are fed a low-calcium, high-phosphorus diet, with subsequent hypocalcaemia and hyperphosphataemia (Bas *et al.*, 2004). Further work is required, but uraemic rabbits fed on a low-calcium and low-phosphorus diet did not develop hyperparathyroidism in one study (Tvedegaard *et al.*, 1983); this is also the experience of the authors.

Specific treatments: Systemic antibiotics are indicated for pyelonephritis. Fenbendazole (20 mg/kg orally q24h for 4 weeks) has been show to eliminate *Encephalitozoon cuniculi* tissue stages; however, a poor response to treatment is seen in severe cases, which is thought to be due to the severity of the associated inflammatory lesions (Suter *et al.*, 2001).

Surgical removal of nephroliths is generally not recommended because further renal tissue will be damaged and it is difficult fully to assess the function of the affected kidney. In addition, surgery does not address the underlying cause and therefore recurrence of the nephrolith is likely. Nephroliths carry a guarded prognosis. Successful surgical removal of bilateral ureteroliths, one forming 3 months after the first one was removed, has been reported (White, 2001). Benign embryonal nephromas, lymphosarcomas, carcinomas and leiomyomas have been reported to affect rabbits (Klaphake and Paul-Murphy, 2012). Surgical removal of unilateral benign renal tumours should be curative. Chemotherapy (using a protocol designed for cats) of lymphoma could be considered, although, if chronic renal failure is seen, the prognosis is very grave. In addition, chemotherapy is not considered very effective in renal carcinomas in other species (Knapp, 2001).

Bladder disease

Cystitis is common and may be one of the predisposing factors for urolithiasis in rabbits. Incomplete voiding (e.g. due to lumbosacral vertebral fractures or subluxations, behavioural or micturition disorders) or excessive production of urinary sediment (due to hypercalcaemia) and presence of cystoliths, may cause damage to the bladder lining and subsequent secondary bacterial infection. Less frequently diagnosed diseases of the bladder include neoplasia (e.g. leiomyoma) and bladder eversion and prolapse in postparturient does.

Clinical features

Historical features of lower urinary tract disease include stranguria, polyuria with or without polydipsia, urine scalding, and either increased frequency or lack of urination. Discomfort or pain may also be present, resulting in bruxism or vocalization during urination, urination outside the rabbit's latrine, haematuria, anorexia, depression and reluctance to move. Incontinence can be difficult to distinguish from polyuria on the basis solely of the clinical history, although careful observation of the rabbit usually aids differentiation of the two conditions. Polyuric rabbits show an increased frequency and volume of urine, which is consciously voided, although some may show loss of litter training. Incontinent rabbits dribble urine constantly or intermittently with abnormal urine voiding in most cases. Palpation of the abdomen may enable detection of a large or small firm bladder, or cystoliths, and may elicit obvious signs of discomfort. Perineal alopecia, erythema and secondary pyoderma may all be associated with the urine scalding that may occur.

Diagnosis

A presumptive diagnosis is usually made, based on the case history and clinical signs.

Urinalysis: Routine urinalysis and bacterial culture should be carried out. Haematuria can be differentiated from red urine due to plant porphyrin pigments by a positive reaction for blood on a dipstick or finding >5 red blood cells per high-power field on urine sediment examination. Urine containing porphyrins may fluoresce in the ultraviolet light of a Wood's lamp but this is not a reliable method. Other less frequent causes of red urine include urobilinuria and uroporphyria, seen with porphyria.

Cystocentesis can usually be carried out in the conscious rabbit, although sedation is recommended for fractious patients (see Chapter 10). It is the route of choice for obtaining a urine sample for submission for bacterial culture. Free-catch urine samples can be obtained relatively easily from litter-

trained rabbits, using sterilized aquarium gravel or commercial non-absorbable products designed for cats as a replacement for litter in their tray. Urethral catheterization is easily accomplished in both male (Figure 13.5) and female rabbits and can be both diagnostic and therapeutic, as removal of sludgy urine sediment and flushing with sterile saline often alleviates the clinical signs. Sedation or general anaesthesia is required.

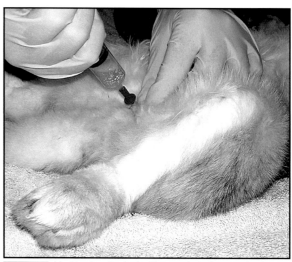

13.5 Urethral catheterization and drainage of urine with sediment in a male rabbit presented with lower urinary tract signs.

Imaging: Plain and contrast (Figure 13.6) radiography and ultrasonography will usually reveal bladder wall, neck or urethral abnormalities and identify cystoliths or urethroliths. In rabbits it can be difficult to distinguish between haematuria and other sources of bleeding, especially vaginal or uterine, because the urethra opens into the ventral aspect of the vaginal body. Urine can be retained in the vagina and mix with the blood coming from the uterus, complicating the identification of the source of haemorrhage. An endoscope, inserted into the vaginal opening, can aid the diagnosis as it

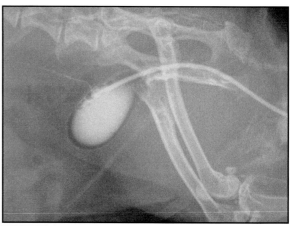

13.6 Lateral abdominal radiograph showing a double-contrast pneumocystogram. The ureter is also outlined and its irregular course suggests spasmodic flow, inflammation of the ureteral mucosa or the presence of small ureteroliths within the ureter.

permits access to both the urinary and reproductive tracts. Cystoscopy has been used in female rabbits, allowing further complementary assessment of the lower urinary tract and indirect assessment of the upper urinary tract by evaluation of urine production by each ureter. Small semi-flexible endoscopes in the 7–12 Fr size range or, more commonly, rigid endoscopes of 2.7 or 1.9 mm diameter can be used for transurethral examination of female rabbits. Selection of the size depends mostly on the patient's size and gender. Care must be taken to avoid iatrogenic trauma to the vagina or urethra. If this occurs, an indwelling Foley catheter should be placed to decompress the bladder and bypass the defect, because such injuries heal within 24–48 hours in cats, and may well also heal rapidly in rabbits. These procedures may not be feasible in smaller patients, and especially in males.

Treatment

Broad-spectrum antibiotics, such as enrofloxacin (10–30 mg/kg orally or s.c. q24h), trimethoprim/sulfadoxine (48 mg/kg s.c. q24h) or trimethoprim/sulfamethoxazole (30 mg/kg orally q12h) should be started if infection is suspected, while awaiting urine culture and sensitivity. If signs of pain are present, analgesia should be provided, using non-steroidal anti-inflammatory drugs (NSAIDs, e.g. meloxicam) or opioids (e.g. buprenorphine). NSAIDs should be used with caution if significant renal dysfunction is suspected.

Treatment of urine scalding is described in Chapter 17. If the rabbit is overweight, a programme of weight reduction is recommended, because obesity will exacerbate urine scalding (Figure 13.7) and urolithiasis has been seen in many overweight rabbits.

If excess sediment is detected on radiography then urethral catheterization and gentle bladder lavage to remove this may be indicated (see Chapter 7). Some cases may require cystotomy (see *BSAVA Manual of Rabbit Imaging, Surgery and Dentistry*). Potassium citrate, given orally, may be useful in rabbits with calcium oxalate crystals, because citrate combines with calcium to form soluble calcium citrate. However, since calcium oxalate solubility is increased in urine with pH above 6.5, oxalate crystals should be a rare occurrence owing to the naturally alkaline urine of rabbits.

Dietary modification to reduce dietary calcium is recommended for long-term management to prevent excess sediment formation or retention and urolith formation. Timothy grass-based pellets may be fed in small quantity. The majority of the diet should be mixed meadow or timothy hay, moderate amounts of green leafy vegetables and small amounts of root vegetables. In general, items to be avoided include all vitamin and mineral supplements, alfalfa (pellet or hay), excess kale, carrot tops, dandelion and clover.

Urohydropulsion: This is a non-surgical technique used in cats and dogs to remove small, round urocystoliths and this technique can also be used in rabbits. Diazepam is recommended as pre-anaesthetic medication in order to relax the urethral smooth muscle, and pre-emptive analgesia is recommended. After induction of general anaesthesia, a urethral catheter is placed and sterile saline (4–6 ml/kg) administered to distend the bladder moderately. The urethral catheter is then removed. The rabbit is held in an upright position and the bladder is manually expressed using firm steady digital pressure. The procedure should be repeated until all of the uroliths have been removed. This can be confirmed by radiographic examination. Haematuria and dysuria can be expected for up to 2 days following this procedure. Particular care must be taken in bucks to ensure that the uroliths are small enough to pass through the urethra, to avoid urethral obstruction. If uroliths are lodged in the distal urethra in male rabbits, they can be removed via a urethrotomy using a similar approach to that used in dogs (Paul-Murphy, 1997). A dorsolateral approach is indicated because of the close proximity of the penile urethra to the anus. To avoid urethral stricture formation, the urethra should be allowed to heal by second intention. This will occur in less than a week, and urethral catheterization is required during this healing period to prevent fistula formation.

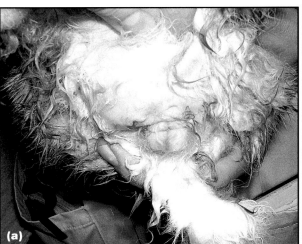

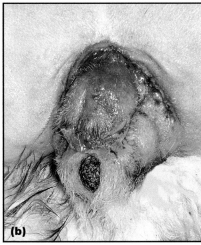

13.7

(a) Severe obesity in this rabbit caused secondary urine scalding as the vulva was covered by the large skin fold. **(b)** The vulva can now be seen in the rabbit after corrective surgery, and the urine scalding has been resolved.

Reverse urohydropulsion is recommended to return large urethral uroliths to the bladder for removal by cystotomy. Cystotomy is also recommended for the removal of all medium-sized, large or irregular cystoliths, as well as for large amounts of thick sediment that cannot be removed by bladder lavage.

Disorders of micturition

Disorders of micturition include both urine retention and urine leakage (incontinence).

Causes and clinical features

Causes of incontinence can be grouped according to their effect on bladder size. Causes of incontinence associated with a large distended bladder include neurogenic disorders such as lower and upper motor neuron lesions, reflex dyssynergia (e.g. with *E. cuniculi* infection, *Toxoplasma* infection, lumbosacral vertebral fractures or subluxation) and paradoxical incontinence due to an outflow obstruction (see Chapter 15). Paradoxical incontinence occurs because the intravesicular pressure exceeds the pressure within the urethra, and urine usually leaks past the obstruction before rupture of the bladder and urethra. Common causes of partial outflow obstruction in rabbits are calculi. Other potential causes include bladder or urethral neoplasia, bladder polyps, urethral strictures, severe urethritis and, in the male, prostatic disease. The authors have seen a case of partial outflow obstruction in a female rabbit due to advanced uterine adenocarcinoma.

Experimental studies of chronic partial outlet obstruction in rabbits have shown that the bladder responds to a mild partial outflow obstruction with an increase in bladder mass and wall thickness, which allows higher pressures to be generated to overcome the increased resistance (Schoor *et al.*, 1994). The rabbit can remain stable in this compensated condition for a long time. If urethral resistance increases progressively, however, further hypertrophy of the bladder occurs, with decreased capacity and a reduced ability of the bladder to contract and empty. The bladder capacity of normal rabbits is approximately 20 ml/kg. Rabbits with severe bladder dilatation (up to 50 ml/kg) may appear to have an extremely thin-walled bladder, but it is usually greatly hypertrophied (Schoor *et al.*, 1994). Overdistension of the bladder also separates smooth muscle tight junctions, which interferes with normal detrusor muscle function. If the damage is severe, fibrosis of the bladder wall and bladder atony may be permanent. Clinical signs of outflow obstruction are dysuria or stranguria, urine dribbling and haematuria (e.g. when bladder polyps or uroliths are present). On palpation the bladder may be distended and be difficult to express and catheterize.

The causes of incontinence seen with a small or normal bladder size include urethral sphincter mechanism incontinence (USMI), detrusor hyper-reflexia or instability or congenital disorders (e.g. ectopic ureters, although this has not been reported in the rabbit). Oestrogen and testosterone are believed to contribute to the maintenance of

urethral muscle tone therefore ovariohysterectomized rabbits are more likely to develop USMI. A clinical sign that may be seen is dribbling of urine when relaxed or asleep, but urine may be voided normally at other times. Detrusor hyper-reflexia or instability is the inability to control voiding because of a strong urge to urinate due to cystitis or urethritis. Rabbits with this condition show clinical signs of cystitis, as described earlier.

Polyuric and polydipsic disorders, such as chronic renal failure, may initially be difficult to differentiate from incontinence and will exacerbate the condition in rabbits. Potential causes of polydipsia and polyuria are listed in Figure 13.8.

Primary polydipsia
• Psychogenic (boredom) • Pain (seen commonly with dental disease) • Anorexia, food deprivation, stress

Primary polyuria
• Renal insufficiency, chronic renal failure • Chronic or severe liver disease (e.g. hepatic lipidosis) • Hypercalcaemia • Hypokalaemia • Pyometra • Endotoxaemia • Pyelonephritis • Post-obstructive diuresis • Hyperviscosity syndrome (polycythaemia, hyperproteinaemia) • Pregnancy toxaemia and ketoacidosis • Diabetes mellitus (very rare) • Iatrogenic (diuretics, corticosteroids)

13.8 Potential causes of polydipsia and polyuria.

Diagnosis and treatment: A presumptive diagnosis can often be made based on the case history and clinical signs. Hospitalization is usually required to allow evaluation of urination, including observation of posture and, where possible, urine stream flow and character. Most rabbits with dysuria tend also to have polyuria, making observation of urination more feasible than in normal rabbits, which are naturally secretive in hospital surroundings. Immediately after the rabbit has attempted to void, the bladder should be palpated to estimate the residual volume. Normally almost all urine should be passed with each voiding, including urine sediment. If the bladder is large, the rabbit should be sedated for catheterization. Cystocentesis and urinalysis with bacterial culture and sensitivity are recommended.

Neurological examination is indicated in all rabbits with large bladders (see Chapter 15). Ultrasonography has been shown to estimate bladder hypertrophy accurately in rabbits (Schoor *et al.*, 1994), and contrast radiography and cystoscopy may also aid diagnosis. Serology for *E. cuniculi* should be carried out in all cases, and a positive titre in addition to neurological signs supports a diagnosis of *E. cuniculi* infection.

A 24-hour water measurement test is recommended to confirm polydipsia. In rabbits this is generally defined as water consumption of >120 ml/kg/day, and an average measured over 3 days in the rabbit's home environment usually provides the most reliable indication of fluid consumption. The urine output is usually estimated to be approximately 130 ml/kg. Further investigation of the aetiology of the polyuria should then be carried out, including haematology, serum biochemistry and urinalysis. Response to therapy frequently aids the diagnosis of micturition disorders. A positive response to diethylstilbestrol (0.5 mg/rabbit orally once or twice a week) is suggestive of USMI. Hormonal treatment of rabbits for this condition is still under investigation in scientific studies rather than clinical trials aimed at therapeutic relief. NSAIDs can be used to provide analgesia and reduce inflammation, if there is no evidence of impaired renal function.

The prognosis is dependent on the severity of the lesion, and chronic overdistension or severe hypertrophy of the bladder carries a poor prognosis for recovery. *E. cuniculi*-associated disease that is unresponsive to fenbendazole treatment also carries a poor prognosis. Psychogenic polyuria and polydipsia have also been reported (Potter and Borkowski, 1998).

Diseases of the female genital tract

The normal anatomy and physiology of the female reproductive tract are discussed in Chapters 1 and 4. Disorders of the reproductive system are now seen less commonly in pet rabbits because owners often elect to have their rabbit neutered in order to prevent ovarian and uterine disease. Nevertheless, older entire females need to be evaluated carefully for detection of reproductive tract disease and any suspected abnormality should be promptly investigated.

Ovarian disease
Ovarian abscesses and pyometra may be caused by *Pasteurella multocida* (Johnson and Wolf, 1993). Ovarian cysts and neoplasia (granulosa cell tumour, haemangiosarcoma and lymphoma) are infrequently reported in rabbits (Iyer and Majumdar, 1979; Heatley and Smith, 2004). Clinical signs include infertility, abdominal distension and weight loss, and large abdominal masses can be detected on palpation. Ultrasonography with or without FNA and radiography will confirm the presence of an ovarian mass. Cytology of an aspirate or histopathology of the tissue is required for a definitive diagnosis. Thoracic radiography and abdominal ultrasound examination for metastases are recommended. Treatment and prevention is by ovariohysterectomy. The prognosis is poor if metastasis has occurred.

Uterine neoplasia
Uterine adenocarcinoma (Figure 13.9) is the most common tumour of female rabbits. It has been reported in most breeds including Dutch, Havana, Tan, French Silver, English, Chinchilla, Beveran,

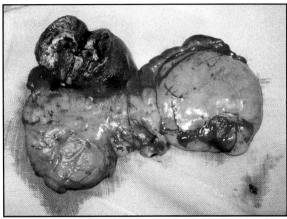

13.9 Rabbit uterine adenocarcinoma after surgical removal.

Sable, Himalayan and Polish. An incidence of 50–80% in intact does >3 years of age has been reported (Heatley and Smith, 2004). Parity has no effect on incidence. The endometrium undergoes progressive and age-related changes that can include increased collagen content and reduced cellularity. Endometrial hyperplasia may therefore progress following the process of polyp formation, cystic hyperplasia, adenomatous hyperplasia and uterine adenocarcinoma (Saito *et al.*, 2002). Asakawa *et al.* (2008) evaluated the expression of oestrogen receptor-alpha and progesterone receptors in normal, hyperplastic and neoplastic endometrium using immunohistochemistry in 88 pet rabbits. Adenocarcinomas were divided into papillary and tubular/solid adenocarcinomas, which had different receptor expression and different endometrium invasiveness, suggesting that rabbits may present two developmental pathways of adenocarcinoma formation. Leiomyomas and leiomyosarcomas are less frequently found in rabbits but can occur concurrently with uterine adenocarcinoma. Adenomas were found to be the second most common uterine tumour of pet rabbits (Saito *et al.*, 2002). Spontaneous choriocarcinoma and a malignant Müllerian tumour have also been reported in rabbits (Goto *et al*, 2006; Kaufmann-Bart and Fischer, 2008).

Clinical features and diagnosis
Uterine tumours may cause reproductive abnormalities including infertility, fetal reabsorption, abortion, stillbirths, fetal retention and smaller litters. As the disease progresses, the rabbit may become depressed and anorexic and develop haematuria. Animals may develop a bloody vulvar discharge, cystic mammary glands and partial urethral obstruction. Advanced pulmonary metastases may cause dyspnoea and other signs of respiratory dysfunction (see Chapter 11). Uterine tumours are generally slow growing, with both local metastasis to the peritoneal cavity and haematogenous metastasis to lung, liver, brain and bone occurring within 1–2 years (Weisbroth, 1994).

On clinical examination, tumours may be palpated in the caudal abdomen and fluid pocketing within the uterus and ascites may also be detected. Affected rabbits may be anaemic. Ultrasonography, with or without FNA, and radiography (Figure 13.10) will confirm the presence of a uterine mass. Cytology of the aspirate or histopathology of the tissue is required for a definitive diagnosis and to rule out other causes of uterine enlargement. Thoracic radiography and abdominal ultrasound examination for evaluation of metastases are recommended.

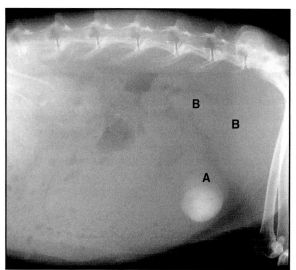

13.10 Lateral abdominal radiograph of rabbit with large uterine mass (B), displacing the bladder (A) cranioventrally. Ultrasound-guided fine-needle aspiration and cytology confirmed the mass to be a uterine adenocarcinoma. Note the normal radiodense urine sediment in the bladder.

Treatment, prevention and prognosis
Ovariohysterectomy can be curative and can prevent metastasis if carried out before any occurs. Early peritoneal metastasis is usually not apparent on imaging or at surgery; therefore a guarded prognosis and routine 3-monthly follow-up screening is recommended for 2 years after surgery. Pulmonary metastasis carries a grave prognosis, and successful chemotherapy for this tumour has not been reported.

Endometrial hyperplasia
Despite endometrial hyperplasia being a common condition in pet rabbits, it is still controversial whether endometrial changes progress from polyp formation to cystic hyperplasia, adenomatous hyperplasia and to adenocarcinoma, as seen in humans, or whether adenocarcinomatous endometrial changes are simply a result of age-related atrophy of the endometrium with no association with cystic hyperplasia (Baba and von Haam, 1972; Elsinghorst et al., 1984; Kraus et al., 1984). The condition is most frequently seen in animals aged 4 years or older (Saito et al., 2002). Clinical signs include intermittent haematuria, anaemia, lethargy, anorexia and palpation of a firm irregular uterus. Cystic mammary glands and ovaries may be present concurrently. Radiography and ultrasonography aid diagnosis, although ovariohysterectomy and histopathology are required for a definitive diagnosis. Ovariohysterectomy is the treatment of choice.

Hydrometra
This involves accumulation of transudate fluid in the uterus. A retrospective study of uterine disorders diagnosed by ovariohysterectomy and histopathology, carried out in 47 pet rabbits, revealed that hydrometra was the third most common uterine lesion (Saito et al., 2002). Endometrial hyperplasia and adenocarcinoma were the first and second most common lesions found. The average age of affected rabbits was 4 years. Clinical features that may be seen are abdominal enlargement, with a fluid thrill being readily detected on abdominal percussion, anorexia, weight loss and an increased respiratory rate. A presumptive diagnosis can usually be made on clinical findings, although ultrasonography may confirm a large, fluid-filled uterus. Surgery for ovariohysterectomy is both diagnostic and therapeutic (Figure 13.11). Mortality was reported to be as high as 50% in the rabbits with hydrometra, although this was thought to be mainly due to the degree of morbidity prior to surgery and chronic high pressure exerted on the abdominal organs (Saito et al., 2002).

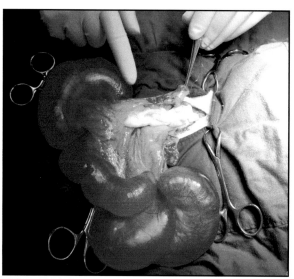

13.11 Hydrometra in a rabbit. The rabbit was in overt good health at the time of surgery. (Courtesy of the University of Newcastle)

Uterine infection
Endometritis, metritis and pyometra may all be seen in rabbits, although infrequently. It is thought that infection may be introduced at the time of mating, although infection in non-breeding does may occur by the haematogenous route. A retrograde infection may develop secondary to vaginitis. Infection may also occur postpartum or following pseudopregnancy. Bacteria that have been isolated include *Pasteurella multocida*, *Staphylococcus aureus* and, less frequently, *Chlamydophila* spp., *Listeria monocytogenes*, *Moraxella bovis*, *Brucella melitensis*, *Salmonella* spp. and *Actinomyces pyogenes*. Hobbs and Parker (1990) also reported hydrometra and endometritis associated with uterine torsion.

Clinical features and diagnosis

Mucopurulent vaginal discharge, anorexia, weight loss, abdominal distension and reduced fertility may be seen. In some cases, the clinical signs may be subtle. On physical examination a large doughy uterus may be detected on careful palpation. Radiography and ultrasonography may be useful in ruling out other potential causes of enlargement of the uterus. Cytology of the vaginal discharge may also aid diagnosis. Haematology in some cases reveals heterophilia, with a slight leucocytosis. Serum biochemistry may reveal azotaemia; this can be pre-renal (dehydration) or renal (due to renal amyloid deposition secondary to chronic inflammation; Hofmann and Hixson, 1986). Exploratory surgery is required for a definitive diagnosis.

Treatment and prognosis

Supportive care, including analgesia, fluid therapy and therapy to prevent gastric stasis and ileus, is recommended to stabilize the rabbit prior to ovariohysterectomy. Broad-spectrum antibiotics should be started while awaiting the results of bacteriological culture of the uterine wall. Prostaglandin therapy to assist uterine contraction and drainage has not been reported in the rabbit and so is not recommended. Medical management of mild endometritis in a breeding animal may be considered, although owing to the caseous nature of pus in the rabbit, even prolonged antibiotic therapy may not achieve full resolution of the infection.

Other female genital tract disease

Uterine torsion, endometrial aneurysms, ectopic pregnancy and dystocia have all been reported infrequently in the rabbit. Torsion of the uterus is usually associated with pregnancy, hydrometra or endometritis. Clinical signs of shock and signs specific to the associated condition are seen. Caesarean section and/or ovariohysterectomy are the recommended treatments.

Rabbits with endometrial aneurysms may present with intermittent haematuria. Passage of blood clots in the urine is highly suggestive of this condition (Figure 13.12). Fatal haemorrhage can occur, and therefore ovariohysterectomy is recommended.

Ectopic pregnancy in the rabbit is not uncommon but is often subclinical (Beddow, 1999; Gil *et al.*, 2004). Extrauterine implantation (in the peritoneum) of fertilized ova leads to the development of fetuses, which are often near to term, that undergo mummification (primary abdominal pregnancy). This condition can also result from uterine rupture and subsequent release of embryos within the abdominal cavity (secondary abdominal pregnancy). Uterine rupture can also occur secondary to trauma (false abdominal pregnancy).

Dystocia is unusual in rabbits. Predisposing factors include obesity, large fetuses, small pelvic canal and uterine inertia. Straining, persistent contractions with no fetal passage and greenish-brown vaginal discharge may be indicative of dystocia or retained fetuses. If uterine inertia is suspected, 5–10 ml of oral 10% calcium gluconate

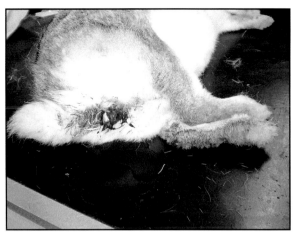

13.12 A rabbit with acute haematuria. The main differential diagnoses would be endometrial aneurysm and rabbit haemorrhagic disease.

given 30 minutes prior to oxytocin (1–2 IU i.m.) may resolve the condition; otherwise a Caesarean section is recommended if there is no response within 30–60 minutes. The prognosis is usually guarded.

Two cases of suspected congenital uterine developmental abnormalities have been reported in two domestic rabbits in which parts of the reproductive tract were found to be absent (Thode and Johnston, 2009).

Pregnancy toxaemia

The cause of this condition is uncertain, but it is most frequently seen in obese animals. Stress and inadequate calorie intake during the last week of gestation also appear to be predisposing factors. Clinical signs include depression, weakness, collapse, abortion, seizures and death. A presumptive diagnosis is usually made on the basis of the case history and clinical findings. Urine is usually colourless with a reduced pH (pH 5–6) and positive for ketones and protein. Ketoacidosis and hepatic lipidosis are usually present. Aggressive supportive therapy, including nutritional support, is required to reverse the negative energy balance in these animals. This condition carries a grave prognosis.

Pseudopregnancy

Unsuccessful mating is the most common cause of pseudopregnancy, although it has also been seen in female pet rabbits that are mounted by another doe, and in does kept alone. Clinical signs include nest building, with hair pulling and mammary development. The condition usually resolves spontaneously within 16–17 days, although it may progress to hydrometra or pyometra. Medical treatment with progestins, androgens and cabergoline is of unproven effectiveness for pseudopregnancy treatment. Cabergoline, a potent prolactin inhibitor, was found to be well tolerated in female rabbits at doses of 5–50 µg/kg/day, with signs of toxicity only seen at very high doses (500 µg/kg/day) (Beltrame *et al.*, 1996). Ovariohysterectomy is the treatment of choice.

Vaginal and vulval disease

Congenital absence of the vagina and cervix has been reported in the rabbit, but is very rare. Squamous cell carcinoma of the vaginal wall has been reported in rabbits that also had concurrent uterine adenocarcinoma (Greene and Strauss, 1949). Vaginal prolapse has been reported in the rabbit and may occur as a result of straining secondary to other urogenital disease. Clinical signs are a friable haemorrhagic soft tissue mass protruding from the vulva. Affected animals may rapidly develop hypovolaemic shock from severe associated haemorrhage. Treatment involves correction of the hypovolaemic shock, surgical reduction of the prolapse and resection of devitalized tissue.

Vulvitis with papules, ulcers or hyperkeratosis may be seen, due to *Treponema cuniculi* infection (rabbit syphilis; see Chapter 17). Oedematous vulval swelling may be due to myxomatosis (see Chapter 17).

Mammary gland disease

Mammary masses

Mammary carcinoma is a common progression from cystic mastitis and has been reported frequently in many breeds including the Belgian, English Belgian and New Zealand White pure and crossbreed does (Heatley and Smith, 2004). Cystic mammary glands may be associated with uterine hyperplasia and adenocarcinoma. Clinical signs of both benign and neoplastic disease are the development of irregularly sized, fluctuant, subcutaneous nodules that discharge milk or amber fluid. They are seldom painful. Mammary adenocarcinoma is usually more invasive and ulceration may be seen. Diagnosis is usually made on the basis of FNA and cytology. Ovariohysterectomy is recommended for treatment of cystic mastitis, and usually results in resolution of the clinical signs within 3–4 weeks. Partial or complete mastectomy and ovariohysterectomy are the treatments of choice for mammary carcinoma or adenocarcinoma; the technique is dependent on the number of tumours and location in the mammary glands. Metastases to regional lymph nodes, lungs, abdominal organs and bone marrow have been reported (Heatley and Smith, 2004), and therefore thorough presurgical investigation of possible metastasis is recommended. Considering the association between mammary and uterine disorders, ovariohysterectomy of young healthy does should reduce the risk of developing mammary neoplasia at an older age. Mammary dysplasia has also been reported concurrently with prolactin-secreting pituitary adenoma (Percy and Barthold, 2001; Sikoski *et al.*, 2008).

Mastitis

This usually occurs in lactating or pseudopregnant does, and may be predisposed to by mammary gland trauma or poor hygiene. *Staphylococcus aureus*, *Pasteurella* and *Streptococcus* spp. are frequently isolated. Clinical signs include: hot, swollen, firm, painful, erythematous mammary glands; pyrexia, anorexia, depression and lethargy; and rejection of young. A presumptive diagnosis is usually made on the basis of the clinical features. Samples of expressed milk should be submitted for culture and antibiotic sensitivity testing. Treatment consists of general supportive therapy, analgesia, broad-spectrum antibiosis, hot packing and expression of milk. Early weaning of the young is often required in lactating does. The use of a foster doe is highly discouraged to avoid transmission of the infection. Surgical excision or mastectomy may be required in severe cases.

Male genital tract disease

The normal anatomy of the genital tract is discussed in Chapters 1 and 4.

Tumours of the testicle

Testicular neoplasia (Figure 13.13) is rare in rabbits. Seminomas, interstitial cell tumours, Sertoli cell tumours and lymphoma have been reported (Roccabianca *et al.*, 1999; Heatley and Smith, 2004). Clinical features typically include non-painful firm nodular testicular enlargement, reproductive failure, change in libido and weight loss. A testicular nephroma has been found in a cryptorchid testis (Meier *et al.*, 1970) and two distinct forms of collagenous hamartomas have been described in middle-aged male rabbits with testicular tumours (Von Bomhard *et al.*, 2008). Castration with histopathology is both diagnostic and therapeutic. The prognosis can be good if metastasis has not occurred.

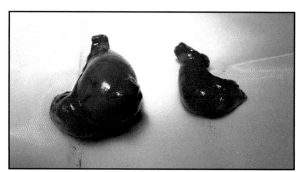

13.13 The testicle on the left of the picture is neoplastic. For comparison, the testicle shown on the right is normal. (Courtesy of Dr Paolo Selleri)

Cryptorchidism

The testes normally descend by 12 weeks of age. Failure of one or both testes to descend into the scrotal sac by 16 weeks of age is defined as cryptorchidism, which may be unilateral or bilateral. The scrotal sac does not develop on the side of the cryptorchid testicle; therefore, if the scrotal sac is present, normal intra-abdominal retraction of the testis is most likely. As neoplasia of a cryptorchid testicle has been reported in the rabbit, removal using a midline abdominal approach is the recommended treatment.

Orchitis and epididymitis

Causes of orchitis and epididymitis include *Pasteurella multocida* and other bacteria, myxomatosis and trauma. Immune complex orchitis has been reported in vasectomized rabbits (Bigazzi *et al.*, 1976). Clinical signs include swollen testes and scrotum, depression, anorexia, pyrexia and reproductive failure. A presumptive diagnosis is usually made on the basis of the case history and clinical signs. Treatment of the specific cause is recommended. In most cases, except for myxomatosis, antibiotic therapy, castration and scrotal ablation, if indicated, are recommended.

Miscellaneous male genital diseases

Treponema paraluis cuniculi infection causes inflammation, papules, ulcers and hyperkeratosis of the perineum and genitalia (Figure 13.14; see also Chapter 17). Preputial trauma due to bite wounds, with secondary infection, may be seen in rabbits. Diseases of the prostate gland have not been recognized in the rabbit, but experimentally induced prostatic ischaemia in the rabbit has resulted in increased prostatic tissue contraction around the urethra, causing bladder outflow obstruction (Azadzoi *et al.*, 2003).

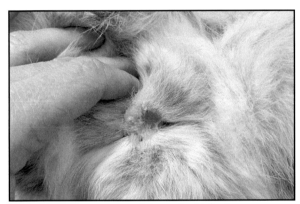

13.14 *Treponema paraluis cuniculi* infection can cause testicular lesions.

References and further reading

Addie D and Ramsey I (2001) The laboratory diagnosis of infectious diseases. In: *BSAVA Manual of Canine and Feline Infectious Diseases*, ed. IK Ramsey and BJ Tennant, pp.1–18. BSAVA Publications, Gloucester

Alvarez A, Martul E, Veiga F and Forteza J (1994) Functional, histological, and ultrastructural study of the protective effects of verapamil in experimental ischemic acute renal failure in the rabbit. *Renal Failure* **16**, 193–207

Asakawa MG, Goldschmidt MH, Une Y, *et al.* (2008) The immunohistochemical evaluation of estrogen receptor-alpha and progesterone receptors of normal, hyperplastic and neoplastic endometrium in 88 pet rabbits. *Veterinary Pathology* **45**, 217–225

Azadzoi KM, Babayan RK, Kozlowski R and Siroky MB (2003) Chronic ischemia increases prostatic smooth muscle contraction in the rabbit. *Journal of Urology* **170**, 659–663

Baba M and von Haam E (1972) Animal models: spontaneous adenocarcinoma in aged rabbits. *American Journal of Pathology* **68**, 653–656

Bas S, Bas A, Estepa JC, *et al.* (2004) Parathyroid gland function in the uremic rabbit. *Domestic Animal Endocrinology* **26**, 99–110

Beddow BA (1999) Ectopic pregnancy in a rabbit. *Veterinary Record* **144**, 624

Beltrame D, Longo M and Mazué G (1996) Reproductive toxicity of cabergoline in mice, rats, and rabbits. *Reproductive Toxicology* **10**, 471–483

Bigazzi PE, Kosuda LL, Hsu KC and Andres GA (1976) Immune complex orchitis in vasectomized rabbits. *Journal of Experimental Medicine* **143**, 382–404

Bush BM (1991) *Interpretation of Laboratory Results for Small Animal Clinicians.* Wiley-Blackwell, Oxford

Carroll JF, Dwyer TM, Grady AW, *et al.* (1996) Hypertension, cardiac hypertrophy, and neurohormonal activity in a new animal model of obesity. *American Physiology Society* **271**, H373–H378

Elsinghorst TA, Timmermans HJE and Hendrix HG (1984) Comparative pathology of endometrial carcinoma. *Veterinary Quarterly* **6**, 200–208

Enriquez JI, Schydlower M, O'Hair KC, *et al.* (1992) Effect of vitamin B6 supplementation on gentamicin nephrotoxicity in rabbits. *Veterinary and Human Toxicology* **34**, 32–35

Erlich JH, Holdsworth SR and Tipping PG (1997) Tissue factor initiates glomerular fibrin deposition and promotes major histocompatibility complex class II expression in crescentic glomerulonephritis. *American Journal of Pathology* **150**, 873–880

Ferguson MA, Vaidya VS and Boventre JV (2008) Biomarkers of nephrotoxic acute kidney injury. *Toxicology* **245**, 182–193

Gil PS, Palau BP, Martinez JM, *et al.* (2004) Abdominal pregnancies in farm rabbits. *Theriogenology* **62**, 642–651

Girling SJ (2003) Preliminary study into the possible use of benazepril on the management of renal disease in rabbits. *British Veterinary Zoological Society Proceedings: Infectious diseases of exotics*, Edinburgh Zoo, p.44

Goto M, Nomura Y, Une Y, *et al.* (2006) Malignant mixed mullerian tumour in a rabbit (*Oryctolagus cuniculus*): case report with immunohistochemistry. *Veterinary Pathology* **43**, 560–564

Greene H and Strauss J (1949) Multiple primary tumors in the rabbit. *Cancer* **2**, 673–691

Heatley J and Smith A (2004) Spontaneous neoplasms of lagomorphs. *Veterinary Clinics of North America: Exotic Animal Practice* **7**, 561–577

Hinton M (1980) Gastric ulceration in the rabbit. *Journal of Comparative Pathology* **90**, 475–481

Hobbs BA and Parker RF (1990) Uterine torsion associated with either hydrometra or endometritis in two rabbits. *Laboratory Animal Science* **40**, 535–536

Hofmann JR and Hixson CJ (1986) Amyloid A protein deposits in a rabbit with pyometra. *Journal of the American Veterinary Medical Association* **189**, 1155–1156

Iyer PKR and Majumdar G (1979) Note on spontaneous granulosa-cell tumor of ovary in a rabbit (*Oryctolagus cuniculus*). *Indian Journal of Animal Sciences* **49**, 242–244

Jeklova E, Jekl V, Kovarcik K, *et al.* (2010) Usefulness of detection of specific IgM and IgG antibodies for diagnosis of clinical encephalitozoonosis in pet rabbits. *Veterinary Parasitology* **170**(1–2), 143–148

Jenkins JR (2008) Rabbit diagnostic testing. *Journal of Exotic Pet Medicine* **17**(1), 4–15

Johnson JH and Wolf AM (1993) Ovarian abscesses and pyometra in a domestic rabbit. *Journal of the American Veterinary Medical Association* **203**, 667–669

Kaufmann-Bart M and Fischer I (2008) Choriocarcinoma with metastasis in a rabbit (*Oryctolagus cuniculus*). *Veterinary Pathology* **45**, 77–79

Keeble EJ and Shaw DJ (2005) An investigation into the possible predisposing factors for infection with *Encephalitozoon cuniculi* in domestic rabbits in the United Kingdom. *Proceedings, British Small Animal Veterinary Association Congress, Birmingham*, pp.551

Kim SY, Ham SC, Yoo HJ and Kim YK (1998) Beneficial effect of verapamil against ischaemic acute renal failure in rabbits. *Korean Journal of Nephrology* **17**(4), 533–544

Klaphake E and Paul-Murphy J (2012) Disorders of the reproductive and urinary systems. In: *Ferrets, Rabbits and Rodents: Clinical Medicine and Surgery, 3rd edn*, ed. KE Quesenberry and JW Carpenter, pp.217–231. Elsevier, St. Louis

Knapp D (2001) Tumors of the urinary system. In: *Small Animal Clinical Oncology*, ed. S Withrow and E MacEwen, pp.490–499. WB Saunders, Philadelphia

Kraus AL, Weisbroth SH, Flatt RE, *et al.* (1984) Biology and diseases of rabbits. In: *Laboratory Animal Medicine*, ed. JG Fox *et al*, pp.207–240. Academic Press, San Diego

Mader DR (1997) Basic approach to veterinary care. In: *Ferrets, Rabbits and Rodents: Clinical Medicine and Surgery*, ed. EV Hillyer and KE Quesenberry, pp.160–169. WB Saunders, Philadelphia

Mancinelli E, Shaw DJ and Meredith AL (2012) γ-Glutamyl-transferase (GGT) activity in the urine of clinically healthy domestic rabbits (*Oryctolagus cuniculus*). *Veterinary Record* **171**(19), 475

Maurer KJ, Fox JG, Marini RP and Rogers AB (2004) Polycystic kidney syndrome in New Zealand White rabbits resembling human polycystic kidney disease. *Kidney International* **65**, 482–489

McLaughlin RM and Fish RE (1994) Clinical biochemistry and hematology. In: *The Biology of the Laboratory Rabbit, 2nd edn*, ed. PJ Manning *et al.*, pp.123–124. Academic Press, London

Meier H, Myers DD, Fox R and Laird CW (1970) Occurrence, pathological features, and propagation of gonadal teratomas in inbred mice and in rabbits. *Cancer Research* **30**, 30–34

Melillo A (2007). Rabbit clinical pathology. *Journal of Exotic Pet Medicine* **16**(3), 135–145

Paul-Murphy J (1997) Reproductive and urogenital disorders. In: *Ferrets, Rabbits and Rodents: Clinical Medicine and Surgery*, ed. EV Hillyer and KE Quesenberry, pp.202–211. WB Saunders, Philadelphia

Percy DH and Barthold SW (2001) *Pathology of Laboratory Rodents and Rabbits, 2nd edn*, pp.253–307. Iowa State University Press, Ames, IA

Potter MP and Borkowski GL (1998) Apparent psychogenic polydipsia and secondary polyuria in laboratory housed New Zealand white rabbits. *Contemporary Topics in Laboratory Animal Science* **37**, 87–89

Reusch B, Murray JK, Papasouliotis K and Redrobe SP (2009) Urinary protein:creatinine ratio in rabbits in relation to their serological status to *Encephalitozoon cuniculi*. *Veterinary Record* **164**, 293–295

Roccabianca P, Ghisleni G and Scanziani E (1999) Simultaneous seminoma and interstitial cell tumour in a rabbit with a previous cutaneous basal cell tumour. *Journal of Comparative Pathology* **121**, 95–99

Saito K, Nakanishi M and Hasegawa A (2002) Uterine disorders diagnosed by ventrotomy in 47 rabbits. *Journal of Veterinary Medical Science* **64**, 495–497

Schoor RA, Canning DA, Bella RD, et al. (1994) Ultrasound diagnosis of bladder outlet obstruction in rabbits. *Neurourology and Urodynamics* **13**, 559–569

Sikoski P, Trybus J, Cline JM, et al. (2008) Cystic mammary adenocarcinoma associated with prolactin-secreting pituitary adenoma in a New Zealand white rabbit (*Oryctolagus cuniculus*). *Comparative Medicine* **58**, 297–300

Suter C, Müller-Doblies UU, Hatt J–M and Deplazes P (2001) Prevention and treatment of *Encephalitozoon cuniculi* infection in rabbits with fenbendazole. *Veterinary Record* **148**, 478–480

Thode HP and Johnston MS (2009) Probable congenital uterine developmental abnormalities in two domestic rabbits. *Veterinary Record* **164**, 242–244

Tvedegaard E, Ladefoged O, Nielsen M and Kamstrup O (1983) Effect of 1 alpha-hydroxyvitamin D3 and dietary calcium and phosphate on the aortic mineral content of rabbits with mild azotemia. *Nephron* **34**, 185–191

Van Den Buuse M and Malpas SC (1997) 24-Hour recordings of blood pressure, heart rate and behavioural activity in rabbits by radio-telemetry: effects of feeding and hypertension. *Physiology and Behavior* **62**, 83–89

Vella D and Donnelly TM (2012) Rabbits: basic anatomy, physiology and husbandry. In: *Ferrets, Rabbits and Rodents: Clinical Medicine and Surgery, 3rd edn*, ed. KE Quesenberry and JW Carpenter, pp.157–173. Elsevier Saunders, St. Louis

Von Bomhard W, Mauldin EA and Pleghaar S (2008) Disseminated collagenous hamartomas in rabbits – a new entity. *Kleintierpraxis* **53**, 224–230

Weisbroth S, Flatt RE and Kraus AL (1974) Anatomy, physiology, and biochemistry of the rabbit. In: *The Biology of the Laboratory Rabbit, 2nd edn*, ed. PJ Manning et al., p.65. Academic Press, London

Weisbroth SH (1994) Neoplastic disease. In: *The Biology of the Laboratory Rabbit, 2nd edn*, ed. PJ Manning, DH Ringler and CE Newcomer, pp.259–292. Academy Press, New York

White RN (2001) Management of calcium ureterolithiasis in the French lop rabbit. *Journal of Small Animal Practice* **42**, 595–598

14

Cardiovascular disease

Connie Orcutt

Cardiovascular disease appears to be increasingly recognized in pet rabbits as they live longer and their owners present them for more sophisticated medical care. Veterinary clinicians should be able to recognize clinical signs consistent with cardiovascular disease in this species, formulate a differential diagnosis, perform relevant diagnostic evaluations and be familiar with appropriate treatments.

Anatomical considerations

The rabbit's thoracic cavity is small in relation to the rest of its body (Figure 14.1). Obesity, cardiomegaly, pleural effusion, intrathoracic masses and pulmonary disease can rapidly compromise respiration. The mediastinum in normal rabbits contains fat,

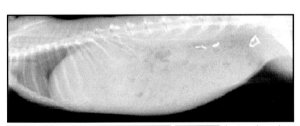

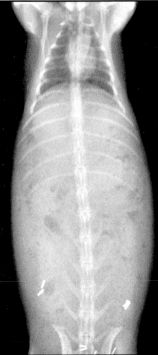

14.1 Lateral and ventrodorsal radiographs of a clinically normal rabbit. Note the small size of the thorax relative to the rest of the body. The metallic densities are surgical clips used in a previous ovariohysterectomy.

which can mimic cardiomegaly, and this effect is more pronounced in obese animals. The rabbit's heart has several unique anatomical features, some of which are clinically very important. Chief among these is the fact that the collateral circulation in the rabbit's myocardium is limited, predisposing the heart to ischaemia subsequent to coronary vasoconstriction. The pulmonary artery and its branches in the rabbit are relatively muscular. The rabbit's right and left auricles are also large relative to the atria, and the coronary sinus is also proportionately large. The left atrioventricular (AV) valve is tricuspid rather than bicuspid.

History and physical examination

History
A thorough history is a very important aspect of the medical evaluation of rabbits with clinical signs consistent with cardiovascular disease. Specific abnormalities noted by the owner may include dyspnoea, tachypnoea, syncopal episodes and cyanosis. However, just as often the case history may include only non-specific signs, such as a reduced appetite or lethargy. In fact, many rabbits with cardiovascular disease have no history of clinical signs, and abnormalities may not be apparent until the rabbit is presented for routine clinical evaluation. In some cases, cardiovascular lesions are only discovered on post-mortem examination as incidental findings.

Observation
The rabbit's behaviour and respiratory character should first be evaluated while the animal is at rest in its carrier. Dyspnoea may be indicated by sternal recumbency, slight elbow abduction or neck extension, which can progress to open-mouthed breathing in severe cases. Rabbits are obligate nasal breathers, and any rabbit extending its head in an attempt to breathe through its mouth is in severe respiratory distress. Examination of a rabbit with respiratory abnormalities must be undertaken very cautiously and may need to be carried out in stages if the rabbit becomes distressed. In some cases, rabbits may need to be sedated for thorough examination and/or diagnostics. If this is necessary, midazolam at a dose of 0.5–1 mg/kg i.v. or i.m. is an effective sedative with minimal cardiovascular effects.

Physical examination

For physical examination, the author prefers first to auscultate the heart rate and respiratory character before stress alters the findings. Use of a paediatric stethoscope facilitates auscultation of focal irregularities. The normal heart rate for a rabbit in the clinic is 150–300 beats per minute (bpm), and only a regular sinus rhythm is considered normal. Cardiac and respiratory sounds may be muffled by pleural effusion, pericardial effusion (rare in rabbits), subcutaneous or intrathoracic fat, areas of pulmonary consolidation or intrathoracic masses. In the author's experience, the most common auscultation irregularity in rabbits with cardiovascular disease is a murmur or gallop rhythm. Abnormal heart sounds are commonly most intense immediately to either side of the sternum. Although the rabbit's normal respiratory rate is reported to be 30–60 breaths per minute, stressed rabbits in the clinic often breathe much more rapidly. Airway sounds superimposed on heart sounds can mimic a murmur, so the clinician should auscultate the thorax until respiratory and valvular sounds can be distinguished. Brief manual occlusion of the nares can facilitate cardiac auscultation, but care must be taken to ensure that this does not overly stress the animal. Excessive pressure of the stethoscope against the compliant chest wall can put pressure on the right ventricular outflow tract and create an artefactual murmur. Respiratory abnormalities noted in rabbits with cardiovascular disease can include rapid superficial respiration, muffled lung sounds or crackles, although the latter are often not as easy to detect as in larger species because of the rabbit's relatively small lung field.

The mucous membranes in rabbits are normally light pink. Cyanosis may be easiest to appreciate by examining the tongue colour. Pulses may be evaluated by palpating the femoral artery (on the proximal medial thigh), the metatarsal artery (along the medial aspect of the metatarsus) or the central artery of the ear (along the longitudinal axis of the pinna).

Older rabbits can have occult cardiovascular disease, which may become apparent only after an exacerbating incident, such as aggressive fluid therapy. Clinical signs of iatrogenic fluid overload are most commonly lethargy and tachypnoea, and findings on clinical examination usually include a heart murmur or gallop rhythm and crackles. If clinical signs develop after fluid administration, thoracic radiographs should be obtained. If radiographic abnormalities are referable to the cardiovascular system, an echocardiographic examination, complete blood count and serum biochemical analysis are warranted.

Diagnostic tests

Radiography

Positioning for radiography may be tolerated in the unsedated rabbit with physical restraint alone, but health and safety considerations preclude direct handling during radiography. In any event, anxious individuals will need to be sedated or anaesthetized. Thoracic radiographs of a clinically normal rabbit are shown in Figure 14.2. The thoracic cavity of the rabbit is very small relative to the large abdomen, and intrathoracic abnormalities can be difficult to assess. The use of digital radiography will allow focal magnification and facilitate radiographic evaluation. The heart normally extends from either the 2nd to the 5th rib or from the 3rd to the 6th rib. The cranial border of the heart is usually not well defined in rabbits owing, in large part, to the wide mediastinum. The lung tissue cranial to the cardiac silhouette cannot be evaluated as in dogs or cats, and radiopacity in this area can mask true lesions.

Radiographic abnormalities in a rabbit with cardiovascular disease may include cardiomegaly, tracheal elevation, pulmonary oedema (usually indicated by an increased pulmonary interstitial pattern), enlarged (congested) pulmonary vessels (Figure 14.3), pleural effusion (Figure 14.4) and mineralized soft tissues (see Figure 14.10). Rabbits with right-sided heart failure may also have hepatomegaly, ascites or pericardial effusion, although the last two findings are rare in rabbits. Anterior mediastinal masses and other intrathoracic pathology can mimic cardiomegaly (Figure 14.5), as can increased amounts of fat in the mediastinum;

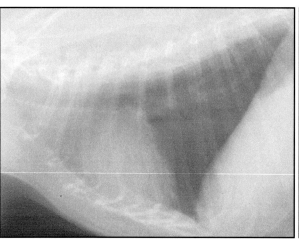

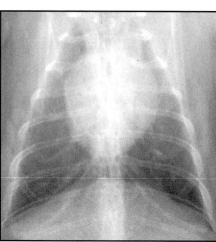

14.2

Lateral and ventrodorsal thoracic radiographs of a clinically normal rabbit.

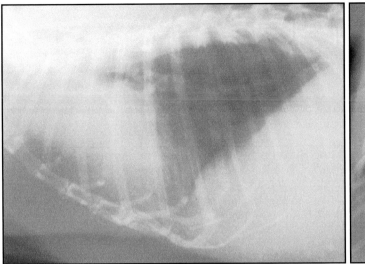
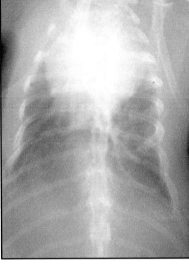

14.3 Lateral and ventrodorsal radiographs of an 11-year-old rabbit presented for weakness and subcutaneous oedema involving the hindlimbs. The ventrodorsal radiograph was difficult to interpret owing to malpositioning. Radiographic abnormalities included cardiomegaly, enlargement of the vena cava, decreased abdominal detail (consistent with ascites) and a diffuse increased pulmonary interstitial pattern. The diagnosis was severe decompensated intermediate/dilated cardiomyopathy.

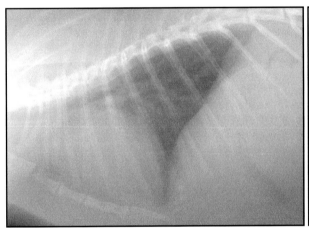
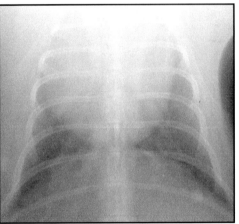

14.4 Lateral and ventrodorsal radiographs of a 5-month-old rabbit taken 2 weeks postpartum. The rabbit was presented for extreme lethargy, anorexia and weight loss. A gallop rhythm was noted during physical examination. Radiographic abnormalities included marked cardiomegaly with a globoid cardiac silhouette and an increased pulmonary interstitial pattern indicating pulmonary oedema. The echocardiographic diagnosis was decompensated dilated cardiomyopathy.

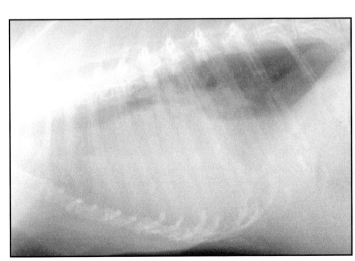

14.5 Lateral radiograph of a 7-year-old rabbit presenting with lethargy, tachypnoea, increased respiratory effort and coughing at night. A large amount of pleural effusion was evident on radiography and prevented evaluation of the cardiac silhouette, cranial mediastinum and pulmonary vasculature. Pleurocentesis yielded a total of 90 ml of fluid from the right and left pleural cavities. The echocardiographic diagnosis was severe dilated cardiomyopathy. (Courtesy of Joan Ogden DVM)

echocardiography can usually provide the definitive diagnosis. Thoracic radiography is discussed further in the *BSAVA Manual of Rabbit Surgery, Dentistry and Imaging*.

Electrocardiography

Electrocardiographic recordings are best used to assess arrhythmias auscultated during physical examination. Rabbits usually tolerate the procedure awake and in sternal recumbency. Alligator clips can be made more tolerable by bending the tips outward and filing off the teeth. Because of the rabbit's relatively high heart rate and small atrial and ventricular complexes, electrocardiograms (ECGs) are easiest to interpret if recorded at a speed of 50 mm/s and an amplitude of 2 cm/mV. Reference ranges in clinically normal pet rabbits have been published (Figure 14.6). The P wave and QRS complexes in rabbits are similar to those in cats and dogs. Reportedly, the rabbit's high-potassium and low-sodium diet, resulting primarily from grasses, causes peaked T waves and a longer S–T segment relative to carnivores (Figure 14.7; Reusch, 2005).

Parameter	Range (mean)
Bodyweight (kg)	1.1–7.9 (2.57)
Heart rate (beats/minute)	190–320 (264)
P wave duration (s)	0.02–0.03 (0.03)
P wave amplitude (mV)	0.01–0.14 (0.08)
P--R interval (s)	0.04–0.08 (0.06)
QRS duration (s)	0.02–0.07 (0.04)
R wave amplitude (mV)	0.08–0.33 (0.21)
Q--T interval (s)	0.08–0.23 (0.12)
T wave amplitude (mV)	0.05–0.21 (0.11)
Mean electrical axis (degree)	−60 to 90 (19)

14.6 Lead II electrocardiographic parameters in 46 clinically normal rabbits. (Data from Lord *et al.*, 2010.)

Echocardiography

Echocardiography is also usually well tolerated by the unanaesthetized rabbit and is the single most useful modality for diagnosing cardiac disease. The rabbit is placed in sternal recumbency with the thorax positioned over a hole in the table, allowing transducer access. A 7.5 MHz transducer and high frame rate ultrasound machine are essential for optimal studies. The echocardiographic anatomy of the rabbit is similar to that of dogs and cats with the exception of the rabbit's large coronary sinus, which is visible at the AV junction and should not be mistaken for a congenital defect or a sign of right-sided heart failure. Echocardiographic reference ranges have been published for several rabbit breeds (Figure 14.8).

Blood pressure measurement

Blood pressure can be measured indirectly in rabbits by using a Doppler ultrasound unit, a paediatric pneumatic cuff and an infant flat probe.

1. The rabbit is placed in lateral recumbency, and the fur is clipped on the ventral aspect of the carpus just above the foot.
2. A small cuff with a width equivalent to 30–40% of the limb circumference is placed proximal to the elbow while the probe crystal is placed on a bed of ultrasound gel over the shaved skin.
3. The cuff is inflated until the Doppler signal is extinguished.
4. As the cuff is slowly deflated, the first sound heard represents the systolic pressure.
5. Several readings should be taken to obtain a mean value.

Cardiovascular parameters follow a normal circadian rhythm in rabbits, with both the heart rate and blood pressure increasing at night. Because blood pressure in rabbits can increase significantly with stress, normal values vary widely. The direct systolic blood pressure measured by telemetry in unrestrained rabbits is 96.0 ± 2.6 mmHg (Sato *et al.*, 1995); however, the systolic pressure for rabbits measured using the Doppler technique in clinical situations is 120–180 mmHg.

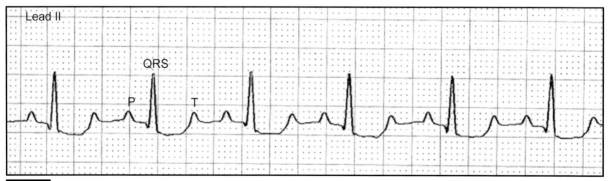

14.7 Electrocardiogram from a clinically normal rabbit. (Reproduced from *In Practice*, with permission)

Parameters	Unsedated (n=20) (Stypmann et al., 2007)	Sedated with ketamine and xylazine (n=20) (Stypmann et al., 2007)	Sedated with ketamine and midazolam (n=26) (Fontes-Souza et al., 2009)
Age (weeks)	16	16	16--20
Mean bodyweight (kg)	2.92	2.92	2.3 ± 0.4
Left ventricular end-diastolic dimension (cm)	1.510 ± 0.112	1.480 ± 0.081	1.35 ± 0.11
Left ventricular end-systolic dimension (cm)	1.009 ± 0.091	1.074 ± 0.089	0.86 ± 0.08
Percentage left ventricular fractional shortening (%)	34.5 ± 4.9	28.5 ± 3.8	36.01 ± 4.31
Interventricular septal thickness at end of diastole (cm)	0.217 ± 0.056	0.199 ± 0.033	0.27 ± 0.03
Left ventricular posterior wall thickness at end of diastole (cm)	0.274 ± 0.041	0.267 ± 0.047	0.23 ± 0.03
Left atrial diameter (cm)	no data	no data	0.75 ± 0.11
Aorta diameter (cm)	no data	no data	0.66 ± 0.05
Left atrium-to-aorta ratio	no data	no data	1.15 ± 0.19
E point to septal separation (cm)	no data	no data	0.14 ± 0.03
Left ventricular outflow tract velocity (m/s)	0.749 ± 0.195	0.723 ± 0.170	0.86 ± 0.12
Right ventricular outflow tract velocity (m/s)	no data	no data	0.78 ± 0.12
Left ventricular ejection time (s)	0.126 ± 0.014	0.146 ± 0.017	0.096 ± 0.010
Mitral valve E wave (m/s)	0.715 ± 0.138	0.556 ± 0.103	0.78 ± 0.15
Mitral valve A wave (m/s)	0.514 ± 0.145	0.379 ± 0.092	0.55 ± 0.11
Mitral valve E-to-A ratio	1.44 ± 0.28	1.51 ± 0.31	1.44 ± 0.16
Stroke volume (ml)	1.8 ± 0.46	1.6 ± 0.6	no data
Cardiac output (ml/min)	421 ± 100	307 ± 99	no data

14.8 Echocardiographic parameters in clinically normal sedated and unsedated New Zealand White rabbits. Values are mean ± SD.

Blood tests

Results of complete blood count and serum biochemical analysis are useful for assessing organs and electrolytes directly affected by cardiovascular disease (e.g. in cases of chronic renal failure involving arteriosclerosis) and to monitor parameters after initiating treatment (e.g. when using furosemide, angiotensin-converting enzyme (ACE) inhibitors or digoxin).

Diseases and medical management

Congestive heart failure

Because the rabbit is a prey species, clinical signs may be hidden until disease has reached a serious stage. This is often the case with congestive heart failure (CHF). Historical abnormalities noted by the owner can include hindlimb weakness progressing to generalized weakness, exercise intolerance, a decreased appetite, weight loss, dyspnoea or signs of specific organ dysfunction (e.g. polyuria and polydipsia indicating renal compromise).

Clinical examination findings can include pallor, cyanosis, muffled heart sounds, tachycardia, a murmur, a gallop rhythm or other arrhythmias, crackles and weak pulses. Contrary to findings with CHF in other animals, coughing is not common in rabbits. On rare occasions, right-sided heart failure may result in distension of the abdominal veins or engorgement of retrobulbar vessels and secondary exophthalmos, although the latter is more commonly seen in rabbits with intrathoracic masses such as thymomas. As with other animals, CHF in the rabbit is usually confirmed radiographically. Most affected rabbits have significant cardiomegaly and some degree of pulmonary oedema with left-sided heart failure (see Figure 14.3) and pleural effusion with right-sided heart failure. When pleural effusion is clinically significant (see Figure 14.5) it should be treated

209

with thoracocentesis. The procedure is similar to that used with dogs and cats but keeping in mind the rabbit's small chest size. Pericardial effusion, ascites, hepatomegaly and peripheral oedema are less commonly present in cases of right-sided heart failure. CHF should be considered when any adult rabbit, especially one over the age of 3 years, develops tachycardia or dyspnoea, particularly when purulent nasal or ocular discharge is absent. Subclinical cardiac disease may also be exacerbated with aggressive fluid administration and may result in CHF.

The dyspnoeic rabbit in CHF must be subjected to minimal stress. No medications are authorized for the treatment of cardiac disease in rabbits, and drugs and dosages are extrapolated from those for dogs and cats (Figure 14.9). Medical care during the acute stage of CHF includes oxygen supplementation in a quiet cage, parenteral furosemide administration, topical application of glyceryl trinitrate 2% ointment, and thoracocentesis in cases of significant pleural effusion and if the rabbit is sufficiently stable for the procedure. Pimobendan has been used anecdotally in small mammals for treatment of CHF secondary to dilated cardiomyopathy (DCM) and valvular disease. Long-term therapy usually includes oral furosemide, often in conjunction with an ACE inhibitor (e.g. enalapril) and treatment tailored to the primary cardiovascular disease. Renal and electrolyte levels should be evaluated during therapy.

Congenital cardiac disease

Congenital heart defects are rare in rabbits. Reported abnormalities include ventricular septal defects, pulmonary hypertension, and defects of the great vessels (e.g. an absent or vestigial pulmonary arterial trunk, pulmonary valve stenosis or a vestigial or absent ascending aorta).

Arrhythmias

Cardiac arrhythmias are not as commonly appreciated in rabbits as in dogs or cats. ECG abnormalities such as atrial fibrillation, a rapid ventricular response rate and ventricular premature complexes have been found in rabbits with CHF and underlying cardiomyopathy or valvular disease. Syncope has been anecdotally reported in some arrhythmic rabbits. A diagnostic work-up should be undertaken to investigate the cause of the arrhythmia, and therapy should be instituted if the animal shows clinical signs. Anti-arrhythmic therapies that have been used in rabbits include atropine, glycopyrrolate, lidocaine, digoxin and diltiazem (Figure 14.9). Glycopyrrolate may be a more effective chronotrope than atropine in the rabbit, because some rabbits produce atropinase. To date, there have been no published reports of pacemaker implantation in rabbits for treatment of spontaneous arrhythmias.

Medication	Dosage	Clinical indications	Comments
Atropine	0.1–1 mg/kg i.m.	Acute bradycardia Used to decrease airway secretions	Many rabbits have high levels of atropinase, so high doses of atropine may be necessary
Benazepril	0.1 mg/kg orally q24h	Congestive heart failure Hypertension	Less nephrotoxic than enalapril. Rabbits may be very sensitive to hypotensive effects. Monitor blood pressure, BUN, creatinine and electrolytes
Digoxin	0.005–0.01 mg/kg orally q12–24h	Myocardial failure Supraventricular tachycardia Atrial fibrillation	Low therapeutic index can result in anorexia, gastrointestinal signs, or development of arrhythmias. Measure serum levels after several days of treatment, 6–8 hours after last dose
Diltiazem	0.5–1 mg/kg orally q12–24h	Supraventricular tachycardia Hypertrophic cardiomyopathy	Monitor heart rate, ECG and blood pressure
Enalapril	0.1–0.5 mg/kg orally q12–48h	Congestive heart failure Hypertension	Monitor blood pressure, electrolytes, BUN and creatinine
Furosemide	Acute: 1–4 mg/kg i.v., i.m. or s.c. q4–6h Chronic: 1–3 mg/kg orally q8–24h	Congestive heart failure	Monitor BUN, creatinine and electrolytes
Glyceryl trinitrate 2% ointment	3 mm transdermally q6–12h	Congestive heart failure	Monitor blood pressure and clinical signs
Glycopyrrolate	0.01–0.1 mg/kg i.m. or s.c.	Acute bradycardia Used to decrease airway secretions	Positive chronotrope of choice in rabbits. Often used as premedicant to prevent bradycardia and excess salivation
Lidocaine	1–2 mg/kg i.v. bolus as needed	Ventricular tachyarrhythmia	Serum potassium level must be normal
Pimobendan	0.2–0.4 mg/kg orally q12h	Dilated cardiomyopathy Congestive heart failure Degenerative valvular disease	Vasodilator and stronger inotrope than digoxin, with higher therapeutic index

14.9 Medications used in treating rabbits with cardiovascular disease. (Data from Reusch (2005); Mitchell *et al.*, (2008); Pariaut (2009); Fiorello and Divers (2012).

Myocardial disease

Cardiomyopathy is a relatively common post-mortem finding from older rabbits. Large breeds are anecdotally reported to be most susceptible. Cardiomyopathies are classified as dilated, hypertrophic or restrictive depending on the echocardiographic and/or post-mortem findings. Definitive diagnosis is made by using echocardiography. Electrocardiography can also be used to assess electrical conductivity secondary to myocardial changes.

Causes

The primary causes of myocardial disease in the rabbit are, for the most part, unknown. Hypovitaminosis E produces a nutritional muscular dystrophy primarily evidenced by degeneration of skeletal muscles, but the myocardium may be affected as well. Clinical signs are usually referable to the skeletal system (hindlimb paralysis) or the reproductive system (infertility, abortion, stillbirths and high neonatal mortality). Plasma vitamin E (alpha-tocopherol) levels <23.2 μmol/l are considered low, and levels <11.6 μmol/l indicate a deficiency (Cheeke, 1994). Treatment involves vitamin E supplementation.

Although taurine deficiency has not been reported in rabbits, taurine dosed at 100 mg/kg orally once daily resulted in increased myocardial contractility and alleviation of CHF in rabbits with artificially induced aortic regurgitation (Takihara et al., 1986). The mechanism remained unknown, but the researchers speculated that improvement resulted from taurine's inotropic action. There are no published reports of taurine supplementation in pet rabbits.

Myocardial disease caused by infectious agents is rarely seen in pet rabbits. Bacterial organisms reported as causative agents of myocarditis include *Pasteurella multocida*, *Salmonella* spp. and *Clostridium piliforme* (the causative organism of Tyzzer's disease). In rabbits severely affected by *Encephalitozoon cuniculi*, focal inflammatory lesions have been found in the myocardium. Coronavirus has also been implicated in 'pleural effusion disease' in laboratory rabbits. The primary clinical abnormality is pleural effusion secondary to right ventricular dilation, but fever, pulmonary oedema and anterior uveitis are also part of the clinical syndrome. Hypergammaglobulinaemia is a feature of chronic cases. While rabbits experimentally inoculated with coronavirus have been used as laboratory models for the study of virus-induced cardiomyopathy, no spontaneous cases have been reported in pet rabbits. Any type of myocarditis can result in myocardial fibrosis, which is not uncommonly found in the myocardium of older rabbits at necropsy.

A left atrial thrombus was found on echocardiographic analysis of a 7-year-old pet rabbit presenting with CHF. The thrombus was confirmed on post-mortem examination, along with gross and histopathological findings consistent with hypertrophic cardiomyopathy (increased ventricular wall thickness bilaterally, bi-atrial dilatation, myocardial fibrosis and the absence of ventricular dilatation) (Lord et al., 2011).

Anaesthetic combinations containing the alpha-2 agonist detomidine have been associated with myocardial necrosis and fibrosis in rabbits (Hurley et al., 1994). The proposed pathophysiology was impaired coronary blood flow causing myocardial ischaemia and subsequent necrosis. Myocardial fibrosis and hypertrophy of pulmonary arteries were also noted in rabbits anaesthetized with ketamine and xylazine several times over a period of 1 year (Marini et al., 1999).

Catecholamine-induced cardiomyopathy in rabbits can result in left ventricular dysfunction (Simons and Downing, 1985). Stress-induced cardiomyopathy and sudden death in rabbits has also been associated with crowded housing conditions (Weber and Van der Walt, 1975). The proposed mechanism involves alpha-adrenergic mediated coronary vasoconstriction in the presence of increased myocardial work. This pathophysiology may play a part in unexplained rabbit deaths in which post-mortem lesions are absent. Reducing stress is essential in helping to prevent such fatalities in rabbits. Steps the clinician and nursing staff can take to reduce stress in hospitalized patients include keeping rabbits away from the sight and smell of predators, reducing environmental noise and hurried activity during treatment and induction of anaesthesia, minimizing the use of stressful devices (e.g. Elizabethan collars), providing familiar cage bedding and accessories, administering analgesic therapy when indicated, handling animals in a quiet and gentle manner and even housing a bonded companion with a hospitalized rabbit.

Dilated cardiomyopathy

Dilated cardiomyopathy (DCM) is the most common form of myocardial disease diagnosed in rabbits in the author's practice. Rabbits often do not present with clinical signs until myocardial function is significantly compromised. Treatment has traditionally included digoxin for inotropic support and enalapril to decrease afterload. However, digoxin is a weak positive inotrope with a relatively low therapeutic index, and rabbits need to be monitored carefully for side effects. Pimobendan is a novel cardiotonic vasodilator, or inodilator, with stronger inotropic action and fewer adverse effects than digoxin, and it also provides peripheral vasodilation along with exerting anti-inflammatory effects. Pimobendan use has been reported anecdotally in rabbits with CHF secondary to DCM.

Valvular disease

Endocardiosis involving the mitral and/or tricuspid heart valves is not uncommon in rabbits and most often affects older animals. The most common clinical finding is a systolic parasternal murmur. The diagnosis is made with echocardiography; abnormal findings include valvular thickening (most often involving one or both atrioventricular valves), dilatation of heart chambers and regurgitation/turbulent blood flow confirmed by Doppler echocardiography. Spontaneous bacterial endocarditis appears to be uncommon in rabbits but is relatively easily induced in animals used as laboratory models. Pimobendan has been used anecdotally in small mammals for treatment of CHF secondary to degenerative AV valvular disease that is refractory to other treatments.

Vascular disease

Several syndromes can produce mineralized soft tissue lesions in the rabbit. Spontaneous arteriosclerosis, predominantly involving the aorta, has been observed in nearly all rabbit breeds and even in wild rabbits. New Zealand White rabbits appear to be particularly at risk, with an incidence of disease of ≥40%. Lesions of aortic arteriosclerosis have been seen in animals as young as 6 weeks of age. Clinical signs are usually non-specific (lethargy, anorexia and weight loss). Definitive diagnosis is difficult ante-mortem; mineralized vessels, which occur in some cases, may be visible on radiographs (Figure 14.10). The aetiology of spontaneous arteriosclerosis in the rabbit is unknown, but genetic factors appear to play a role.

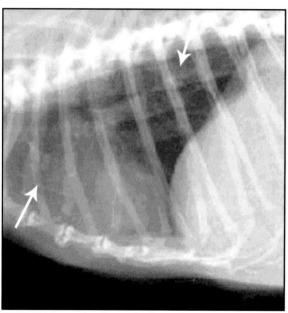

14.10 Lateral radiograph of a geriatric rabbit, showing a calcification of the aorta (arrowed). The aetiology was unknown.

Vitamin D toxicity can result in lesions similar to those seen in cases of spontaneous arteriosclerosis. Excessive dietary levels of vitamin D are usually implicated. Clinical signs are varied and may be non-specific (progressive emaciation and weakness, decreased appetite, diarrhoea, intense thirst, ataxia, paralysis and death). The primary lesion is calcification of soft tissues, including the liver, kidney, arterial walls and muscle.

Chronic renal failure has been implicated in the development of soft tissue mineralization as well as excessive calcium deposition in bone (Harcourt-Brown, 2002). Rabbits rely on renal excretion of calcium for homeostasis; if the kidneys are unable to perform this function adequately, excess calcium may be laid down in body tissues.

The New Zealand White rabbit and related genetically altered strains, e.g. the Watanabe heritable hyperlipidaemic rabbit, have been used for years as laboratory models for the study of diet-induced and familial hypercholesterolaemia, respectively, and the subsequent development of atherosclerotic lesions. Among the species of animals studied as laboratory models of atherosclerosis, the rabbit is the only one that tends to exhibit hypercholesterolaemia within a few days after being fed a high-cholesterol diet. In fact, the plasma cholesterol level in New Zealand White rabbits can increase 2- to 8-fold within 20 days after the administration of a 0.25–2% cholesterol-supplemented diet (Bocan et al., 1993). Female rabbits are less prone to diet-induced atherosclerotic lesions than males because of the atheroprotective effect of 17-β-oestradiol. The extent of disease caused by naturally occurring atherosclerosis in pet rabbits is unknown.

Conclusion

Because of the rabbit's tendency to hide clinical signs, cardiovascular abnormalities may be clinically silent until the disease process has become well established or compensatory mechanisms are over-ridden by other events such as fluid overload or stress. Cardiomyopathy and valvular disease are the most clinically significant forms of cardiovascular disease seen in pet rabbits; treatment is similar to that used in other small mammals. Perhaps the single most cardioprotective action the clinical staff can take towards any rabbit patient is to make every effort to reduce the animal's stress, since catecholamine-induced myocardial dysfunction has been implicated in sudden death. Much more work needs to be done to understand the aetiology of cardiovascular disease in rabbits in order to treat them, and ultimately work towards prevention.

References and further reading

Beaufrère H and Pariaut R (2009) Pinobendan. *Journal of Exotic Pet Medicine* **18**, 311–313

Bocan TMA, Mueller SB, Mazur MJ, et al. (1993) The relationship between the degree of dietary-induced hypercholesterolemia in the rabbit and atherosclerotic lesion formation. *Atherosclerosis* **102**, 9–22

Carmel B (2013) Radiographic interpretation of the thorax. In: *BSAVA Manual of Rabbit Surgery, Dentistry and Imaging*, ed. F Harcourt-Brown and J Chitty, pp.69–75. BSAVA Publications, Gloucester

Carpenter JW, Mashima TY, Rupiper DJ and Morrisey JK (2001) *Exotic Animal Formulary, 2nd edn.* WB Saunders, Philadelphia

Cheeke PR (1994) Nutrition and nutritional diseases. In: *The Biology of the Laboratory Rabbit, 2nd edn*, ed. PJ Manning et al., pp.321–333. Academic Press, San Diego

Crary DD and Fox RR (1975) Hereditary vestigial pulmonary arterial trunk and related defects in rabbits. *Journal of Heredity* **66**, 50–55

DeLong D and Manning PJ (1994) Bacterial diseases. In: *The Biology of the Laboratory Rabbit, 2nd edn*, ed. PJ Manning et al., pp.129–170. Academic Press, San Diego

DiGiacomo RF and Maré CJ (1994) Viral diseases. In: *The Biology of the Laboratory Rabbit, 2nd edn*, ed. PJ Manning et al., pp.190–192. Academic Press, San Diego

Finking G and Hanke H (1997) Nikolaj Nikolajewitsch Anitschkow (1885–1964) established the cholesterol-fed rabbit as a model for atherosclerosis research. *Atherosclerosis* **135**, 1–7

Fiorello CV and Divers SJ (2012) Rabbits. In: *Exotic Animal Formulary, 4th edn*, ed. JW Carpenter, pp.517–559. Elsevier Saunders, St. Louis

Fontes-Sousa AP, Moura C, Santos Carneiro C, et al. (2009) Echocardiographic evaluation including tissue Doppler imaging in

New Zealand white rabbits sedated with ketamine and midazolam. *The Veterinary Journal* **181**, 326–331

Harcourt-Brown F (2002) Cardiorespiratory disease. In: *Textbook of Rabbit Medicine*, pp.324–334. Butterworth Heinemann, Oxford

Hurley RJ, Marini RP, Avison DL, *et al.* (1994) Evaluation of detomidine anesthetic combinations in the rabbit. *Laboratory Animal Science* **44**, 472–477

Huston SM and Quesenberry KE (2004) Cardiovascular and lymphoproliferative diseases. In: *Ferrets, Rabbits and Rodents: Clinical Medicine and Surgery, 2nd edn*, ed. KE Quesenberry and JW Carpenter, pp.211 220. WB Saunders, Philadelphia

Koller LD (1969) Spontaneous *Nosema cuniculi* infection in laboratory rabbits. *Journal of the American Veterinary Medical Association* **155**, 1108–1114

Li X, Murphy JC and Lipman NS (1995) Eisenmenger's syndrome in a New Zealand White rabbit. *Laboratory Animal Science* **45**, 618–620

Lindsey JR and Fox RR (1994) Inherited diseases and variations. In: *The Biology of the Laboratory Rabbit, 2nd edn*, ed. PJ Manning *et al.*, pp.293–319. Academic Press, San Diego

Lord B, Boswood A and Petrie A (2010) Electrocardiography of the normal domestic pet rabbit. *Veterinary Record* **167**, 961–965

Lord B, Devine C and Smith S (2011) Congestive heart failure in two pet rabbits. *Journal of Small Animal Practice* **52**, 46–50

Marini RP, Li X, Harpster NK and Dangler C (1999) Cardiovascular pathology possibly associated with ketamine/xylazine anesthesia in Dutch belted rabbits. *Laboratory Animal Science* **49**, 153–160

Martin MWS, Darke PGG and Else RW (1987) Congestive heart failure with atrial fibrillation in a rabbit. *Veterinary Record* **121**, 570–571

Maxwell MP, Hearse DJ and Yellon DM (1987) Species variation in the coronary collateral circulation during regional myocardial ischaemia: a critical determinant of the rate of evolution and extent of myocardial infarction. *Cardiovascular Research* **21**, 737–746

Mitchell EB, Zehnder AM, Hsu A and Hawkins MG (2008) Pimobendan: treatment of heart failure in small mammals. *Proceedings of the Association of Exotic Mammal Veterinarians Scientific Program, Savannah, Georgia*, pp.71–79

Orlandi A, Francesconi A, Marcellini M, *et al.* (2004) Role of ageing and coronary atherosclerosis in the development of cardiac fibrosis in the rabbit. *Cardiovascular Research* **64**, 544–552

Pariaut R (2009) Cardiovascular physiology and diseases of the rabbit. *Veterinary Clinics of North America: Exotic Animal Practice* **12**, 135–144

Plumb DC (2002) *Veterinary Drug Handbook, 4th edn*. Iowa State Press, Ames

Reusch B (2005) Investigation and management of cardiovascular disease in rabbits. *In Practice* **27**, 418–425

Sato K, Chatani F and Sato S (1995) Circadian and short-term variabilities in blood pressure and heart rate measured by telemetry in rabbits and rats. *Journal of the Autonomic Nervous System* **54**, 235–246

Simons M and Downing SE (1985) Coronary vasoconstriction and catecholamine cardiomyopathy. *American Heart Journal* **109**, 297–304

Stypmann J, Engelen MA, Breithardt A-K, *et al.* (2007) Doppler echocardiography and tissue Doppler imaging in the healthy rabbit: differences of cardiac function during awake and anaesthetized examination. *International Journal of Cardiology* **115**, 164–170

Takihara K, Azuma J, Awata N, *et al.* (1986) Beneficial effect of taurine in rabbits with chronic congestive heart failure. *American Heart Journal* **112**, 1278–1284

Weber HW and Van der Walt JJ (1975) Cardiomyopathy in crowded rabbits. *Recent Advances in Studies on Cardiac Structure and Metabolism* **6**, 471–477

Yanni AE (2004) The laboratory rabbit: an animal model of atherosclerosis research. *Laboratory Animals* **38**, 246–256

15

Nervous system and musculoskeletal disorders

Emma Keeble

Neurological disease, such as head tilt and hindlimb paresis/paralysis, is a common clinical finding in pet rabbits. In older animals, arthritis is a frequent cause of lameness and crouched posture. The most common causes of nervous system disorders in rabbits include bacterial infections such as pasteurellosis, encephalitozoonosis, trauma and toxaemia. Obtaining a final diagnosis can be challenging in these cases. The increased availability of advanced diagnostic procedures, such as computed tomography (CT) and magnetic resonance imaging (MRI), combined with recent advances in serological testing and interpretation, make case evaluation and definitive diagnosis easier for the veterinary surgeon in practice.

History-taking and clinical examination

A thorough clinical history should be taken (see Chapter 7), to include details such as:

- Access to toxins, for example ingestion of lead-based paint from walls
- Recent in-contact animals and recent new additions that could increase the likelihood of infectious diseases
- Recent stressors, such as changes in diet.

In cases of neurological disease a detailed description of the presenting complaint should be ob-tained, including how and when it was first noticed, whether it is associated with pain and whether the condition has altered since onset. This will help to ascertain the chronicity and severity of the condition.

Assessment of pain in rabbits is difficult because an afflicted animal may attempt to disguise signs of pain to avoid being singled out by a predator. In severe cases patients may vocalize. Rabbits have similar pain receptors and nerve pathways to those of other mammals and therefore do feel pain, but their behavioural response is different to that of dogs and cats (see Chapter 10).

A routine clinical examination should be performed (see Chapter 7). This should include observation of posture and gait, and assessment of mental status. In cases of neurological disease, other body systems may also be involved that could affect the final prognosis. For example, a bacterial sinusitis may occur concurrently with a head tilt secondary to otitis media. A full ophthalmological examination (see Chapter 16) should form part of the neurological ex-amination of each case since assessment of eye position, eye movement, tear production and vision allows cranial nerve function to be evaluated (see Figure 15.2). Ocular examination may also reveal lesions such as phacoclastic uveitis following lens rupture associated with *Encephalitozoon cuniculi* infection.

Clinical signs associated with neuromuscular disease in the rabbit are outlined in Figure 15.1. Head tilt is the most common clinical sign and in a recent study this was found to be overwhelmingly associated with inflammatory lesions, primarily caused by *E. cuniculi*. Paresis was the second most common clinical presentation reported, again primarily associated with inflammatory lesions (Gruber *et al.*, 2009).

Clinical presentation	Differential diagnoses
Head tilt (vestibular dysfunction)	**Central (cerebellum, medulla oblongata):** Bacterial infection (e.g. listeriosis); herpesvirus encephalitis; visceral larval migrans; encephalitozoonosis; toxoplasmosis; neoplasia; cerebrovascular incident; degenerative changes; trauma; rabies virus – not UK; toxins; metabolic disease
	Peripheral (vestibular nerve – CN VIII, inner ear): Bacterial otitis interna/media (e.g. *Pasteurella multocida, Bordetella bronchiseptica, Pseudomonas aeruginosa, Staphylococcus aureus*); toxins (e.g. aminoglycosides); 'idiopathic vestibular syndrome'?
Paresis/ paralysis (may be central or peripheral in origin)	Vertebral fracture/luxation; spondylosis; osteoarthritis; intervertebral disc disease; encephalitozoonosis; toxoplasmosis; splay leg; hypovitaminosis A; neoplasia; ulcerative pododermatitis; toxins; metabolic disease; idiopathic
Seizures	Pasteurellosis; bacterial encephalitis; lead toxicosis; heat stroke; pregnancy toxaemia; hypoxia; azotaemia; electrolyte imbalance; terminal systemic disease (e.g. rabbit haemorrhagic disease); neoplasia; toxaemia; cardiovascular disease; hypovitaminosis A; hereditary ataxia (glycogen storage disease?); idiopathic epilepsy (blue-eyed white rabbits); vascular disease; degenerative disease; idiopathic

15.1 Differential diagnoses according to neurological/musculoskeletal presentation.
(continues) ▶

Clinical presentation	Differential diagnoses
Muscular weakness	Hypovitaminosis E/selenium deficiency; cerebrovascular incident; spinal lesions; bacterial infection; metabolic disease (e.g. hypocalcaemia, hypokalaemia); hepatic lipidosis; myasthenia gravis?
Lameness/ abnormal gait	Fracture; luxation; traumatic injury/sprain; osteoarthritis; septic arthritis; splay leg; hip dysplasia; pododermatitis; spinal disease; neoplasia; osteomyelitis; mycobacteriosis

15.1 (continued) Differential diagnoses according to neurological/musculoskeletal presentation.

Neurological examination

A full neurological examination should be performed, including cranial nerve assessment (Figure 15.2), postural reaction testing, spinal reflexes and sensory evaluation (Figure 15.3). Results should be interpreted with care in rabbits, because owing to their natural prey status they may not react as anticipated in stressful situations. In the author's experience rabbits tend to react to postural changes by remaining immobile. Proprioceptive positioning and placing responses are most useful and result in a satisfactory response in normal animals (Figure 15.4). Hopping, hemi-walking and wheel-barrowing postural reaction tests are usually resented, with

Cranial nerve (CN)	Function test	Assessment useful in rabbits?
CN I (Olfactory)	Response to noxious-smelling substance	No
CN II (Optic)	Menace response	No – rabbits remain stationary
	Pupillary light reflex	Yes, though response may be slow/delayed
	Visual placing reflex	Yes – observation of navigation around obstacles
CN III (Oculomotor)	Observe eye position and movements at rest and on movement of head (vestibulo-ocular reflex)	Lateral eye position makes assessment difficult at rest. Physiological nystagmus observed with head movement
CN IV (Trochlear)	As for CN III	As for CN III
CN V (Trigeminal): motor function	Size and symmetry of masticatory muscles	No – atrophy and facial swelling common with dental disease
	Test resistance to jaw opening	Partly – minimal vertical jaw movement only possible and manipulation often resented
CN V (Trigeminal): sensory function	Corneal reflex	Yes
	Palpebral reflex	Yes
	Facial skin pinching and observation of facial twitch/whisker movement	Yes
CN VI (Abducent)	As for CN III	As for CN III
CN VII (Facial)	Observe facial symmetry, blinking and nostril movement	Yes
	Palpebral reflex	Yes
	Corneal reflex	Yes
	Menace response	No
	Facial pinching	Yes
CN VIII (Vestibulocochlear)	Response to sudden noise	Yes – become stationary, ears twitch (though reduced if stressed)
	Vestibulo-ocular reflex (nystagmus induced by head movement)	Yes
CN IX (Glossopharyngeal)	Observation of swallowing	Yes
	Gag reflex	No
CN X (Vagus)	Oculocardiac reflex	Yes – though accurate assessment difficult with rapid heart rate in stressed animal
CN XII (Hypoglossal)	Inspection of tongue	Yes – use otoscope
	Observation of licking	Yes – place food on lips

15.2 Assessment of cranial nerve function.

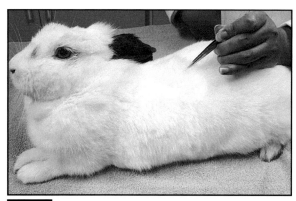

15.3 Assessing the panniculus reflex.

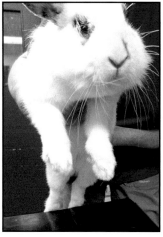

15.4 Postural reaction tests such as the placing response shown here can be useful in rabbits. Results should be interpreted with care, however, as rabbits do not react in the same way as cats and dogs. It should be noted that these reflexes detect neurological dysfunction, but do not provide detailed information for exact lesion localization.

the animal struggling, resulting in a risk of traumatic injury to the rabbit during the examination. Spinal reflex testing is primarily of use in rabbits presenting with paresis/paralysis and is used to classify the neurological disorder as either LMN (lower motor neuron) or UMN (upper motor neuron) and thereby to localize the lesion. Sensory evaluation for conscious pain perception in rabbits is, in the author's experience, difficult to perform compared with cats and dogs because rabbits do not respond with vocalization or attempting to bite. This makes assessment of deep pain perception in cases with severe spinal cord damage problematic and can make determination of prognosis and case management difficult in rabbits with hindlimb paralysis secondary to spinal trauma.

Diagnostic procedures

Clinical pathology
Complete blood count, serum biochemistry and urinalysis should be performed in all cases to identify systemic diseases that may result in neurological disorders.

- Systemic infections with *Pasteurella multocida*, *E. cuniculi* and *Toxoplasma gondii*: Chronic systemic disease may cause a non-regenerative anaemia; in acute disease a heterophilia and lymphopenia may be observed; elevated serum renal parameters may be noted associated with *E. cuniculi* infection, as well as elevations in the gamma globulin fraction on serum protein electrophoresis and a lower albumin/globulin (A/G) ratio. Increased urinary protein:creatinine ratio has not been demonstrated in association with seroconversion to *E. cuniculi* infection in pet rabbits (Reusch *et al.*, 2009).
- Toxins: Lead poisoning is classically associated with basophilic stippling and a non-regenerative anaemia.
- Metabolic disorders: Renal failure/uraemic encephalopathy is associated with elevated levels of blood urea nitrogen, creatinine and serum phosphate, hyperkalaemia and hyponatraemia; liver failure/hepatoencephalopathy is associated with elevated serum alkaline phosphatase (ALP), alanine aminotransferase (ALT) and bile acids. Chronic renal failure can also result in a non-regenerative anaemia.

Radiography
Standard radiographic views should be taken in cases of lameness, abnormality of gait, spinal disease and head tilt. In addition, the author routinely takes skull radiographs (lateral, dorsoventral, left and right 45-degree oblique and open-mouth views) to assess for evidence of dental disease and increased radiodensity of the tympanic bulla(e) that may be seen associated with otitis media/interna. Bony changes to the bulla may be seen in chronic cases (Figure 15.5). It should be noted, however, that normal skull radiographs do not rule out otitis media/otitis externa, and additional imaging techniques such as CT (see below) should be carried out in suspect cases. Orthopaedic abnormalities are a common radiographic finding and include fractures, luxations, hip dysplasia (Figure 15.6), scoliosis (Figure 15.7), kyphosis and lordosis of the spine, and vertebral spondylosis and osteoarthritis (Figure 15.8) in older animals.

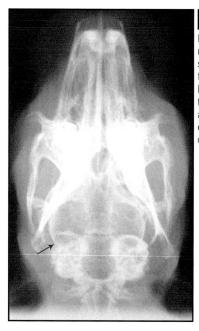

15.5 Dorsoventral skull radiograph showing severe changes to the tympanic bullae, especially the right (arrowed), associated with chronic bacterial otitis interna.

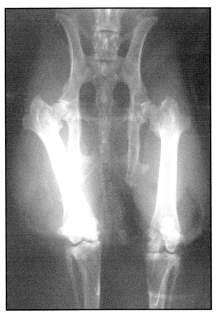

15.6 Ventrodorsal radiograph showing hip dysplasia in a young rabbit.

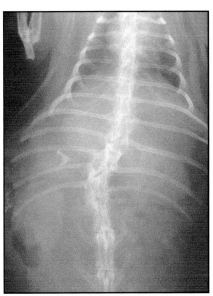

15.7 Dorsoventral radiograph showing vertebral scoliosis in a rabbit. The owner had not noted any abnormalities.

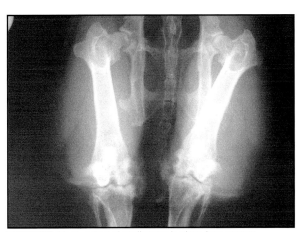

15.8 Ventrodorsal radiograph showing severe osteoarthritis of the stifle joints.

Magnetic resonance imaging and computed tomography

CT is the diagnostic imaging technique of choice for evaluation of the ear, skull, vertebral column and all calcified structures and is an essential tool, in the author's experience, in the diagnosis of otitis media (Figure 15.9). Prognosis and case management decisions can be better determined following use of this imaging technique as it allows full assessment of the extent of the disease process. This is important when deciding on the surgical approach and technique. It will also allow assessment of whether the condition is unilateral or bilateral (the latter being commonly seen in the author's practice). MRI is more useful in cases with central nervous system disease and associated clinical signs, such as epilepsy, as soft tissue abnormalities and fine detail can be clearly visualized.

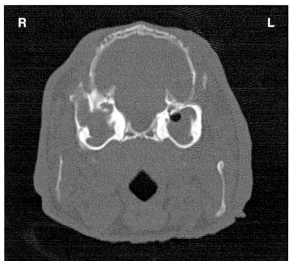

15.9 CT image of the head of a rabbit with bilateral otitis media. There is complete obliteration of the right tympanic bulla by fluid-attenuating material and partial obliteration of the left tympanic bulla.

Serology

Serological measurement of antibody titres is indicated in neurological disease associated with infectious agents.

Encephalitozoon cuniculi

Specific antibody assays are available in the UK, and measurement of both IgG and IgM antibody titres is now possible. Indirect enzyme-linked immunosorbent assay (ELISA) tests are used to measure serum antibody levels. IgM levels increase early on (1 week post-infection), but by day 17 after infection IgG antibodies become more dominant, with IgM levels declining to zero by 35 days. IgG levels continue to rise steadily from 30 days after infection and at this time spores may also be detected in the urine (Figure 15.10). IgG antibodies remain elevated and peak at 70 days (Cox *et al.*, 1979). Excretion of *E. cuniculi* spores mimics the trend in IgG levels. A wide individual variation in humoral response has however been reported in rabbits, with some animals having persistently high levels of IgG for a prolonged

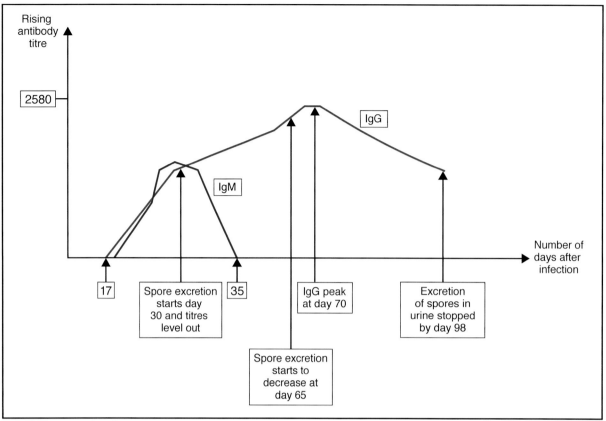

15.10 Humoral antibody response in rabbits infected with *E. cuniculi*. Note that considerable individual variation in antibody response has been recorded in rabbits (Kunstyr *et al.*, 1986).

period and others becoming seronegative after 8 weeks. No correlation was found between the antibody titre and the severity of the clinical signs or the presence of the parasite within the brain (Kunstyr *et al.*, 1986). Rabbits infected with *E. cuniculi* exhibit an abnormal humoral response to other concurrent infections, with lowered IgG levels and elevated IgM (Cox, 1977).

Early acute active infection is indicated if both IgM and IgG antibodies are elevated. However, if testing early on in the disease process (<30 days after infection), IgM may be elevated and IgG titres may be negative. This has been demonstrated in a small number of cases (Jeklova *et al.*, 2010). In this case affected animals should be treated and retested after 4 weeks, when IgM titres should have decreased and IgG titres increased, confirming an active infection. The situation is less clear where IgG titres are elevated and IgM titres are negative, owing to the considerable individual variation in duration of the IgG antibody response. Elevations in IgG indicate chronic exposure to the parasite or latent infection, but are commonly found in clinically normal rabbits. A positive IgG titre in an individual animal only detects the presence of antibody at that particular time, indicating exposure to the parasite; it does not reflect the course of clinical disease, because carrier status may occur. IgM antibodies may also be elevated in cases with reactivation of existing infection with *E. cuniculi* or in cases that become reinfected. Elevations in IgM and IgG antibodies have been found in clinically healthy

rabbits as well as rabbits with clinical signs of disease not associated with *E. cuniculi* infection (Jeklova *et al.*, 2010). This may be due to disease or stress precipitating reactivation of the parasite or predisposing an individual to infection with the parasite. In healthy animals, elevations in IgM as well as IgG indicate a subclinical acute infection, possibly as a result of a low infective dose of parasite, host response or variations in parasite pathogenicity.

Serum IgG titres can remain elevated for years, with or without clinical signs (Csokai *et al.*, 2009b). In cases with elevation of both IgM and IgG, treatment should be instigated, particularly if there are associated clinical signs. It should be noted however that concurrent disease is commonly seen in these cases, in particular toxoplasmosis and otitis media/interna (Jeklova *et al.*, 2010). In cases with elevated IgG not associated with clinical signs it would be prudent to monitor serum antibody levels over a period of time in case IgM becomes elevated, indicating reinfection or reactivation.

A positive IgM result with a negative IgG test indicates very early infection; however, in a clinical situation this result is rarely encountered because rabbits presenting with clinical signs associated with the disease are more likely to be chronically infected. Elevations in IgM and IgG antibodies occur 2 weeks prior to parasitic organisms being present in the kidneys, 4 weeks prior to pathological changes being seen in the kidneys associated with parasite infection and 8 weeks prior to pathological changes occurring in the brain. More commonly, in the author's experience, either IgM and IgG are simultaneously elevated, or just IgG titres are elevated, associated with classic clinical signs. This is similar to the situation reported by Jeklova *et al.* (2010), where the highest detection rate for both IgM and IgG antibodies was in rabbits with neurological signs (primarily vestibulitis). If elevation of antibody titres occurs associated with clinical signs the animal should be treated. Antibody titres should be retested 4 weeks later and if both are still elevated and associated with clinical signs a repeat treatment course is recommended by the author. If IgM levels are normal and IgG still elevated, with resolution or significant improvement of clinical signs at this stage, the author recommends monitoring with serological sampling, initially on a monthly basis, but increasing the time period between samples if IgG levels remain static or decrease, with no recurrence or further worsening of clinical signs.

In cases associated with neurological clinical signs, however, a single negative IgM/IgG result rules out *E. cuniculi* as a cause of clinical disease, as clinical signs are associated with chronic infection with the parasite (Figure 15.11).

Clinical stage of infection	Serological test result	Action
Acute infection	↑IgM, ↑IgG	Treat with fenbendazole, retest after 4 weeks and if still elevated with clinical signs present, repeat treatment course
Acute infection (<30 days after infection)	↑IgM, IgG negative	Start treatment, but retest in 4 weeks when IgG should be elevated
Chronic infection	↑IgG, IgM negative	Indicates exposure to parasite. If no clinical signs present, repeat serology. If clinical signs present start treatment
Neurological signs present	IgG and IgM negative	Rules out *E.cuniculi* as cause of disease

15.11 Interpretation of *E. cuniculi* serological test results.

Polymerase chain reaction (PCR) testing is available commercially to aid the diagnosis of *E. cuniculi* infection in pet rabbits; however recent studies have shown PCR testing of both cerebrospinal fluid and urine for this parasite to be unreliable in both clinical and subclinical cases. Conversely, PCR analysis of phacoemulsified lens material from suspect ocular cases of *E. cuniculi* is a reliable diagnostic tool (Csokai *et al.*, 2009b).

Pasteurella multocida
Antibody assays are available in the UK, but their value is questionable in pet rabbits, in which this organism is thought to be endemic. A rising titre does not necessarily prove that the organism is responsible for clinical signs, such as head tilt, as other bacteria are increasingly being isolated in these cases. Many clinicians now question whether this organism is truly responsible for all the various infectious disease conditions with which it is often associated in the literature. The assay may, however, be useful as a herd health indicator in specific-pathogen-free rabbits in a laboratory situation.

Toxoplasma gondii
Detection of IgG antibodies may be useful in the diagnosis of neurological disease in rabbits. In one study 19% of rabbits were found to be positive on serological examination for this parasite (this included both clinically healthy rabbits and those with clinical disease; Jeklova *et al.*, 2010).

Cerebrospinal fluid analysis
Cerebrospinal fluid (CSF) may be collected in small volumes from both the cisterna magna and the lumbosacral epidural space in rabbits (see Chapter 7 for technique and Chapter 9 for normal values). This procedure is indicated when there is disease affecting the central nervous system. In cases of meningitis, injection of contrast material may exacerbate clinical signs and therefore CSF analysis should ideally be carried out prior to myelography. Samples may be submitted for cytological examination and PCR testing. Cytological changes are often non-specific and associated with inflammatory/infectious diseases such as protozoal, viral or bacterial encephalitis, or lymphoma.

Microbiology
In cases of suspected bacterial (e.g. *Listeria*) or fungal meningitis, urine, blood and CSF culture are indicated. Otitis media/interna may be associated with sinusitis in rabbits and in these cases deep bilateral nasal swabs should be obtained for bacteriological culture (see Chapter 7). Nasal endoscopy is also used by the author with this technique to aid visualization, with the rabbit under general anaesthesia. Samples may also be collected via endoscopic biopsy for culture. Unless care is taken, contaminants from the external nares are common. A pure growth of a single organism is likely to be significant; mixed cultures are likely to represent normal bacterial flora. Normal nasal flora in healthy rabbits includes *Moraxella catarrhalis*, *Bordetella bronchiseptica*, *Pasteurella multocida*, *Staphylococcus* spp., *Streptococcus* spp. and *Bacillus* spp. (see Chapter 11).

Common neurological and musculoskeletal conditions

Head tilt/vestibular disease
Pet rabbits commonly present with acute-onset head tilt/torticollis (Figure 15.12), resulting in loss of balance, rolling and, in severe cases, inability to eat. In mild cases the rabbit may cope well with the head tilt, maintain their balance and continue to eat. The lesion is related to either central or peripheral nervous system disease and it is important to distinguish between the two in order to obtain a diagnosis (Figure 15.13).

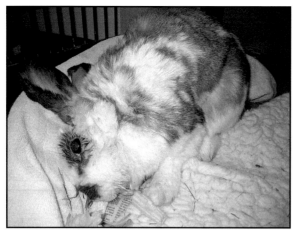

15.12 Head tilt in a rabbit secondary to bacterial otitis interna.

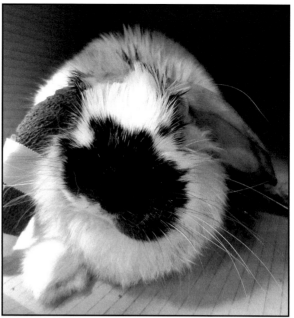

15.14 Facial nerve paralysis in a rabbit secondary to otitis interna. Note the severely drooped left side of the rabbit's face.

Clinical observation	Central vestibular disease	Peripheral vestibular disease
Concurrent signs of CNS disease	Yes	No
Nystagmus	Horizontal, vertical, rotatory. Fast phase in any direction and changes with changing head position	Horizontal, rotatory. Fast phase away from side of lesion and does not change with changing head position
Facial nerve paralysis	No	Yes
Horner's syndrome	No	Yes

15.13 Differentiating central from peripheral vestibular disease.

- Nystagmus may or may not be associated with either central or peripheral disorders. With diseases affecting the central nervous system, nystagmus is likely to be horizontal, vertical or rotary, the fast phase may be in any direction and it may change with alterations in head position. In peripheral disease, nystagmus is usually horizontal or rotary, with the fast phase away from the side of the lesion, and the direction is not altered by altering position of the head.
- Concurrent neurological signs, such as head tremors, proprioceptive deficits and hypermetria, are usually associated with central disease. With peripheral disease, these are usually absent.
- Facial nerve paralysis (Figure 15.14) and Horner's syndrome may be seen associated with peripheral disease. Horner's syndrome, resulting from damage to the sympathetic nerve supply, is associated with unilateral constriction of the pupil, protrusion of the third eyelid, retraction of the globe and a slight drooping of the eyelid.

Clinical signs may gradually resolve, with affected rabbits adapting to the head tilt over a few weeks. The rabbit should be housed in a safe environment during this time to avoid self-injury. In severe cases associated with rolling, euthanasia may be indicated. The two major differential diagnoses for head tilt in rabbits are bacterial otitis media/interna (e.g. *Pasteurella multocida* or *Staphylococcus aureus* infection) causing peripheral vestibular disease, and encephalitozoonosis causing central vestibular disease.

Bacterial otitis media/interna

Causes and clinical signs: Bacterial otitis media/interna is a common condition in pet rabbits and may be associated with the following organisms: *Staphylococcus aureus*, *Pasteurella multocida*, *Pseudomonas aeruginosa*, *Bordetella bronchiseptica*, *Escherichia coli* and *Proteus mirabilis* (although in the author's experience culture of samples taken deep within the external acoustic meatus at the time of surgery may be negative). An aural examination should be carried out to check for a primary or secondary otitis externa and for rupture of the tympanic membrane. The ear should be carefully and thoroughly palpated, particularly at the base of the vertical ear canal which is a common location for abscesses. The author often finds soft tissue lesions here on routine clinical examination that have been missed by the owner. Other clinical signs which may be noted include head shaking or scratching the base of the ear. A primary otitis media may be caused by infection spreading to the middle ear from the upper respiratory tract via the Eustachian tubes. Concurrent sinusitis/rhinitis and associated clinical signs are suggestive of this. Approximately 80% of rabbits with upper respiratory tract disease also have changes associated with the tympanic bulla (Deeb *et al.*, 1990). In severe cases otitis interna may spread further, resulting in encephalitis and seizures.

Diagnosis: Diagnosis is based on clinical signs, skull radiography (see Figure 15.5), microbial culture and sensitivity (deep nasal swabs or aural swabs) and CT scanning (see Figure 15.9) or MRI. In the author's experience CT imaging is essential in the diagnosis of otitis media because cases are often subclinical and bilateral disease occurs in approximately 70% of cases diagnosed. In one study, approximately 11% of clinically healthy rabbits had middle ear infections on post-mortem examination (Deeb *et al.*, 1990). The author recommends surgery in cases with confirmed otitis media; however the potential complications and intensive nursing required postoperatively should be carefully discussed with the owner first.

Treatment: Systemic antibiotics should be given for at least 4–6 weeks, ideally based on culture and sensitivity testing. Antibiotics with good penetration of the CNS and activity against the commonly isolated bacteria involved should ideally be used. Antibiotics such as fluoroquinolones (ciprofloxacin, marbofloxacin, enrofloxacin), penicillin, cefalexin or potentiated sulphonamides may be beneficial in these cases (see Figure 15.26).

If otitis externa is present the rabbit should be anaesthetized and the affected ear canal gently flushed with saline. Extreme care should be taken with this technique if rupture of the tympanic membrane has occurred because iatrogenic damage with associated neurological signs may occur, in the author's experience. Topical antibiotic drops, such as enrofloxacin, may also be used. Surgical treatment with total ear canal ablation and lateral bulla osteotomy (LBO) is indicated in cases with both otitis media and externa (for further details see the *BSAVA Manual of Rabbit Surgery, Dentistry and Imaging*). However, surgery is associated with a high risk of postoperative complications such as cellulitis, abscess formation and facial nerve paralysis. At the author's practice the technique has been modified to a partial ear canal ablation and LBO, with good success. Long-term administration of systemic antibiotics should help reduce the incidence of postoperative complications. Spasm of the neck muscles is commonly associated with head tilt and owners should be encouraged to massage these muscles regularly.

Antiemetic drugs may be useful to prevent suspected nausea secondary to vestibular damage, for example metoclopramide at 0.5 mg/kg orally or s.c. q8h. It is not known, however, whether this sensation occurs in rabbits because they cannot vomit and lack a vomiting centre in the medulla oblongata. Phenothiazine derivatives and antihistamines may prove useful in head tilt cases, as they act on vestibular pathways and are dopamine antagonists. An example is prochlorperazine, which is used in humans for diseases of the inner ear (such as labyrinthitis) and is formulated as an oral suspension, which is convenient for dosing. A suggested dose rate (extrapolated from human medicine) is 0.2–0.5 mg/kg orally q8h. The use of meclizine has been anecdotally reported in the USA to be beneficial in head tilt cases at a dose rate of 12.5–25 mg/kg orally q8h.

Encephalitozoon cuniculi infection

E. cuniculi is an obligate intracellular protozoal parasite, belonging to the phylum Microsporidia. This parasite is widespread in the domestic rabbit population in the UK, with a seroprevalence of 52% in clinically healthy pet rabbits (Keeble and Shaw, 2006). Infections occur primarily in rabbits, but have also been diagnosed in sheep, goats, pigs, dogs, cats, foxes, rodents and monkeys. The infection is zoonotic and can cause severe life-threatening disease in immunocompromised humans. Close contact between owners and susceptible pet species may lead to an increase in human exposure to this parasite. Infections in humans have been shown to involve the same strain that infects rabbits (Deplazes *et al.*, 1996) and in some cases previous contact with rabbits is reported (Weber *et al.*, 1997). Transfer of human strains to rabbits is possible (Mathis *et al.*, 1997). Infection in humans is primarily through environmental spore contamination from infected humans or animals, such as via contaminated water sources.

Infective spores are shed in the urine and transmission usually occurs by ingestion of contaminated food and water. Transplacental infection and infection following inhalation have also been reported. The spores can remain viable in extreme environmental conditions for some time; in dry conditions at normal temperatures (22°C), their survival time is 4 weeks, on average. They are easily destroyed by most routine disinfectants (including a 0.1% solution of bleach for 10 minutes exposure time, 70% ethanol for 30 seconds exposure time) as well as boiling and autoclaving.

Once ingested the parasite infects the intestinal epithelium, where it replicates, and infective spores are carried in circulating macrophages to the liver, kidney, central nervous system, lungs and heart. Cell rupture eventually occurs, releasing infective spores and causing inflammation and granuloma formation in these target organs. In the central nervous system there is focal non-suppurative granulomatous meningoencephalitis. Infected rabbits may be asymptomatic, and carrier status occurs. Clinical signs associated with this disease are listed in Figure 15.15.

Active infection has been diagnosed in healthy asymptomatic animals, based on IgM and IgG serology (Jeklova *et al.*, 2010). Concurrent disease (such as dental, respiratory, intestinal or neoplastic disease) was also a common finding in *E. cuniculi*-positive rabbits in this study.

Diagnosis: Diagnosis in the live rabbit is difficult because the organism is hard to isolate. On post-mortem examination, histopathology of the kidney or brain typically demonstrates granulomatous changes. It should be noted that clinically healthy rabbits have been found to be infected with the parasite and to exhibit granulomatous changes on post-mortem histopathological examination of the brain. Organisms may be identified within target tissues. Serum antibody titres can be measured using ELISA in the UK (see previous discussion

Clinical signs
• Head tilt • Torticollis • Hindlimb paresis • Paralysis • Urinary incontinence • Renal failure • Cataracts and lens-induced uveitis • Retarded growth • Collapse • Tremors • Convulsions • Death
Differential diagnoses (Gruber *et al.*, 2009)
• Otitis media/interna • Spinal fracture, trauma • Bacterial central abscess (e.g. *Pasteurella* infection) or encephalitis • Splay leg • Metabolic/toxic disease (e.g. lead toxicity, hepatic lipidosis) • Toxoplasmosis • Herpes simplex viral encephalitis • Listeriosis, CNS neoplasia (e.g. lymphoma) • CNS hypoxia secondary to vascular disease • Degenerative CNS lesions • (Borna disease virus, rabies and *Baylisascaris* infections should also be considered in rabbits that have recently travelled)

15.15 Clinical signs associated with *E. cuniculi* infection in rabbits and differential diagnoses.

under diagnostic techniques). Seroconversion precedes renal shedding by 4 weeks (see Figure 15.10), so antibody assay tests could be used in a multi-rabbit household to screen in-contact animals following a clinical case and remove any seropositive animals before they become infective. A presumptive diagnosis is made on the basis of elevated IgM and IgG antibody titres, or elevated IgG on its own in conjunction with clinical signs. Clinical signs may also be associated with concurrent bacterial infection, in which case systemic antibiotics are indicated. Serum/plasma protein electrophoresis may be used to measure the A:G ratio in suspected cases of *E. cuniculi* infection. A lower A:G ratio, lower beta-globulin fraction and a higher gamma-globulin fraction is found in *E. cuniculi*-infected rabbits compared with clinically normal animals (Rich, 2010). *E. cuniculi*-positive rabbits with neurological signs often have elevations in serum urea (>8.38 mmol/l) and lowered serum phosphorus levels (<1.28 mmol/l). *E. cuniculi*-positive rabbits with renal disease (azotaemia, polyuria/polydipsia, pollakiuria) often have lowered PCV (<33%), increased absolute neutrophil (heterophil) counts (>8 × 10⁶/l), and lowered serum phosphorus (<1.28 mmol/l) and potassium levels (<3.2 mmol/l) (Jeklova *et al.*, 2010).

Analysis of CSF from infected rabbits reveals non-specific changes such as elevated protein levels and lymphomonocytic pleocytosis; these changes may also be seen with other infections (Jass *et al.*, 2008) and are not diagnostic. They do, however, increase the likelihood of infection as a cause of the associated clinical signs.

PCR detection of spore DNA is available commercially for urine and CSF samples. However excretion in urine is sporadic and both urine and CSF samples can be negative in clinically affected animals. This test is therefore not reliable, except for diagnosis of *E. cuniculi*-associated phacoclastic uveitis (Csokai *et al.*, 2009b).

Kidney biopsy and histopathological examination of tissue is used in human medicine to diagnose infection and has been used by the author for diagnosis of this disease in pet rabbits using laparoscopy. Preliminary results are being analysed; however in theory this should give a definite diagnosis in cases presenting with renal disease from 9 weeks post infection. Care must be taken to evaluate renal function fully prior to this technique. Liver biopsy may also be helpful in detecting the parasite in the early stage of infection (<98 days after infection), as was found in experimentally infected animals in one study (Csokai *et al.*, 2009a).

Treatment: Treatment aims to reduce inflammation and prevent formation of spores. In suspected clinical cases the author typically prescribes a 28-day course of oral fenbendazole at 20 mg/kg q24h, together with broad-spectrum systemic antibiosis such as trimethoprim–sulfamethoxazole at 15–30 mg/kg orally q12h or enrofloxacin at 10 mg/kg orally q12h for 7–10 days. Antibiotics are prescribed to treat a primary bacterial cause (which may be concurrent) or any secondary bacterial infections. In cases that present in the acute stage of the disease, particularly those with severe acute neurological signs, dexamethasone at 0.1–0.2 mg/kg s.c. q48h for up to three doses may also be given; however it should be noted that this may affect the host's immune response and is not routinely used by the author. Animals with severe neurological signs, such as head tilt and rolling, may require sedation with diazepam at 0.5 mg/kg s.c., i.m. or i.v. or midazolam at 0.07–0.22 mg/kg i.m. or i.v. Prochlorperazine at 0.25–0.5 mg/kg orally q8h may also be helpful in animals with head tilt. The animal should be housed in a quiet stress-free environment and supportive care instigated with supplemental feeding, fluid therapy and prokinetic drugs as required. Physiotherapy and hydrotherapy may be indicated. Once neurological signs have developed it is unlikely that these will resolve completely. Acute cases with urinary incontinence as the presenting clinical sign may resolve with fenbendazole. The prognosis for ophthalmic disease is good following lens removal (see Chapter 16).

New research shows that microsporidians are related to fungi. Treatment of *E. cuniculi* infection in humans includes the use of albendazole and this drug has also been used in rabbits. Fumagillin, sparfloxacin, oxytetracycline, polyoxin D, nikkomycin Z, oxibendazole and tiabendazole are effective *in vitro*, but there is no information on their use in pet rabbits.

Control: As this parasite is widespread in pet rabbits, prevention of infection may not be possible. Infection may also be present in wild rabbits and rodents, which could be a source of environmental contamination with spores (Meredith *et al.*, 2013). Establishment of an *E. cuniculi*-free breeding colony is possible, but requires time and expense. Healthy seronegative young rabbits should be housed in complete isolation from other rabbits and in separate rodent-proof cages. Serum antibody levels are then tested every 2 weeks for 2 months and all seropositive animals, however low the titre, are removed. Testing continues until all animals are negative for 1 month. These animals are then used to set up the breeding colony, but testing should continue on a monthly basis to confirm the disease-free status (Cox *et al.*, 1977). If this is not practically feasible, measures that may reduce the incidence of infection are prophylactic fenbend-azole in feed, testing and isolation of positive animals, good hygiene with routine disinfection practices, raised food dishes, and use of water bottles rather than bowls to reduce the risk of uri-nary transmission. Direct or indirect contact with wild rabbits and rodents should be avoided. If contact between rabbits not normally housed together is necessary, for example at rabbit shows and studs, then stringent hygiene practices should be followed and urine contact between rabbits at shows should be avoided.

The author recommends prophylactic treatment of all new rabbits recently acquired by owners and presented to the veterinary clinic with a 28-day course of fenbendazole where animals may have previously been exposed to the parasite by contact with other rabbits at the source. This will prevent infection and treat any infection that may have been acquired. It is important to stress to owners, how-ever, that it will not prevent infection at a later date.

Less common causes of head tilt
The clinical approach to a case of head tilt in a rabbit is illustrated in Chapter 22.

Human herpes simplex virus: This has been re-ported in pet rabbits as a rare cause of meningo-encephalitis (Weissenbock *et al.*, 1997, Muller *et al.*, 2009). Clinical signs include initial conjunctivitis, fol-lowed by ataxia, circling, seizures and collapse. Euthanasia is usually indicated. Diagnosis is based on histology of neural tissues at post-mortem exami-nation, with non-suppurative meningoencephalitis of the cerebral grey matter, neuronal cell necrosis and neuron and glial cell intranuclear inclusions being typically present. Definite diagnosis is obtained using immunohistochemistry and *in situ* hybridiza-tion, or PCR analysis. The source of infection is thought to be close contact with a person with her-pes labialis (cold sores). Horizontal transfer of infec-tion between rabbits has also been demonstrated.

Rabies: Rabies virus can rarely affect rabbits and primarily causes paralysis. The virus has been reported in pet rabbits in the USA (Karp *et al.*, 1999). Initial clinical signs are non-specific and include anorexia, pyrexia, lethargy and lameness, progressing to paresis or paralysis of one or more limbs, particularly the forelimbs, head tremor, coma and death. Cases have been described following skunk or raccoon bites. Control is through limiting exposure to these wildlife reservoirs by housing rabbits indoors in rabies-enzootic areas. There is no approved vaccine for rabbits in the USA. If diag-nosed on post-mortem examination, post-exposure rabies prophylaxis may be indicated for in-contact humans, especially if syringe feeding has occurred leading to contact with the rabbit's saliva.

Toxoplasmosis: Exposure to *Toxoplasma gondii* infection is reported to be widely prevalent in do-mestic rabbits (Dubey *et al.*, 1992; Leland *et al.*, 1992); however infection is usually subclinical and latent. A recent study found a 19% seroprevalence in pet rabbits (Jeklova *et al.*, 2010). In this study a signif-icant percentage of *T. gondii*-seropositive rabbits were also seropositive for *E. cuniculi*. Clinical toxo-plasmosis is rare, but it has been reported to be associated with pyrexia, lethargy, paresis, posterior paralysis, head tremor, ataxia and acute death follow-ing ingestion of feed or water contaminated with infected cat faeces. Post-mortem examination reveals a granulomatous meningoencephalitis with focal areas of necrosis and tachyzoites present in multiple organs. The kidneys are rarely affected however, in contrast to infections with *E. cuniculi*. Serological IgG antibody testing is available and treatment with tri-methoprim/sulphonamide and pyrimethamine or doxy-cycline is indicated. Prevention is by covering feed containers and preventing cats from accessing hay stores or rabbit grazing areas. The disease can be transmitted transplacentally in rabbits.

Nematodiasis: Cerebrospinal nematodiasis (cere-bral larval migrans) secondary to *Baylisascaris* spp. migration is seen in pet rabbits in the USA, following ingestion of feed contaminated by raccoon or skunk faeces. Clinical signs such as head tilt, ataxia, circling, tremors, nystagmus and, in advanced cases, seizures, rolling and paralysis, are seen. Motor function is impaired, although spinal reflexes remain intact. Some resolution of clinical signs may be seen following use of oxibendazole at 60 mg/kg orally q24h indefinitely. Control is by limiting access to contaminated materials, although *Baylisascaris* eggs are highly resistant in the environment and can remain infective for over a year. Rabbits are thought to be paratenic hosts for this parasite.

Listeriosis: Listeriosis occurs in pet rabbits, where it primarily results in metritis, abortion, infertility, liver disease and death. Central nervous system lesions are rare, in contrast with *Listeria* septicaemia in ruminants, where central nervous system disease is common (Watson and Evans, 1985).

Cuterebra *species* infection: Larvae of *Cuterebra* spp. (rabbit botfly) may be found as subcutan-eous infections (see Chapter 17). Aberrant intra-cranial migration resulting in neurological clinical signs has also been reported in the rabbit (Hendrix *et al.*, 1989).

Neosporosis: This has not, to the author's knowledge, been reported in pet rabbits. It causes neurological disease in dogs, such as head tilt and paralysis. It is present, however, in the wild rabbit population in the UK with a 10% reported prevalence (Hughes *et al.*, 2008).

Other causes: Other potential causes of head tilt in rabbits include cerebrovascular accidents, degenerative changes, toxins, metabolic disease, trauma and neoplasia, such as pituitary adenoma, with clinical signs dependent on the site of the lesion.

Paresis/paralysis

Pet rabbits commonly present with paresis or paralysis. Paresis implies reduced voluntary motor function and can be secondary to neuromuscular junction, muscular, skeletal, nerve or spinal cord dysfunction, drug toxicities and systemic or metabolic disorders. Causes in pet rabbits include lumbar vertebral fracture or dislocation, intervertebral disc disease, spondylosis, encephalitozoonosis (Figure 15.16), toxoplasmosis, hypovitaminosis A, toxins, metabolic disease, neoplasia, osteoarthritis, splay leg and ulcerative pododermatitis. The latter three conditions are discussed later under Lameness.

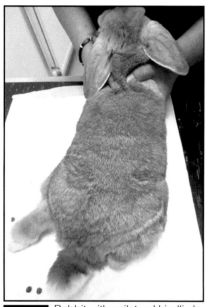

15.16 Rabbit with unilateral hindlimb paresis secondary to infection with *E. cuniculi*. This animal showed a delayed placing reflex of the left hindlimb on neurological examination.

Lumbar vertebral fracture or luxation/subluxation

This is a common condition in pet rabbits and usually results from trauma to the spine following incorrect handling. If the rabbit struggles while being restrained it may kick out with the hindlegs, resulting in spinal dislocation or fracture, usually involving the lumbosacral region (L6–L7). In the rabbit there is minimal cauda equina and the spinal cord extends well into the sacral region, thus damage at any level will affect both upper and lower motor neurons. Urinary and faecal incontinence and loss of skin sensation (panniculus reflex) are often seen.

Diagnosis is based on clinical signs, neurological examination, radiography and myelography. Advanced imaging techniques are extremely useful in the author's experience to evaluate spinal cord compression (Figure 15.17) and identify bone lesions which may not be apparent on survey radiographs.

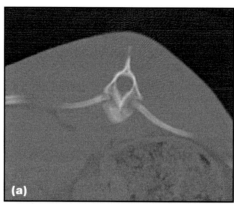

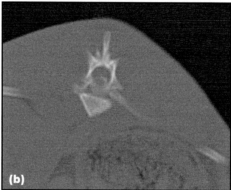

15.17 CT images of the thoracic spine showing transverse sections at **(a)** T11 (normal) and **(b)** T12 (showing compression of the spinal cord).

Prognosis depends on the site and severity of the lesion. A poor prognosis is associated with absence of deep pain reflexes (Figure 15.18); it should be noted, however, that this reflex is not always a reliable indicator because rabbits hide signs of pain, and that a withdrawal reflex is purely local and does not confirm an intact cord.

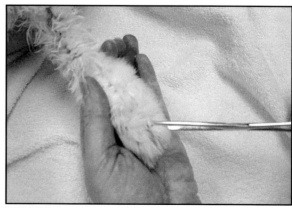

15.18 Assessment of deep pain reflexes is performed as for dogs and cats. A poor prognosis is associated with the absence of deep pain reflexes. This test is not always reliable, however, because rabbits hide signs of pain.

Treatment: Treatment aims to minimize secondary tissue damage by reducing hypotension and hypoxaemia. Administration of neuroprotective therapy such as glucocorticoids is of questionable value. Treatment should be instigated as soon as possible because the majority of secondary tissue damage occurs within the first 24 hours following injury. The use of high-dose methylprednisolone (30 mg/kg i.v.) within the first 8 hours post-injury is controversial since in clinical studies in dogs and humans no significant beneficial effects have been found and there are potential severe side effects such as gastrointestinal haemorrhage and immunosuppression. Appropriate fluid therapy should be instigated to increase perfusion to the injured area and supplemental oxygen therapy provided. Analgesia should be provided using opiate and non-steroidal anti-inflammatory (NSAID) therapy.

In chronic cases, if the prognosis for a return to normal function is poor, euthanasia is indicated. Surgical stabilization has been described in rabbits and is an option in cases with spinal instability or compression. It should be noted, however, that this procedure is technically difficult in rabbits owing to their small size, fragile skeleton and unique anatomy. Complications such as wound infection, seroma and nerve damage are common.

If the defect is stable, cage rest for 6 weeks is indicated (Figure 15.19). Affected animals may require intensive long-term nursing with manual bladder expression 3–4 times daily and administration of NSAIDs. There is a risk of bladder wall damage due to overdistension, and urinary tract infection. Diazepam at 0.25–0.5 mg/kg orally may be useful to relax the external urethral sphincter and aid manual expression. Daily baths to remove urine and faeces, application of barrier creams and rotation of the animal's position every 4–6 hours to prevent pressure sores are also indicated. Physiotherapy can be instigated with calm rabbits, for example hindlimb muscle massage, kinesiotherapy (passive) and hydrotherapy (Figure 15.20) may be of benefit in the recovery of stable spinal injury cases.

Owners should be made fully aware of the nursing commitment required at the onset and the prognosis for return to function vs. the stress and

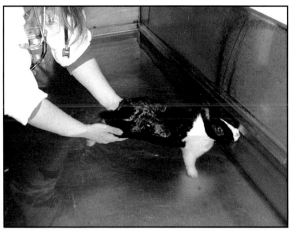

15.20 Hydrotherapy can be useful in the rehabilitation of rabbits with stable spinal trauma and is well tolerated by this species.

discomfort to the animal. In one report treatment of a severe spinal fracture in a rabbit was partially successful using a body bandage as external support and confining the animal to a small cage for 3 weeks. A return to full function was not achieved; however the animal was able to move around by itself and had a reasonable quality of life (Hammons, 1980). Carts adapted to rabbits for support of the hindlimbs have been used, although the welfare implications of using these in a highly stress-susceptible animal should be considered.

Intervertebral disc disease

This is rare in rabbits but has been reported associated with posterior paralysis and urinary and faecal incontinence (Baxter, 1975). The lumbar vertebrae are usually affected. Disc protrusion and extrusion of nuclear material, leading to compression of the spinal cord, occur following forceful hyperflexion of the spine. Pedal and patellar reflexes may still be intact. Clinical signs are similar to cases with lumbar vertebral fracture or luxation/subluxation and diagnostic imaging may be required to reach a diagnosis. The cases described did not respond to treatment and the animals were euthanased.

Hypovitaminosis A

Hypovitaminosis A secondary to dietary deficiency may cause circling, paralysis, convulsions and opisthotonus in rabbits. Affected does may give birth to young with hydrocephalus.

Seizures

The most common causes of seizures in pet rabbits are secondary to inflammatory changes associated with encephalitozoonosis and bacterial encephalitis or meningitis (e.g. due to *Pasteurella*) (Gruber *et al.*, 2009). Other causes include pregnancy toxaemia, trauma, heat stroke, lead toxicosis, hypoxia, azotaemia, electrolyte imbalances, terminal systemic disease (e.g. rabbit haemorrhagic disease), neoplasia, advanced hepatic lipidosis, toxaemia, cardiovascular disease, hypovitaminosis A and hereditary ataxia (glycogen storage disease). Idiopathic epilepsy is

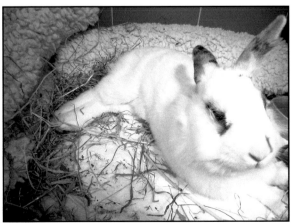

15.19 Cage rest is essential when nursing rabbits with spinal trauma.

reported in blue-eyed white rabbits. Initial stabilization with diazepam is indicated (see Supportive care) in addition to addressing the underlying cause. If no causative agent is identified symptomatic treatment with oral phenobarbital at 1–2 mg/kg/day and systemic antibiotics may be useful. The prognosis is generally poor.

Pregnancy toxaemia

Pregnancy toxaemia may be associated with clinical signs such as lethargy, incoordination, seizures, coma and death, typically late in the gestation period, although these signs may also be seen in the postpartum period and in non-gravid does with pseudopregnancy. Immediate treatment is indicated with intravenous fluid therapy (lactated Ringer's with 5% glucose) and supportive care. The condition is more common in obese animals undergoing a period of anorexia, and providing a high-energy diet in late pregnancy may reduce the incidence.

Heat stress

Rabbits are unable to sweat and are consequently very susceptible to heat stress and heat stroke. Clinical signs include seizures, depression, incoordination and coma. Rectal temperature reaches 40.5°C or higher. Slow cooling by immersing in tepid water, sedation with diazepam (see Supportive care), administration of intravenous fluids and mannitol to reduce cerebral oedema, and general supportive care can be attempted, but the prognosis is generally very poor.

Lead toxicity

Lead toxicity is commonest in rabbits housed indoors, following ingestion of lead-based paint. Clinical signs consist of chronic weight loss, lethargy, anorexia and associated intestinal ileus, anaemia (Figure 15.21), with neurological signs such as mild tremors, hindlimb ataxia and seizures being less common. Radiography may reveal radiodense particles, although usually ingested particles are not visible. Classically haematology reveals nucleated red blood cells, hypochromasia, poikilocytosis and cytoplasmic basophilic stippling. Heteropenia, lymphocytosis and a reduced haematocrit may also be present. A serum heparin blood sample is

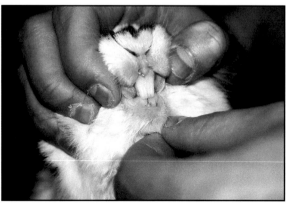

15.21 Anaemia of the oral mucous membranes in a rabbit with chronic lead toxicity.

required to demonstrate elevated blood lead levels (>1.45 μmol/l; >0.03 mg/dl; Roscoe *et al.*, 1975) and confirm the diagnosis.

The treatment of choice is chelation with edetate calcium disodium at 27.5 mg/kg s.c. twice daily for 5 days on, 5 days off, 5 days on, with retesting of blood lead levels after a further 5 days off treatment. Motility modifiers such as metoclopramide may also be useful. The author has given blood transfusions in cases where the haematocrit was significantly decreased (<15%).

Other toxicities

Seizures may occur secondary to pyrethrin/permethrin or fipronil toxicity, following an initial period of anorexia and lethargy. Response to treatment is poor; however removal of topical ectoparasiticides by bathing, oral administration of activated charcoal, fluid therapy, supportive care and diazepam to control seizures may be attempted.

Neoplasia

Neoplasia of the central nervous system has been reported in rabbits, the most commonly reported tumour being lymphoma. Pituitary adenoma, teratoma and ependymoma have also been reported. Clinical signs depend on the size and site of the lesion. Diagnosis is possible with MRI; however the prognosis is poor (see Chapter 18 for further details).

Hereditary ataxia

Hereditary ataxia is a glycogen storage disease that causes opisthotonus, paddling movements and nystagmus. It has been rarely reported in rabbits.

Muscle weakness

Causes of generalized muscle weakness in rabbits include hypovitaminosis E/selenium deficiency, toxoplasmosis, sarcocystosis, coccidiosis, bacterial infection, spinal lesions, cerebrovascular accident and metabolic disease, such as hypokalaemia, hypocalcaemia and hepatic lipidosis. Myasthenia gravis has been postulated as a cause of muscle weakness, but no cases in which a definitive diagnosis was made have been reported. The term 'floppy rabbit syndrome' is sometimes used to describe the clinical appearance of a rabbit with varying degrees of sudden-onset generalized weakness, flaccidity, paresis or paralysis. There are many proposed causes of this syndrome, including those listed above and described under Paresis/paralysis. Additional possible causes include plant toxins (e.g. woolly pod milkweed (*Asclepius eriocarpa*) in the USA, 'lettuce poisoning' – some species of lettuce contain lactucarium, an opioid compound), triazine herbicide toxicity and botulism. Treatment is aimed at the underlying cause, but in some cases a cause cannot be found and these patients often respond well to general supportive therapy.

Nutritional muscular dystrophy

Nutritional muscular dystrophy secondary to vitamin E deficiency has been described in rabbits and is associated with feed that has been stored too long

(Ringler and Abrams, 1970). Clinical signs include neonatal mortality, infertility, weakness and coma. On post-mortem examination skeletal muscles are pale and atrophic. If fresh food is available at all times it is unlikely that this condition will develop.

Sarcocystis
Myositis secondary to *Sarcocystis cuniculi* infection with cyst formation in skeletal muscle occurs in rabbits in the USA. When these cysts rupture, an intense inflammatory response occurs. There is no treatment and contact with wild rabbits, the natural host, should be avoided.

Lameness/abnormal gait
Assessment of gait should be part of any routine clinical examination. Common causes of lameness include fractures, luxations, traumatic injury, osteo-arthritis, septic arthritis, splay leg, pododermatitis, spinal disease, neoplasia and osteomyelitis (including mycobacterial bone infection).

Spinal disease
Vertebral spondylosis, scoliosis, kyphosis and lordosis are common radiographic findings in pet rabbits and may be incidental in mild cases (see Figure 15.7). Lesions may, however, be painful, leading to anorexia and intestinal ileus and resulting in clinical signs ranging from mild gait abnormalities to severe lameness, perineal caecotroph accumulation and urinary scalding. These spinal abnormalities may be predisposed by small cage size, sex of the animal (more common in females owing to high calcium requirements during pregnancy and lactation) and lack of exercise. Congenital hemivertebrae are seen in pet rabbits and may be asymptomatic.

Neoplasia
Osteosarcoma affecting the long bones has been reported in older rabbits and limb amputation should improve the rabbit's chance of survival.

Splay leg
Splay leg is a non-specific general term describing a number of developmental conditions occurring in young rabbits from birth up to a few months old, where the animal is unable to adduct one or more limbs (Figure 15.22). The condition is also sometimes referred to as hip dysplasia. The hindlimbs are more often involved, with femoral shaft torsions, neck anteversions and hip and patellar luxations/subluxations. Generalized joint laxity and primary acetabular dysplasia are not implicated in this condition. Abnormalities primarily involve only the bony structures of the femoral neck and subtrochanteric region (see Figure 15.6). It is an inherited simple autosomal recessive condition and therefore breeding from the same parent pair and affected offspring is not recommended. Euthanasia should be considered where multiple limbs are affected. In milder cases the animal may be able to cope with the deformity. Environmental factors, such as bedding type and floor structure, have been implicated in the pathogenesis of this disease

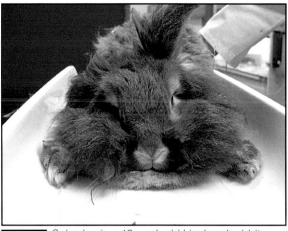

15.22 Splay leg in a 12-week-old Lionhead rabbit. Note the abduction of both forelimbs.

in young rabbits. In one study 22% of animals housed on smooth perspex-type flooring developed this condition, whereas those housed on a rough floor did not (Owiny *et al.*, 2001). High calcium intake has been suggested as a cause of osteochondrosis in young rabbits.

Other hereditary skeletal abnormalities
Hereditary chondrodystrophy has been described, with shortening of the scapulae, long bones and ribs and normal cranium development. Of the cases described all died shortly after birth. Spina bifida associated with a lethal recessive gene has also been documented in the rabbit.

Osteoarthritis
Age-related diseases, such as spondylosis and osteoarthritis, are now more commonly encountered in pet rabbits as longevity increases with improved husbandry and diet. Clinical signs include abnormal gait, reluctance to move, hunched posture (Figure 15.23) and urine scalding of the perineum. Affected animals are usually in a degree of discomfort, although this may be difficult to assess clinically. Diagnosis is made on radiographic examination (see Figure 15.8).

Treatment options include long-term analgesic and anti-inflammatory drug administration (e.g. oral meloxicam, oral tramadol), deep bedding material to

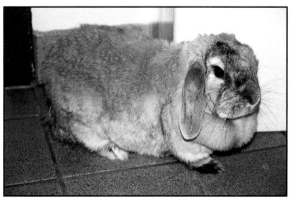

15.23 Elderly female rabbit with crouched posture secondary to severe osteoarthritis of the stifle joints.

prevent pressure sores, clipping of hair around the perineum with daily bathing of this area, barrier creams, and antibiosis if indicated.

Ulcerative pododermatitis

Severe ulcerative pododermatitis may present with similar clinical signs to those described for spondylosis and osteoarthritis in rabbits. Classically this condition involves the plantar metatarsus, resulting in a chronic granulomatous ulcerative dermatitis. It often occurs secondary to poor hygiene, abrasive flooring or wire-floored cages. Obese rabbits, giant breeds and Rex rabbits with thin plantar fur pads are predisposed to develop the condition.

Necrotic sores ulcerate, become infected and may lead to osteomyelitis of the underlying metatarsal and tarsal bones. A diagnosis is made on the basis of clinical signs, radiography and bacterial culture and sensitivity. Surgical treatment consists of debridement of necrotic tissue, saline and antiseptic flushing, and application of antibiotic impregnated polymethylmethacrylate beads. Alternatively, the area may be bandaged daily with antibiotic-impregnated dressings. In severe cases of osteomyelitis amputation may be necessary. Systemic antibiotics, NSAIDs and analgesics should be given. The underlying cause should always be addressed.

Neurological disorders of the urogenital system

Urinary incontinence is a common condition in pet rabbits and may have an underlying neurological aetiology. Loss of bladder control can occur secondary to spinal fracture/luxation (UMN or LMN dysfunction) or as a result of central nervous system disease, such as *E. cuniculi* infection (Figure 15.24).

Perineal dermatitis (Figure 15.25) and secondary infection are common sequelae, and treatment involving clipping of hair, topical antiseptic flushing, application of barrier creams, systemic antibiotics and analgesia is indicated. The underlying cause should always be identified.

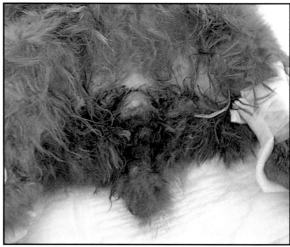

15.25 Severe urine scald secondary to infection with *Encephalitozoon cuniculi.*

Neurological disorders of the gastrointestinal tract

Dysautonomia occurs in rabbits affecting the gastrointestinal tract and is associated with mucoid enteropathy and caecal impaction (see Chapter 12). The condition affects the autonomic nervous system with degeneration of neurons in the autonomic ganglia. There is a resultant loss of parasympathetic and sympathetic function.

Differential diagnosis	Diagnostic tests and factors	Treatment options
Lumbosacral vertebral fracture or dislocation	Neurological examination. Radiography, myelography, MRI, CT	Acute cases: intravenous fluids, oxygen therapy, analgesia and supportive care Chronic cases: supportive care/euthanasia. Intensive nursing (manual bladder expression) and long-term NSAIDs
Encephalitozoon cuniculi	Neurological examination. Concurrent CNS signs. Elevated antibody titres. CT to rule out middle ear disease	See Figure 15.26
Hormone-responsive urinary incontinence	Ovariohysterectomized rabbit. Response to treatments that increase urethral sphincter tone	Estriol (0.5 mg/rabbit q24h) and/or phenylpropanolamine (1.5 mg/kg orally q12h)
Urinary calculi/hypercalciuria	Radiography, ultrasonography. Urinalysis and culture	Fluid therapy. Catheterization and flushing of bladder. Cystotomy. Nephrectomy, depending on size and location of calculus
Ectopic ureter (NB Never described in rabbits)	Bladder contrast studies, excretory urography. Retrograde cystoscopy	Surgical correction indicated
Urinary tract infection	Radiography, ultrasonography. Sterile urine culture (bacterial and fungal) and sensitivity testing. Urine cytology. Full urinalysis	Appropriate systemic antibiotics, NSAIDs, glycosaminoglycans
Neoplasia	Radiography, contrast studies, ultrasonography. Bladder biopsy	Meloxicam at standard dose rates in cases of transitional cell carcinoma may have an apoptotic effect on tumour cells. Surgical resection. Euthanasia

15.24 Differential diagnoses for urinary incontinence in pet rabbits.

Supportive care

Initial therapy and stabilization is essential in cases of neurological disease, prior to performing diagnostic tests. The rabbit should be housed away from potential predators (dogs and cats) to reduce external stressors, and to allow assessment of normal behaviour. Animals presenting with seizures should be treated with either diazepam (0.5–2 mg/kg i.v. or per rectum) or midazolam (0.07–0.22 mg/kg i.v., i.m.) repeated three times in refractory cases.

Affected rabbits are usually anorexic, and supportive care (fluid therapy, analgesia, gastro-intestinal motility drugs, probiotics, vitamins and provision of a high-fibre diet) is indicated. Rabbits tolerate oral fluids and food via syringe well and this will also promote normal gut motility. Commercial high-fibre critical-care diets for rabbits are available. Appetite may be stimulated by the provision of fresh greens such as grass, dandelion leaves, parsley and kale. Provision of analgesia is essential for the debilitated rabbit even if there are no obvious signs of pain, because response to treatment and recovery rate are generally improved.

Prophylactic systemic antibiotic treatment may be instigated pending further diagnostic tests. In cases of head trauma, oxygen administration, intravenous fluid therapy, furosemide (0.7 mg/kg i.v.) and mannitol (0.25–1 g/kg i.v.) may be indicated. If infection with *E. cuniculi* is suspected, treatment with fenbendazole at 20 mg/kg orally q24h for 28 days may be commenced.

Ethical considerations and prognosis

The prognosis should be discussed early on in the initial consultation with the owner for any rabbit presenting with advanced neurological signs. These cases are clinically challenging and definite final diagnosis may not be possible. Financial constraints and lack of availability of advanced diagnostic techniques, such as MRI and CT scanning, should be taken into account. In cases where quality of life or welfare is significantly compromised, euthanasia should always be considered.

Formulary

Figure 15.26 provides a summary of drugs used in treatment of rabbits with neuromuscular disease. The drugs mentioned in this chapter are not authorized for use in rabbits, unless indicated, and the legal implications of this should be borne in mind when prescribing them.

Drug	Dose rate, route and frequency	Comments
Antibiotics active against **Pasteurella**		
Cefalexin	15 mg/kg s.c. q12h	Oral route not recommended in rabbits
Chloramphenicol	25–50 mg/kg orally q8h 30–50 mg/kg s.c., i.m., i.v. q8h	
Enrofloxacin	5–10 mg/kg orally, s.c., i.m. q12h	Irritant drug; muscle necrosis/sterile abscess formation with s.c. or i.m. injection. **Authorized for use in rabbits in the UK**
Tetracycline	50–100 mg/kg orally q8–12h	
Trimethoprim/sulphonamide	15–30 mg/kg orally, s.c., i.m. q12h	Irritant s.c.; causes tissue necrosis
Treatment of **E. cuniculi** *infection*		
Glucocorticoids	Dexamethasone 0.1–0.2 mg/kg s.c. q48h × 3 doses	Reduces granulomatous inflammation. Prednisolone may alleviate clinical signs, but use with extreme care in rabbits, because immunosuppressive. CNS signs treated with glucocorticoids may resolve in 50% of cases
Albendazole	7.5–20 mg/kg orally q24h for 3–14 days	Use in rabbits is experimental, with the long-term side effects unknown. Evidence exists that it is teratogenic and embryotoxic in rabbits, and anecdotal deaths reported in rabbits
Fenbendazole	20 mg/kg orally q24h for 28 days	Fenbendazole reportedly effective in reducing clinical signs in less advanced cases and also in preventing infection in exposed rabbits
Oxibendazole	15–30 mg/kg orally q24h for 30–60 days	
Ophthalmological infections	Albendazole orally (see above) Topical 1% prednisolone acetate drops q12h for 8 weeks 1% atropine drops q12h	Phacoclastic uveitis may be treated medically or in severe cases enucleation may be indicated. Lens removal using phacoemulsification has also been described. Corticosteroid treatment may be necessary postoperatively

15.26 Dose rates of drugs used in treatment of neuromuscular disease. (continues) ▶

Drug	Dose rate, route and frequency	Comments
Anticonvulsants		
Diazepam	0.5–2 mg/kg i.v., per rectum. Repeat 3 times in refractory cases	Control of seizures, circling, rolling
Midazolam	0.07–0.22 mg/kg i.v., i.m. Repeat 3 times in refractory cases	Control of seizures, circling, rolling
Phenobarbital	1–2 mg/kg orally q24h	Control of seizures
Miscellaneous		
Methylprednisolone	30 mg/kg i.v. once	Indicated in spinal trauma within 8 hours of initial insult. **Use is controversial and not advocated by the author**
Furosemide	0.7 mg/kg i.v. once	Used in head trauma to lower intracranial pressure
Mannitol	0.25–1 g/kg slow intravenous infusion over 30-60 minutes	Used in head trauma; reduces brain oedema and increases cerebral blood flow and oxygenation. *Use only in critical or deteriorating animals*
Metoclopramide	0.5 mg/kg orally, s.c. q6–8h	Prevention of nausea secondary to vestibular disease
Prochlorperazine	0.2–0.5 mg/kg orally q8h	Prevention of nausea secondary to vestibular disease
Meclizine	12.5–25 mg/kg orally q8–12h	Anecdotal reports; reduces motion sickness in vestibular disease

15.26 (continued) Dose rates of drugs used in treatment of neuromuscular disease.

References and further reading

Baxter JS (1975) Posterior paralysis in the rabbit. *Journal of Small Animal Practice* **16**, 267–271

Birchard SJ and Sherding RG (1994) *Saunders Manual of Small Animal Practice*. WB Saunders, Philadelphia

Broome RL and Brooks DL (1991) Efficacy of enrofloxacin in the treatment of respiratory pasteurellosis in rabbits. *Laboratory Animal Science* **41**, 572–576

Capello V (2004) Surgical treatment of otitis externa and media in pet rabbits. *Exotic DVM* **6**(3), 15–21

Carpenter JW (2013) *Exotic Animal Formulary, 4th edn.* Elsevier Saunders, Missouri

Chow EP (2011) Surgical management of rabbit ear disease. *Journal of Exotic Pet Medicine* **20**(3), 182–187

Chow EP, Bennett RA and Dustin L (2009) Ventral bulla osteotomy for treatment of otitis media in a rabbit. *Journal of Exotic Pet Medicine* **18**(4), 209–305

Cox JC (1977) Altered immune responsiveness associated with *Encephalitozoon cuniculi* infection in rabbits. *Infection and Immunity* **15**(2), 392–395

Cox JC, Gallichio HA, Pye D and Walden NB (1977) Application of immunofluorescence to the establishment of an *Encephalitozoon cuniculi*-free rabbit colony. *Laboratory Animal Science* **27**(2), 204–209

Cox JC, Hamilton RC and Attwood HD (1979) An investigation of the route and progression of *Encephalitozoon cuniculi* infection in adult rabbits. *Journal of Protozoology* **26**(2), 260–265

Csokai J, Gruber A, Kunzel F, Tichy A and Joachim A (2009a) Encephalitozoonosis in pet rabbits (*Oryctolagus cuniculus*): pathohistological findings in animals with latent infection versus clinical manifestation. *Parasitology Research* **104**, 629–635

Csokai J, Joachim A, Gruber A, *et al.* (2009b) Diagnostic markers for encephalitozoonosis in pet rabbits. *Veterinary Parasitology* **163**(1–2), 18–26

Deeb BJ, DiGiacomo RF, Bernard BL and Silbernagal SM (1990) *Pasteurella multocida* and *Bordetella bronchiseptica* infections in rabbits. *Journal of Clinical Microbiology* **28**, 70–75

Deplazes P, Mathis A, Baumgartner R, Tanner I and Weber R (1996) Immunologic and molecular characteristics of encephalitozoon-like Microsporidia isolated from humans and rabbits indicate that *Encephalitozoon cuniculi* is a zoonotic parasite. *Clinical Infectious Diseases* **22**, 557–559

Dubey JP, Brown CA, Carpenter JL and Moore JJ (1992) Fatal toxoplasmosis in domestic rabbits in the USA. *Veterinary Parasitology* **44**, 305–309

Ewringmann A and Göbel T (1999) Untersuchungen zur Klinik und Therapie der Encephalitozoonose beim Heimtierkaninchen. *Kleintierpraxis* **44**, 357–372

Franssen FFJ, Lumeij JT and van Knapen F (1995) Susceptibility of *Encephalitozoon cuniculi* to several drugs *in vitro*. *Antimicrobial Agents and Chemotherapy* **39**, 1265–1268

Gruber A, Pakozdy, A, Weissenböck H, Csokai J and Kunzel F (2009) A retrospective study of neurological disease in 118 rabbits. *Journal of Comparative Pathology* **140**, 31–37

Hammons JR (1980) Vertebral fracture in a rabbit. Clinical reports. *Modern Veterinary Practice* **61**, 779–780

Harcourt-Brown FM (2002) *Textbook of Rabbit Medicine*. Butterworth-Heinemann, Oxford

Harcourt-Brown FM and Holloway HKR (2003) *Encephalitozoon cuniculi* in pet rabbits. *Veterinary Record* **152**, 427–431

Hendrix CM, DiPinto LN, Cox NR, Sartin EA and Clemons-Chevis CL (1989) Aberrant intracranial myiasis caused by larval Cuterebra migration. *Compendium on Continuing Education for the Practicing Veterinarian* **11**, 550–559

Hughes JM, Thomasson D, Craig PS, *et al.* (2008) *Neospora caninum*: Detection in wild rabbits and investigation of co-infection with *Toxoplasma gondii* by PCR analysis. *Experimental Parasitology* **120**(3), 255–260

Jass A, Matiasek K, Henke J, *et al.* (2008) Analysis of cerebrospinal fluid in healthy rabbits and rabbits with clinically suspected encephalitozoonosis. *Veterinary Record* **162**, 618–622

Jeklova E, Jekl V, Kovarcik K, *et al.* (2010) Usefulness of detection of specific IgM and IgG antibodies for diagnosis of clinical encephalitozoonosis in pet rabbits. *Veterinary Parasitology* **170**, 143–148

Karp BE, Ball NE, Scott CR and Walcoff JB (1999) Rabies in two privately owned domestic rabbits. *Journal of the American Veterinary Medical Association* **215**(12), 1824–1827

Katiyar SK and Edlind TD (1997) In vitro susceptibilities of the AIDS-associated microsporidian *Encephalitozoon intestinalis* to albendazole, its sulfoxide metabolite and 12 additional benzimidazole derivatives. *Antimicrobial Agents and Chemotherapy* **41**, 2729–2732

Keeble EJ (2011) Encephalitozoonosis in rabbits – what we do and don't know. *In Practice* **33**(9), 426–435

Keeble EJ and Shaw DJ (2006) Seroprevalence of antibodies to *Encephalitozoon cuniculi* in domestic rabbits in the United Kingdom. *Veterinary Record* **158**, 539–544

Kotler DP and Orenstein JM (1999) Clinical syndromes associated with microsporidiosis. In: *The Microsporidia and Microsporidiosis*, ed. M Wittner and LM Weiss, pp.285–292. ASM Press, Washington DC

Kunstyr I, Lev L and Naumann S (1986) Humoral antibody response of rabbits to experimental infection with *Encephalitozoon cuniculi. Veterinary Parasitology* **21**, 223–232

Leland MM, Hubbard GB and Dubey JP (1992) Clinical toxoplasmosis in domestic rabbits. *Laboratory Animal Science* **42**(3), 318–319

Manning PJ, Ringler DH and Newcomer CE (1994) *The Biology of the Laboratory Rabbit, 2nd edn.* Academic Press, London

Mathis A, Michel M, Kuster H, *et al.* (1997) Two *Encephalitozoon cuniculi* strains of human origin are infectious to rabbits. *Parasitology* **114**, 29–35

Meredith AL, Cleaveland SC, Brown J, *et al.* (2013) Seroprevalence of *Encephalitozoon cuniculi* in wild rodents, foxes and domestic cats in three sites in the United Kingdom. *Transboundary and Emerging Infectious Diseases* doi:10.1111/tbed.12091

Mortiz C (2004) Reactions in albendazole-treated rabbits. *Exotic DVM* **6**(4), 21–22

Muller K, Fuchs W, Heblinski N, *et al.* (2009) Encephalitis in a rabbit caused by human herpesvirus-1. *Journal of the American Veterinary Medical Association* **235**, 66–69

Owiny JR, Vandewoude S, Painter JT, Norrdin RW and Veeramachaneni DNR (2001) Hip dysplasia in rabbits: association with nest box flooring. *Comparative Medicine* **51**(1), 85–88

Prescott JF and Baggot JD (1993) *Antimicrobial Therapy in Veterinary Medicine.* Iowa State University Press, Ames, IA

Quesenberry KE and Carpenter JW (2004) *Ferrets, Rabbits and Rodents: Clinical Medicine and Surgery, 2nd edn.* WB Saunders, St. Louis

Reusch B, Murray JK, Papasouliotis K and Redrobe SP (2009) Urinary protein:creatinine ratio in rabbits in relation to their serological status to *Encephalitozoon cuniculi. Veterinary Record* **164**, 293–295

Rich G (2010) Clinical update on testing modalities for *Encephalitozoon cuniculi* in clinically sick rabbits. *Journal of Exotic Pet Medicine* **19**(3), 226–230

Ringler DH and Abrams GD (1970) Nutritional muscular dystrophy and neonatal mortality in a rabbit breeding colony. *Journal of the American Veterinary Medical Association* **157**(11), 1928–1934

Roscoe D, Nielsen S, Eaton H and Rousseau J (1975) Chronic plumbism in rabbits: a comparison of three diagnostic tests. *American Journal of Veterinary Research* **36**, 1225–1229

Stiles J, Didier E, Ritchie B, Greenacre C, Willis M and Martin C (1997) *Encephalitozoon cuniculi* in the lens of a rabbit with phacoclastic uveitis: confirmation and treatment. *Veterinary and Comparative Ophthalmology* **7**, 233–238

Suter C, Muller-Doblies UU, Hatt J-M and Deplazes P (2001) Prevention and treatment of *Encephalitozoon cuniculi* infection in rabbits with fenbendazole. *Veterinary Record* **148**, 478–480

Watson GL and Evans MG (1985) Listeriosis in a rabbit. *Veterinary Pathology* **22**, 191–193

Weber R, Deplazes P, Flepp M, *et al.* (1997) Cerebral microsporidiosis due to *Encephalitozoon cuniculi* in a patient with human immunodeficiency virus infection. *New England Journal of Medicine* **336**, 474–478

Weissenbock H, Hainfellner JA, Berger J, Kasper I and Budka H (1997) Naturally occurring herpes simplex encephalitis in a domestic rabbit (*Oryctolagus cuniculus*). *Veterinary Pathology* **34**, 44–47

16

Ophthalmology

Tim Knott

Rabbits are herbivorous crepuscular prey mammals with both terrestrial and airborne predators in the wild. As such, they require large visual fields both horizontally and dorsally, good distance vision, good sensitivity to movement and the ability to detect camouflaged predators. These visual requirements need to be achieved in the low light levels present at their commonest periods of activity, dawn and dusk. Given that much of the night is spent in the total darkness of the warren, their requirement for vision in *very* low levels of light is arguably less than that of surface prey animals. This should be borne in mind both when assessing vision and when counselling the owners of bilaterally blind rabbits, which seem to make the transition to blindness very readily.

Ocular anatomy and vision

The large laterally placed globes provide a near 300-degree lateral visual field and near 180-degree dorsal visual field. The dorsal visual field is enhanced by the dorsally positioned optic nerve head and the dorsoventrally ovoid pupil (Figure 16.1), a useful adaption for identification of airborne predators. A blind spot is present just cranial to the nose where the sensitive vibrissae allow detection of near objects prior to prehension with the cleft upper lip. A larger 60-degree caudal blind spot is also present, which is reduced when the rabbit is standing on its hindlimbs and elevating the ears, perhaps explaining the typical intermittent 'sentinel' posture seen in wild rabbits presumed to be scanning the horizon for predators (Figure 16.2). Rabbits possess a relatively small area of binocular overlap, estimated at some 10–20 degrees.

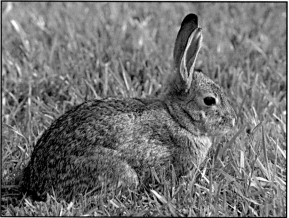

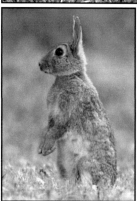

16.2 Repetitive 30-degree lateral movements of the head in the alert standing rabbit can produce a near total hemispherical survey of the environment, and this behaviour can be observed in the wild rabbit in response to auditory or visual stimuli.

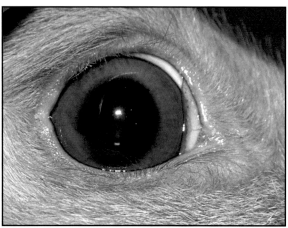

16.1 The rabbit pupil is a vertical ovoid when half dilated; the accompanying arrangement of pupillary muscle fibres allows more rapid and complete dilation than a circular pupillary motor arrangement. The lateral upper eyelashes and the more medial lower eyelashes overlap when the lids close; this may help to protect the eye from dirt during burrowing. Note the pigmented nodules on the leading edge of the third eyelid; these are a normal finding of uncertain significance.

The rabbit globe is foreshortened in the anterior–posterior axis. This is likely to contribute to the somewhat hypermetropic (long-sighted) peripheral vision and the strongly axial myopia (short sightedness) reported by Jekl (2012). This may confer a selective visual advantage, with peripheral vision being useful for the detection of distant predators while central, binocular vision is used for used for identification of conspecifics and food sources.

The close relationship between the retrobulbar venous plexus and the caudal globe means that engorgement of this plexus (due to an increase in mean arterial pressure or decreased venous drainage) leads to posterior pressure on the globe. Physiological engorgement of this plexus can be seen as a stress response in some rabbits, which is likely to shorten the axial length of the globe further, exacerbating the axial myopia, but can also lead to exophthalmos. This may both increase peripheral vision and widen the field of binocular overlap, a potentially useful visual strategy for identification of distant predators (Figure 16.3).

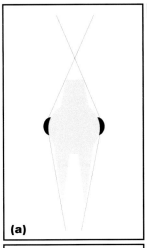
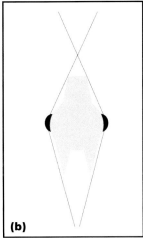
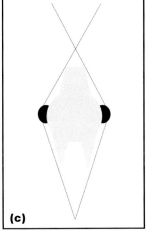

16.3 Lateral visual fields in the rabbit, illustrating the effect of ear elevation **(b)** and exophthalmos **(c)**.

(a)

(b)

(c)

The rabbit's retina has a large, dorsally placed optic nerve head with horizontally radiating myelinated ganglion cells and superficial blood vessels (a merangiotic vascular pattern). This arrangement results in a large horizontal retinal blind spot in the ventral part of the visual field.

The rabbit retina is dominated by rods (estimated at 95% of photoreceptor numbers) and lacks a tapetum lucidum. Rods are particularly sensitive to movement, are maximally stimulated in low light levels and are of great importance in detecting movement, vital for visual detection of predators.

Cones are active in high light levels and have the highest degree of convergence on to the ganglion cells, and thus are essential for visual acuity. The rabbit appears to have dichromatic vision with two separate cone populations: 'blue' cones with a peak sensitivity of 425 nm and green cones with a sensitivity of 520 nm. A horizontal linear cone-rich area present some 5 mm ventral to the optic nerve head is termed the visual streak and represents the area of greatest visual acuity, with both green and blue sensitive cones present, in a ratio of approximately 10:1. Unusually, the rabbit has a second horizontal area of high cone density in the ventral retina adjacent to the ora ciliaris. This second streak of high cone density contains almost exclusively blue sensitive cones and is termed the 'blue streak' (Juliusson *et al.*, 1994). This area of the retina corresponds to the most dorsal part of the rabbit's visual field, i.e. the sky above, and may be an adaption to detect airborne predators in high light levels, as peripheral rods would be rapidly bleached by high ambient light levels in daylight.

The very large crystalline lens has a limited accommodative capacity, estimated at 1.5 dioptres (D) in the adult rabbit (Gwon, 2008). Key features of rabbit ocular anatomy are listed in Figure 16.4.

- Aspherical globe with large cornea (Figure 16.5)
- Very large crystalline lens (Figure 16.6)
- Dorsal rectus muscle visible (Figure 16.7)
- Single large ventral lacrimal punctum
- Multiple retrobulbar glands including a Harderian gland
- Small nictitans: full excursion across the eye is difficult; the placement of third eyelid flaps is technically challenging and is contraindicated when the corneal integrity is uncertain
- Multiple small, often pigmented, nodules on the outer surface of the distal third eyelid are normal, although of uncertain function (see Figure 16.1)
- Floor of orbit contains roots of premolar arcade. Eruption of tooth roots due to dental disease is a major risk factor for retrobulbar abscessation
- Large retrobulbar venous plexus: difficult to ligate, rabbits can exsanguinate very quickly if bleeding occurs
- Merangiotic fundus: large extensively myelinated optic disc with natural pit in centre; retinal vessels radiate medially and laterally
- Normal bacterial conjunctival flora: *Staphlycoccus* spp. most commonly isolated (57% in study by Cooper *et al.*, 2001, compared with only 6% *Pasteurella*)

16.4 Key features of rabbit ocular anatomy.

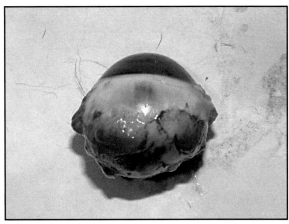

16.5 The globe is aspherical, with an anterior–posterior length some 15% less than the globe diameter. Note the large cornea, which covers approximately 75% of the globe.

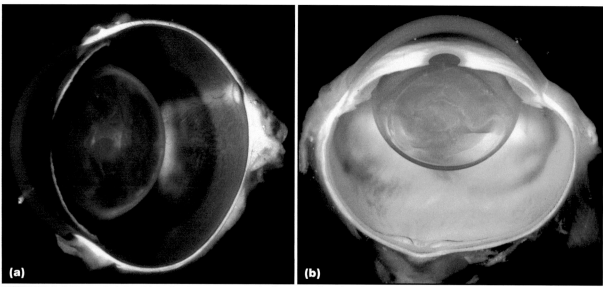

16.6 **(a)** Normal globe. Note the large cornea, shallow anterior chamber, marked anterior bowing of the iris, very large lens (43% of axial lens length), the dorsally located optic nerve head and the adjacent horizontal myelination and superficial retinal vessels. **(b)** Normal albinotic rabbit globe. Note the absence of pigment throughout the uveal tract. (Courtesy of John Mould)

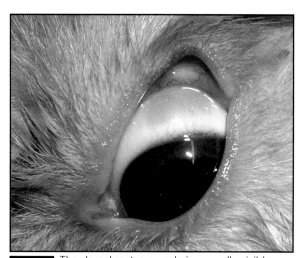

16.7 The dorsal rectus muscle is normally visible through the dorsal bulbar conjunctiva.

Orbital anatomy

The rabbit orbit contains several anatomical peculiarities. The complex orbital anatomy has a direct impact on the function of the eye, both in health and in disease. The normal rabbit globe protrudes significantly past the protective orbital rim, increasing the available field of view (see Figure 16.3) but also increasing the chances of ocular injury.

Orbital glands
The orbit contains large amounts of glandular tissue. Anatomical nomenclature varies but some six separate glandular structures can be identified:

- The superior lacrimal gland is found ventral to the dorsal orbital rim (analogous to the temporal lacrimal gland in dogs, cats and horses)

- The inferior lacrimal gland is found ventral and ventrolateral to the globe, where it extends lateral to the zygomatic arch
- The accessory lacrimal gland is found caudal to the lateral canthal ligament in the temporal foramen
- The bilobed Harderian gland (Figure 16.8) is relatively large and is found ventromedial to the globe. Both lobes are secretory, with the dorsal white lobe producing higher quantities of porphyrins, which are believed to have a pheromone function, and large numbers of plasma cells suggesting an immune function. The ventral pink lobe produces significantly more lipid, which is believed to have a role in maintaining the remarkably stable pre-corneal tear film (Bayraktaroğlu and Ergun, 2010)
- The nictitans gland is found loosely attached to the anterior surface of the proximal nictitans cartilage and is thought to produce aqueous tears
- The infraorbital salivary gland is found in the lateral orbit beneath the anterior part of the zygomatic arch.

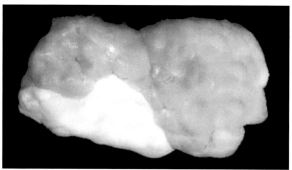

16.8 The bilobed Harderian gland. Both the white and pink lobes produce a mixture of protein, lipid and carbohydrate. The function of the Harderian glands is believed to be complex, including ocular lubrication, pheromone production and immune modulation. (Courtesy of R Dubeilzig)

Orbital vascular plexus

The retrobulbar venous plexus (or orbital sinus) extends from the orbital apex past the globe equator to sit immediately caudal to the peribulbar orbital fascial membrane, just below the conjunctival fornices. Communicating directly with several major orbital veins, some of which drain into the intracranial cavernous sinus, this allows a theoretical route for retrobulbar infection to enter the cranial vault, as well as presenting surgical challenges during orbital surgery in this species.

The orbits are connected by a small (approximately 5 mm) foramen, which allows the potential spread of infection or neoplasia from one side to the other.

Ocular surface

The ocular surface is a continuous epithelial layer consisting of the corneal and conjunctival epithelia. New epithelial cells are produced from stem cells located at the limbus, and the corneal epithelium is completely replaced every 7–10 days. The conjunctival epithelium plays an important role in the production of a healthy tear film and in immune defence of the whole ocular surface.

Corneal thickness is 386 ± 20 μm, reducing by 1–2 μm peripherally (Wang and Wu, 2013), significantly thinner than the corneas of humans, cats and dogs. This is of clinical significance when considering corneal surgery and in the interpretation of intraocular pressure (IOP) measurements obtained using applanation tonometers such as the Tonopen.

Eyelids

The naturally prominent rabbit globe protrudes past the orbital rim and is protected by tightly fitting lids. Both upper and lower eyelids are mobile. Eyelashes are present in both upper and lower lids and are more developed medially on the upper lids and ventrally on the lower lids, allowing the cilia to overlap, which may provide better protection from dirt when digging underground.

Meibomian glands are present on both upper and lower lids and are a common location for pathology. The thin eyelids allow transillumination of the meibomian glands, which can allow the identification of very subtle lesions (Jester *et al.*, 1982).

Ocular examination

Assessment of vision can be challenging in a species that freezes when it perceives threat, and visual assessment is notably easier in 'humanized' house rabbits. The menace response is unreliable, but the dazzle reflex is a very useful baseline test of visual function and potential. Pupillary reflexes are often sluggish and incomplete in the consulting room environment, owing to high catecholamine levels. Obstacle courses are of limited use; blind rabbits are often able to negotiate obstacles, presumably relying on use of their vibrissae. Visual placing reflexes can be of use, as can a visual cliff made from a sheet of glass or Perspex placed on top of low blocks.

Pain assessment

Assessment of ocular pain can be challenging. Signs of pain such as increased blink rate and photo-phobia, reliable in other species, are less so in the rabbit. Blink rate is very low, with recorded rates as low as 1 per 10 minutes (Wei *et al.*, 2013). This low blink rate is matched by a very long fluorescein break-up time, of up to 30 minutes (in contrast to 5–8 seconds in humans), illustrating the remarkable stability of the rabbit tear film. It is postulated that this may be due to the large quantities of lipid produced by the Harderian gland and that the milky appearance of tears sometimes observed in the rabbit is due to high levels of these same lipids. The large lacrimal punctum means that increased lacrimation caused by ocular pain does not always present with epiphora, unless there is concomitant nasolacrimal duct obstruction or wicking of tears from periorbital hair. Quantifying lacrimation using the Schirmer tear test can be a useful method of documenting increased tear production associated with ocular pain, particularly that due to ocular surface disease (Figure 16.9). Chronic ocular pain, e.g. due to glaucoma, may present as poor appetite and behavioural changes. Once again these behavioural changes are most notable in 'humanized' house rabbits that are less prone to concealing signs of chronic pain.

Characteristic	Normal values
Inter-blink interval [a]	10 minutes
Schirmer tear test [b]	5.30 mm/min (± 2.96), range 0–15
Fluorescein break-up time [a]	29.8 ± 3.4 minutes
Corneal thickness	300 μm (axial) to 450 μm (peripheral)
Normal globe measurements: [c, d]	
Axial globe length	17.12 mm (± 0.41 mm)
Globe height	17–18 mm
Globe width	18–20 mm
Anterior chamber depth	2.70 mm (± 0.22 mm)
Aqueous volume	0.25–0.3 ml
Pupil diameter	7 mm (range 5–11 mm)
Axial vitreal chamber length	7.32 mm (± 0.45 mm)
Cornea:	
Corneal diameter: horizontal	13.5–14 mm
Corneal diameter: vertical	15 mm
Corneal radius of curvature	7–7.5 mm

16.9 Normal pre-corneal tear film and corneal parameters. [a] (Wei *et al.*, 2013); [b] (Abrams *et al.*, 1990); [c] (Gwon, 2008); [d] (Toni *et al.*, 2010). (continues) ▶

Characteristic	Normal values
Cornea: continued	
Corneal refractive power (dioptres, D):	
Birth	60 D
30 weeks	50 D
60–80 weeks	40–43 D
Corneal thickness:	
Centre	0.3–0.4 mm
Peripheral	0.45 mm
Lens:	
Axial lens length	7.20 mm (± 0.40 mm)
Lens diameter	11 mm
Anterior radius	5.3 mm
Posterior radius	5 mm
Anterior lens capsule thickness (axial)	30 μm
Posterior lens capsule thickness (axial)	3.4 μm

16.9 (continued) Normal pre-corneal tear film and corneal parameters.

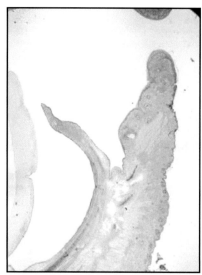

16.10 Normal lower eyelid and nictitating membrane. Note the tight adherence of the anterior nictitans to the lower lid. H&E stain. (Courtesy of R Dubeilzig)

Distant hands-off examination

Distant hands-off examination is important in the assessment of visual responses and signs of ocular pain such as altered blink rate or pattern. The face should be examined straight on, assessing globe and lid position. Normal ear and nares position and movement should be noted to rule out facial paralysis – a commonly missed clinical sign in the rabbit. Ocular and nasal discharge should be assessed at this time.

Note should be taken of globe and third eyelid position by examining the head in a rostral-to-caudal direction. The prominently curved cornea should be visible, as should the leading edge of the third eyelid. Little or no sclera should be visible in the normal rabbit eye and 'scleral show' (visible sclera) is associated with exophthalmos. Similarly, the normal resting position of the nictitans (third eyelid) should be noted because prolapse of this structure is also associated with increased retrobulbar volume, for example caused by retrobulbar abscesses, tumours or vascular engorgement. The rabbit's nictitans is relatively smaller than that of the dog or cat and more tightly adherent to the lower eyelid, resulting in a shallower ventral conjunctival fornix (Figure 16.10). This means that changes in nictitans position are often less obvious in the rabbit.

The globe and third eyelid position should be assessed with the head in the neutral position and then again with the head lowered beneath the level of the heart, when abnormalities affecting venous return (e.g. mediastinal masses) lead to rapid engorgement of the retrobulbar vascular plexi, causing a dynamic exophthalmos (Figure 16.11).

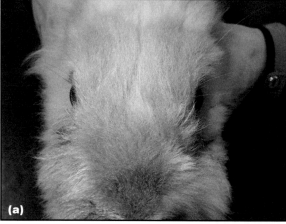

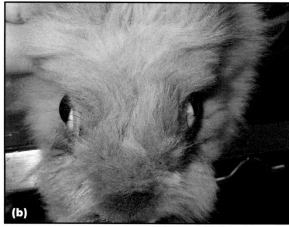

16.11 The position of the globe and third eyelid should be assessed with the head: **(a)** in the neutral position; and **(b)** lowered beneath the level of the heart.

Hands-on examination

Where there are no deep corneal ulcers or suspicion of globe penetration or rupture, gentle palpation of the globes through the closed upper eyelids is useful for assessment of the retrobulbar space (is there resistance to retropulsion?), ocular pain (is there an aversive reaction to palpation?) and, to a lesser degree, intraocular pressure (does the globe feel hard or soft?). In very soft (hypotonous) eyes, observation of the globe during palpation may reveal indentation of the cornea. This should not be attempted deliberately.

Intraoral examination should be performed in all cases of ophthalmic disease, given the common association between dental disease and both orbital and nasolacrimal diseases (see *BSAVA Manual of Rabbit Surgery, Dentistry and Imaging*). Globe retropulsion should be performed gently through the upper lids, assessing globe pressure, ocular pain, ability to retropulse the globe and the third eyelid position. Note that, in contrast to other species, retrobulbar abscessation may not be demonstrably painful in the rabbit and can thus be difficult to differentiate from other orbital space-occupying lesions.

The lid margins should be everted and the caudal margins examined for meibomian gland disease and ectopic cilia. Examination of the single ventral lacrimal punctum is facilitated by everting the lower medial lid to part the mucosal 'lips' of the punctum. The lacrimal sac should be palpated in the medial canthal region and the puncta examined for lacrimal discharge. Ocular and nasal discharge should be sampled using small-tipped bacteriology swabs and submitted for culture and cytological examination.

The conjunctival surfaces should be examined, taking special note of the location of hyperaemia. Lid margin conjunctival hyperaemia is associated with marginal blepharitis, often due to meibomian gland disease. Hyperaemia of the bulbar surface of the globe may indicate intraocular disease. While the marked dilatation of the episcleral vessels associated with glaucoma in the dog (episcleral congestion) is less obvious in the rabbit, 'ciliary flush' (circumcorneal dilatation of conjunctival and episcleral vessels) is often observed in the presence of uveitis. Note that the insertion of the dorsal rectus muscle is clearly visible through the conjunctiva of the dorsal globe and is a normal finding (see Figure 16.7).

The entire cornea should be examined for reflectance (a marker of corneal surface health) and transparency (cellular infiltration and vascularization are best highlighted against the red reflex, the reflected light from the retina). Oblique illumination of the corneal surface is a useful technique for highlighting subtle stromal or endothelial opacities and should be routinely performed. Where anterior corneal opacity is seen, corneal scrapes should be performed and stained using Gram and Giemsa for cell examination.

The globe should be examined systematically from anterior to posterior, first assessing the visual axis for transparency using a light source coaxial with the observer's pupil (e.g. a direct ophthalmoscope set at 0 D). Examination of the peripheral lens and anterior peripheral vitreous for transparency should be performed by directing the examination light oblique to the pupil.

Pupillary dilation with tropicamide allows diagnostic mydriasis. Topical phenylephrine used concurrently can give more rapid dilation, particularly in rabbits with non-pigmented irises. The pigment-dependent mydriatic effect of atropine in the eye is well documented, with irises in albino rabbits remaining dilated for only 96 hours compared with 8–10 days in pigmented eyes. A number of rabbits have a serum atropine esterase which markedly reduces the duration of activity of atropine from 8–10 days to 12 hours (Salazar *et al.*, 1976). This limitation should be borne in mind when using topical atropine to treat anterior uveitis.

Retinal examination can be performed using both direct and indirect ophthalmoscopy with a 20 D lens. Imaging the striking optic nerve head requires an acute dorsal viewing angle. The tapetal retina is variably pigmented, with choroidal vessels being readily seen in most patients (Figure 16.12). Retinal photography can be readily performed in the clinic using smartphone cameras, where the light-emitting diode (LED) is sufficiently close to the lens and can be illuminated continuously (Knott, 2012; www.theeyephone.co.uk).

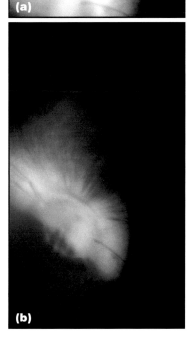

16.12
(a) Normal fundus of a pigmented wild rabbit (*Oryctolagus cuniculus*). Note the visible choroidal vasculature. (Retinal images photographed using iPhone 4S using technique described by Knott, 2012). **(b)** Normal merangiotic optic nerve head with prominent lateral nerve fibre layer and physiological nerve head cupping.

Ophthalmic disease

Ophthalmic disease is both a common cause for presentation to the veterinary surgeon and a common incidental finding at examination. The incidence of ophthalmic disease has been reported at nearly 10% in commercial rabbits: predominant findings are blepharitis followed by cataract and conjunctivitis, with dacryocystitis being found in only 0.2% of affected rabbits (Jeong *et al.*, 2005). This contrasts starkly with the pet rabbit population, where a similar rate of ophthalmic disease (10%) was seen in a study of rabbits presented with eye problems, but 73% of rabbits were diagnosed with dacryocystitis (Florin *et al.*, 2009).

Systemic diseases with ophthalmic involvement

Pasteurellosis ('snuffles')
Commonly presenting as upper respiratory tract (URT) infection (see Chapter 11), *Pasteurella multocida* infection may lead to bacteraemia, causing abscesses (which may involve the retrobulbar space), uveitis, iridal abscesses and endophthalmitis (Kern, 1997; Harcourt-Brown, 2002) The intraocular signs of pasteurellosis can be difficult to differentiate from other causes of uveitis and endophthalmitis such as other septicaemic disease (e.g. staphylococcal disease), phacoclastic uveitis and uveal lymphosarcoma. These intraocular signs may be seen during the recovery phase from the acute URT infection or concomitantly.

Diagnosis can be challenging, and while culture and cytology demonstrating short Gram-negative rods is diagnostic, obtaining appropriate samples can be difficult. Samples of aqueous and, if involved, vitreous from enucleated eyes should be taken where endophthalmitis is suspected. Aspiration of iridal abscess material from enucleated eyes for cytology and culture or histology may be required to obtain a definitive diagnosis. Serology may be of some use; however, it is an indicator of exposure rather than acute infection. Culture of aqueous humour samples is unlikely be diagnostic where iris abscesses have formed and aspiration of iridal abscesses is not recommended.

Treatment of all in-contact animals may limit the spread of disease. Culling should be considered where appropriate. Various antibiotics are effective, e.g. enrofloxacin, cephalosporins, ampicillin, gentamicin and possibly tetracyclines.

Encephalitozoon cuniculi infection
See Diseases of the uveal tract and lens.

Myxomatosis
See Eyelid disease.

Neuro-ophthalmological disease

Facial paralysis
Facial paralysis is the commonest neuro-ophthalmic disease seen in rabbits in the author's clinic. The lateral globe placement and low blink rate of the rabbit mean that it can easily be overlooked if the patient is not examined from a distance for facial symmetry and blink reflexes are not specifically tested in all patients. The facial nerve can be damaged as it traverses the lateral zygomatic arch following trauma such as dog bites to the head (Figure 16.13) or road traffic accidents, and more commonly as it passes through the middle ear. Chronic cases may develop ipsilateral facial contracture resulting in the contralateral side appearing to droop.

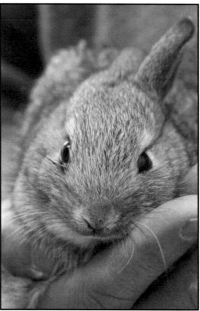

16.13 Wild rabbit (*Oryctolagus cuniculus*) with right-sided facial paralysis following peripheral facial trauma (dog bite). Note the obvious change in ear carriage but the normal palpebral aperture and very subtle position change of the right-sided naris. No blink could be induced by touching the medial or lateral canthus (negative palpebral reflex) and the right naris was paralysed.

The inherently stable rabbit tear film means that not all cases lead to keratitis; however, exposure keratitis may ensue with chronicity. Where keratitis is very severe it is important to rule out concomitant sensory denervation of the cornea (see Trigeminal paralysis). Treatment is aimed at identifying and correcting the underlying cause, supporting the cornea with topical lubrication and in severe cases partial tarsorrhaphy.

Horner's syndrome
Horner's syndrome is caused by interruption in the sympathetic supply to the eye. A three-neuron pathway originates in the hindbrain, passing down the spinal cord to exit in the cranial thoracic spine, then via the mediastinum and the ventral cervical region to synapse with the third neuron in the chain in the cranial cervical ganglion, prior to passing through the middle ear and the retrobulbar space before entering the eye. Damage at any point in the pathway results in clinical signs, and the prognosis will depend on the cause of the damage. The most obvious clinical signs of Horner's syndrome in the rabbit are miosis and

conjunctival hyperaemia due to vasodilatation; ptosis and third eyelid protrusion are less apparent. Middle ear disease appears to be the commonest cause of Horner's syndrome in the rabbit.

Localization of the Horner's syndrome lesion to either proximal ('preganglionic') or distal ('postganglionic') to the cranial cervical ganglion is the first diagnostic step (Skarf and Czarnecki, 1982). This should be performed by assessment of the response of the clinical signs to topically administered phenylephrine (pharmacological localization). Advanced imaging techniques may be required to locate the site of damage.

Trigeminal paralysis

Trigeminal nerve damage results in denervation of the ocular surface and facial skin. Partial lesions are common and are consistent with peripheral damage. Loss of ocular surface sensation results in a rapid onset of severe keratitis ('neurotropic keratopathy'). Assessment of corneal sensation should be performed by evaluating the response to a fine wisp of sterile cotton wool stroked across the corneal surface: the corneal reflex. It should be noted that false-negative results may be seen in rabbits in the clinical setting, owing to heightened stress levels.

Nystagmus

Nystagmus, usually accompanied by head tilt, is a common presenting sign in the rabbit. Differentiation between peripheral and central patterns of nystagmus should be attempted at an early stage; however it is not possible to differentiate central from peripheral vestibular signs reliably in all rabbits (see Chapter 15).

Neurogenic dry eye

Experimental preganglionic parasympathetic denervation of the lacrimal gland in rabbits results in a profound sudden-onset dry eye. While no published case reports exist to the author's knowledge, it is expected that pathological damage to this pathway, e.g. due to middle ear disease, may lead to neurogenic keratoconjunctivitis sicca (KCS). Tear production should be assessed in all cases of suspected cranial nerve and middle ear disease. Treatment of the underlying pathology (e.g. otitis) is important. The use of parasympathomimetics (pilocarpine) is palliative in canine patients and may be of use in rabbits.

Orbital disease

Exophthalmos

Exophthalmos (globe protrusion) should be differentiated from globe enlargement (hydrophthalmos, buphthalmos). Ultrasonography is a useful method for measuring globe diameter although interpretation of images of the retrobulbar space can be challenging unless fluid-filled structures are present. The presence of scleral show can help to differentiate exophthalmos from buphthalmos. Retrobulbar space-occupying lesions readily lead to protrusion of the globe and increased scleral exposure, initially in the same quadrant as the position of the space-occupying lesion (Figure 16.14), while the sclera

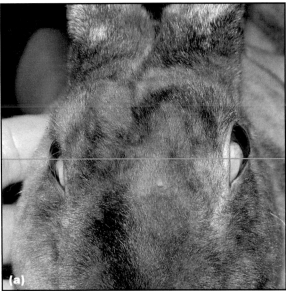

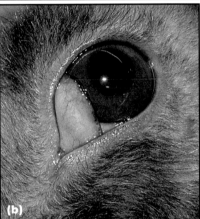

16.14 Retrobulbar abscess in the left eye. **(a)** Drawing a line between the pupils illustrates the marked dorsal displacement of the globe. **(b)** Note partial third eye lid prolapse caused by a retrobulbar mass and the ventromedial scleral show caused by dorsolateral displacement of the globe, localizing the mass to the ventromedial orbit.

only becomes visible in very severe cases of buphthalmos when it is usually seen circumferentially (Figure 16.15). The position of the third eyelid remains normal in buphthalmos but it becomes prolapsed when extraconal (outside the muscle cone) retrobulbar masses are present.

Masses inside the muscle cone (intraconal) are unusual in the rabbit and would present with increased scleral show and normal third eyelid position. Retrobulbar abscessation is the commonest cause of exophthalmos in the rabbit; other differentials are listed in Figure 16.16. Retrobulbar infection is usually differentiated from neoplasia in other species by being painful and rapid in onset whereas neoplasia is often slowly progressive and well tolerated. However in the rabbit this differentiation is not clear with many cases of retrobulbar abscessation growing slowly while the rabbit retains normal appetite. Globe position should be assessed and deviation of the globe may help in localizing orbital lesions.

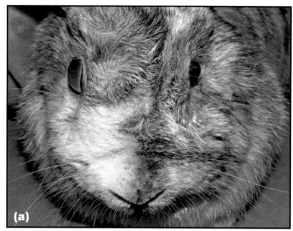

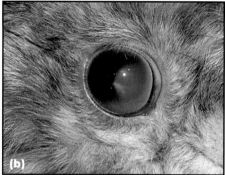

16.15 **(a)** Glaucoma causing marked globe enlargement (buphthalmos) in the right eye. **(b)** Note the absence of nictitans prolapse and the circumferential visible sclera.

- Retrobulbar abscess:
  - Dental disease
  - Pasteurellosis
- Idiopathic retrobulbar adenitis (Knott, 2003)
- Neoplasia (lymphosarcoma) (Wagner and Fehr, 2007)
- Tapeworm cyst (O'Reilly, 2002)
- Congestion of retrobulbar venous sinus:
  - Physiological
  - Mediastinal mass e.g. thymic lymphoma or adenocarcinoma
  - Vascular anomaly

16.16 Causes of exophthalmos.

Retrobulbar abscessation

Retrobulbar abscesses are a common cause of unilateral exophthalmos in the rabbit. Although progression to bilateral involvement is possible because of the potential connection between the two orbital spaces in the rabbit, it is uncommon. Underlying dental disease is a common primary cause, with eruption of molar roots through the base of the orbit secondary to apical dental abscesses and maxillary osteomyelitis. In contrast to dogs and cats, rabbits generally show a slowly progressive and apparently comfortable exophthalmos. Resistance to globe retropulsion is often marked, with flattening of the globe often readily demonstrable on ocular ultrasonography.

The inspissated nature of rabbit pus makes drainage challenging in this species. Drainage is sometimes possible caudal to the zygomatic arch, but care is needed to avoid the auriculopalpebral branch of

the facial nerve as it runs over the arch. Flushing and topical antibiotics, combined with systemic antibiotics and non-steroidal anti-inflammatory drugs (NSAIDs) occasionally bring remission. Systemic antibiotics and NSAIDs on their own may bring temporary improvement and can be a useful approach to management in older rabbits or those with a short life expectancy owing to severe dental disease.

However, most cases require enucleation and orbital exenteration (see below) if the severity of the underlying dental disease does not necessitate euthanasia; therefore, radiographic or computed tomography (CT) evaluation of the skull and teeth is very important. Given that some abscesses yield no bacteria on culture, cytological examination with Gram staining should be performed alongside culture of the abscess cavity. In a review of cases of maxillary and mandibular dental-associated abscesses, bacterial isolates included anaerobic Gram-negative rods (particularly *Fusobacterium nucleatum*), anaerobic Gram-positive spore-forming rods (especially *Actinomyces* spp.) and aerobic cocci, particularly from the *Streptococcus milleri* group, but not *Pasteurella multocida* (Tyrrell *et al.*, 2002).

Idiopathic retrobulbar adenitis

Bilateral exophthalmos not associated with retrobulbar infection, neoplasia or vascular changes is occasionally seen and may be caused by inflammation of the retrobulbar glandular tissue, of uncertain aetiology. Concurrent dental disease and neoplasia should be ruled out where possible. Cases are sporadic and appear to respond when treated with systemic NSAIDs and broad-spectrum antibiotics, although recurrence may be seen (Knott, 2003). These cases often present with a fluctuating, bilateral, non-painful exophthalmos (Figure 16.17). Ultrasonography shows multilobulated retrobulbar masses.

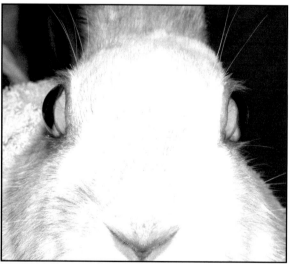

16.17 Presumed retrobulbar adenitis. This rabbit was clinically well, with no evidence of dental disease, but presented with sudden-onset bilateral exophthalmos. Bilateral multilobular masses were identified on ocular ultrasonography. Resolution with no recurrence was seen following 7 days' treatment with systemic meloxicam and enrofloxacin.

Retrobulbar neoplasia

As a consequence of the potential connection between the orbital spaces in the rabbit, slow-growing retrobulbar masses may present as bilateral exophthalmos. Retrobulbar neoplasia is rare, with malignant lymphosarcoma being the commonest tumour at this site. A single case of lymphoma of the Harderian gland has been reported which presented as unilateral exophthalmos (Volopich *et al.*, 2005).

Vascular exophthalmos

Enlargement or engorgement of the retrobulbar vascular plexus can result in marked exophthalmos in the rabbit (Figure 16.18). Physiological engorgement is seen as a stress response in some rabbits and

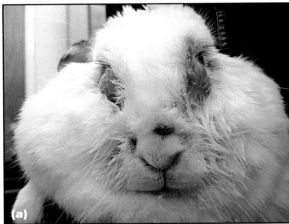
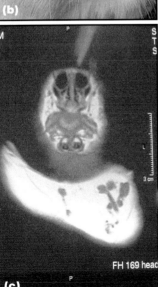

16.18 **(a)** Chronic bilateral vascular exophthalmos due to abnormal venous drainage. **(b)** Engorged vessels visible subconjunctivally caudal to the prolapsed third eyelid. **(c)** Magnetic resonance image: transverse slice showing bizarre vascular pattern in dewlap. These vessels were contiguous with the vena cava; congenital or post-traumatic lesions were suspected. (Images courtesy of Kevin Eatwell)

may have a role in altering the visual fields and focal ability. Any lesion causing chronic or intermittent obstruction of the vena cava may lead to vascular engorgement of this plexus. Mediastinal mass lesions are the commonest cause. Congenital, post-traumatic or post-inflammatory changes may lead to vascular abnormalities, which can lead to chronic or stress-exacerbated vascular engorgement.

Surgical treatment options for orbital disease

Enucleation: Orbital surgery carries a high risk of haemorrhage which can be difficult to control owing to the large retrobulbar venous plexus. This is very difficult to ligate and patients can exsanguinate quickly. For this reason the transconjunctival approach is recommended because it allows the surgeon to remain closer to the sclera, reducing the risk of bleeding and allowing more of the orbital contents to be retained. (For further details of ocular surgery see the *BSAVA Manual of Rabbit Surgery, Dentistry and Imaging*). Should orbital haemorrhage occur, the head should be elevated above the level of the heart and tamponade applied using swabs to stem the orbital bleeding prior to three-layer closure of the socket. The use of silicone orbital implants can aid in the control of orbital haemorrhage if continued bleeding is seen.

Evisceration: Evisceration and intraorbital silicone implant placement (Figure 16.19) can be safely performed in the rabbit and carries a reduced risk

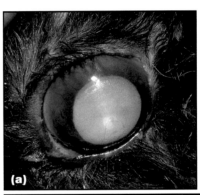
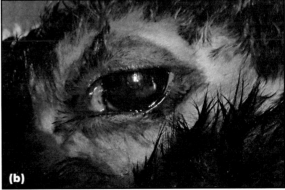

16.19 **(a)** Mature cataract and glaucoma (IOP 84 mmHg) prior to evisceration. Note the circumferential scleral show and normal nictitans position. **(b)** Intrascleral silicone implant placed following removal of all globe contents (evisceration) via a dorsolateral scleral incision parallel to the limbus; immediate postoperative photo.

of intraoperative haemorrhage. This is a technically challenging procedure which leaves the ocular surface intact and at risk of chronic and recurrent corneal disease. Usually reserved for cases of bilateral enucleation due to glaucoma, it is contraindicated where infection or neoplasia are suspected and should be considered a specialist surgical procedure.

Orbital exenteration for the treatment of retrobulbar abscessation: Where retrobulbar abscessation is present or suspected, greater care should be taken with dissection because the orbital anatomy is often abnormal, with orbital vascular structures displaced rostrally. Once the globe has been removed the abscess can be better visualized and an attempt made to resect it *en bloc*. Retrobulbar abscesses in the rabbit do not always form a discrete capsule, despite the usual chronicity of the disease, and thus surgical excision without contamination of the orbit is challenging. It is common to find connection with abnormal maxillary bone on the floor of the orbit, associated with periapical dental abscessation and rupture of the subalveolar bone into the orbit. This area should be curetted, flushed, sampled (for Gram stain and culture), and removal of any suspect loose molars should be attempted orally by levering them out with curved mosquito forceps or rabbit molar extractors. Preoperative plain radiography is helpful to confirm generalized dental disease but, in the author's experience, is rarely useful in identifying the specific tooth or teeth involved. CT of the skull may prove to be of more use in these cases.

Careful examination of the ventral orbit while putting gentle oral pressure on the caudal maxillary molar teeth may identify apical abscesses and the roots of cheek teeth that have erupted into the orbital space. Oral, and occasionally orbital, extraction of the affected teeth appears to improve the long-term prognosis in these cases. Thorough flushing of the orbital cavity with dilute iodine (1% in normal saline) or metronidazole (1%) prior to closure, and postoperative systemic antibiosis with an appropriate antibiotic, is recommended. Topical application of antibiotics to the abscess cavity prior to wound closure appears to be well tolerated, and given the difficulties in obtaining a margin of normal tissue, appears to reduce the risk of recurrence. Methylmethacrylate beads impregnated with enrofloxacin, gentamicin or clindamycin have been widely used and appear to be well tolerated.

Appropriate postoperative systemic antibiotics, selected on the basis of culture, should be continued for at least 10–14 days. Long-term systemic antibiosis given continuously or as pulse therapy may be required in recurrent cases.

Surgical orbitotomy: A dorsal approach to the orbit that potentially allows surgical exploration of the dorsal orbital space has been described, and may provide a safe route for enucleation especially when orbital floor abscesses are present (Li *et al.*, 2009).

Lacrimal and nasolacrimal disease

Epiphora

Epiphora may be caused by increased tear production due to ocular pain or to abnormal drainage of tears. Normal tear drainage requires normal lid anatomy, normal location, size and patency of the lacrimal puncta and a patent lacrimal duct of the correct size. Assessment of tear production using the Schirmer tear test can help to confirm increased tear production and is consistent with ocular pain, particularly ocular surface pain.

Assessment of tear drainage can be made using topical fluorescein. In the normal eye, fluorescein collects in the meniscal tear film layer between the lower eyelid and the ventral cornea (the 'lacrimal lake'); it should not spill on to the eyelid skin and should appear at the nose within 2–5 minutes. Where nasolacrimal obstruction or increased tear production is present, fluorescein is often seen to spill out of the lacrimal sac and to run down the medial canthal area. Where fluorescein is seen to spill along the whole length of the lid, an abnormal relationship between the globe and eyelids should be suspected. Common examples include: entropion, where the lid hairs wick fluorescein on to the lid skin; ectropion, where stain collects in a conjunctival pocket tending to overflow on to the central lid skin; buphthalmia and exophthalmia, where the angle between cornea and lower lid is altered sufficiently to allow the lacrimal lake to spill on to the lid margin.

Differential diagnoses for ocular pain in the rabbit include:

- Conjunctivitis
- Dacryocystitis
- Ulcerative keratitis
- Conjunctival or corneal foreign body
- Acute uveitis
- Acute glaucoma.

Dacryocystitis

Dacryocystitis is arguably the most important ophthalmic disease in the pet rabbit, owing to both its incidence and its association with chronic dental disease. Disease incidence has been reported as 7% of rabbits presenting to a university clinic (Burling *et al.*, 1991); this is likely to approximate to the incidence in most general practice populations.

Obstruction of the lacrimal duct by foreign material, inflammation (e.g. conjunctivitis) or distal duct narrowing (e.g. associated with dental disease) will lead to pooling of tears in the lacrimal sac and reduced drainage of IgA-rich secretion into the duct system, and is likely to predispose the entire lacrimal duct to chronic or recurrent bacterial infection.

Chronic lacrimal sac infection results in thickening of the mucosa which may exacerbate drainage from the lacrimal sac contributing to the challenges in treatment of chronic dacryocystitis. Chronic dacryocystitis leads to thickening of the distal duct mucosa and further narrowing of the duct.

Acute dacryocystitis: Conjunctivitis or blepharo-conjunctivitis (e.g. in myxomatosis) may lead to temporary obstruction of the lacrimal sac and inflammation of the sac wall. This reduces transit of tears and predisposes to the development of dacryocystitis. Secondary dacryocystitis should be suspected if there is a poor response to medical treatment of conjunctivitis.

Chronic dacryocystitis: Chronic dacryocystitis may develop following primary bacterial infection of the nasolacrimal duct; however it is more commonly due to lacrimal duct stenosis or obstruction associated with periductal osteomyelitis or apical dental disease, as a result of the close association of the duct with the tooth roots and its passage through the lacrimal and maxillary bones. The clinical signs include:

* Epiphora
* Conjunctivitis
* Variable purulent ocular discharge
* Variable pain on palpation of the lacrimal sac at the medial canthus
* Purulent material expressed from lacrimal puncta on palpation of the lacrimal sac region. In severe cases large quantities (≥1–2 ml) may be expressed (Figure 16.20)

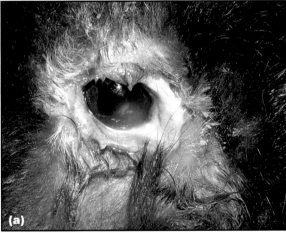

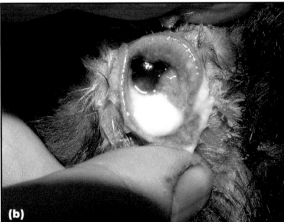

16.20 **(a)** Dacryocystitis with secondary blepharoconjunctivitis. **(b)** Dacryocystitis: massaging pus from the lacrimal sac.

* Secondary blepharitis
* Loss of hair (depilation) overlying the lacrimal sac
* Excoriation of medial canthal region in severe cases
* Nasolacrimal duct obstruction
* Stenosis or cicatricial closure of the lacrimal puncta in severe cases
* The nasolacrimal flush ranges from a milky appearance (due to inflammatory cells) to clots of purulent material and, in severe cases, blood.

Diagnostic work-up:

* Early assessment of concomitant dental disease is important in order to make early decisions regarding the likely long-term prognosis.
* Palpate the ventral border of the mandible for erupted molar roots; check the quality of incisor enamel; examine the oral surface of the molars; move the jaws laterally feeling for a smooth movement; and directly examine the molar arcades.
* A full ophthalmic examination should be performed to rule out predisposing or coexisting disease.
* Massage of the lacrimal sac should be performed to detect lacrimal sacculitis.
* Nasolacrimal flushing (see Chapter 7) should be attempted.
* Samples for Gram staining and culture should be taken from both the lacrimal sac and nasal discharge following flushing.
* Where dental disease is evident, early skull radiography should be considered to assess severity.
* Dilatation of the duct at the natural stenosis at the base of the incisors is not always associated with overt dental disease.
  Dacryocystorhinography is a simple and effective technique for demonstrating narrowing and associated dilatations in the lacrimal duct: 0.5–1 ml of an iodine-based contrast medium is used to fill the ducts after flushing. If the disease is unilateral, perform the technique on the affected side first because the lateral view may be confused by overlying ducts. Both dorsoventral and oblique views are useful.
* In cases refractory to treatment contrast radiography (dacryocystography) should be performed at an early stage to assess prognosis.
* Where available, contrast computed tomographic dacryocystography (CCTD; Figure 16.21) is the gold standard for assessing both the duct and dental and skull anatomy, and is indicated early in the disease process.

Treatment:

* Ensure adequate analgesia.
* Deliver appropriate antibiotics (on the basis of Gram staining and ideally culture and sensitivity testing) to the conjunctiva, the lacrimal sac, the lacrimal duct lumen and surrounding tissues. A

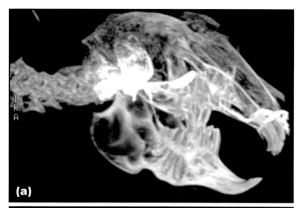

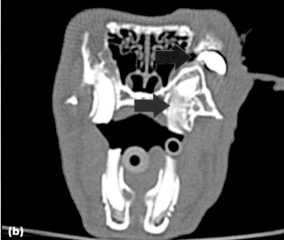

16.21 **(a)** Contrast computed tomographic dacryocystogram. (Courtesy of Vim Katarunga) **(b)** Cross-sectional CT view of the head, showing overgrowth of all the molar tooth roots, particularly the right maxillary molar teeth (blue arrow). Disruption of the tooth-root architecture and mild osteolytic changes the bony tooth sockets are seen. Proximity of the nasolacrimal duct (seen as a pool of bright white contrast material) to the maxillary, molar tooth roots can be appreciated (purple arrow).

combination approach of systemic antibiotics and instillation directly into the duct is advised. Where Gram-positive infections are present, fusidic acid is a good choice for duct instillation because it penetrates pus and inflamed tissue rapidly. Where Gram-negative bacteria or mixed infections are present, instillation of ofloxacin appears well tolerated. Gentamicin should be used with caution in this way owing its epitheliotoxic nature. Injectable enrofloxacin should not be instilled into the duct because of its alkalinity.
- Treat any conjunctivitis with appropriate topical antibiotics, ocular hygiene and in severe cases topical dexamethasone. Combination antibiotic/steroid products (e.g. Maxitrol, Alcon) may be used with care initially; prolonged treatment is not advised owing to the risk of ulcerative keratitis in these cases.
- Support the ocular surface: chronic secondary conjunctivitis often causes tear film changes which will compromise corneal health. Maintain ocular hygiene (regular cleaning of the periorbital area and conjunctival sac with ocular cleaner) and corneal lubrication.

- Treat lacrimal sacculitis with back-flushing of the sac to remove accumulated debris, appropriate antibiotics and systemic non-steroidal agents. Severe cases may benefit from topical and instilled steroids; dexamethasone is recommended owing to its reduced systemic absorption compared with prednisolone.
- Treat lacrimal duct infection.
- Re-establish duct patency by performing nasolacrimal duct lavage. Surgical dacryo-buccostomy, involving trephination through the hard palate to connect the dilated duct at the base of the incisors to the oral cavity, has been performed successfully by the author in refractory cases (Knott, 2003). This should be considered a high-risk procedure owing to the proximity of the greater palatine artery to the stoma site. Surgical removal of the incisors has been suggested as a method of reducing the narrowing of the duct at the incisor base and improving lacrimal duct drainage. This technique has been unsuccessful in the author's hands.
- Physically remove nasolacrimal duct debris by thorough and regular flushing as often as tolerated.
- Address underlying confounding factors – specifically dental disease and maxillary osteomyelitis.

Prognosis: Permanent duct changes in chronic disease mean that control of symptoms, rather than cure, is often the aim. Occasional spontaneous or iatrogenic rupture of the lacrimal duct into the nasal cavity occurs, leading to secondary rhinitis and, rarely, resolution of signs, presumably due to the formation of a dacryonasal fistula. Severe cases may warrant euthanasia.

Prolapse of the deep gland of the orbit
Spontaneous prolapse of the deep gland of the orbit (PDOG, 'cherry eye') is an uncommon condition in the rabbit. Cases usually present unilaterally with no history of antecedent trauma and are often, but not always, apparently comfortable. The deep gland prolapses through the circumferential orbital fascia (the orbital ligament) which separates the base of the conjunctival fornices from the retrobulbar space. The prolapsed tissue is found caudal to the nictitans subconjunctivally and often results in eversion of the third eyelid cartilage (Figure 16.22). The aetiology is uncertain and in many cases it is likely to be idiopathic; however, trauma to the orbital fascia following blunt ocular trauma may be a contributing factor.

PDOG should be differentiated from orbital space-occupying lesions such as vascular distension (see Figure 16.18b), orbital neoplasia or abscess formation. Prolapse leads to excessive conjunctival exposure and secondary conjunctivitis, justifying surgical repair in most cases. The gland can be returned to the normal retrobulbar position using the modified pocket technique described for treatment of prolapse of the nictitans gland in the dog (Morgan *et al.*, 1993). Magnification, appropriate microsurgical instrumentation and absorbable

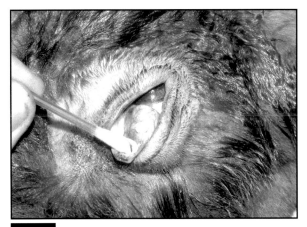

16.22 Prolapse of the deep gland of the orbit.

multifilament polyglycolic acid suture no larger than 0.7 metric (6/0 USP) on a 9 mm ($^3/_8$ inch) curved reverse cutting needle are recommended. Two curved conjunctival incisions are made 2–3 mm from each side of the prolapsed gland, parallel to the nictitans margin. The suture should be secured on the outer surface of the nictitans prior to passing the suture through the third eyelid to exit within one of the wounds. A two-layer continuous subconjunctival suture pattern should be used, ensuring that no suture is visible in the conjunctival wound. Owing to the vascular nature of the deep gland of the orbit and the presence of the orbital vascular plexus, surgical procedures that involve tacking the prolapsed tissue to the orbital rim are strongly discouraged.

Eyelid disease

Marginal blepharitis
The thin eyelid skin of the rabbit predisposes it to the development of marginal blepharitis and this is therefore a common sequel to conjunctivitis or blepharitis regardless of the cause. Inflammation of the thin lid margin often leads to a striking folded appearance (Figure 16.23a) which usually resolves once the underlying inflammation settles down. Chronic marginal blepharitis may result in scarring of the lid margin and cicatrization (Figure 16.23b).

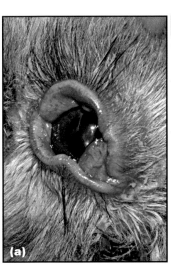

16.23

(a) Acute marginal blepharitis. There is marginal lid folding, in this case secondary to blepharoconjunctivitis. Dacryocystitis was the underlying pathology in this dwarf-breed rabbit. (continues)

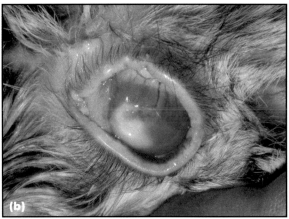

16.23 (continued) **(b)** Chronic marginal blepharitis in a case of long-standing corneal abscessation. Note the multiple lid margin folds; these remained after the corneal disease had been treated successfully.

Chalazion formation
Any chronic ocular surface inflammatory condition runs the risk of affecting the epithelial lining of the meibomian glands, resulting in cystic meibomian gland changes and the formation of lipid granulomas or chalazia (Figure 16.24). Chalazia are also a common incidental finding in rabbits and should be treated by curettage if any deformation of the lid contour or corneal change is present. Eversion of

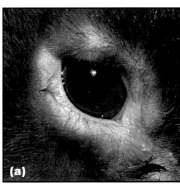

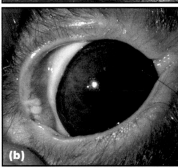

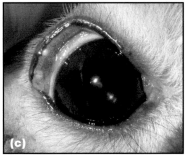

16.24

(a,b) Incidental finding of chalazia in a rabbit with active chronic dacryocystitis. The lid swelling can be seen in the upper lateral lid. Everting the lid is an important part of the examination and reveals the grossly abnormal meibomian glands laterally. **(c)** Multiple chalazia identified incidentally in another rabbit following a history of dacryocystitis.

the eyelids should be performed as a routine part of the ophthalmic examination in the rabbit. A solitary chalazion in the absence of overt conjunctival or lid swelling or inflammation is a common finding but this rarely requires treatment.

Bacterial blepharitis

The thin rabbit eyelid skin readily develops secondary bacterial blepharitis in cases of chronic ocular infection, e.g. dacryocystitis. Subclinical myxomatosis should be excluded early by checking for other compatible nasal or genital lesions. Eyelid margin involvement readily leads to the development of an undulating lid margin, and secondary entropion is not uncommon. Identification of the underlying cause and treatment with systemic antibiotics, NSAIDs, topical lubrication and topical antibiotics is required. Staphylococcal infection appears to be most common, making fusidic acid a useful topical medication; however, application should be no more than twice daily owing to the irritant nature of the drug. Prolonged treatment is often required.

Myxomatosis

Affected rabbits present with severe blepharoconjunctivitis (Figure 16.25), depression, pyrexia, and oedematous and ulcerative lesions of the lids, lips and genitalia. The eyelids are a common site for myxoma formation in rabbits vaccinated against myxomatosis but presumed to have been exposed (Figure 16.26). Other sites include the genitalia, ear

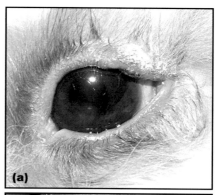
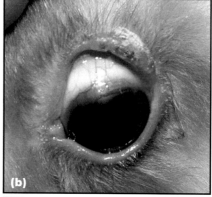

16.26 (a) Eyelid margin myxoma in a vaccinated rabbit. (b) Note the dorsal keratitis present. This lesion resolved uneventfully, the keratitis was treated with ocular lubricants and a full recovery was seen.

and nares (Figure 16.27). Myxoma lesions usually slough after 6–8 weeks, although surgical removal may be indicated should secondary ocular effects be seen, such as notable keratitis. Some cases can develop necrotic crusting lesions which also tend to resolve with symptomatic treatment (see Chapter 17).

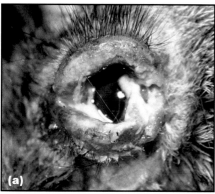
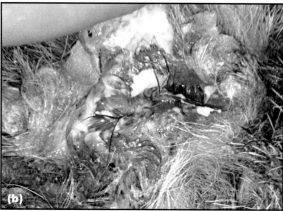

16.25 Acute myxomatosis. (a) Ulcerative, oedematous blepharitis with markedly purulent conjunctivitis in a wild rabbit. Ulcerative keratitis is a common sequel. (b) Severe ulcerative blepharitis and a secondary bacterial keratoconjunctivitis in a domestic rabbit.

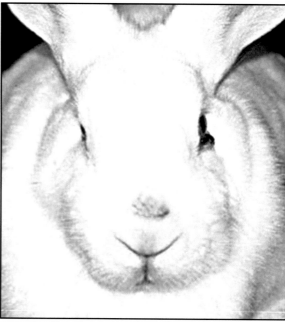

16.27 Chronic myxoma formation on the eyelid and nose of a vaccinated rabbit. Both lesions sloughed and the rabbit made an uneventful recovery. (Courtesy of David Nutbrown-Hughes) (continues) ▶

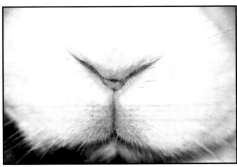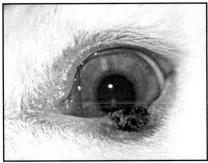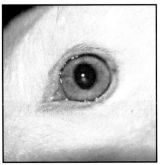

16.27 (continued) Chronic myxoma formation on the eyelid and nose of a vaccinated rabbit. Both lesions sloughed and the rabbit made an uneventful recovery. (Courtesy of David Nutbrown-Hughes)

Ringworm

Trichophyton spp. infections are often asymptomatic and do not fluoresce. *Microsporum canis* fluoresces under ultraviolet light and more commonly causes disease, presenting with alopecia and scaling of lids, nose, ears and paws. Hair plucks for microscopic examination and fungal culture are useful. Treatment with topical medication should be undertaken with care to minimize corneal exposure. Topical antifungals should be used with care around the eye; oral antifungals are preferred when the eyelids are involved.

Syphilis

Rabbit syphilis is caused by the venereally transmitted spirochaete *Treponema paraluis cuniculi.* Neonates may become infected at birth from infected dams. Infection causes genital and facial papular crusting and in some cases ulcerative lesions which may involve the eyelids (treponemal blepharitis; Figure 16.28). Treatment involves weekly injections of high-dose penicillin (40,000 IU, with caution to avoid gastrointestinal side effects), tetracycline or chloramphenicol (see Chapter 17).

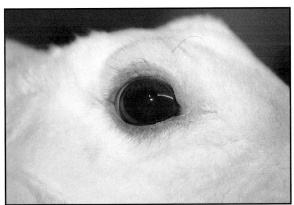

16.28 *Treponema paraluis cuniculi* blepharitis in a domestic rabbit. Crusting skin lesions were present on the nares, pinna, feet and vulval regions. Lesions often become more extensive and ulcerative.

Note the similarity in clinical signs seen with myxomatosis, ringworm and syphilis. A poor response to treatment of blepharitis in the rabbit is an indication for skin biopsy; whereas cytology, hair plucks and ultraviolet lamp examination should be considered early in the presentation.

Combined entropion–ectropion

This condition is analogous to the 'diamond eye' syndrome seen in large-breed dogs and is caused by a relative lid overlength and an overlarge orbit, leading to enophthalmos. The overlong lids develop an obvious kink in the middle of the upper and lower lid, giving a diamond-shaped palpebral aperture (Figure 16.29). The condition is seen most commonly in the giant breeds such as the French Lop and the Flemish Giant. Surgical correction is advised if ocular discomfort or corneal changes are present; however the condition may remain asymptomatic until later in life when other ocular disease causing ocular discomfort (e.g. dacryocystitis) leads to a secondary spastic entropion. This often remains after the primary cause is treated, and requires surgical correction. Shortening of the lids using simple wedge resection is usually sufficient, but occasionally requires a Holtz–Celsus technique to evert the lower lid. Use of 0.7 metric (6/0 USP) multifilament polyglycolic acid suture with a 9 mm (3/8th) inch curved reverse cutting needle is recommended.

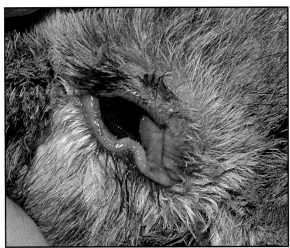

16.29 Lid overlength leading to combined entropion and ectropion in a giant-breed rabbit. Note the upper lid notch and the striking marginal folding of the lower lid due to secondary marginal blepharitis.

Eyelid tumours

Neoplastic lid lesions are not a common presentation and include squamous cell carcinoma, non-viral squamous papilloma, meibomian adenoma, Shope fibroma and malignant melanoma (Figure 16.30; von

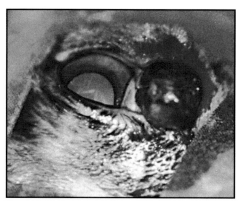

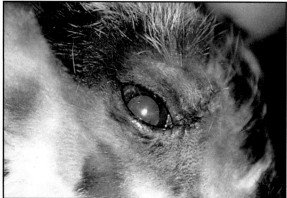

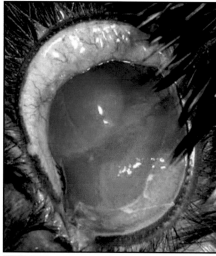

16.32 A large well circumscribed pink fleshy mass arising from the ventrolateral limbus. Perilesional corneal oedema, corneal vascularization, and moderate conjunctival hyperaemia are present. (Reproduced from Keller *et al.* (2007) with the permission of Wiley)

16.30 Eyelid melanoma. Upper medial lid, middle-aged Dwarf Lop. Resected *en bloc* and closed in two layers using 0.7 metric (6/0 USP) polyglycolic acid.

Bomhard *et al.*, 2007). Lid masses can be resected *en bloc* with up to one-third of the lid length in most patients, and with up to half of the lid in large-breed rabbits. A figure-of-eight suture pattern, magnification and fine dissolvable suture material (e.g. 0.7 metric (6/0 USP) polyglycolic acid) can all aid in the critical maintenance of a normal lid margin. Imperfect lid apposition can lead to ulcerative keratitis (Figure 16.31).

Although rare, ocular fibromas associated with infection with Shope fibroma virus have been reported, involving the eye lids, sclera and cornea. Corneal and scleral lesions present as pink fleshy nodules with associated corneal opacity (Figure 16.32; Keller *et al.*, 2007).

Ectopic cilia

Ectopic cilia are unusual in the rabbit but do occur. Aberrant cilia are most commonly significant when on the upper lid, owing to greater upper lid mobility, and they typically present as superficial dorsal corneal ulcers with a vertical pattern. Treatment is surgical removal *en bloc*. No sutures are required (Figure 16.33).

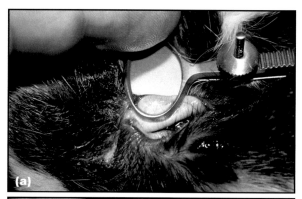

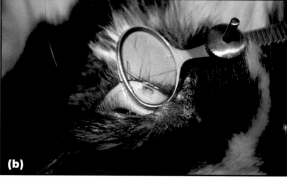

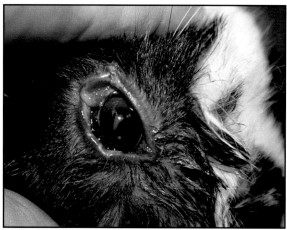

16.31 Lid margin repair with secondary superficial ulcer. Note the vertical pattern of ulceration.

16.33 **(a)** Ectopic cilium visible as a black dot on the conjunctival lid margin surface at the base of the tarsal plate. Visualization is often difficult, requiring high magnification. **(b)** Ectopic cilium removal. The lid margin is stabilized with a chalazion clamp and the hair removed together with a section of overlying conjunctiva. Removal of all hair follicles is essential, making magnification mandatory.

Diseases of the ocular surface and conjunctiva

Conjunctivitis

In the rabbit, conjunctivitis is usually secondary to another ophthalmic condition or to respiratory disease (Figure 16.34).

Primary conjunctivitis:
• Irritant, e.g. poor quality bedding, wood stains and ammonia associated with poor hygiene • Allergic, e.g. bedding
Secondary conjunctivitis (usually bacterial):
• Dacryocystitis • Pasteurellosis • Myxomatosis • Trichiasis (e.g. entropion) • Conjunctival sac foreign bodies

16.34 Causes of conjunctivitis.

Where bacterial infection is present, commensal bacteria are most frequently isolated, suggesting that opportunistic infection by commensal organisms is the primary source of bacterial infection (Figure 16.35; Cooper *et al.*, 2001). A similar pattern is seen in clinical cases of conjunctivitis, where again the commonest isolates are staphylococci, with a significant number of Gram-negative isolates noted (Figure 16.36; Cobb, 1999). Thus a broad-spectrum topical antibiotic is advised as a first-line treatment in cases of suspected secondary bacterial infection. Identification and, where possible, correction of the underlying cause is key to a successful outcome. It should be noted that it is not uncommon for the tear film of the rabbit to be milky in appearance; this is thought to be due to Harderian gland secretions and should be differentiated from purulent discharge by cytological examination. Bacterial conjunctivitis can be differentiated from dacryocystitis by straightforward flushing of the nasolacrimal ducts; no clots of purulent material will be seen around the cannula or at the nose.

Bacteria isolated	Percentage of cases	Microscopic characteristics
Staphylococcus spp.	57%	Gram-positive cocci
Micrococcus spp.	25%	Gram-positive cocci
Bacillus spp.	19%	Gram-negative bacilli
Stomatococcus spp.	8%	Gram-positive cocci
Neisseria spp.	8%	Gram-negative diplococci
Pasteurella spp.	6%	Gram-negative bacilli
Corynebacterium spp.	6%	Gram-positive bacilli
Streptococcus spp.	6%	Gram-positive cocci
Moraxella spp.	4%	Gram-negative short bacilli

16.35 Conjunctival flora of clinically normal rabbits. (Data from Cooper *et al.*, 2001)

Bacteria isolated	Percentage of cases	Microscopic characteristics
Staphylococcus spp.	34%	Gram-positive cocci
Pasteurella spp.	16%	Gram-negative bacilli
P. multocida	5%	Gram-negative bacilli
Other Gram-negative bacteria	30%	
Other Gram-positive bacteria	5%	

16.36 Bacteria isolated from cases of superficial ocular infection in the rabbit. (Data from Cobb, 1999)

While cases of primary conjunctivitis (where inflammation is limited to the conjunctiva) may go on to develop secondary bacterial infection, initial signs include increased lacrimation and conjunctival hyperaemia. Once a bacterial conjunctivitis is established a profound purulent discharge develops, at which point identification of an underlying cause can be challenging until the bacterial infection is under control.

Indolent ulcer

Indolent ulceration is typified by non-adherence of the corneal epithelium to the underlying corneal stroma, identified clinically by a rim of unattached epithelium at the edge of a corneal erosion (superficial ulcer). The epithelium in affected corneal areas is readily debrided with a sterile cotton bud. Abnormality or absence of the epithelial basement membrane is the common pathology and any disease process or medication which is damaging to the basement membrane may potentially lead to the formation of an indolent ulcer.

Primary indolent ulceration is commonly recognized in the dog and described as 'Boxer ulcer' or 'spontaneous chronic corneal epithelial deficit' (SCCED; Campbell and Murphy, 1999). SCCED is a diagnosis of exclusion made by eliminating all factors that can be detrimental to the epithelial basement membrane. Whilst not commonly recognized in the rabbit, primary indolent ulceration or SCCED appears to occur sporadically; however, a careful ophthalmic examination must be performed and history obtained to exclude other causes of indolent ulceration.

More commonly, indolent ulceration is caused by a recurrent or ongoing trauma to the corneal surface. This may be caused by an underlying disease process such as trichiasis, corneal exposure or poor tear film quality, or may be iatrogenic, e.g. resulting from topical steroid use or the chronic use of any topical medication, particularly those containing preservatives or which are epitheliotoxic in nature.

The indolent ulcer can be frustrating to treat and should be approached in a logical and stepwise manner:

1. Identification and correction of an underlying cause.

2. Debridement of non-attached epithelium.
3. Tear film support (the author's preference is a topical preservative-free hyaluronate).
4. Broad-spectrum antibiotic cover with a well tolerated topical antibiotic such as chloramphenicol.
5. If required, therapeutic bandage contact lenses.

Healing of indolent ulcers is expected to be slower than for a normal corneal erosion; however, if significant healing is not seen by day 14 with this approach, further interventions should be considered. Given the thin rabbit cornea, the author strongly suggests that surgical keratotomy or keratectomy techniques are reserved until medical management alone has failed, and should only be attempted with the correct equipment and expertise. Phenol cautery is a relatively safe procedure and in the author's hands is very successful (Figure 16.37).

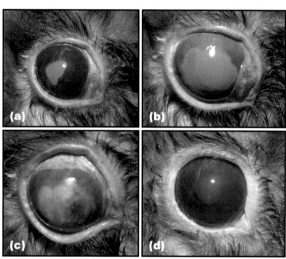

16.37 (a) Indolent ulcer prior to debridement; a rim of non-adherent epithelium is present. (b) The same ulcer following debridement with a sterile cotton bud, revealing the true area of corneal abnormality. (c) Phenol has been applied sparingly to the exposed corneal stroma where coagulated corneal stromal protein can be seen as a white plaque. (d) Healed indolent ulcer, day 10 after phenol cautery.

While keratotomy techniques can often be performed in conscious patients with local anaesthesia, great care should be taken when using magnification, and sedation or general anaesthesia is advised. Punctate keratotomy is the preferred technique owing to the reduced risk of corneal stromal damage when compared with grid keratotomy or superficial keratectomy. The use of the Alger brush (a 3.5 mm rotating diamond burr) has recently been advocated in the dog because of its association with reduced stromal damage, and this may prove a useful technique in the rabbit.

Topical cyanoacrylate glue has been used successfully when applied to the dried cornea after all non-adherent epithelium has been removed; this glue degrades to form formaldehyde and may cause a similar effect to phenol cautery. However, the resultant roughened corneal surface can cause significant ocular discomfort as a consequence of abrasion of the lid and conjunctiva, and for this reason it is not recommended.

Stromal ulceration

Deep corneal (stromal) ulceration is usually traumatic in origin and it is important to rule out causes of ongoing trauma, e.g. foreign bodies in the conjunctival sac. It should be noted that an intense white change to the exposed stroma is often seen and, while this may be caused by superficial corneal stromal infection (Figure 16.38a), it may also reflect deposition of tear film lipids in the exposed corneal stroma. Interestingly, melting ulcers appear to occur rarely in the rabbit.

Surgical treatment is often required for deep ulcers. Debridement of damaged stroma with a fine-tipped sterile bacteriology swab should be carried out routinely (when a low risk of corneal rupture allows this to be done safely) and samples submitted for cytology and Gram staining. Surgical support should be considered early and especially where the stromal deficit is suspected to be >50%. Conjunctival grafting techniques are probably to be preferred in the rabbit (e.g. rotational conjunctival pedicle graft) owing to the challenges of performing lamellar corneal dissection in the rabbit cornea and the propensity for the thin rabbit conjunctiva to become transparent following healing of the corneal stromal deficit (Figure 16.38b,c). Corneal surgery must be undertaken with good magnification, the correct microsurgical instruments, the correct suture material (0.4 metric (8/0 USP) or preferably 0.3 metric (9/0 USP) polyglycolic acid) and the correct suture needle (a micropoint spatulated 9 mm (³/₈ inch) curved needle).

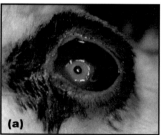
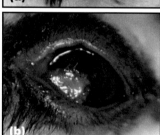
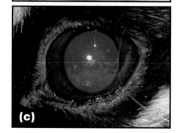

16.38 (a) Descemetocele: note the white colour of the exposed stroma. (b) Conjunctival pedicle graft in place, repairing the stromal deficit. (c) Appearance on day 45 after surgery: rapid corneal remodelling and a transparent conjunctival graft are seen.

Third eyelid flaps can be used but are of limited utility in the rabbit, reducing the efficacy of topical medication and precluding examination of the progression or otherwise of the corneal pathology. The external third eyelid conjunctiva should be sutured to bulbar conjunctiva with 0.7 metric (6/0 USP) polyglactin 910 using two or three mattress sutures. It should be noted that the third eyelid of the rabbit is smaller and less mobile than that of other domestic species, making the placement of third eyelid flaps technically challenging, and they are contraindicated when the corneal integrity is uncertain.

Therapeutic bandage contact lenses can be used safely in the rabbit and are preferred to the third eyelid flap for the treatment of non-healing superficial ulcers. Aqueous topical treatments such as gentamicin, chloramphenicol or ofloxacin can be used with a bandage lens in place.

Lipid keratopathy

Lipid keratopathy presents as a white to yellow corneal opacity and should be differentiated from corneal lipidosis, where corneal vascularization is seen associated with the corneal lipid. Lesions are often most obvious in the cooler central cornea where liquid-phase corneal lipids are more readily able to precipitate (Figure 16.39).

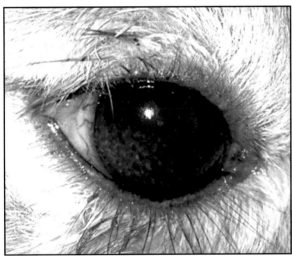

16.39 Lipid keratopathy in a dwarf-breed rabbit. Note the linear central distribution matching the cooler regions of the cornea, where lipids precipitate in the anterior corneal stroma. (Courtesy of Vim Katarunga)

Ocular lesions associated with hyperlipidaemia are well documented in the rabbit. An inherited hyperlipidaemia is seen in the Watanabe heritable hyperlipidaemic (WHHL) rabbit and is used as a model for human familial hypercholesterolaemia; ocular manifestations include lipid accumulation in the cornea, ciliary body and iris. The earliest visible lesions are yellow granules at the limbus (Kouchi *et al.*, 2006), with severely affected animals becoming visually affected as a result of central corneal involvement (Garibaldi and Goad, 1988).

Spontaneous cases of diet-induced lipid keratopathy have been reported (Sebesteny *et al.*, 1985).

Where lipid keratopathy is suspected, serum lipid and lipoprotein levels should be measured, as well as examining the composition of the diet for high-fat components (e.g. fish meal, milk chocolate or cheese). Total low and very low density lipoproteins (TLDL and TVLDL), types of cholesterol, appear to be responsible for the accumulation of corneal lipid in these cases (Reddy *et al.*, 1987) and should be critically assessed on serum lipoprotein profiles in affected animals.

Aberrant overgrowth of conjunctiva

A rare condition, aberrant conjunctival stricture and overgrowth (ACS) presents as a 360-degree double thickness growth of conjunctiva originating at the limbus. The ingrowing conjunctival plica gradually extends towards the central cornea, eventually impinging on vision. While it shares similarities to pterygoid membrane formation in humans, the peripheral cornea remains unattached to the overlying plica of the conjunctiva in ACS. A predisposition in young male dwarf rabbits has been suggested. This disease should be differentiated from symblepharon, where conjunctiva becomes adherent to the peripheral cornea following damage to the epithelial limbal stem cells.

Resection of the folded conjunctival tissue brings only temporary improvement with rapid regrowth being the norm. Definitive treatment has involved resection of the conjunctival membrane 1–2 mm beyond the limbus and postoperative immunosuppression with ciclosporin with or without topical steroids, which appears to delay recurrence; however, the prognosis with respect to recurrence is guarded. A technique involving division of the corneal conjunctival folds with centrifugal cuts, inverting the folded tissue and suturing the folds in the dorsal and ventral fornix has been described by Allgoewer *et al.* (2008), with good success rates.

Punctate superficial keratitis

A punctate superficial keratopathy is seen on occasion in the rabbit, similar to that seen in equine patients. There may be a viral or immune-mediated aetiology. The author has noted little response to topical antiviral therapy but good response to ciclosporin. In the first instance tear film supplementation with a mucinomimetic tear supplement (e.g. hyaluronate) and topical antibiotics, e.g. chloramphenicol q6h, is recommended. If there is a poor response the addition of ciclosporin q12h should be considered.

Diseases of the uveal tract and lens

Acute uveitis

Acute uveitis can be seen in association with any systemic bacterial, septicaemic or thromboembolic disease. Systemic infections such as pasteurellosis readily lead to acute uveitis in the rabbit. Clinical signs are similar to those in other species, i.e. aqueous flare, hypopyon, hyphaema, iridal hyperaemia and swelling, miosis and reduced intraocular pressure. Symptomatic treatment relies on atropine, topical steroids and systemic antibiotics. Identifying and addressing an underlying cause is important. Topical atropine may need to be given 4 times daily to maintain a dilated pupil and at this dose paralytic ileus becomes a very real risk.

Iris abscess

Iris abscess formation is a potential result of haematogenous spread of *Pasteurella* spp. but may also be due to focal lens rupture (associated with *Encephalitozoon cuniculi*). Long-term topical steroids combined with systemic antibiotics (and/or fenbendazole) can lead to these lesions remaining static for long periods.

Phacoclastic uveitis

Lens rupture causes a dramatic response in the rabbit eye with the formation of white iris abscesses, which often grow aggressively leading ultimately to secondary glaucoma.

The commonest cause appears to be encephalitozoonosis. With infection *in utero* the organisms are believed to travel via the uterine vascular supply to the developing lens, where they become isolated following regression of the lenticular vascular supply in the last stages of pregnancy. Both sessile cataracts and spontaneous lens rupture with secondary lens-induced uveitis may be seen. Young dwarf-breed rabbits appear to be predisposed to spontaneous lens rupture. Elimination of the putative causative organism does not appear to arrest progression of this aggressive disease and probably reflects the limited intraocular penetration of drugs active against the parasite and the highly immunogenic nature of lens proteins. Removal of the lens by phacoemulsification can save vision and the globe (Felchle and Sigler, 2002) and carries a good prognosis if performed early in the disease process.

Small focal lens ruptures can cause a localized granulomatous response limited to the iridal tissue overlying the rupture, and the phacoclastic uveitis can sometimes be controlled with long-term topical steroids (prednisolone). Definitive diagnosis of *E. cuniculi* lens disease relies on identification of protozoal DNA or microscopic identification of the parasite in lens tissue following phacoemulsification or enucleation.

If intraocular *E. cuniculi* infection is suspected, systemic treatment should be given because central nervous system lesions are likely to be present. Systemic steroids may act to suppress granulomatous inflammation although care must be taken owing to the risk of immunosuppression. For further discussion of *E. cuniculi* including treatment options, please refer to Chapter 15.

Cataract

Cataracts are commonly seen in the rabbit. Causes include congenital inherited and teratogenic cataracts, developmental inherited cataract, developmental intralenticular *E. cuniculi* infection, lens trauma and spontaneous *E. cuniculi*-associated lens rupture. Persistence of the embryonic vascular system such as the hyaloid artery and the tunica vasculosa lentis may result in posterior capsular and subcapsular cataract (Figure 16.40). The position of the opacity

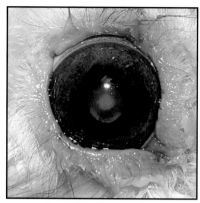

16.40 Posterior capsular and subcapsular cataract associated with a persistent hyaloid remnant.

within the lens can help to identify the likely time of injury to the lens, with nuclear opacities generally being formed prenatally, epinuclear opacities being formed at or around parturition (Figure 16.41) and equatorial cortical opacities being formed more recently.

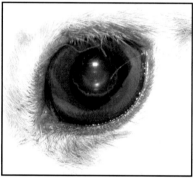

16.41 Epinuclear cataract in a 3-year-old domestic rabbit. The epinuclear region of the lens develops at or around birth; thus lens opacities in this position are thought to reflect metabolic insults to the lens at this time.

Phacoemulsification can be successfully used in rabbit cataracts, in cases of both lens rupture and spontaneous cataract formation (Figure 16.42). The size of the rabbit eye and the lateral placement makes positioning more straightforward than in dog

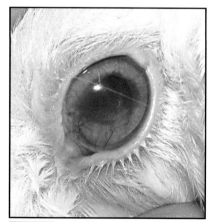

16.42 Aphakic eye immediately following cataract removal by phacoemulsification for *E. cuniculi*-associated lens rupture and lens-induced uveitis. The edge of the posterior rhexis is just visible. Corneal neovascularization is present, associated with a pre-existing chronic lens-induced uveitis.

and cat patients. Intraocular lenses are of uncertain utility, owing to the high incidence of lens fibre regrowth and posterior capsular opacification, thus a planned posterior capsulorrhexis should be considered by the cataract surgeon to maximize the prognosis for long-term vision. Currently there are no commercially available intraocular lenses of the correct refractive power for the rabbit

Glaucoma

Glaucoma is caused by obstruction of the normal outflow of aqueous humour from the eye and can either be due to a primary abnormality of this pathway or can be secondary to other intraocular diseases such as uveitis, neoplasia or hyphaema resulting from uveitis or globe trauma. Primary glaucoma is the commonest presentation in the rabbit, where acute painful episodes are rarely recognized until they progress to secondary corneal ulceration. In contrast to the dog, grossly identifiable changes in the irido-corneal drainage angle are not always visible. Gonioscopy can be readily performed in the rabbit and may be of use in identifying primary angle closure, infiltrative diseases of the angle and occult anterior uveitis (Figure 16.43).

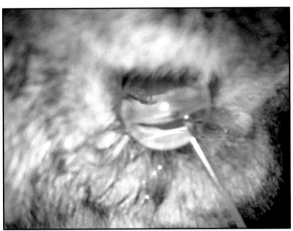

16.43 Chronic glaucoma of unknown cause. Gonioscopic view of the iridocorneal drainage angle shows haemorrhage in the drainage angle consistent with anterior uveitis.

Primary glaucoma is not uncommon in the rabbit and has been well researched (Tesluk *et al.*, 1982). Known to be inherited in the New Zealand White, it can be seen in any breed. The gene for glaucoma (*bu*) is recessive and semi-lethal, with heterozygotes giving birth to small litters of unthrifty young (Williams, 2007). Globe enlargement occurs more readily than in other species, particularly in young rabbits, and can be striking; hence the colloquial name 'bull's eye'. Haabs striae (linear breaks in Descemet's membrane), severe corneal oedema and episcleral congestion are seen rarely in buphthalmic rabbit eyes. Secondary lens luxation caused by progressive globe enlargement is commonly seen (Figure 16.44) and may be seen in eyes retaining demonstrable vision, whereas optic disc cupping and retinal

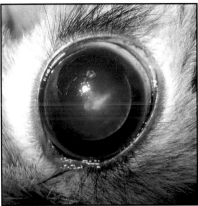

16.44 Chronic glaucoma. Secondary lens luxation due to progressive globe enlargement.

degeneration are more commonly associated with blindness (Figure 16.45). Intraocular pressure may not uncommonly return to near normal as the globe enlarges. There is a slow progression to blindness and often secondary corneal ulceration due to chronic corneal oedema.

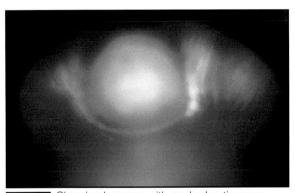

16.45 Chronic glaucoma with marked optic nerve head cupping and complete vascular attenuation.

Medication can delay the disease process, in some cases for up to several years. Timolol and dorzolamide are both tolerated and effective in short-term management of intraocular pressure and appear to have a synergistic effect, making the use of a combination drop (e.g. CoSopt; administered q8h) the formulation of choice. Care should be taken to identify systemic side effects of both of these drugs (bradycardia and electrolyte disturbances, which often present as ileus) and to reduce the dose accordingly.

Given the chronic course of this disease and the rabbit eye's tolerance to raised intraocular pressure, the use of glaucoma surgery in this species might be expected to be a useful long-term strategy. Critical assessment of the impact of glaucoma on the quality of life of a natural prey species such as the rabbit can be difficult; however, enucleation is recommended in cases of blind buphthalmic eyes where the intraocular pressure cannot be maintained in the normal range using medication. Bilateral enucleation is the long-term outcome for many rabbits with glaucoma and appears to be tolerated well (Figure 16.46).

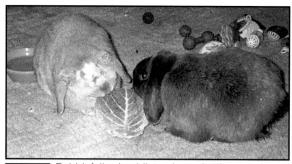

16.46 Rabbit following bilateral enucleation, playing 'tug-of-war' with a sighted companion.

Ocular therapeutics

Dosages for topical ophthalmic medications are given in Chapter 21.

References

Abrams KL, Brooks DE, Funk RS and Theran P (1990) Evaluation of the Schirmer tear test in clinically normal rabbits. *American Journal of Veterinary Research* **51**(12), 1912–1913

Allgoewer I, Malho P, Schulze H and Schäffer E (2008) Aberrant conjunctival stricture and overgrowth in the rabbit. *Veterinary Ophthalmology* **11**(1), 18–22

Bayraktaroğlu AG and Ergun E (2010) Histomorphology of the Harderian gland in the Angora rabbit. *Anatomia Histologia Embryologia* **39**(6), 494–502

Burling K, Murphy CJ, Da Silva Curiel J, Koblik P and Bellhorn RW (1991) Anatomy of the rabbit's nasolacrimal duct and its clinical implications. *Progress in Veterinary and Comparative Ophthalmology* **1**(1), 33–40

Campbell S and Murphy C (1999) Clinical characterization of spontaneous, chronic, non-septic corneal epithelial defects in dogs. *Investigative Ophthalmology and Visual Science* **40**(4), S337 [Abstract 1786]

Cobb MP (1999) A survey of the conjunctival flora in rabbits with clinical signs of superficial ocular infection. *British Association of Veterinary Ophthalmology – Spring Congress, Birmingham*, p.17

Cooper SC, McLellan GJ and Rycroft AN (2001) Conjunctival flora observed in 70 healthy domestic rabbits (*Oryctolagus cuniculus*). *Veterinary Record* **149**(8), 232–235

Felchle LM and Sigler RL (2002) Phacoemulsification for the management of *Encephalitozoon cuniculi* induced phacoclastic uveitis in the rabbit. *Veterinary Ophthalmology* **5**(3), 211–215

Florin M, Rusanen E, Haessig M, Richter M and Spiess BM (2009) Clinical presentation, treatment, and outcome of dacryocystitis in rabbits: a retrospective study of 28 cases (2003–2007). *Veterinary Ophthalmology* **12**(6), 350–356

Foster CS, Lass JH, Moran-Wallace K and Giovanoni R (1981) Ocular toxicity of topical antifungal agents. *Archives of Ophthalmology* **99**(6), 1081–1084

Garibaldi BA and Goad ME (1988) Lipid keratopathy in the Watanabe (WHHL) rabbit. *Veterinary Pathology* **25**(2), 173–174

Gwon A (2008) The rabbit in cataract/IOL surgery. In: *Animal Models in Eye Research*, ed. PA Tsonis, pp.184–204. Elsevier, New York

Harcourt-Brown F (2002) Ophthalmic diseases. In: *Textbook of Rabbit Medicine*, ed. F. Harcourt-Brown, pp.292–306. Butterworth-Heinemann, Oxford

Hernandez V, Albini T, Lee W, *et al.* (2012) A portable, contact animal fundus imaging system based on Rol's GRIN lenses. *Veterinary Ophthalmology* **15**(3), 141–144.

Ishikawa M, Kubo M, Maeda S, *et al.* (2011) Structural changes in the lacrimal sac epithelium and associated lymphoid tissue during experimental dacryocystitis. *Clinical Ophthalmology* **5**, 1567–1574

Jekl VHR (2012) Rabbit ophthalmology. *Proceedings, British Association of Veterinary Ophthalmology, Birmingham*, pp.10–12

Jeong MB, Kim NR, Yi NY, *et al.* (2005) Spontaneous ophthalmic diseases in 586 New Zealand white rabbits. *Experimental Animals* **54**(5), 395–403

Jester JV, Rife L, Nii D, *et al.* (1982) In vivo biomicroscopy and photography of meibomian glands in a rabbit model of meibomian gland dysfunction. *Investigative Ophthalmology and Visual Science* **22**(5), 660–667

Juliusson B, Bergstrom A, Rohlich P, *et al.* (1994) Complementary cone fields of the rabbit retina. *Investigative Ophthalmology and Visual Science* **35**(3), 811–818

Keller RL, Hendrix DV and Greenacre C (2007) Shope fibroma virus keratitis and spontaneous cataracts in a domestic rabbit. *Veterinary Ophthalmology* **10**(3), 190–195

Kern T (1997) Rabbit and rodent ophthalmology. *Seminars in Avian and Exotic Pet Medicine* **6**(3), 138–145

Knop E and Knop N (2001) Lacrimal drainage-associated lymphoid tissue (LDALT): a part of the human mucosal immune system. *Investigative Ophthalmology and Visual Science* **42**(3), 566–574

Knott T (2003) Small mammal ophthalmology. *Proceedings, British Association of Veterinary Ophthalmologists, Birmingham*, pp.18–22

Knott T (2012) Phoneoscopy: the use of smart phone cameras in ophthalmoscopy. *Proceedings, British Association of Veterinary Ophthalmologists, Selsdon, Surrey*, pp.18–22

Kouchi M, Ueda Y, Horie H and Tanaka K (2006) Ocular lesions in Watanabe heritable hyperlipidemic rabbits. *Veterinary Ophthalmology* **9**(3), 145–148

Künzel F and Joachim A (2012) Encephalitozoonosis in rabbits. *Parasitology Research* **106**(2), 299–309

Li X, Cai C, Li L, Chai X and Ren Q (2009) Low-hemorrhage-risk surgical approach to expose the optic nerve. *Veterinary Ophthalmology* **12**(4), 227–223

Morgan RV, Duddy JM and McClurg K (1993) Prolapse of the gland of the third eyelid in dogs: a retrospective study of 89 cases (1980-1990). *Journal of the American Veterinary Medical Association* **201**, 1861–1867

O'Reilly A, McCowan C, Hardman C and Stanley R (2002) *Taenia serialis* causing exophthalmos in a pet rabbit. *Veterinary Ophthalmology* **5**(3), 227–230

Pirie CG and Pizzirani S (2012) Anterior and posterior segment photography. An alternative approach using a dSLR camera adaptor. *Veterinary Ophthalmology* **15**(4), 280–287

Reddy C, Stock EL, Mendelsohn AD, *et al.* (1987) Pathogenesis of experimental lipid keratopathy: corneal and plasma lipids. *Investigative Ophthalmology and Visual Science* **28**(9), 1492–1496

Saito K, Tagawa M and Hasegawa A (2003) RPR test for serological survey of rabbit syphilis in companion rabbits. *Journal of Veterinary Medical Science* **65**(7), 797–799

Salazar M, Shimada K and Patil PN (1976) Iris pigmentation and atropine mydriasis. *Journal of Pharmacology and Experimental Therapeutics* **197**(1), 79–88

Sebesteny A, Sheraidah GA, Trevan DJ, Alexander RA and Ahmed AI (1985) Lipid keratopathy and atheromatosis in an SPF laboratory rabbit colony attributed to diet. *Laboratory Animals* **19**(3), 180–188

Skarf B and Czarnecki JS (1982) Distinguishing postganglionic from preganglionic lesions: studies in rabbits with surgically produced Horner's syndrome. *Archives of Ophthalmology* **100**(8), 1319–1322

Tesluk GC, Peiffer RL and Brown D (1982) A clinical and pathological study of inherited glaucoma in New Zealand white rabbits. *Laboratory Animals* **16**(3), 234–239

Toni MC, Meirelles AÉ, Gava FN, *et al.* (2010) Rabbits' eye globe sonographic biometry. *Veterinary Ophthalmology* **13**(6), 384–386

Tyrrell KL, Citron DM, Jenkins JR and Goldstein EJ (2002) Periodontal bacteria in rabbit mandibular and maxillary abscesses. *Journal of Clinical Microbiology* **40**(3), 1044–1047

Volopich S, Gruber A, Hassan J *et al.* (2005) Malignant B-cell lymphoma of the Harder's gland in a rabbit. *Veterinary Ophthalmology* **8**(4), 259–263

von Bomhard W, Goldschmidt MH, Shofer FS, *et al.* (2007) Cutaneous neoplasms in pet rabbits: a retrospective study. *Veterinary Pathology* **44**(5), 579–588

Wagner F and Fehr M (2007) Common ophthalmic problems in pet rabbits. *Journal of Exotic Pet Medicine* **16**(3), 158–167

Wang X and Wu Q (2013) Normal corneal thickness measurements in pigmented rabbits using spectral-domain anterior segment optical coherence tomography. *Veterinary Ophthalmology* **16**(2), 1–5

Wei XE, Markoulli M, Zhao Z and Willcox MD (2013) Tear film break-up time in rabbits. *Clinical and Experimental Optometry* **96**(1), 70–75

Williams DL (2007) Rabbit and rodent ophthalmology. *European Journal of Companion Animal Practice* **17**(3), 242–252

17

Dermatoses

Anna Meredith

Skin disease is a common clinical problem in rabbits. Abnormalities are generally easily detected by the owner, even in individuals that are not regularly handled. There are a number of particular problems encountered with the diagnosis and treatment of skin disease in rabbits. These include the necessity for sedation or general anaesthesia for obtaining diagnostic samples in some animals and limitations of topical medication because of the rabbit's fastidious grooming habits. In addition, there are few authorized drug preparations, and some drugs, particularly antibiotics and corticosteroids, may have adverse effects.

Approach to the skin case

The general principles of diagnosing skin disease in cats and dogs are equally applicable to rabbits, and the same diagnostic techniques may be used (Figure 17.1). The diagnostic approach consists of:

- Obtaining a history – general; presenting complaint
- General clinical examination
- Skin examination
- Differential diagnosis
- Specific diagnostic tests
- Definitive diagnosis and appropriate treatment.

History
Important details to obtain are:

- Source and length of time owned
- Source and sex of any companions
- Husbandry – outdoor or house rabbit, type of housing, flooring, bedding and cleaning regimes
- Diet
- Water presentation – bottle or bowl
- Vaccination status
- Insect control
- Presence of other pets
- General health and previous problems
- Presenting problem:
  - How long has it been present?
  - Are any other rabbits affected?
  - Are any other pets or the owner affected?
  - Is pruritus present?
  - Have any parasites been seen?

Clinical examination
A thorough clinical examination should always be undertaken (see Chapter 7) before concentrating on the skin lesions. It is important to examine the ventral surface of the rabbit, especially the genitalia, perineal area and the plantar aspects of the feet, because lesions here are commonly missed by the owner. An illuminated hand lens will aid the detection of ectoparasites.

Test	Technique/comments	Indications
Skin scraping	Clip affected area carefully. Moisten skin with liquid paraffin. Scrape gently – avoid excessive trauma	Ectoparasites, dermatophytes
Cellophane tape	Clip affected area carefully. Apply tape several times. Use fresh tape – more adhesive	Ectoparasites, dermatophytes, assessment of self-trauma
Fine-needle aspirate	Clip and clean lesion. Use 21 G needle – exudate may be thick	Subcutaneous abscesses, possible neoplasia
Wood's lamp examination	Allow lamp to warm up. Perform test in dark room. Allow enough time to examine carefully	*Microsporum canis* (not all strains fluoresce)
Bacterial culture	Standard aerobic culture	Possible infection with *Pseudomonas* spp.
Fungal culture	Take plenty of hairs or use Mackenzie brush tehnique	Dermatophytes including *Trichophyton mentagrophytes* and *M. canis*
Skin biopsy	Sedation or general anaesthesia usually required	Possible neoplasia or infection with *Treponema* spp.

17.1 Special diagnostic tests for skin.

Parasitic skin disease

Fur mites

Cheyletiella parasitovorax is the rabbit fur mite. It is a non-burrowing mite, just visible to the naked eye. Many rabbits carry the mites with no overt clinical signs. Lesions are generally not severe and generally present as crusting and scaling along the dorsum, with mild pruritus and partial alopecia in heavy infestations (Figure 17.2). Severe infestations are more commonly seen in young or immunosuppressed rabbits, or those that have difficulty grooming. *Cheyletiella* is zoonotic, causing a pruritic papular dermatitis in humans. The life cycle is 14–21 days, and adult females can survive for at least 10 days off the host. Diagnosis is easily made with the cellophane tape test. Treatment is with ivermectin at 0.4 mg/kg s.c. once every 10–14 days for three doses. Alternatively, selamectin at 12 mg/kg has also been shown to be highly effective (Kim *et al.*, 2008). Other treatments include lime/sulphur dips and topical permethrin products. All in-contact animals should be treated and the environment thoroughly cleaned. Any lesions on the owner will resolve if the mites are eliminated from the rabbit.

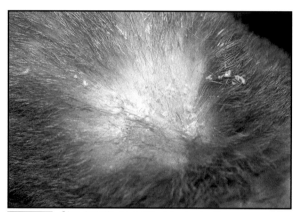

17.2 *Cheyletiella parasitovorax* typically causes scaling of the skin, with minimal pruritus.

Listrophorus (*Leporacarus*) *gibbus* is a non-burrowing fur mite that is commonly described as non-pathogenic even when heavy infestations are present. However, infection can be associated with hair loss, seborrhoea and abnormal moult (Pinter, 1999; Jenkins, 2001). It is not zoonotic. Both imidacloprid + permethrin and topical selamectin have been shown to be effective against *L. gibbus*, although treatment with selamectin more rapidly eliminated the infestation (Birke *et al.*, 2009).

Ear mites

Psoroptes cuniculi is the rabbit ear mite. It is a large non-burrowing mite that causes intense irritation, resulting in head shaking and scratching of the ears with consequent hyperaemia and the production of exudates. This can lead to a thick crust of exudate filling the auditory canal (Figure 17.3). Lesions can spread to the face and neck, and the ear drum can be perforated, leading to a purulent otitis media due to secondary bacterial infection

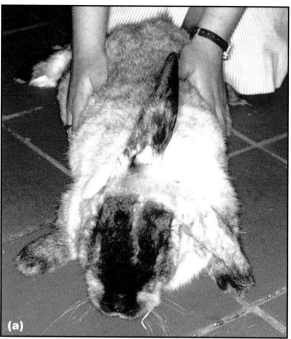

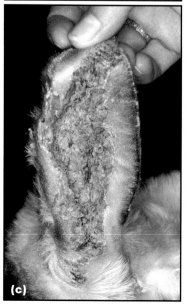

17.3
(a) Rabbit with *Psoroptes cuniculi* infection in one ear. **(b)** Normal ear. **(c)** Affected ear. Note tightly adherent crusts. (Courtesy of D Scarff)

and to neurological signs such as a head tilt. Mites can be seen on otoscopic examination, or by microscopic examination of debris removed from the ear. The life cycle is less than 3 weeks, and adult mites can survive away from the host for up to 21 days, depending on ambient temperature and humidity. Transmission is by direct contact or via fomites. Various treatments can be used, including ivermectin (0.4 mg/kg s.c. once every 10–14 days for 3 treatments), selamectin (6–18 mg/kg topically every 4 weeks for 1–2 treatments), or moxidectin (alone, or combined with imidacloprid, at 0.2 mg/kg s.c. once every 10 days for 2 treatments) (White *et al.*, 2003; Hansen *et al.*, 2005).

All in-contact animals should be treated and the environment also cleaned and treated with flea products. Mild infections may be treated with acaricidal ear drops. The thick crusts in the ear canals will resolve with systemic treatment but, if necessary, they can be softened with mineral oil before being removed. Care must be taken not to damage the lining of the ear canal. The pain and intense irritation can be reduced by the administration of non-steroidal anti-inflammatory drugs (NSAIDs; e.g. carprofen or meloxicam).

Other mites
Demodex cuniculi is rarely found, and its pathological significance is unknown (Harvey, 1990). Affected rabbits can show variable levels of pruritus, or it can cause non-pruritic alopecia in immunosuppressed animals. Treatment is with systemic ivermectin or topical amitraz (0.05%).

Sarcoptes scabiei var. *cuniculi* and *Notoedres cati* var. *cuniculi* are occasionally reported. They are associated with a pruritic dermatosis characterized by yellow discharge. Treatment is with ivermectin or selamectin (Farmaki *et al.*, 2009) as for other mites.

A new subspecies of *Psorobia lagomorphae* has been reported as causing mild pruritus and alopecia in a 6-month-old dwarf rabbit (Bourdeau *et al.*, 2001).

Fleas
Spilopsyllus cuniculi (the 'stick-tight' flea) is the flea most frequently seen in wild rabbits in the UK and is important as a vector for myxomatosis. In pet rabbits, cat and dog fleas (*Ctenocephalides felis* and *C. canis*) are more commonly found. In the USA the Eastern rabbit flea (*Cediopsylla simplex*), giant Eastern rabbit flea (*Odontopsyllus multispinosus*) and the 'stick-tight' flea (*Echidnophaga gallinacea*) may also be found. Treatment of the rabbit is rarely required if cats and dogs and the environment are treated in the usual way. However, imidacloprid (Hutchinson *et al.*, 2001) and selamectin are effective flea treatments in rabbits. Topical selamectin at a dosage of 20 mg/kg every 7 days has been shown to be efficacious for treatment of flea infestation in rabbits (Carpenter *et al.*, 2012). Long-term use of lufenuron is also reported to be safe (Jenkins, 2001). Adverse reactions to fipronil have been reported, and it should not be used.

Lice
Haemodipsus ventricosus, the rabbit louse, can cause anaemia and pruritus, but is rare in pet rabbits. Systemic ivermectin can be used as treatment; imidacloprid seems to be effective in dogs and so could also be used in rabbits.

Ticks
Many species of tick can parasitize rabbits, the most common being the continental rabbit tick *Haemaphysalis leporis-palustris*. Heavy infestation can cause anaemia, and ticks can act as vectors for myxomatosis, papillomatosis and tularaemia. Ticks can be manually removed or treated with systemic ivermectin at 0.4 mg/kg (Jenkins, 2001).

Myiasis
Fly strike is common in rabbits in the summer months (Figure 17.4). In the UK it is caused mainly by the greenbottle fly (*Lucilia* spp.). Strike is usually primary (i.e. affecting intact skin) and flies are attracted by caecotroph accumulation around the perineum and especially in the skin folds on either side of the genitals. This is invariably due to lack of caecotrophy, which can be associated with a number of conditions: dental disease; obesity; back problems such as spondylitis or arthritis; and old age. True diarrhoea and urine scalding due to urinary incontinence will also attract flies. Eggs can hatch within 12 hours to L1 maggots, which are not harmful. Within 3 days L1 larvae moult to L2 and L3; these then cause the tissue damage. Environmental conditions of at least 60% humidity and 9–11°C are required for larval development. It is thought that the maggots may secrete a local anaesthetic and so the damage is rarely observed to be painful to the rabbit. In the USA the flesh fly (*Wohlfahrtia vigil*) is most common, with eggs being laid at the edges of wounds.

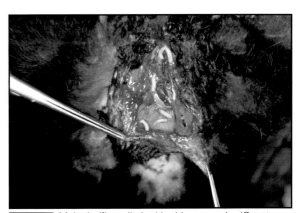

17.4 Myiasis (fly strike) with skin necrosis. (Courtesy of D Scarff)

Initial treatment involves clipping of the fur and cleaning of the area, with manual removal of the maggots and flushing of the area with dilute antiseptic solution. Supportive therapy should be given immediately for toxic shock (warmth, fluids, corticosteroids in severe cases). Systemic ivermectin at 0.4 mg/kg s.c. may also be given, which will kill any subcutaneous or internal maggots, and any that subsequently hatch. Secondary bacterial (often clostridial) infection of the necrotic tissue often occurs and appropriate antibiotic cover should also be given. Topical silver sulfadiazine cream has also been recommended (Jenkins, 2001). The underlying cause of the accumulation of caecotrophs or urine must then be addressed. A healing wound is pictured in Figure 17.5.

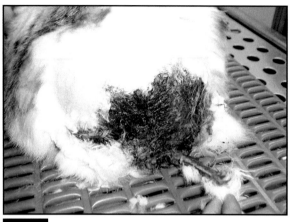

17.5 A healing fly strike wound.

Cyromazine is an insect growth inhibitor authorized for prevention of fly strike in rabbits. It does not repel flies but prevents the moult from L1 to L2. Permethrin spot-on products can also be applied every 2 weeks as a preventive measure. Some products also contain a fly repellent.

Cuterebra spp. larvae can also affect rabbits, causing fistulous nodules. The larvae should be individually removed. The rabbit should be sedated or anaesthetized and the affected area clipped and disinfected. The breathing hole is then enlarged using haemostats and the larva gently removed. Great care should be taken not to crush the larva during removal, as this can cause anaphylaxis. Debridement of the necrotic fistulous tract is necessary, and antibiotic treatment should be given for secondary bacterial infection.

Other parasites

Coenurus serialis cysts caused by the tapeworm *Taenia serialis* have been reported to cause fluctuant subcutaneous swellings (Fountain, 2000; Bennett, 2001; Wills, 2001) which can be surgically removed.

The rabbit pinworm *Passalurus ambiguus* is common in laboratory rabbits and can occasionally be associated with pruritus of the anal area, leading to self-trauma and rectal prolapse.

Harvest mites (*Trombicula autumnalis*) can be found on outdoor rabbits and cause intense pruritus and the formation of macules and pustules.

Bacterial skin disease

Abscesses

Subcutaneous abscesses may result from entry of bacteria via a skin wound, or, more rarely, are secondary to bacteraemia. Facial abscesses are frequently associated with dental or nasolacrimal duct disease. A variety of bacteria may be isolated, including *Pasteurella multocida*, *Staphylococcus aureus*, *Fusobacterium* spp., *Proteus* spp., *Pseudomonas aeruginosa*, *Bacteroides* spp. and *Actinomyces* spp. Rabbit pus is thick, tenacious and very difficult to remove, and there is usually a thick abscess capsule (Figure 17.6). Successful culture is most likely from a swab of the inside of the capsule wall or a piece of this wall, because the pus itself is frequently sterile. Samples should be submitted for both aerobic and anaerobic culture.

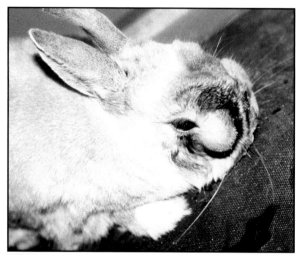

17.6 Rabbit with facial abscess. Abscesses have thick capsules and, when on the face, are typically related to dental disease. (Courtesy of D Scarff)

Abscesses may form single or multiple subcutaneous nodules with or without a discharging sinus or associated wound. If associated with dental disease or nasolacrimal duct disease, facial swelling, lacrimation and anorexia are common presenting signs.

Ultrasonography or computed tomography (CT) may be useful in determining the extent of an abscess, and radiography of the skull is vital if a facial abscess is present in order to obtain a prognosis. All abscesses are best treated by complete surgical excision wherever possible. If this is not possible, lancing and aggressive flushing with antiseptic solutions, plus appropriate systemic antibiotic therapy, can be employed, but the prognosis for resolution is more guarded. Dental abscess treatment is covered in the *BSAVA Manual of Rabbit Surgery, Dentistry and Imaging*.

Cellulitis

Acute cellulitis is usually due to infection with *Staphylococcus aureus*, *Pasteurella multocida* or *Bordetella bronchiseptica* (Jenkins, 2001), and may develop secondary to respiratory infection. Clinical signs are of painful oedematous skin swelling, usually of the head, neck or thorax (Figure 17.7). The rabbit is usually febrile (40–42°C), depressed and anorexic. Treatment consists of aggressive antibiosis based on bacterial culture and sensitivity. Supportive care, including cool

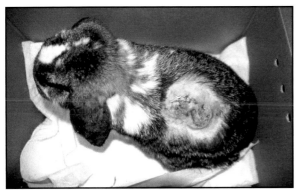

17.7 Cellulitis on the dorsum due to bite wounds from another rabbit.

water baths to reduce body temperature, must be provided. In rabbits that survive the initial stage of the condition, the cellulitis may progress to form an abscess or may develop a necrotic eschar in the affected area.

Moist dermatitis
This may be seen in overweight rabbits and in females with a large dewlap, in animals with severe dental disease and excess salivation, or as a result of urine scalding. The wet fur becomes infected with *Pseudomonas aeruginosa*, or other bacteria. If *Pseudomonas* is involved the fur turns a characteristic blue colour. Treatment involves clipping the affected area, and applying antiseptic or antibiotic preparations, plus investigating and addressing the underlying cause. Systemic antibiosis is generally not required, but may be necessary in some cases.

Rabbit syphilis/venereal spirochaetosis
This is caused by the spirochaete *Treponema paraluis cuniculi*. Clinical signs are relatively uncommon, and subclinical infection is believed to be common, with serological screening suggesting that up to 25% of rabbits are infected (Jenkins, 2001). Lesions begin as redness and oedema, progressing to vesicles, ulcers, scabs and proliferative lesions around the perineum, and also around the face from autoinoculation (Figure 17.8). Transmission is venereal and by direct contact. Affected does can infect kits as they pass through the birth canal. The incubation period is long, with lesions generally appearing 3–6 weeks after exposure and a positive serological titre developing after 8–12 weeks. Rabbits can be asymptomatic carriers, with overt disease precipitated by stress, sometimes months or years after initial exposure. Clinical signs are very characteristic, but definitive diagnosis involves microscopic visualization of the organism from scrapings of the lesion on a dark-field background, or with special silver stains on biopsy. Serological tests developed for detection of human syphilis (*Treponema pallidum*) can be used. Lesions can be self-limiting, but effective treatment is with penicillin G (42,000–84,000 IU/kg) once every 7 days for 3 doses. Treated rabbits should be monitored closely for signs of antibiotic-associated enterotoxaemia. All exposed rabbits should be treated. Rabbit syphilis is not zoonotic.

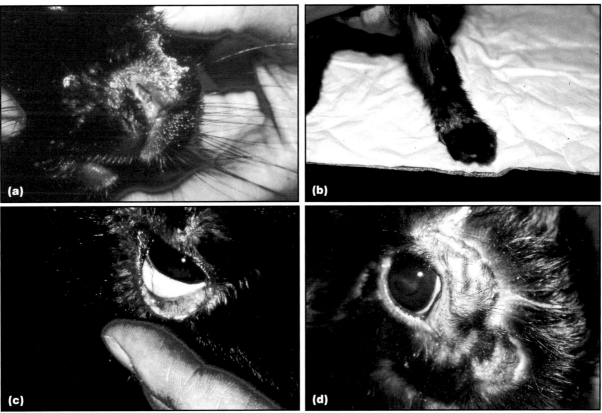

17.8 Lesions of rabbit syphilis (*Treponema paraluis cuniculi*) on **(a)** the muzzle, **(b)** the foreleg and **(c)** the eyelids. **(d)** The same rabbit 1 week after treatment with systemic penicillin.

Necrobacillosis (Schmorl's disease)

This is an uncommon skin infection caused by *Fusobacterium necrophorum*. This organism is commonly found in rabbit faeces, and disease results from faecal contamination of wounds. Swelling, inflammation, abscessation, ulceration and necrosis occur, usually on the face and neck, and occasionally the feet. Underlying bone can sometimes be involved. Diagnosis is by bacterial culture. Treatment involves debridement and antibiosis. One suggested regime is penicillin at 40,000 IU/kg/day s.c. for 10–30 days (Jenkins, 2001). Tetracycline (Scott *et al.*, 2001) and antibiotic-impregnated polymethylmethacrylate (PMMA) beads have also been used (Jenkins, 2001).

Fungal skin disease

Trichophyton mentagrophytes is the dermatophyte most commonly isolated from guinea pigs and rabbits, but *Microsporum canis* has also been reported (Donnelly *et al.*, 2000). Other dermatophytes cultured from the skin of rabbits are *T. verrucosum*, *M. nanum*, *M. gypseum*, *M. persicolor* and *M. distortum*. Infection can cause hair loss and crusting lesions, especially around the eyes and nose and on the extremities. Asymptomatic carriage appears to be uncommon: a recent study by Kraemer *et al.* (2012) of 1021 rabbits with suspected dermatophytosis found that *T. mentagrophytes* was the most common fungal species isolated (72.3% of 83 positive cultures), but they did not isolate any dermatophytes from healthy animals. In another study, *T. mentagrophytes* was cultured from the coat of 4 out of 104 healthy rabbits (Vangeel *et al.*, 2000).

Diagnosis is made by microscopic examination of the hair shaft and by fungal culture. Although most infections are self-limiting, treatment is generally recommended owing to the zoonotic risk. Treatment options are similar to those for other domestic animals, and topical treatment of the affected areas only is not recommended because the dermatophyte will not necessarily be confined to these areas. Rabbits often find therapies that involve bathing stressful, so systemic treatments may be preferable. Oral itraconazole (5–10 mg/kg q24h) and terbinafine (10 mg/kg q24h) are anecdotally reported to be successful. Oral griseofulvin is also effective (15–25 mg/kg q24h) but it is teratogenic and high doses have been associated with bone marrow suppression and panleucopenia (Donnelly *et al.*, 2000). Topical treatments include lime/sulphur dips (1:32 dilution), and enilconazole 0.2% twice weekly. As in other species, treatment should be continued until monthly fungal cultures are negative twice in succession. Disinfection of the environment is also important, by vacuuming, cleaning with sodium hypochlorite or fogging with enilconazole or F10.

Focal topical treatment of visibly affected areas alone is not recommended, as the dermatophytes can also be present in areas that appear unaffected. Although most dermatophyte infections will ultimately be self-limiting in rabbits, treatment is recommended because of the zoonotic implications.

Viral skin disease

Myxomatosis

Myxomatosis is caused by the myxoma virus, a double-stranded DNA poxvirus. The natural hosts are wild jungle rabbits (*Sylvilagus brasiliensis*) in South and Central America, and wild brush rabbits (*Sylvilagus bachmani*) in California. In these rabbits, myxoma virus causes a cutaneous fibroma, and no systemic disease. However, in the domestic rabbit (*Oryctolagus cuniculus*) myxomatosis is a severe and almost invariably fatal systemic disease. It was first described in laboratory rabbits in Uruguay in 1896. In 1950 the virus was released into Australia as a means of controlling wild *Oryctolagus cuniculus*. It was initially highly effective but subsequent emergence of attenuated strains and genetically resistant rabbits have reduced its impact. In 1952 the disease was introduced to France to control rabbits, and it spread to continental Europe and the UK. It has also been released by humans on sub-Antarctic islands, in Chile, Argentina, and unsuccessfully in New Zealand. The disease is not generally seen as a clinical problem in domestic rabbits in the USA, although it has been described in California and Oregon.

The incubation period is 8–21 days. Clinical signs depend on viral strain, route of inoculation and host immune status, and include swelling of the eyelids and genitals, a milky ocular discharge, pyrexia, lethargy, depression and anorexia. More generalized swelling of the face and ears occurs, and skin nodules up to 1 cm in diameter may be found on the face and body (Figure 17.9). Death usually occurs within 14 days and is thought to be due to overwhelming bacterial infection. There are anecdotal reports of

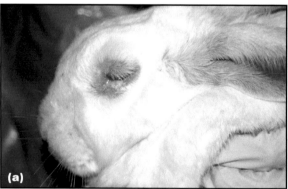

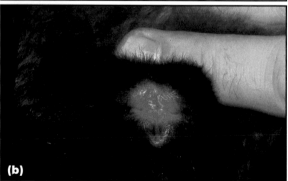

17.9 Myxomatosis, showing typical lesions of **(a)** facial swelling and **(b)** vulval swelling.

successful treatment of some carefully selected cases. Antibiotics, NSAIDs, high ambient temperature and good nursing care have been used. However, given the severe and distressing nature of the condition and the very poor prognosis, euthanasia is generally recommended on humane grounds.

In rabbits infected with attenuated, less virulent strains of the virus, the lesions seen can be similar to those described above, but are more variable, generally milder and the time course may be delayed and prolonged. Many rabbits will survive and the cutaneous lesions gradually scab and slough, leaving scarring.

A milder form of the disease is also seen in previously vaccinated rabbits. These often present with a scabbing lesion on the bridge of the nose and around the eyes (Figure 17.10), or multiple cutaneous masses over the body. Affected animals often survive with nursing care. Diagnosis is based on clinical signs and histopathology. Virus isolation can confirm the diagnosis.

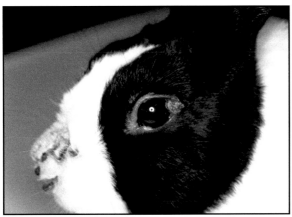

17.10 Vaccinated rabbit with milder form of myxomatosis. (Courtesy of D Scarff)

The virus is transmitted passively by blood-feeding arthropods, usually the rabbit flea and the mosquito. The virus does not replicate within the vector. The virus replicates at the inoculation site and spreads within leucocytes to the regional lymph node, where it replicates further and disseminates to the skin, spleen, other lymph nodes, mucosal surfaces, testes, lungs and liver. Although the virus is also shed in discharges, transmission by close contact is very unusual.

Control is mainly by vaccination, and a variety of vaccines are available depending on country. In the UK and Europe a novel bivalent vectored vaccine is available for protection against both myxomatosis and rabbit haemorrhagic disease (RHD). Attention should also be given to control of vectors, with the use of insect-proof screening for outdoor rabbits, and flea control. Fleas brought in by cats may infect indoor rabbits. Contact with wild rabbits should be avoided.

Shope papilloma virus
The Shope papilloma virus occurs in wild Californian brush rabbits (*Sylvilagus bachmani*) and cottontails (*S. floridanus*). Infection of domestic rabbits

(*Oryctolagus cuniculus*) is rare but has been reported, causing multiple horn-like lesions around the ears and eyelids. Manual removal results in healing in wild rabbits, but in domestic rabbits experimental infection resulted in approximately 75% of inoculation sites undergoing malignant transformation to squamous cell carcinoma.

Shope fibroma virus
The Shope fibroma virus is a naturally occurring poxvirus of North and South American wild rabbits (*Sylvilagus* spp.). Domestic rabbits are occasionally infected via mosquito vectors and develop fibromas which slough away about 30 days after inoculation. Newborn and young animals develop more extensive lesions. A live attenuated Shope fibroma virus can be used as a myxomatosis vaccine but this has been largely superseded by a new bivalent vectored vaccine for both myxomatosis and RHD.

Environmental and behavioural conditions

Ulcerative pododermatitis
This is a chronic ulcerative granulomatous dermatitis of the metatarsal area (Figure 17.11) seen generally in overweight inactive rabbits kept on wet bedding or grid floors. Occasionally the metacarpal area can be affected. Hereditary factors are also thought to be involved and Rex rabbits are particularly affected because they lack protective guard hairs. Increased pressure on the skin closely overlying bone leads to ischaemia and necrosis. Secondary bacterial infection, commonly with *Staphylococcus aureus*, occurs, which can progress to an osteomyelitis. Infection of the synovial structures can result in displacement of the superficial flexor tendon. Treatment involves addressing the initiating cause, combined with surgical debridement and cleaning of the lesions. Topical and systemic antibiotic therapy should be administered and protective dressings applied, although these may not be well tolerated. Analgesic and anti-inflammatory medications should also be provided. Lesions are difficult to resolve and a guarded prognosis should be given for rabbits suffering from osteomyelitis and tendon displacement.

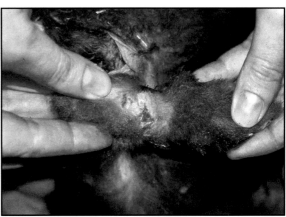

17.11 Pododermatitis on the plantar surface of the hindlimb.

Barbering and excessive grooming

These can occur in rabbits but are not common problems. Rabbits can be barbered by dominant animals (Hillyer, 1997; Scarff, 2000) but it is more likely to be performed by a subordinate companion (Jenkins, 2001). Self-barbering may occur in does in oestrus or rabbits on a low-fibre diet. Excessive grooming is a rare behavioural problem.

Self-mutilation

Compulsive self-mutilation has been seen as a genetic problem in highly inbred Checkered cross rabbits (Iglauer *et al.*, 1995) and subsequent to intramuscular ketamine and xylazine use (Beyers *et al.*, 1991).

Reproductive behaviour

It is normal for does to pluck hair from the dewlap to line the nest and from around the nipples to expose them.

Neoplasia

Shope fibroma virus and Shope papilloma virus are oncogenic (see Viral skin disease and Chapter 18). Spontaneous non-viral cutaneous neoplasia is rare in rabbits. In one study, trichoblastomas (basal cell tumours) were the most common cutaneous neoplasm (Mauldin and Goldschmidt, 2002). Cutaneous lymphoma has been described in rabbits (Hinton and Regan, 1978; White *et al.*, 2000; Mauldin and Goldschmidt, 2002).

Squamous cell carcinoma, sebaceous gland carcinoma, basal cell carcinoma, malignant melanoma and papilloma are other cutaneous neoplasms reported in the rabbit (Scott *et al.*, 2001; Mauldin and Goldschmidt, 2002).

Miscellaneous conditions

Urine scald

Urine scald is a common problem, due to urinary incontinence or the rabbit adopting an incorrect stance to urinate owing to musculoskeletal problems (e.g. spondylosis, spondylitis, arthritis, pododermatitis; see Chapter 13). Once urine scalding is present a vicious circle can develop, where painful perineal skin will make the rabbit reluctant to adopt the normal stance for urination, and it will sit in a pool of urine, thus exacerbating the scalding effect. Initial treatment should be to clip the soiled fur from the perineum, tail and hindlegs. The rabbit may require sedation during this procedure. The affected skin should then be cleaned and dried and topical dermatological antibiotic, anti-inflammatory and barrier products applied. Systemic antibiotic therapy should be provided if there is associated secondary pyoderma. Analgesics should be administered and the animal provided with clean dry bedding. The underlying cause of the urine scalding must then be investigated and addressed.

Eosinophilic granuloma

An eosinophilic granuloma-like lesion, identified as a type II eosinophilic plaque, has been reported in a New Zealand White rabbit (Henriksen, 1983). The author has seen one confirmed case of eosinophilic granuloma in a mixed-breed house rabbit (unpublished; Figure 17.12). The clinical presentation involved self-mutilation of the ventral abdomen, weight loss, and an erythematous, necrotic, ulcerative well-demarcated lesion stretching from the umbilicus to the perineum. *Cheyletiella* mites and eggs were found in scrapings taken from the edge of the lesion. Complete resolution was achieved with a depot injection of methylprednisolone acetate and treatment of the mites with ivermectin.

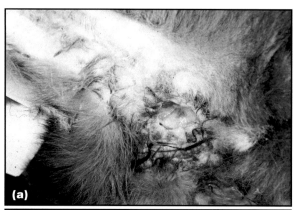

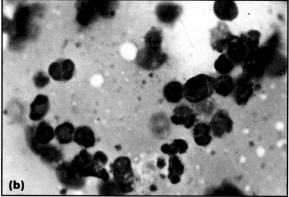

17.12 **(a)** Eosinophilic granuloma on the ventral abdomen. **(b)** Impression smear of the lesion, showing large numbers of eosinophils.

Sebaceous adenitis

Sebaceous adenitis has been reported in rabbits (White *et al.*, 2000; Jassies-van der Lee, 2008). Non-pruritic scaling, flaking and alopecia occur. Histopathology shows absence of sebaceous glands and replacement with perifollicular lymphocytic infiltrate, hyperkeratosis, follicular keratosis and dystrophy, and perifollicular fibrosis. The aetiology is unknown, but it is most likely due to an autoimmune reaction directed at the sebaceous glands and a defect in lipid metabolism. In one report (White *et al.*, 2000) treatment was attempted in two cases with retinoids and essential fatty acids, but was not effective. Treatment with ciclosporin and medium-chain triglyceride solution, combined with essential fatty acids and topical propylene glycol sprays, resulted in regression of skin lesions (Jassies-van der Lee, 2008). Sebaceous adenitis has been linked to the presence of thymoma in rabbits (Florizoone, 2005).

Cutaneous asthenia

Cutaneous asthenia due to a collagen defect similar to Ehlers–Danlos syndrome has been reported in the rabbit (Harvey *et al.*, 1990). The skin had increased extensibility and was prone to tearing.

Raised skin patches

Raised skin patches can occur during hair growth as rabbits age (Collins, 1987). Hair growth waves become less frequent and patchy and these irregular patches appear as thickened islands of skin that are redder and more vascular than surrounding areas. These changes are due to increasing follicular size and enlargement of the cutaneous vascular phase during anagen.

Dermal fibrosis

Dermal fibrosis has been reported in two entire male rabbits exhibiting cutaneous thickening on the dorsum (Hargreaves and Hartley, 2000; Mackay, 2000). No associated pruritus or alopecia was present. The histological appearance in one case was similar to that seen in biopsy samples from the cheek skin of entire male cats, and the lesion may be hormonally related.

Nutritional skin disease

This is extremely rare in pet rabbits but experimentally induced zinc and copper deficiency have been associated with alopecia, scaling and depigmentation of the hair.

References and further reading

Bennett H (2001) *Coenurus* cyst in a pet rabbit. *Veterinary Record* **147**, 428

Beyers TM, Richardson JA and Prince MD (1991) Axonal degeneration and self-mutilation as a complication of intramuscular use of ketamine and xylazine in rabbits. *Laboratory Animal Science* **41**(5), 519–520

Birke LL, Molina PE, Baker DG, *et al.* (2009) Comparison of selamectin and imidacloprid plus permethrin in eliminating *Leporacarus gibbus* infestation in laboratory rabbits (*Oryctolagus cuniculus*). *Journal of the American Association of Laboratory Animal Science* **48**(6), 757–762

Bourdeau PG, Fain A and Fromeaux-Cau C (2001) An original dermatosis in a rabbit (*Oryctolagus cuniculus*) due to a newly discovered mite *Psorobia lagomorphae* nov. subsp. In: *Proceedings of the 17th European Society of Veterinary Dermatology and European College of Veterinary Dermatology Congress*, p.188. [abstract]

Carpenter JW, Dryden MW and Kukanich B (2012) Pharmacokinetics, efficacy, and adverse effects of selamectin following topical administration in flea-infested rabbits. *American Journal of Veterinary Research* **73**(4), 562–566

Collins BR (1987) Dermatologic disorders of common small nondomestic animals. In: *Contemporary Issues in Small Animal Practice, vol. 8 Dermatology*, ed. GH Nesbitt, pp.235–294. Churchill Livingstone, New York

Donnelly TM, Rush EM and Lackner PA (2000) Ringworm in small exotic pets. *Seminars in Avian and Exotic Pet Medicine* **9**, 82–93

Farmaki R, Koutinas AF, Papazahariadou MG, Kasabalis D and Day MJ (2009) Effectiveness of a selamectin spot-on formulation in rabbits with sarcoptic mange. *Veterinary Record* **164**(14), 431–432

Florizoone K (2005) Thymoma-associated exfoliative dermatitis in a rabbit. *Veterinary Dermatology* **16**, 281–284

Fountain K (2000) *Coenurus serialis* in a pet rabbit. *Veterinary Record* **147**, 340

Hansen O, Gall Y, Pfister K and Beck W (2005) Efficacy of a formulation containing imidacloprid and moxidectin against naturally occurring acquired ear mite infestations (*Psoroptes cuniculi*) in rabbits. *International Journal of Applied Research in Veterinary Medicine* **3**, 281–286

Hargreaves J and Hartley NJW (2000) Dermal fibrosis in a rabbit. *Veterinary Record* **147**, 400

Harvey RG (1990) *Demodex cuniculi* in dwarf rabbits (*Orytolagus cuniculus*). *Journal of Small Animal Practice* **31**, 204–207

Harvey RG, Brown PF, Young RD and Whitbread TJ (1990) A connective tissue defect in two rabbits similar to the Ehlers-Danlos syndrome. *Veterinary Record* **126**, 130–132

Henriksen P (1983) Eosinophilic granuloma like lesion in a rabbit. *Nordic Veterinary Medicine* **35**, 243–244

Hillyer EV (1997) Dermatologic diseases. In: *Ferrets, Rabbits and Rodents: Clinical Medicine and Surgery*, ed. EV Hillyer and KE Quesenberry, pp.212–219. WB Saunders, Philadelphia

Hinton H and Regan M (1978) Cutaneous lymphoma in a rabbit. *Veterinary Record* **103**, 140–141

Hutchinson MJ, Jacobs DE, Bell GD and Mencke N (2001) Evaluation of imidacloprid for the treatment and prevention of cat flea (*Ctenocephalides felis felis*) infestations on rabbits. *Veterinary Record* **148**, 695–696

Iglauer F, Beig C, Dimigen J, *et al.* (1995) Hereditary compulsive self-mutilating behaviour in laboratory rabbits. *Laboratory Animals* **29**, 385–393

Jassies-van der Lee A, von Zeeland Y, Kik M and Schoemaker N (2008) Successful treatment of sebaceous adenitis in a rabbit with ciclosporin and triglycerides. *Veterinary Dermatology* **20**(1), 67–71

Jenkins JR (2001) Skin disorders of the rabbit. *Veterinary Clinics of North America: Exotic Animal Practice* **4**(2), 543–563

Kim SH, Lee JY, Jun HK, *et al.* (2008) Efficacy of selamectin in the treatment of cheyletiellosis in pet rabbits. *Veterinary Dermatology* **19**(1), 26–27

Kraemer A, Mueller RS, Werckenthin C, Straubinger RK and Hein J (2012) Dermatophytes in pet guinea pigs and rabbits. *Veterinary Microbiology* **157**(1–2), 208–213

Kurtdede A, Karaer Z, Acar A, *et al.* (2007) Use of selamectin for the treatment of psoroptic and sarcoptic mite infestation in rabbits. *Veterinary Dermatology* **18**(1), 18–22

Mackay R (2000) Dermal fibrosis in a rabbit. *Veterinary Record* **147**, 252

Mauldin EA and Goldschmidt MH (2002) A retrospective study of cutaneous neoplasms in domestic rabbits (1990–2001). *Veterinary Dermatology* **13**, 214

Pinter L (1999) *Leporacarus gibbus* and *Spilopsyllus cuniculi* infestation in a pet rabbit. *Journal of Small Animal Practice* **40**, 220–221

Scarff DH (2000) Dermatoses. In: *BSAVA Manual of Rabbit Medicine and Surgery*, ed. PA Flecknell, pp.69–79. BSAVA Publications, Gloucester

Scott DW, Miller WH and Griffin CE (2001) Dermatoses of pet rodents, rabbits and ferrets. In: *Muller and Kirk's Small Animal Dermatology, 6th edn*, pp.1415–1458. WB Saunders, Philadelphia

Vangeel I, Pasmans F, Vanrobaeays M, De Herdt P and Haesebrouck F (2000) Prevalence of dermatophytes in asymptomatic guinea pigs and rabbits. *Veterinary Record* **146**, 440–441

White S, Campbell T, Logan A, *et al.* (2000) Lymphoma with cutaneous involvement in three domestic rabbits. *Veterinary Dermatology* **11**, 61–67

White SD, Bourdeau PJ and Meredith A (2003) Dermatologic problems of rabbits. *Compendium on Continuing Education for the Practicing Veterinarian* **25**(2), 90–101

White SD, Linder KE, Schultheiss P, *et al.* (2000) Sebaceous adenitis in four domestic rabbits. *Veterinary Dermatology* **11**, 53–60

Wills J (2001) Coenurosis in a pet rabbit. *Veterinary Record* **148**, 188

Zrimsek P, Kos J, Pinter L and Drobnic-Kosork M (1999) Detection by ELISA of the humoral immune response in rabbits naturally infected with *Trichophyton mentagrophytes*. *Veterinary Microbiology* **70**, 77–86

18

Neoplasia

Molly Varga

Neoplasia has previously been reported as being a rare finding in rabbits. With the increase in numbers of rabbits being kept as pets, and longer life spans, as well as the high expectations of owners regarding the veterinary care provided, more reports of neoplastic disease and its treatment are being published. Nevertheless, much of the information available currently is based on extrapolation from other species and anecdotal reports. One study suggested that 20% of rabbits over 3 years old had some type of neoplastic disease (Heatley and Smith, 2007).

Neoplasia is defined as the abnormal proliferation of cells, which is uncontrolled and not synchronized with surrounding tissues (Figure 18.1). This leads either to a solid mass of abnormal cells within a tissue (tumour or neoplasm), or a population of abnormal cells in the circulation. Neoplastic disease can be further categorized according to the expected behaviour of the disease. Benign neoplasia (e.g. squamous papilloma) refers to an abnormal proliferation of cells that is localized, well circumscribed and does not spread around the body. Benign tumours do not transform into malignancies (cancer). Pre-cancerous neoplasia (e.g. carcinoma *in situ*) does not invade local tissue; however, given time it will transform into malignant disease. Malignant neoplasia often invades and destroys local tissues and has the potential to form secondary metastases at distant locations (e.g. uterine adenocarcinoma).

Types of neoplasia

Rabbits can suffer from many types of neoplastic disease. Those that have been reported are shown in Figure 18.2.

Term	Definition
Hypertrophy	An increase in cell size not cell numbers. This change is reversible. Does not progress to neoplasia
Hyperplasia	An increase in cell numbers but not size. Cells remain differentiated and tissue architecture is defined. Occurs in response to physiological demands or injury and does not usually progress to neoplasia. This change is reversible
Metaplasia	A preneoplastic change that involves transformation of one differentiated cell type into another. This type of preneoplastic change can be retained during the progression to neoplasia
Dysplasia	An abnormal pattern of cell growth. This preneoplastic change may progress to true neoplasia

18.1 Terms used in the description of abnormal cell proliferation.

Body system	Tissue of origin	Tumour types reported
Integument	Skin; ears; eyelids; lips	Squamous cell carcinoma; basal cell carcinoma; sebaceous adenocarcinoma; trichoepithelioma; malignant melanoma; squamous papilloma; apocrine carcinoma. Skin tumours also associated with Shope papilloma virus, Shope fibroma virus, myxoma virus
Gastrointestinal tract	Stomach, intestines; exocrine pancreas; liver	Bile duct adenoma/adenocarcinoma; tumours of stomach, intestine
Musculoskeletal/ mesenchymal tissue	Bones; muscles; joint tissue; ligaments; tendons; subcutaneous connective tissue	Osteosarcoma; infiltrative myxoma of joint capsule; lipoma/liposarcoma; peripheral nerve sheath tumour; fibrosarcoma; leiomyosarcoma
Blood and lymphatic systems	Blood; lymph nodes; spleen; thymus; bone marrow	Lymphoma/lymphosarcoma; thymoma/thymosarcoma; haemangioma/ haemangiosarcoma; leukaemia

18.2 Neoplasms reported in rabbits. (continues) ▶

Body system	Tissue of origin	Tumour types reported
Nervous system	Brain; spinal cord; peripheral nerves; eyes	Neurofibrosarcoma; plasma cell tumours/myeloma; intraocular sarcoma
Endocrine system	Pituitary gland; adrenal gland; thyroid gland; endocrine pancreas	Pituitary gland eosinophilic adenoma; adrenal gland adrenocortical carcinoma; thyroid carcinoma
Respiratory system	Nasal cavities; sinuses; trachea; lungs	Adenocarcinoma of nasal mucosa; metastatic disease (metastases of any tumour, but particularly uterine adenocarcinoma)
Urogenital system	Kidney; ureters; bladder; urethra; uterus; cervices; vagina; vulva; testicles; prostate; mammary glands	Renal carcinoma; benign embryonal nephroma; uterine endometrial adenocarcinoma; uterine myometrial leiomyoma/leiomyosarcoma; mammary gland carcinoma/carcinosarcoma; testicular interstitial cell tumours; testicular Leydig cell tumours; testicular adenocarcinoma; testicular teratoma

18.2 (continued) Neoplasms reported in rabbits.

Diagnosis of neoplasia

Clinical history and physical examination

The history of a rabbit with neoplasia can be very variable and is often non-specific. Almost all potential presenting signs can also be associated with other conditions; a robust work-up is therefore indicated. Significant concerns can include:

- Inappetence
- Unexplained weight loss
- Mass lesion noted
- Gut stasis (anorexia, lack of droppings)
- Lameness/reduced mobility
- Dyspnoea
- Exercise intolerance.

Abnormalities can be coincidental findings when a rabbit is presented for routine examination. A signalment and thorough history must be completed. When obtaining a history it is important to clarify a timeframe for the changes noted, any alterations in diet (offered and eaten), any other recent illness, and to confirm neutering and vaccination status. A comparison of recent weights and gain/loss is useful and particular attention should be paid to the presence of muscle wastage (cachexia).

A full physical examination should be performed and a problem list generated, including differential diagnoses. Baseline laboratory samples (including blood and urine) should be obtained in order to have a complete overview of the health/disease status of the patient.

Diagnostic tests and imaging

The diagnostic modalities available are the same as those utilized in cats and dogs.

Haematology and biochemistry

Blood analysis should be performed as part of the initial baseline information gathering. It can also be useful in:

- Primary diagnosis of leukaemias
- Evaluation of paraneoplastic changes, e.g. hypercalcaemia (NB hypercalcaemia must be interpreted with care owing to the rabbit's usually high blood calcium levels)
- Assessment of organ function and general health.

Imaging

Radiology can be a helpful adjunct to other diagnostic methods (Figure 18.3). It is useful for:

- Assessing the extent of a lesion, as a preparation for surgery
- Screening for metastases as part of the staging process.

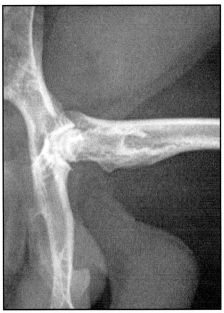

18.3 Radiograph of the proximal femur in a rabbit that had become acutely lame. The tumour eventually proved to be an osteosarcoma.

Advanced imaging (computed tomography (CT) and magnetic resonance imaging (MRI); Figure 18.4) can also be very valuable in assessing the extent and invasiveness of a lesion, and the information gained using these modalities can be far more detailed than that gained by radiography alone.

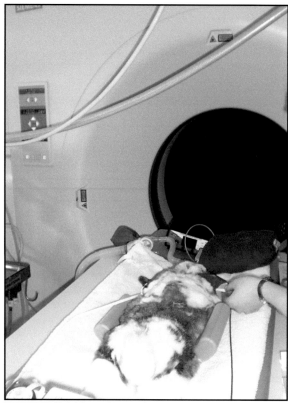

18.4 Rabbit positioned for an MRI scan. (Courtesy of K Eatwell)

Cytology

The advantages of cytological evaluation are that it is non-invasive, associated with low morbidity and provides rapid results. The disadvantages include low yield of diagnostic cells, so a diagnosis can be missed, and an inability to assess tissue architecture and invasiveness, and the mitotic index. Cytological samples may be obtained in several ways.

Fine-needle aspiration: This is a technique in which cells are aspirated from a solid mass using negative pressure applied to a needle/hypodermic syringe inserted into the mass. In most cases this technique does not require chemical restraint, and is well tolerated by rabbits. A suitably sized syringe and needle should be used for the size of both the mass and the patient.

1. After aseptic surface preparation, the mass is stabilized and the needle inserted into it.
2. Negative pressure is applied to the syringe plunger. Cells/blood may be seen in the hub of the syringe; however, even if nothing is visible, cells may have been aspirated.
3. The pressure is then gently released from the syringe plunger, the needle withdrawn slightly from the mass and redirected into another area.
4. The plunger is again pulled back.
5. This procedure is repeated four or five times, with the redirections made in a 'fan' shape.
6. At the end of the procedure, the plunger is released and the needle removed from the mass without any negative pressure being applied.

This allows the cells to remain in the hub of the needle, rather than being sucked back into the body of the syringe.

7. The needle is then removed from the syringe, the syringe filled with air and the needle replaced on the syringe.
8. The air in the syringe is used to blow the cells in the needle hub on to a microscope slide.
9. The cells blown on to the slide can then be spread using a 'squash prep' technique (see *BSAVA Guide to Procedures in Small Animal Practice*).
10. The slides can then be dried, fixed and stained before examination.

Impression smears: This technique involves exfoliating cells from the surface of an ulcerated lesion.

1. The lesion should be gently cleaned and dried and a dry microscope slide applied multiple times to the surface of the lesion.
2. The slide is touched to the lesion surface and rapidly removed.
3. The slide is then moved slightly and the procedure repeated. This is done many times (often in excess of 20) so that the resulting samples left on the microscope slide are not bloody (excess blood can make diagnosis more difficult by diluting the relevant cells) and thin enough to read newsprint through.
4. The slides can then be dried, fixed and stained prior to being evaluated (Figures 18.5 and 18.6).

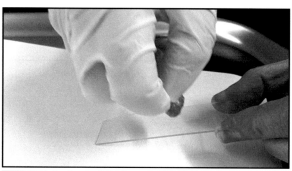

18.5 A piece of tissue removed from a lesion is being used to make an impression smear. The cut surface of the tissue is pressed on to the slide multiple times. This procedure can also be used on an ulcerated lesion on a live animal.

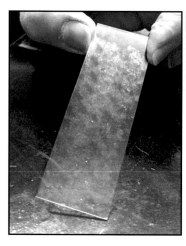

18.6 A slide with completed impression smears. This will subsequently be stained and examined under a microscope.

Cell brushing: This technique is employed when a lesion is found endoscopically. It is very suitable for use in rabbits because it is less likely to cause iatrogenic damage to delicate viscera than more invasive procedures.

1. The endoscope is used to visualize the lesion and a brush is inserted through the auxiliary port.
2. Once the tip of the brush is visualized it is manipulated towards the lesion and used to exfoliate cells from the lesion surface.
3. Once this is accomplished, the brush is withdrawn and the cells harvested are wiped off on to a clean microscope slide.
4. They can be spread using a 'squash prep' technique.

Wash/flushing techniques: These are often used for lesions in the lungs or hollow viscera.

1. The lesion is viewed endoscopically and a sterile catheter inserted in the auxiliary port of the endoscope.
2. Sterile fluid (e.g. saline) is then flushed into the area, and the animal rotated to allow the fluid to have as much contact with abnormal cells as possible.
3. The fluid is then aspirated through the catheter.
4. The resultant sample should be divided between plain and EDTA blood tubes, submitted for bacterial culture and also smeared on to a clean microscope slide for cytological evaluation.

This technique can also be attempted 'blindly'; however, the chances of sampling relevant cells are reduced if the lesion is not visualized. While the technique is suitable for rabbits in some situations it should be remembered that the rabbit lung volume is much smaller than that of a dog or cat of similar weight, so the amount of fluid instilled should be reduced accordingly.

Histology
If cytology is inconclusive then histological examination should be performed. The goal of histological examination is to harvest sufficient tissue to allow the architecture and the interface with adjacent normal cells to be evaluated. Sampling for histology requires chemical restraint in most instances and is associated with a higher morbidity and mortality than less invasive procedures. It is the 'gold standard' for diagnosis of neoplastic disease. Histological samples may be obtained in various ways.

Excisional biopsy: This is the surgical removal of a mass lesion. It is usual to attempt to remove a margin of normal tissue around the mass to reduce the likelihood of neoplastic cells being left behind. The whole mass can then be submitted for histological evaluation. The advantage of this method is that the architecture and the relationship with surrounding tissue can be evaluated. In the right case, excisional biopsy can be both diagnostic and

therapeutic. The disadvantage is that in some circumstances the removal of a primary tumour, where metastatic disease is already present, can remove inhibition on the growth of secondary tumours. This can result in clinical worsening of disease. If histology suggests that tumour-free margins have not been obtained, revision surgery is indicated. This method is the 'gold standard' for diagnosis of solid tumours. It is wholly appropriate for use in rabbits.

Incisional biopsy: This involves surgical biopsy of a mass lesion that cannot be removed in its entirety. A wedge of tissue, including both part of the mass and surrounding normal tissue, should be submitted. The advantage of this over excisional biopsy is that the surgery is less invasive. The disadvantage is that it is not therapeutic and wound healing may prove difficult.

Punch biopsy: A biopsy punch, similar to a very wide-bore needle, is used to take a core of a mass lesion. The procedure can be done after local anaesthetic infiltration/nerve blocks rather than sedation. The local anaesthetic should be infiltrated into the skin and subcutis in a ring around the lesion, and not into the lesion itself, because it can alter the architecture and affect the diagnostic value of the sample. This technique can be very useful in rabbits, because it gives maximum information with minimal invasiveness, and reduced postoperative complications.

1. The biopsy punch is pushed into a suitable portion of the lesion, perpendicular to the skin, and rotated to cut the core away from its surroundings.
2. Without withdrawal, the punch is then angled at 45 degrees to the surface of the skin and inserted a little further. This cuts the base of the core.
3. The punch is then withdrawn, with the core inside.
4. The tissue is placed into formol saline prior to histological evaluation.

Surface-biting biopsy: This technique is typically used when a lesion has been located using endoscopy. The advantage of this technique is that it is relatively non-invasive; however, often only the surface of the lesion is sampled, and relevant tissue can be missed.

1. The lesion is visualized using the endoscope and biopsy forceps are inserted through the auxiliary port of the endoscope.
2. Once the tip of the forceps is visualized, the jaws should be opened and the forceps advanced towards the lesion.
3. Once the surface of the lesion is between the jaws, these should be snapped shut and the forceps pulled sharply away, and withdrawn from the endoscope.
4. The tissue sample harvested can be placed into 10% formol saline for histology.
5. The endoscope should remain in position to monitor for bleeding and to allow several samples to be taken.

> **WARNING**
> Rabbits have very thin-walled, delicate hollow viscera, which can make the above technique more risky. Breaching the wall of the gut can cause peritonitis and potentially death.

Jamshidi bone biopsy: This is used to obtain biopsy samples of hard lesions or bone. A Jamshidi bone biopsy punch is essentially a stylet with a trench cut into it, housed inside a hollow needle (Figure 18.7). The trench in the internal stylet provides a space in which the tissue sample can sit.

1. The stylet and needle are inserted into the mass.
2. The internal stylet is advanced out of the end of the outer needle (and thus further into the mass) and the whole apparatus is rotated around its long axis, allowing tissue to be pushed into the trench.
3. The outer needle is then advanced to cover the stylet, trapping the tissue sample in the trench.
4. The whole apparatus is then withdrawn.
5. The internal stylet is advanced out of the external needle to allow the tissue sample to be removed.
6. This tissue can then be submitted for histological examination.

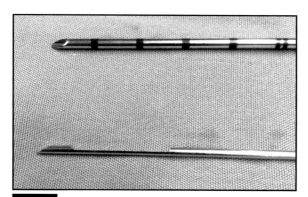

18.7 Jamshidi needle and stylet.

Staging methods
Staging is important to determine whether and where a malignancy has spread. It is usual to combine the results of several tests in order to give the most specific information. Methods include sampling of local lymph nodes, bone marrow, radiography, ultrasonography, CT and MRI (see *BSAVA Manual of Canine and Feline Oncology*).

Treatment of neoplasia

The goal of treatment is to promote the patient's welfare while treating the neoplastic disease. The risks, side effects and recovery period associated with the treatment must be balanced against the potential benefits. These decisions should be made with the owner's input, and a frank discussion of euthanasia in severe cases should take place early in this process. For some cases euthanasia is the best option.

Surgery
Surgery is the commonest treatment for neoplasia in dogs, cats and human patients and results in more cures than all other treatments combined. Surgery is not immunosuppressive, is non-carcinogenic and is more effective for large lesions than either chemotherapy or radiotherapy. Surgery is also the most commonly reported treatment for neoplasia in pet rabbits.

Excision
This technique is indicated where removal of the lesion will be associated with minimal morbidity and will preserve the functional integrity of the underlying tissue where possible, and where knowledge of the underlying tumour type would not alter the clinical decision (i.e. where the tumour is likely to be benign). Surgery should be planned such that a margin of visually normal tissue can be removed, and the overlying skin can be suitably closed. The use of reconstructive techniques including skin advancement flaps may be indicated. The whole tumour should be submitted for histology and revision surgery planned to remove a wider margin of normal tissue if necessary (Figure 18.8).

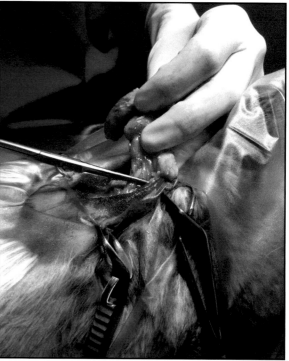

18.8 Surgical removal of a subcutaneous fibroma from the ventral chest. Note the bruising and discoloration of the overlying skin.

Debulking
This should be considered where the mass is large but not amenable to complete removal owing to size or location. It involves removal of a proportion of the mass to allow improved comfort, diagnostics, and improved success of chemotherapy, radiotherapy or intralesional therapy. Surgery should be planned to allow improved mobility, minimal morbidity and reasonable potential for healing to occur.

Chemotherapy

Systemic chemotherapy

This is the administration of antineoplastic drugs either orally or intravenously. The dose given is the maximum dose with the minimum risk of side effects. Most drugs have a therapeutic dose very close to the toxic dose, so careful dose calculation is needed. The therapeutic ratio of a drug is the toxic dose divided by the effective dose, and this value is usually small for chemotherapeutic agents, indicating how close the toxic dose is to the therapeutic dose. Chemotherapeutic doses are usually based on body surface area rather than weight, although some authors feel that dose calculations based on metabolic rate may be more appropriate in exotic species. This sort of dosage calculation is not yet validated.

Intralesional chemotherapy

This involves injecting antineoplastic drugs into and around a tumour. It allows a higher therapeutic index and reduces the likelihood of side effects. It is a simple and direct approach for treating solid tumours. However, aqueous drugs used in this manner may be rapidly cleared from the tumour site so that the length of time the tissue is exposed to the drug is short and there is systemic exposure that may result in toxicity. Currently the drug of choice is cisplatin suspended in a water/sesame oil emulsion or a collagen matrix to allow slow release of the drug locally. Cisplatin has good activity against all histological types of solid tumour and does not cause tissue necrosis.

Side effects

Chemotherapeutic drugs affect cells that are dividing. This is why side effects are often noted as gastrointestinal signs or immunosuppression (the gut lining and bone marrow divide actively at all times). In rabbits, side effects may manifest as inappetence and gut stasis, or immunosuppression allowing the expression of pre-existing subclinical infections such as pasteurellosis or encephalitozoonosis. Patients may exhibit side effects at the time of treatment or up to a few days afterwards. Those rabbits showing inappetence may require parenteral fluids and supportive care (e.g. assisted feeding, prokinetic drugs and anti-ulcer treatments). Subsequent chemotherapy doses may need to be reduced by up to 20% in order to avoid repeated problems. The degree of immunosuppression can be evaluated by monitoring white blood cell counts. Rabbits with very depressed heterophil/lymphocyte counts should have their chemotherapy delayed until the white cell levels return to normal. Concurrent infections should be treated and the animal stabilized prior to continuing chemotherapeutic treatments. Reducing chemotherapy doses or frequency will result in fewer side effects but also less efficient tumour cell destruction.

Monitoring

Routine monitoring should include pre-treatment haematology to allow decision-making regarding the suitability of the patient for treatment at a particular time. Organ function tests should also be carried out regularly (the timing will depend on the baseline parameters, the treatment being given and the site of the tumour); animals with depressed renal or liver function may have prolonged drug clearance and be at increased risk of toxicity occurring. Consideration should also be given to repeat imaging (radiography, CT, MRI) in order to repeat the tumour staging and assess for metastasis. The specifics of timing will depend on the individual patient (Figure 18.9).

Radiotherapy

This refers to the use of ionizing radiation to treat localized solid tumours. Ionizing radiation works by damaging DNA, causing cell death. The radiation will also kill surrounding normal cells, so the radiation is applied using several focused beams set up to intersect at the tumour. This ensures that the abnormal tissue will absorb a much higher radiation

Drug class	Mechanism of action	Side effects	Doses reported for rabbits
Alkylating agents (cyclophosphamide, chlorambucil, melphalan and lomustine)	Work by forming bonds between alkyl groups in biological molecules such as DNA. This affects DNA replication, and the effect is greater in cells that already have faulty DNA replication. The drugs bind directly to DNA and the effect is independent of the replication cycle	Bone marrow suppression, gastrointestinal effects, haemorrhagic cystitis (the latter would indicate that the drug should be permanently discontinued). In other species corticosteroids are given to mitigate the side effects. In rabbits steroids must be used with appropriate caution	Cyclophosphamide (for lymphoma) 50 mg/m^2 orally q24h 2–3 days per week or 100–200 mg/m^2 i.v. weekly to every 3 weeks (often combined with doxorubicin)
Anti-tumour antibiotics (e.g. doxorubicin and mitoxantrone)	Several mechanisms of action: affect DNA and RNA polymerase, can form free radicals and cause direct damage to the DNA/RNA and cell membrane, and can affect topoisomerase I that causes cleavage and rejoining of DNA during synthesis. Independent of the cell cycle	Bone marrow suppression, gastrointestinal effects, cardiomyopathy (doxorubicin). Allergic reactions reported. Corticosteroids and antihistamines can be used to counteract side effects	Doxorubicin 1 mg/kg i.v. slowly every 12 days (for lymphoproliferative disease)

18.9 Chemotherapeutic agents, their mechanism of action and usage. Body surface area may be calculated using the equation: 9.5 × (weight in grams)$^{2/3}$ (Data from Harris, 1994). (continues) ▶

Drug class	Mechanism of action	Side effects	Doses reported for rabbits
Vinca alkaloids (vincristine and vinblastine)	Inhibit intracellular microtubule formation (these are involved in producing the mitotic spindle). Specific to the phase of the cell cycle	Peripheral neuropathy that can result in constipation and ileus	Vincristine 0.5–0.7 mg/m² i.v. every 7–14 days for lymphoma
Platinum products (cisplatin and carboplatin)	Cause cross-linking between DNA strands, and are cell cycle non-specific	Nephrotoxicity (fluid therapy is required before, during and after administration), gastrointestinal effects and myelosuppression (this can be severe)	Carboplatin 150–180 mg/m² i.v. every 3–4 weeks (for carcinoma)
Crisantaspase	Degrades L-asparagine, an amino acid required for protein and DNA synthesis	Anaphylaxis and pancreatitis reported in other species	400 IU/kg i.m. or s.c. Premedicate with antihistamines to prevent anaphylaxis (for lymphoma)

18.9 (continued) Chemotherapeutic agents, their mechanism of action and usage. Body surface area may be calculated using the equation: $9.5 \times$ (weight in grams) $^{2/3}$ (Data from Harris, 1994).

dose than the surrounding tissue (Figures 18.10 and 18.11). If the tumour appears to have already spread to the local lymph nodes then these may also be included in the treatment field, and in most cases a margin of normal tissue around the mass is irradiated in an attempt to remove areas of micro-metastases. The amount of radiation delivered is measured in Greys (Gy). The total radiation dose is divided into multiple small doses (fractions) to reduce the possibility of side effects in surrounding healthy tissues. The time intervals between the fractions allow normal cells to recover, while tumour cells are generally less able to do this.

Radiotherapy can be used in order to cure a tumour, or as part of a multimodal approach that may include surgery and chemotherapy as well. It can be applied either pre- or postoperatively. In cases where the disease is terminal, radiation can be used palliatively in order to prolong good quality life. Chemotherapeutic drugs (e.g. cisplatin) may be used to enhance the sensitivity of tissues to radiation. One of the drawbacks of radiation therapy is that it requires multiple anaesthetic episodes, often within a short period of time. Different tumour types respond differently to radiation. Leukaemias and lymphomas are thought to be very sensitive, epithelial tumours are only moderately sensitive, while renal tumours and melanomas are insensitive.

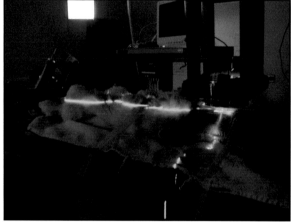

18.11 A rabbit undergoing radiotherapy. The area of interest is at the intersection of the green beams of light. (Courtesy of K Eatwell)

Side effects

Radiotherapy itself is painless; however, pain may occur a few days after treatment, associated with tissue swelling in treated areas compressing nerves. Skin irritation, similar to sunburn, may also be recognized, and may lead to self-trauma. Areas affected by radiation will heal rapidly; however, these are often less elastic than normal tissue owing to the formation of fibrous scarring. Hair loss may also be seen, and regrowth may well be white. Heart damage is reported in human patients with breast cancer because of the proximity of the heart to the irradiated area, and is a possibility in rabbits treated with radiotherapy for thymomas, for example.

Photodynamic therapy

Photodynamic therapy (PDT) involves the use of non-toxic light-sensitive compounds that become toxic on exposure to light, thereby killing malignant cells. Light-sensitive agents accumulate preferentially in neoplastic tissues and light is applied selectively to the affected areas to reduce the effect on normal tissue. PDT is a technique that is recognized as being minimally invasive and minimally toxic. It has been used most often in companion animals to treat squamous cell carcinoma; however,

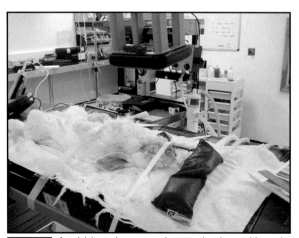

18.10 A rabbit under general anaesthesia positioned for radiotherapy. (Courtesy of K Eatwell)

the success rate has been variable. The disadvantages of PDT are the expense of the equipment required, the limited ability of this modality to treat deep tumours and the fact that the skin of many animals remains sensitive to light for a few weeks after treatment. While rabbits have been used extensively in PDT research, no published examples of its clinical use in rabbits were found.

Cryotherapy

This involves the use of cryogens (nitrous oxide or liquid nitrogen) to freeze tissues, causing cell rupture and death. Tumours found on the skin, lips, eyelids and the perianal region are particularly amenable to this type of treatment. The advantage of this type of treatment is that it does not always require multiple anaesthetic episodes (this depends on the area that is to be frozen). The disadvantage is that there can be post-freezing swelling, pain and self-trauma.

Immunotherapy

Immunotherapy is the treatment of disease by inducing, enhancing or suppressing the immune response. This treatment modality has been used with some success in certain types of cancer. Acemannan (a polysaccharide found in aloe vera) has been used to treat neoplasia in a variety of species. Acemannan causes macrophage activation, leading to release of tumour necrosis factor, interleukin-1 and interferon. Its use has been reported intratumorally and systemically, in combination with surgical debulking. Whilst acemannan has been extensively tested in rabbits and found to be safe, there are few reports of its use in clinical cases. Other immunomodulatory agents such as interferon and retinoids have been used with apparent clinical success in rabbits.

Non-steroidal anti-inflammatory drugs

Many NSAIDs have shown anti-tumour activity *in vivo*. Piroxicam in particular has documented activity against several types of tumour in dogs. The mode of action is thought to be related to the prevention of platelet aggregation or the inhibition of angiogenesis (thus restricting the potential for tumour growth). Meloxicam, a drug very commonly used in rabbit medicine, is undergoing evaluation for its use in neoplastic conditions (Wolfesberger *et al.*, 2006).

Other therapeutic considerations
Nutrition

In all species the alteration of carbohydrate, lipid and fat metabolism is a common paraneoplastic syndrome. Cachexia, the loss of muscle and fat despite adequate nutritional intake, can be the first clinical sign noted before primary signs of neoplasia are evident. Anorexia, lethargy and impaired immune function are possible consequences. Nutritional therapy is therefore very important and should be instituted early in the treatment regime. Rabbits are reliant on long-stem fibre to maintain gut motility and support the bacterial population in the caecum. Provision of *ad libitum* hay, fresh vegetables and a small amount of good quality pellets is a good basic strategy; however, some rabbits will still lose weight despite eating well. Supportive feeding can be instituted (there are several commercial formulas available) but the provision of high levels of simple carbohydrates can support tumour growth even though weight is maintained. Therefore, selection of assisted-feeding products that are higher in fibre and lower in simple carbohydrates should be advocated. In cases where anorexia is a significant problem, the placement of a nasogastric or pharyngostomy tube can be considered for supportive feeding during treatment. Nasogastric tubes are not large enough in most cases to allow the provision of a fibrous diet and, in the author's experience, can be poorly tolerated by many rabbits. Pharyngostomy tubes, being wider, do allow feeding of a more suitable diet; however, there are many reported cases of complications at the insertion site (abscessation in particular) so the expected benefits must outweigh the potential risks.

Analgesia

Many cancers are associated with significant pain, and analgesia is a vital part of the treatment plan. Pain can be mild to severe, acute, chronic or intermittent, and can be associated either with the disease itself or with the treatment given. Mild to moderate pain can be adequately controlled using NSAIDs, while more severe pain may require opiates.

Consideration can also be given to other modalities such as acupuncture. Many rabbits tolerate acupuncture well and appear to benefit from it. The use of acupuncture to relieve pain in humans with cancer is well documented, and its use in animals is becoming more widespread. The author has used acupuncture, delivered by a veterinary surgeon experienced with rabbits, with apparent good success in many cases.

Common neoplasms in rabbits

Uterine adenocarcinoma

Uterine adenocarcinoma is the commonest spontaneously occurring neoplasm of the rabbit (Figures 18.12 and 18.13). Up to 80% of non-neutered does (in those breeds that are most susceptible such as Tan, French Silver and Dutch) are reported to have pre-cancerous or cancerous uterine changes by the age of 3 years. This disease can prove fatal within 5 months of first diagnosis (up to 20 months has been reported) if untreated. Clinical signs can include anorexia, bloody urine or vulvar discharge, cystic or swollen mammary glands and a reduction in fertility in breeding does.

Uterine adenocarcinoma is prevented by ovariohysterectomy, and this also forms the basis of treatment. During the neutering operation (see *BSAVA Manual of Rabbit Surgery, Dentistry and Imaging*), the opportunity should be taken to examine the abdominal cavity for metastases. Cases that are still contained within the uterus (carcinoma *in situ*) may

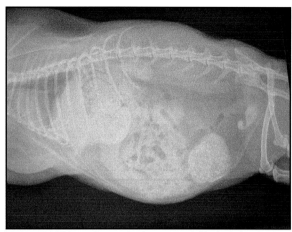

18.12 This radiograph shows a calcified abdominal mass; uterine adenocarcinoma was diagnosed on post-mortem histology.

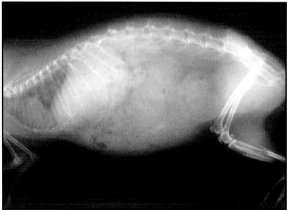

18.13 This rabbit was presented for fracture of the tibia and fibula. Radiography showed a large abdominal mass which proved to be a uterine adenocarcinoma. There were also secondary masses in the thorax.

be definitively treated by surgery, although periodic follow-up for spread should be undertaken. Cases that have spread locally have a poor prognosis, because metastatic disease has already begun. There are few reports of attempted treatment of metastatic uterine adenocarcinomatosis, and chemotherapy is generally felt to be unsuccessful. Palliative treatment with NSAIDs and additional pain relief is warranted; however, euthanasia should be considered for those cases with both local and distant metastases.

Thymoma

In contrast to other species, the thymus gland of the rabbit does not regress with age, and occupies much of the anterior thorax. Disease within the gland that causes swelling rapidly leads to clinical signs. The incidence of thymic neoplasia is low (8% of tumours in a recent survey of 55 rabbits with neoplasia; Morrisey and McEntee, 2005), and clinical signs include dyspnoea (76.9% of cases), bilateral exophthalmos (46.2% of cases) and exercise intolerance (53.9%), or may be inapparent or subtle (Kunzel *et al.*, 2012). The diagnosis relies on a combination of

radiography and cytology in the first instance (ultrasonography may also be helpful). CT imaging can be helpful for surgical planning if this is an option.

Reports of successful surgical treatment have been published, with the caution that rabbits undergoing thoracotomy require a high level of perisurgical support and the morbidity rates are high. Some thymomas appear to be easily removed surgically (see *BSAVA Manual of Rabbit Surgery, Dentistry and Imaging*) while others are not well defined and surgery is much more difficult.

Most thymomas in humans express somatostatin (growth hormone inhibiting hormone) receptors on their surface. Octreotide, a synthetic somatostatin analogue, has been used in the treatment of thymoma in humans and the author has used this in two cases of confirmed thymoma in rabbits. The drug must be given parenterally owing to poor gut absorption. In both cases an initial good response was noted, with a reduction in clinical signs and radiographic evidence of regression. However, both rabbits eventually showed side effects associated with the medication (apparent gut pain after administration, anorexia and gut stasis), to the extent that treatment was discontinued.

Other chemotherapeutic protocols are used with good success in human patients; however, few are reported in rabbits. More recently, good success has been achieved using radiation therapy in the treatment of thymoma (Guzman Sanchez-Migallon *et al.*, 2006).

Thymomas are radiosensitive and a reduction in tumour size has been documented even after a single treatment. However, reports of pulmonary fibrosis and thrombosis local to the radiation have caused long-term problems for these patients.

Lymphoma/lymphosarcoma

Lymphoma is the most common form of neoplasia in juvenile rabbits, and the second commonest in rabbits overall (Heatley and Smith, 2007). Lymphomas may be of either B-cell or T-cell origin. Clinical signs may be very non-specific, including anorexia, lethargy, depression, cutaneous ulcerated nodules, bilateral blepharitis, diarrhoea and peripheral lymphadenopathy. At diagnosis, lymphoma is already believed to be a systemic disease, although a single case of isolated skin lymphosarcoma has been reported (White *et al.*, 2000). A leukaemic form has been recognized, associated with an increase in total white cell count or lymphocytosis in addition to organ infiltration with cells of myelogenous origin (White *et al.*, 2000).

Owing to its systemic nature, lymphoma is treated with a combination of surgery and chemotherapy in other species, and this strategy is suggested for rabbits. Although no specific chemotherapeutic protocols have been published, drugs that have published doses for rabbits (e.g. cyclophosphamide, carboplatin, vincristine) can be used with appropriate caution and supportive care. Interferon and isotretinoin have been used to treat cutaneous lymphoma (with systemic involvement), but without success (White *et al.*, 2000).

Viral associated tumours

Shope fibroma virus, Shope papilloma virus and myxoma virus all cause tumours in rabbits (see also Chapter 17). A 'malignant rabbit fibroma virus' has been isolated that is thought to be a recombinant combination of fibroma and myxoma viruses. This virus leads to immunosuppression and malignant tumours (Strayer *et al.*, 1983).

Shope papilloma virus

Shope papilloma virus causes keratinous carcinomas on or around the head that can be large enough to prevent the rabbit from eating. It can occur in both pet rabbits (*Oryctolagus cuniculus*) and cottontails (*Sylvilagus* spp.). The virus is a member of the Papovaviridae and may be spread by biting insects. The nodules caused may become malignant and should therefore be surgically removed. Insect control is the best way to prevent infection.

Shope fibroma virus

Shope fibroma virus, a poxvirus, is also spread by biting insects. The virus is endemic in wild rabbits in North America. The disease occurs sporadically in pet rabbits. It leads to fibromatous growths on the feet and legs primarily, and to a lesser extent the face and back. These growths can be up to 7 cm in diameter and their size can impede mobility and eating. These tumours do not become malignant and usually resolve in 12–14 months in wild rabbits (*Sylvilagus, Lepus*) but more rapidly in *Oryctolagus* spp. Generalized fibromatosis can occur in immunocompromised or newborn rabbits. The tumours must be differentiated histologically for a definitive diagnosis; however, fibromas are usually flat and subcutaneous, while papillomas are wart-like and keratinized. Supportive care may be required and surgical resection considered if the size or position of the tumour significantly affects the welfare of the rabbit.

Myxoma virus

This poxvirus causes a life-threatening systemic disease in *Oryctolagus cuniculus*, but a mild cutaneous disease in its natural hosts *Sylvilagus brasiliensis* and *S. bachmani*. Transmission is via insect vectors or direct contact. Early skin lesions take the form of oedema which spreads around the eyelids, nose and face. Nodules on the body, face and legs appear after 10–14 days. These nodules can be large and necrotic. In an immunocompetent rabbit these will resolve in 3–4 weeks. Depending on the strain involved death can occur within 4 days to 5 weeks of infection, due to the wide ranging effects of the viraemia and overwhelming secondary infection. Occasionally rabbits will survive this infection, and supportive care, pain relief and appropriate antibiosis are helpful.

Rabbits that have been previously vaccinated against myxomatosis will occasionally contract 'atypical myxomatosis' after exposure to a natural myxoma infection (see Chapter 17). This infection is usually not fatal; however, the rabbit will exhibit scabbing around the eyes and nose and may develop multiple skin nodules over the body. These nodules will often regress over time and do not necessarily require treatment unless they are causing pain or distress to the rabbit, in which case surgical resection can be considered.

References and further reading

Finkelstein A and Cassone L (2007) Testicular interstitial cell neoplasia in a rabbit. *Exotic DVM* 9(3), 15–16
Graham JE, Kent MS and Theon A (2004) Current therapies in exotic animal oncology. *Veterinary Clinics of North America: Exotic Animal Practice* 7, 757–781
Green HSN (1939) Familial mammary tumours in the rabbit. *Journal of Experimental Medicine* 70, 167–188
Guzman Sanchez-Migallon D, Mayer J, Gould J and Azuma C (2006) Radiation therapy for the treatment of thymoma in rabbits (*Oryctolagus cuniculus*). *Journal of Exotic Pet Medicine* 15(2), 138–144
Harris I (1994) The laboratory rabbit. *ANZCCART News*, 7(4), 1–8
Heatley JJ and Smith AN (2007) Spontaneous neoplasms of lagomorphs. *Veterinary Clinics of North America: Exotic Animal Practice* 7, 561–577
Irazarry-Rovira AR, Lennox AM and Ramos-Vara JA (2008) Granular cell tumour in the testis of a rabbit: cytologic, histologic, immunohistochemical and electron microscopic characterisation. *Veterinary Pathology* 45, 73–77
Kent MS (2004) The use of chemotherapy in exotic animals. *Veterinary Clinics of North America: Exotic Animal Practice* 7, 807–820
Kunzel F, Hittmair KM, Hassan J, et al. (2012) Thymoma in rabbits: clinical evaluation, diagnosis and treatment. *Journal of the American Animal Hospital Association* 48(2), 97–104
Lennox AM and Chitty J (2006) Adrenal neoplasia and hyperplasia as a cause of hypertesteronism in 2 rabbits. *Journal of Exotic Pet Medicine* 15(1), 56–58
Lohr CV, Hedge ZN and Pool RR (2012) Infiltrative myxoma of the stifle joint and thigh in a domestic rabbit (*Oryctolagus cuniculus*). *Journal of Comparative Pathology* 147, 218–222
Maratea KA, Ramos-Vara JA and Corriveau LA (2007) Testicular cell tumour and gynaecomastia in a rabbit. *Veterinary Pathology* 44, 513
McPherson L, Newman SJ, McLean N, et al. (2009) Intraocular sarcoma in two rabbits. *Journal of Veterinary Diagnostic Investigation* 21, 547
Meher SJ and Bennet RA (2004) Surgical oncology of exotic animals. *Veterinary Clinics of North America: Exotic Animal Practice* 7, 783–805
Morrisey JK and McEntee M (2005) Therapeutic options for thymoma in the rabbit. *Seminars in Avian and Exotic Pet Medicine* 14(3), 175–181
Nisker JA, Kirk ME and Nunez-Troconis JT (1988) Reduced incidence of rabbit endometrial neoplasia with levonorgestrel implant. *American Journal of Obstetrics and Gynecology* 158(2), 300–303
Shahbazfar AA, Mohammadpour H and Isfahani HRE (2012) Mammary gland carcinosarcoma in a New Zealand White rabbit (*Oryctolagus cuniculus*). *Acta Scientiae Veterinariae* 40(1), 1025
Strayer DS, Skaletsky E, Cabirac GF, et al. (1983) Malignant rabbit fibroma virus: observations on the culture and histopathologic characteristics of a new virus-induced rabbit tumour. *Journal of the National Cancer Institute* 71(1), 105–116
von Bomhard W (2007) Cutaneous neoplasms in pet rabbits: a retrospective study. *Veterinary Pathology* 44, 579
Weiss ATA and Muller K (2011) Spinal osteolytic osteosarcoma in a pet rabbit. *Veterinary Record* 168, 266
White SD, Logan A, Meredith A, et al. (2000) Lymphoma with cutaneous involvement in three domestic rabbits (*Oryctolagus cuniculus*). *Veterinary Dermatology* 11, 61–67
Wolfesberger B, Hoelzl C, Walter I, et al. (2006) Antineoplastic effect of cyclo-oxygenase inhibitor meloxicam on canine osteosarcoma cells. *Research in Veterinary Science* 80(3), 308–316

19

Endocrine disease

Angela M. Lennox and Kellie A. Fecteau

There are few published reports of endocrine disease in pet rabbits, which suggests that endocrine disease is either uncommon or underdiagnosed in this species. Therefore, few endocrine testing procedures and hormone reference intervals have been established for rabbits. The majority of endocrine cases presented in this chapter involve either adrenal gland dysfunction or gonadal issues in neutered rabbits. Other endocrinopathies may exist in rabbits but are not diagnosed owing to a lack of information. The majority of information used for this chapter was obtained from veterinary teaching hospital files and from personal communications with veterinary surgeons who submitted the cases.

Pancreatic endocrine disease

Rabbits are often used as models for diabetes in humans. Diabetes can be experimentally induced in the laboratory rabbit with various agents, including alloxan (Wojtowicz *et al.*, 2004). In rabbits with experimentally induced diabetes, hyperglycaemia is accompanied by marked increases in triglyceride and cholesterol levels. Cases of naturally occurring diabetes in pet rabbits have not been documented in the literature. However, spontaneous diabetes has been described in a female laboratory New Zealand White rabbit with polyuria and polydipsia, and blood glucose levels between 540 and 590 mg/dl (Roth *et al.*, 1980; Conaway *et al.*, 1981). Inbreeding of this rabbit with her offspring produced a colony of diabetic rabbits characterized by loss of beta cell mass and markedly decreased insulin secretion. Of all the offspring, 19% were overtly diabetic with fasting glucose levels between 150 and 620 mg/dl (8.3–34.4 mmol/l). Features of the disease in these rabbits included relatively late onset (1–3 years), severe hyperglycaemia, depressed insulin secretion without ketoacidosis, and lack of obesity. Insulin therapy corrected hyperglycaemia in affected individuals from this group (Conaway *et al.*, 1981).

Glucose levels in normal rabbits can be very high, especially in response to stress, and can result in non-pathological glucosuria. Confirmation of hyperglycaemia requires repeated identification of glucose outside the reference range, ideally with minimization of stress and handling. Measurement of serum fructosamine will help to distinguish stress hyperglycaemia from the persistent hyperglycaemia of diabetes mellitus. A fructosamine reference range (188–349 μm/l) has been established for healthy rabbits (Harpole *et al.*, 2002).

Reference ranges for glucose in rabbits vary. Harcourt-Brown and Harcourt-Brown (2012) determined blood glucose concentrations in non-stressed, non-fasted healthy pet rabbits to range between 4.3 and 15 mmol/l (77.4–270 mg/dl), using a portable glucometer. In this same study, one rabbit with confirmed insulinoma (a pancreatic beta cell tumour resulting in hypoglycaemia) had a blood glucose concentration of 1.2 mmol/l (21.6 mg/dl).

Published reports of insulinoma in pet rabbits are scarce. An insulinoma was identified in the pancreas of a 10-year-old spayed New Zealand White rabbit with sudden onset of grand mal seizures and bilateral cataracts (Cheryl Greenacre, personal communication). Blood glucose was analysed using a hand-held glucometer and was below the detection limit of the device (<10 mg/dl; <0.05 mmol/l). Emergency treatment included an intravenous infusion of a single bolus of dextrose and a 5% dextrose solution. After 6 hours of lateral recumbency, continuing seizures and lack of response to intravenous dextrose (blood glucose never read above 'Lo' on the glucometer), the rabbit was euthanased; the diagnosis was based on post-mortem examination and histopathology.

Adrenal endocrine disease

Six cases of spontaneous adrenal hyperplasia or neoplasia have been described in neutered pet rabbits (Lennox, 2013; Marcy Souza, personal communication). Age of onset was between 6 and 10 years of age, with four male and two female affected rabbits reported. Clinical signs included unusual aggression and chasing and/or mounting other pets or humans; one rabbit also had an enlarged clitoris which may have been influenced by high testosterone concentration. All cases demonstrated elevated serum testosterone and one rabbit also had an elevated progestin concentration.

Reference ranges for sex hormones, including progesterone, testosterone, androstenedione and 17-hydroxyprogesterone, for neutered male and female rabbits were established by Fecteau *et al.* in 2007 (Figure 19.1). The six reported cases were confirmed via histopathology at surgery or post-mortem examination, and the results included adrenocortical

Hormone	Reference interval in ng/ml (nmol/l)
Androstenedione	0.80–4.00 (2.79–13.96)
Cortisol	4.64–11.20 (12.80–30.91)
Progesterone	0.11–0.46 (0.35–1.46)
17-Hydroxyprogesterone	0.75–22.20 (2.27–67.26)
Testosterone	0.02–0.04 (0.07–0.14)

19.1 Serum steroid concentrations in healthy neutered rabbits. (Data from Fecteau *et al.*, 2007)

hyperplasia, possible adrenocortical carcinoma and adenocarcinoma. The right gland was affected in two cases, and the left gland in three cases (Figure 19.2). One rabbit had adrenal hyperplasia of both glands in addition to a phaeochromocytoma of the left adrenal gland, which may have been an incidental finding as the clinical signs were consistent with the increase in sex hormones from the adrenal cortex.

Figure 19.2 also shows the therapy offered in each case, which ranged from surgical excision to administration of the gonadotropin-releasing hormone (GnRH) agonists leuprorelin and deslorelin. One patient that failed to respond to leuprorelin or finasteride responded well to surgical excision for 3 months until clinical signs recurred. Owing to the small number of cases reported, the prognosis and recommended treatment is uncertain.

A review of pathological samples submitted to an exotic animal pathology laboratory produced 110 submissions that included rabbit adrenal glands (Drury Reavill, Zoo/Exotic Pathology Service, personal communication, July 2012). Of these submissions, 24 rabbit adrenal glands were abnormal. The abnormalities included: adrenal cortical hyperplasia (13 cases); adrenal cortical adenoma (3); ectopic adrenal gland (2); and 1 case each of lymphocytic infiltrate (possible lymphoma), cortical hypertrophy and mild multifocal adrenalitis. These submissions are unlikely to reflect the incidence of adrenal disorders in rabbits in general, because they included only abnormal rabbits, or rabbits with visible adrenal abnormalities. Complete histories were unavailable for most of these rabbits; therefore it is unknown how many cases of neoplasia and/or hyperplasia were associated with clinical signs.

Pituitary endocrine disease

Nine cases of prolactin-secreting pituitary adenomas have been described in nulliparous laboratory New Zealand White does (Lipman *et al.*, 1994). The average age of the affected animals was 3.2 years; the clinical findings included enlarged, non-painful, fluid-filled teats, which in most animals were grey, blue or greenish-black in colour. Serum prolactin was measured for each rabbit, and ranged from 22.4 ng/ml to 2.21 µg/ml, which represents a 10–1000-fold increase over normal values for non-pregnant rabbits. Pituitary adenoma was confirmed at necropsy. Neoplastic portions of the pituitary glands were positive for prolactin on immunohistochemistry.

Cystic mammary adenocarcinoma was associated with a prolactin-secreting pituitary adenoma in a 44-month-old laboratory New Zealand White rabbit (Sikoski *et al.*, 2008). The mammary glands were enlarged and discoloured with brown mucoid discharge. Both the elevated serum prolactin levels and computed tomography supported the presence of a prolactin-secreting pituitary tumour, which was confirmed at histopathology to be a pituitary adenoma. Immunohistochemical staining revealed prolactin-secreting neoplastic cells.

Thyroid and parathyroid endocrine disease

Naturally occurring thyroid and parathyroid disease in rabbits is not reported in the literature. Hyperthyroidism can be induced in laboratory rabbits by

Age (years)	Sex	Histopathology, other diagnostics	Testosterone (ng/ml)	Treatment/outcome
9	M	Right adrenocortical hyperplasia	2.67	Attempted removal, unable to remove all; did not respond to deslorelin
7	M	Right adrenocortical hyperplasia	3.96	No response to leuprorelin; responded for 3 months to right adrenalectomy, then recurred; no response to finasteride
8	M	Left adrenocortical neoplasia; possible carcinoma	0.80	Attempted removal of left adrenal gland; elected euthanasia
6	F	Left adrenal adenocarcinoma	0.68 initially; 0.57 after medical therapy; 0.02 after adrenalectomy	No response to deslorelin or trilostane; responded well to adrenalectomy
8	M	Left adrenal hyperplasia	0.52 initially; 0.57 after flutamide and trilostane; 0.04 after leuprorelin; 0.03 after adrenalectomy	Responded to leuprorelin and adrenalectomy
10	F	Adrenocortical hyperplasia; left adrenal phaeochromocytoma	1.02	No treatment; euthanased

19.2 Clinical presentation, signalment and therapy offered in six pet rabbits with histopathologically confirmed adrenal hyperplasia or neoplasia. (Case data provided by Paolo Selleri, Angela Lennox, John Chitty, Robert Wagner and Marcy Souza)

injection of triiodothyronine (Harrison and McLoon, 2002) or L-thyroxine (Nowosadzka *et al.*, 2009). Hypothyroidism can be induced in laboratory animals via administration of various agents such as propylthiouracil (Nowosadzka *et al.*, 2009) or thiamazole (Kowalczyk *et al.*, 2011), or by thyroidectomy (Min *et al.*, 1998). Most research on hyper- or hypothyroidism in rabbits involves the study of isolated tissue or cells (Harrison and McLoon, 2002; Nowosadzka *et al.*, 2009; Kowalczyk *et al.*, 2011) and does not shed light on possible disease presentation *in vivo*.

Endocrine diseases of the reproductive organs

While not specifically an endocrine disorder, pseudopregnancy is common in pet rabbits, and is the result of normal elevations of post-ovulatory prolactin levels. Rabbits are induced ovulators, and induction can occur after sterile mating, mounting by other does, or other stimulation.

Ovarian remnant/retained testicle

Functional ovarian or testicular tissue may be present in a previously neutered rabbit. Common signs in a female rabbit with aberrant ovarian tissue are aggression and sexual behavior. Aggression and sexual behavior are also common in males with retained testicular tissue, along with urine spraying. These signs are similar to those of neutered rabbits with hyperadrenocorticism, therefore analysis of a basal sample may not distinguish the source of sex hormones as gonadal or adrenal; provocative testing should be performed. A test to aid in differentiating functional gonadal tissue from hyperadrenocorticism in the rabbit is the human chorionic gonadotropin (hCG) stimulation test. hCG is similar to luteinizing hormone (LH) in function and, like LH, hCG can stimulate secretion of progesterone and testosterone from the gonads. Protocols for the hCG stimulation test in rabbit are presented in Figure 19.3.

---

hCG stimulation test for detecting presence of testicular tissue [a]

1. Collect blood sample for basal testosterone concentration.
2. Inject 1500 IU hCG i.m.
3. Collect blood sample 3 hours after hCG administration.

Interpretation: significant increase in testosterone post hCG is suggestive of testicular tissue

hCG stimulation test for detecting presence of ovarian tissue [b]

1. Collect blood sample for basal progesterone concentration.
2. Inject 50 IU hCG i.v.
3. Collect blood sample 4 days after hCG administration.

Interpretation: significant increase in progesterone post hCG is suggestive of an ovarian remnant

---

19.3 Protocols for human chorionic gonadotrophin (hCG) stimulation tests in male and female rabbits. [a] Shimamoto and Sofikitis (1998); [b] Kaufmann *et al.* (1992).

Based on samples submitted to the University of Tennessee Clinical Endocrinology Service, the hCG stimulation test has been positive for gonadal tissue in rabbits as old as 10 years. In one case, inoperable aberrant ovarian tissue attached to the dorsal abdomen with major intestinal adhesions was found during an exploratory laparotomy in a 6-year-old spayed female rabbit (Jason Hutcheson, personal communication). This rabbit was displaying aggressive behaviour and hair pulling, and had enlarged mammary tissue. In some cases, leuprorelin or deslorelin (GnRH agonists) have been used with varying effects on behaviour.

References and further reading

Conaway HH, Faas FH, Smith SD, *et al.* (1981) Spontaneous diabetes mellitus in the New Zealand white rabbit: Physiologic characteristics. *Metabolism: Clinical and Experimental* **30**(1), 50–56

Fecteau KA, Deeb BJ, Rickel JM, *et al.* (2007) Diagnostic endocrinology: Blood steroid concentrations in neutered male and female rabbits. *Journal of Exotic Pet Medicine* **16**, 256–259

Harcourt-Brown FM and Harcourt-Brown S (2012) Clinical value of blood glucose measurement in pet rabbits. *Veterinary Record* **170**(26), 674–678

Harpole T, Runyeard V, English K and Archer FJ (2002) Serum fructosamine in hyperglycaemic rabbits. *Journal of Veterinary Clinical Pathology* **31**, 205

Harrison AR and McLoon LK (2002) Effect of hyperthyroidism on the orbicularis oculi muscle in rabbits. *Ophthalmic Plastic and Reconstructive Surgery* **18**(4), 289–294

Kaufmann RA, Savoy-Moore RT, Subramanian MG, *et al.* (1992) Cocaine inhibits mating-induced, but not human chorionic gonadotropin-stimulated, ovulation in the rabbit. *Biology of Reproduction* **46**, 641–647

Keeble E (2001) Endocrine diseases in small mammals. *In Practice* **23**, 570–585

Kowalczyk E, Urbanowicz J, Kopff M, *et al.* (2011) Elements of oxidation/reduction balance in experimental hypothyroidism. *Endokrynologia Polska* **62**(3), 220–223

Lennox AM (2013) Surgical treatment of adrenocortical disease. In: *BSAVA Manual of Rabbit Surgery, Dentistry and Imaging*, ed. F Harcourt-Brown and J Chitty, pp.269–273. BSAVA Publications, Gloucester

Lennox AM and Chitty J (2006) Adrenal neoplasia and hyperplasia as a cause of hypertestosteronism in two rabbits. *Journal of Exotic Pet Medicine* **15**(1), 56–58

Lipman NS, Zhi-Bo Z, Hurley RJ, *et al.* (1994) Prolactin-secreting pituitary adenomas with mammary dysplasia in New Zealand white rabbits. *Laboratory Animal Science* **44**(2), 114–120

Min X, Xiaohui Z, Zhaixiang D, *et al.* (1998) Effect of the Yang tonifying herbs on myocardial β-adrenoceptors of hypothyroid rabbits. *Journal of Ethnopharmacology* **60**(1), 43–51

Nowosadzka E, Szymonik-Lesiuk S and Kurzepa J (2009) The effects of hypo- and hyperthyroidism on nuclear, cytosolic, endoplasmic and mitochondrial fractions of sialoglycoproteins in rabbit hepatocytes. *Folia Biologica* **55**(1), 7–10

Roth SI, Conaway HH, Sanders LL, *et al.* (1980) Spontaneous diabetes mellitus in the New Zealand white rabbit. Preliminary morphologic characterization. *Laboratory Investigation* **42**(5), 571–579

Shimamoto K and Sofikitis N (1998) Effect of hypercholesterolaemia on testicular function and sperm physiology. *Yonago Acta Medica* **41**, 23–29

Sikoski P, Trybus J, Cline JM, *et al.* (2008) Cystic mammary adenocarcinoma associated with a prolactin-secreting pituitary adenoma in a New Zealand White Rabbit (*Oryctolagus cuniculus*). *Comparative Medicine* **58**(3), 297–300

Wilson HK, Boyd III AE, Bolton WE, *et al.* (1982) Somatostatin secretion in diabetic rabbits. *Metabolism: Clinical and Experimental* **31**(5), 428–432

Wojtowicz Z, Wrona W, Kis G, *et al.* (2004) Serum total cholesterol, triglycerides and high density lipoproteins (HDL) levels in rabbits during the course of experimental diabetes. *Annales Universitatis Maria-Curie-Sklodowska Sectio D: Medicina* **59**(2), 258–260

20

Problems of the geriatric rabbit

John Chitty

With improvements in the understanding of a rabbit's dietary and health requirements, pet rabbits are living longer and more geriatric diseases are being seen. Some diseases (e.g. neoplasia) may be related to the aging process itself, whereas other conditions may reflect 'wear and tear' associated with a longer lifespan (e.g. osteoarthritis).

The 'average' rabbit should live to 10–12 years (though some individuals may live longer). Geriatric disease may therefore be seen from approximately 7 years of age. Dwarf and giant breeds do not have the same life expectancy, so diseases associated with older age may often be seen from 4–5 years in these breeds. There will also be an effect of the onset of chronic disease at earlier age; for example, a young rabbit exhibiting dental disease is unlikely to reach a full normal lifespan and may show 'geriatric' disease at an earlier age than a rabbit without dental disease.

Many diseases show an insidious onset and so may not be noticed in their early stages, except by the most observant owners. Importantly, many of these diseases may only be identified as underlying causes of other, more apparent, conditions. For example, cheyletiellosis in the older rabbit may be a consequence of immunosuppression; and pododermatitis may reflect underlying osteoarthritis (Figure 20.1). Such conditions may also directly render the rabbit more susceptible to other acute problems; for example, myiasis may be much more likely in a rabbit with spinal osteoarthritis that is unable to clean itself. It is vital that owners look out for the more subtle signs of underlying disease and, in particular, signs of chronic pain, as many geriatric diseases are associated with pain.

Typical signs of pain include:

- Reduced activity
- Weight loss
- Altered mood – the rabbit may be reluctant to move or come to its owner, or may become aggressive
- Reduced appetite
- Faecal and urinary changes.

However, any deviation from what is known as normal behaviour is worthy of attention as it may be linked to pain.

It is also important that owners of older rabbits understand that many diseases may require a more in-depth approach than in the younger rabbit. Conversely, the clinician must also remember that some diseases will affect rabbits of all ages and, while always being aware of diseases that affect the geriatric rabbit, recognize that these are not the only conditions that may be seen in the older animal.

When treating geriatric pets it is important to be aware that many of these conditions are manageable rather than curable. Therefore, the effects of disease and the ability to control clinical signs (especially pain) must always be discussed with the owner before starting therapy. Where control of clinical signs is not possible such that the animal can maintain a good quality of life, euthanasia should always be considered.

Geriatric diseases

The following is not a complete list of diseases seen in old age. However, it does represent some of the more common and important conditions seen in the older rabbit.

Osteoarthritis

This is one of the most common age-related complaints and can result in periodic bouts of gut stasis or urinary stasis, as well as generalized pain. It can also make grooming more difficult and should be

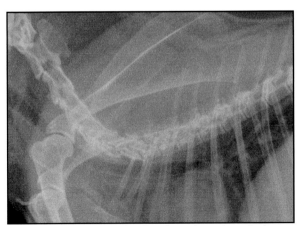

20.1 Radiograph showing thoracic and cervical spinal lesions at C3–C4 and C7–T1 in an older rabbit. The presenting sign was of pododermatitis of the forefeet, which responded well to meloxicam at 1 mg/kg orally q12h.

suspected in any animal that has reduced grooming activity and appears more unkempt or develops a matted haircoat. Problems with prehension of caecotrophs are common in cases of spinal or hindlimb osteoarthritis, and these conditions should always be suspected and investigated in cases where there is an accumulation of uneaten caecotrophs in the perineal area, or the presence of caecotrophs in the environment.

An inability to raise the hindquarters when urinating, as well as reduced ability to groom the hindquarters, may result in urine staining and scalding. Such problems with urine and caecotroph removal may also render the rabbit more susceptible to myiasis. Osteoarthritis can also result in problems due to altered weight-bearing or reduced activity, for example pododermatitis.

Ear problems can also result from an inability to scratch the ear with a hindfoot, or to groom the pinnae with the front feet, because this may result in increased build-up of dry cerumen. In cases of unilateral otitis with dry discharge visible in ear canal, osteoarthritis of the spine or the ipsilateral hindlimb should be suspected.

Rabbits rarely, if ever, vocalize when in pain, but just because they do not complain overtly this does not mean they are not in a great deal of distress. This is important to convey to owners who may not understand that their rabbit is in pain and so may be less compliant in terms of giving analgesics over the long term.

Osteoarthritis should always be suspected in a rabbit showing the signs described earlier, and in any rabbit showing non-specific signs. On clinical examination there may be obviously enlarged or fibrotic joints. It is more likely, though, to see muscle wastage in the affected limb(s) or caudal to a spinal lesion. Certainly if a rabbit shows good body condition over the forequarters and poor condition over the hindquarters, thoracolumbar or hindlimb osteoarthritis must be considered. Given that osteoarthritis is so common, radiography is indicated for any animal showing potential signs of pain, or a disease that may be linked to an underlying focus of pain.

The joints typically affected by osteoarthritis in the older rabbit are:

- Spine (all regions) – changes may be observed at the lumbosacral junction and in the lumbar, thoracic and cervical regions (Figure 20.2)
- Stifle joints
- Hips.

Giant breeds are particularly prone to such problems in all joints. This reflects the increased load-bearing on the joints in such breeds (Figure 20.3).

The following radiographic views should be taken in all cases where osteoarthritis is suspected:

- Lateral and dorsoventral views of the entire spinal column. In terms of owner cost, digital radiography is extremely useful because whole body views may be obtained and images

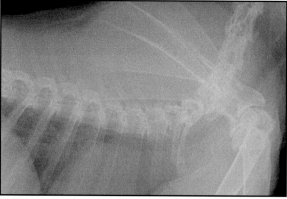

20.2 Radiograph of a rabbit with spinal lesions at T1–T2 and T2–T3. The presenting sign was of a neuropathy of both forelimbs and wastage of the triceps muscle. This corresponded to a lesion of the caudal brachial plexus.

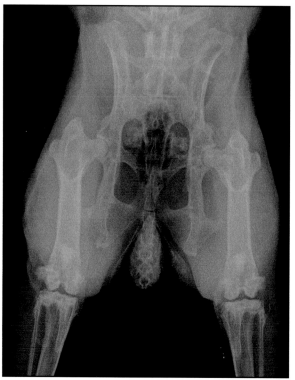

20.3 Radiograph of a giant-breed rabbit showing osteoarthritis of hip joints secondary to dysplasia, and of the stifles secondary to valgal limb deformity.

manipulated to allow assessment of each region. Otherwise, separate views of each region of the vertebral column are required. Good positioning is vital because changes may be subtle
- Lateral views of both stifles
- Dorsoventral view of the hips.

Radiographic changes are similar to those seen in the dog or cat and include:

- Roughening of joint surfaces
- New bone formation around the joints
- Spondylosis in the vertebral column.

In the rabbit it is also common to see displaced vertebrae, particularly in the lumbar spine (Figure 20.4). These are likely to be a sequel to handling injuries (fracture or subluxation of the vertebrae) that occurred when the rabbit was younger. It should be remembered that the changes seen represent advanced long-term changes and the prognosis is affected accordingly. Similarly, if no changes are seen on plain radiographs, this may not mean that there is no osteoarthritic change, merely that the changes occurred too recently to be visible radiographically. In such cases, myelography may be useful for spinal assessment (especially for intervertebral disc lesions), or computed tomography (CT) or magnetic resonance imaging (MRI) may be utilized where available.

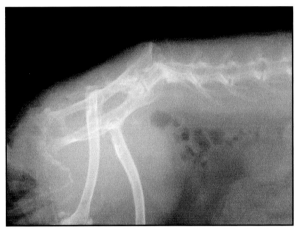

20.4 Subluxation of the lumbar spine. This elderly rabbit presented with muscle wastage and weakness of the hindlimbs.

Therapy

Osteoarthritis is managed, not cured, and many approaches are taken. Pain relief is essential. The mainstay is the use of non-steroidal anti-inflammatory drugs (NSAIDs), and these are effective in most cases. Meloxicam is most commonly used because it is not only effective but is easy to administer, and the dose can be changed easily as required. This author will typically commence treatment with 0.75–1 mg/kg orally twice daily (Turner *et al.*, 2006) and reduce the dose as the clinical signs improve until the lowest effective dose is established. Relapses are treated by increasing again to the starting dose rate, before gradually reducing again. The author has used carprofen at 5 mg/kg orally or s.c. q24h in some cases that did not respond to meloxicam.

Many owners express concern over long-term use of NSAIDs in rabbits with osteoarthritis. These are important concerns because both gastric ulceration and renal failure are potential side effects of NSAID therapy. These problems appear to be rare in the author's experience, though it is important to assess renal function when renal disease is suspected (see later) before starting NSAID therapy. However, measurement of biochemical changes in renal failure is as insensitive as in other species, so normal plasma urea and creatinine levels do not rule out pre-existing renal disease. Anti-ulcer medication such as ranitidine can be given concurrently with NSAID use if gastric ulceration is a concern.

Where renal problems exist alongside osteoarthritis, it is important that analgesia is not denied. Multimodal analgesic plans may be utilized to reduce NSAID doses. Tramadol appears very effective in these cases, though an effective dose has not been established in the rabbit. Souza *et al.* (2008) showed that an oral dose of 11 mg/kg in rabbits did not achieve the plasma levels that are required for adequate analgesia in human patients. However, this does not imply that there is no analgesic effect at this, or lower, doses and further work is required to assess the analgesic effect in the rabbit and to determine a dose rate. Typically the author will use 15 mg/kg orally q12h.

It is important to discuss these cases thoroughly with the owner, because they may find it confusing that a seemingly contraindicated family of drugs (which is not authorized for use in rabbits) is being recommended. However, it must be understood that the primary aim is to improve animal welfare, not just to achieve patient longevity, and therefore a potentially shorter but 'pain-free' lifespan may be acceptable.

Diet is also important, and a good quality high-fibre diet is essential to reduce weight or to avoid obesity. Some clinicians will use nutraceuticals in these cases to reduce NSAID doses. While there is no proven action of such agents in the literature, there is some anecdotal evidence to suggest that essential fatty acids and glucosamine may have some beneficial effect. Acupuncture has also been employed in these cases. The author works alongside a veterinary acupuncturist and has seen beneficial effects from acupuncture in cases of lumbar spinal osteoarthritis.

It is certainly true that owners can assist with daily management to help the osteoarthritic rabbit and paying attention to these factors may have a great effect in reducing drug doses:

- Flooring (for indoor rabbits) should be modified to prevent the animal slipping on smooth surfaces
- Prevent the rabbit climbing up or down steps, and reduce jumping on furniture. Instead the rabbit should be lifted and carried
- Care should be taken when handling and the owner should be particularly careful to support the spine and hindquarters when lifting the rabbit
- Where rabbits are housed in multi-tier hutches these should be altered so they are either single tier or the need to climb is reduced, e.g. by feeding on the ground floor. Where climbing is unavoidable, gentle ramps should be provided
- Rabbits with cervical spine lesions should be fed with the food and water bowls raised off the ground
- Gentle physiotherapy may be of assistance in cases of neurogenic muscle atrophy

- Exercise is important to avoid depletion of muscle mass. These animals should not be overly restricted. However, exercise should be gentle and on the flat. Hydrotherapy may be well tolerated by some rabbits.

Dental disease

Older rabbits may actually be at less risk of dental disease than younger animals: having got this far without problems, they are presumably unlikely to possess the predominant risk factors for dental disease (see the *BSAVA Manual of Rabbit Surgery, Dentistry and Imaging*).

However, many rabbits may enter the geriatric phase of life with pre-existing dental disease and this may require more sensitive or intense management as other concurrent diseases occur. In particular, the altered anaesthetic risk associated with certain geriatric diseases may necessitate more careful attention, or altered regimes, when anaesthetizing older rabbits for regular dental care (see below).

Cardiovascular disease

Cardiac disease is increasingly diagnosed in rabbits (see also Chapter 14). This probably reflects improved diagnostic capabilities and understanding as well as an increasing number of animals living long enough to develop such pathology.

Typical signs are of a quieter animal losing weight (or failing to gain weight). There are often few other signs, although classic signs of lethargy, dyspnoea, abdominal distension or collapse may be seen on occasion. On clinical examination affected rabbits are often slightly thin, and heart murmurs may or may not be present; these are usually soft. If murmurs are present and not associated with anaemia they are generally significant (Figure 20.5). Ultimately the diagnosis depends on imaging using radiography and echocardiography. The latter is especially useful in monitoring disease progression because it can usually be performed in the conscious rabbit.

Serum biochemistry will be of use in determining renal function: cardiac disease and renal disease

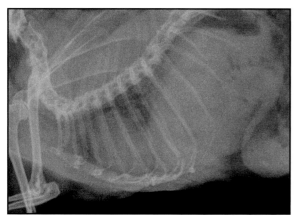

20.5 This case of cardiomegaly was presented with dysphagia and regurgitation, probably due to the extremely large heart and compression of the oesophagus. Hypertrophic cardiomyopathy was confirmed using echocardiography.

are often seen together, and the presence of concurrent renal disease will affect prognosis. Most cases appear to be typical of a hypertrophic cardiomyopathy, and giant breeds appear particularly prone. Long-term prognosis is therefore poor. However, in many cases the quality of life can be significantly improved in the short to medium term.

The author will generally use imidapril (0.25 mg/kg orally q24h) or benazepril (1.25 mg/rabbit orally q24h). Furosemide at 2 mg/kg orally q8–24h may also be used if there is ascites or pleural effusion. Pimobendan (0.1–0.3 mg/kg orally q12–24h) is used in severe cases (Pariaut, 2009).

Hepatic disease

There are few liver diseases specifically associated with older age in the rabbit, although neoplasia has been reported. Primary tumours (e.g. bile duct adenoma/carcinoma) have been observed, and the liver is also a site for multisystemic tumours, e.g. lymphosarcoma.

Most importantly, many overweight rabbits may be suffering from subclinical hepatic lipidosis. Anorexia resulting from any condition may therefore trigger clinical disease.

Renal disease

Renal disease is common in older rabbits. As well as chronic renal failure associated with renal fibrosis, disease may be seen as a result of chronic (or previous) encephalitozoonosis and secondary to urinary flow problems, with the development of uroliths throughout the urinary tract and chronic inflammatory changes that may result in an ascending infection. Renal disease should be suspected in all thin, quiet rabbits, especially if there is polyuria/polydipsia or urinary incontinence or scalding (it can be hard to identify the presence of polyuria) (see also Chapter 13).

Renal disease may be diagnosed on blood biochemistry or radiography (Harcourt-Brown, 2007). However, there appear to be no particularly sensitive tests of renal function. Compared with dogs and cats, creatinine level appears to be particularly insensitive in rabbits, so a rise in urea alone does not necessarily distinguish prerenal failure from renal failure (see also Chapter 9).

Urinalysis can be useful, although specific gravity does not appear as useful in rabbits as in dogs and cats. Measurement of the urinary protein:creatinine ratio to quantify or monitor persistent proteinuria may help to assess the severity of renal disease, disease progression and prognosis (see also Chapter 13). Urine cytology (particularly if there is proteinuria) can be extremely useful (see also Chapter 9). Renal ultrasonography may be of value and guided biopsy can be performed, though it does carry some risks.

Serology for *Encephalitozoon cuniculi* should be performed in all cases of suspected renal failure. Both IgG and IgM should be measured, with only those cases that are positive for both antibody isotypes being given fenbendazole therapy (see also Chapter 15). While the risk is low, radiomimetic effects of fenbendazole have been reported in rabbits (Graham *et al.*, 2012) and many rabbits with renal disease (or any chronic disease or pain) may already have a low-grade non-regenerative anaemia.

The cause of any urinary flow problem must be addressed. Uroliths should be managed medically or surgically as necessary. The rabbit should be encouraged to move around and to drink (water should be provided in both bowls and drinkers to enable the rabbit to choose its own preferred route); these are important aspects of management, as is analgesia, especially because many of cases of renal impairment are secondary to arthritis (Figure 20.6). Once urinary flow is established, diuresis can be a help in many cases in order to prevent urine sludging. In addition to fluid therapy and increased water intake, dandelions, dandelion extracts and thiazide drugs may all be utilized. Dietary modification may be helpful in cases of chronic renal failure or urine sludging (see Chapter 13).

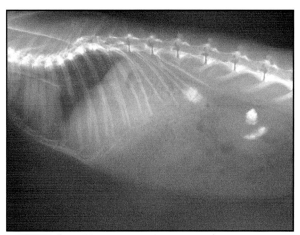

20.6 Renoliths due to reduced urine flow secondary to a thoracic spinal lesion (chronic subluxation).

Benazepril (see above) appears to be an effective aid in rabbits with chronic renal disease. Some authors report the potential for hypotensive episodes due to angiotensin-converting enzyme (ACE) inhibitor use. This has not been this author's experience, but blood pressure may be measured and monitored in the same way as for cats, using an artery located immediately proximal to the hock or carpus for Doppler ultrasonography in order to avoid clipping fur from the feet. Normal systolic pressure for rabbits measured by using the Doppler technique in clinical situations is 120–180 mmHg (see Chapter 14 for further details).

As with cardiac disease, renal conditions are usually managed rather than cured and owners should be advised accordingly. If altered, blood parameters may be monitored at regular intervals.

Ocular disease

Ocular disease, especially cataract formation, is common in rabbits. Some cataracts in larger individuals may be amenable to surgery. Diabetes, and hence diabetic cataract, is rare (see Chapter 19).

Cataracts secondary to encephalitozoonosis are seen but are more likely in younger rather than older animals. They are unlikely to respond to fenbendazole, which should be reserved for cases where encephalitozoonosis has been definitely identified and there is active infection (see above).

Otherwise, many rabbits do very well with reduced or no vision. Care must be taken not to make major changes in the environment as this may cause distress. Food and water bowls must be left in the same familiar places because there will be reduced ability to locate them. Muscle bulk should be monitored regularly as a means of checking how well the rabbit is moving (or how willing it is to move).

Aural disease

Chronic otitis media may result in deafness, which may also result in other sensory deprivation. Environmental changes and moves should be kept to a minimum because the affected rabbit will have reduced ability to cope with such alterations. Assessment of hearing can be difficult in the rabbit (see Chapter 15).

Neoplasia

Tumours are a natural consequence of living longer. Reproductive tumours (e.g. testicular tumours or uterine adenocarcinoma) are avoided by early neutering. However, many other neoplasms are seen: benign or malignant; localized or systemic (see Chapter 18).

Any unusual swelling or mass should be investigated and treated in much the same way as in other species. Detection of a likely malignancy should stimulate investigation for metastases (generally using radiography) before surgery is performed (Figures 20.7 and 20.8).

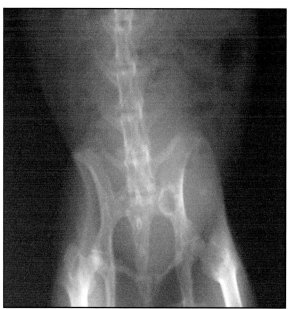

20.7 Radiograph showing metastasis of uterine adenocarcinoma to the ilium. The presenting signs related to lameness of the left hindlimb, not to the primary tumour.

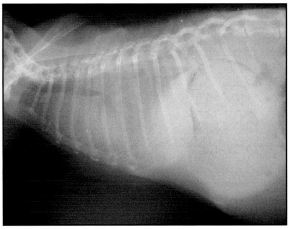

20.8 Pleural effusion and chest masses representing metastatic spread from uterine adenocarcinoma.

Endocrinopathies

These are extremely unusual in the rabbit (see also Chapter 19). In particular, diabetes mellitus is very rarely seen, with glucosuria and hyperglycaemia normally being a consequence of stress or pain. If hyperglycaemia is seen, fructosamine measurement may assist in distinguishing stress from diabetes, apart from in the chronically stressed rabbit, or one fed primarily on a diet high in sugar/simple carbo-hydrates, where this parameter may be altered. Hepatic function and appearance (ultrasonography/ radiography) should also be assessed because con-current hepatic lipidosis may confuse the diagnosis.

Adrenal neoplasia (Figure 20.9) and overproduc-tion of sex hormones has been reported. So far, the author has only seen this in neutered male rabbits, and the signs have been related to a return to repro-ductive (especially aggressive) behaviours. Diag-nosis involves measurement of serum testosterone levels and ultrasonography of the adrenal glands.

Therapy requires surgical removal of the neo-plastic gland (see *BSAVA Manual of Rabbit Surgery, Dentistry and Imaging*). Many tumours are malig-nant, however, so removal is not always possible. Deslorelin implants do not appear to be effective (see Chapter 19).

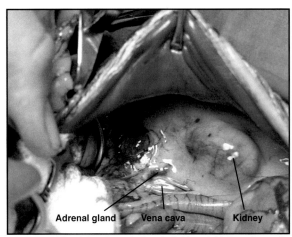

Adrenal gland · Vena cava · Kidney

20.9 The left adrenal gland of this rabbit is enlarged due to neoplasia.

Anaesthesia of the older rabbit

The aged rabbit is more likely than a young animal to have underlying or overt disease that may be worsened by physiological changes induced by anaesthesia. However, many of these disease conditions will require anaesthesia or sedation to enable investigation. As in other species, extra care (as well as discussion with concerned owners) is required when anaesthetizing older animals.

Pre-anaesthetic assessment is particularly impor-tant, and animals to be anaesthetized should have a detailed history taken and receive a full physical examination. Conscious nasal capnography may assist in evaluating respiratory function. Pre-anaesthetic blood panels may be of assistance. However, rather than blanket screening of all older animals, directed tests based on the findings of the clinical examination may be more appropriate.

For 'quick' procedures, such as radiography, chamber induction followed by maintenance using sevoflurane alone may be considered and appears to be effective and 'safe' in the author's practice. Alternatively, use of sedation rather than full anaes-thesia may be considered for non-painful pro-cedures, with midazolam + etomidate or other midazolam combinations being particularly useful. For longer procedures, it is particularly important to monitor and maintain blood pressure to maintain renal blood flow. Hence fluid therapy is mandatory in such cases (see the *BSAVA Manual of Rabbit Surgery, Dentistry and Imaging*).

In all cases the likely risks and sequelae of the procedure should be balanced against the likely benefits and discussed with the owner before proceeding.

Care of the older rabbit

In addition to those described earlier, there are many actions an owner can take to assist in the care of the older rabbit. In particular, it is important to know the individual animal and for owners to be particularly observant for any changes in its normal attitude, activity levels, appetite, drinking, and urine or faecal output because all of these may be indi-cators of disease and, particularly, pain. Routine monitoring of bodyweight should be encouraged.

A good quality high-fibre diet should be provided and, even if the rabbit is used to a water bottle, water should also be provided in a bowl to encourage drinking. Vaccine status should be main-tained and owners should be extra vigilant in summer for signs of myiasis. The environment should not be changed dramatically unless absolutely necessary, in case of reduced sensory perception. Gentle ramps should be provided instead of steps and climbing should be reduced wherever possible in cases of subclinical or overt osteoarthritis. However, careful exercise and play should always be encouraged to enable preservation of muscle mass. This should be on level surfaces, without jumping or climbing, and the rabbit should be able to rest as it desires.

Routine healthcare

As with the owner, the veterinary surgeon should be aware of likely problems in older rabbits, and of the potential importance of subtle signs and changes reported by owners, and the presence of seemingly trivial signs as markers of underlying disease. Regular health checks should be maintained twice a year, although the frequency of these may be increased if required to monitor a chronic illness.

As ever, the history taking and physical examination is the most important part of any health check. Samples (e.g. blood or urine) may be taken and monitored routinely, but the low sensitivity of tests means that these may not be useful unless directed to confirm or deny findings noted on physical examination, or to monitor trends and progression of a disease process.

Care plans

As has been explained, many of the conditions seen in older rabbits may be established or initiated at a much younger age. While increased vigilance of rabbits in older age is of importance, and will enable earlier detection of geriatric disease, it is often too late actually to prevent problems occurring. Therefore, it is vital that care plans for life are established pre-purchase, at the initial contact or at the first vaccination; this is when geriatric disease control starts!

Care plans should include:

- Breed selection: dwarf and giant breeds are certainly much shorter-lived than 'normal' rabbits. Giant breeds are particularly prone to cardiac disease and osteoarthritis. Desirable though such breeds are as pets, the only way to reduce such problems is to reduce their production via reduced demand. Potential owners keen on giant or dwarf breeds should be advised of their likely problems in order to make an informed decision
- Vaccination advice
- Handling advice, to prevent injury
- Neutering advice, especially for does
- Dietary advice: a high-fibre (as near to forage-only as possible) diet should be established as early as possible (see also Chapter 3)
- Weight management
- Husbandry advice: especially with respect to exercise and flooring
- Myiasis control: in particular, observation for the build-up of risk factors for fly strike.

References and further reading

Graham J, Garner M and Reavill D (2012) Benzimidazole toxicity in rabbits. In: *Proceedings of the Association of Avian Veterinarians Annual Conference and Expo*, p.57

Harcourt-Brown F (2007) Radiographic signs of renal disease in rabbits. *Veterinary Record* **160**, 787–794

Lennox AM (2010) Care of the geriatric rabbit. *Veterinary Clinics of North America: Exotic Animal Practice* **13**, 123–133

Pariaut R (2009) Cardiovascular physiology and diseases of the rabbit. *Veterinary Clinics of North America: Exotic Animal Practice* **12**, 135–144

Souza M, Greenacre C and Cox SC (2008) Pharmacokinetics of orally administered tramadol in domestic rabbits (*Oryctolagus cuniculus*). *American Journal of Veterinary Research* **69**(8), 979–982

Turner PV, Chen HC and Taylor WM (2006) Pharmacokinetics of meloxicam in rabbits after single and repeat oral dosing. *Comparative Medicine* **56**(1), 63–67

21

Therapeutics

Richard Saunders

The rabbit has been used as a laboratory animal for many years, and as a result there is a wealth of data on the use of therapeutic agents in this species. However, much of this information pertains to toxicity testing only, and such trials are carried out on healthy young animals of specific breeds, with no pre-existing diseases. Rabbits have been farmed for meat and fur for hundreds of years, and therapeutic agents are also used in these animals; however, these are often used as group prophylaxis against infectious diseases, in particular bacterial and protozoal infections. Although rabbits are the third most commonly kept mammalian pet in the UK, they form a relatively small target market for pharmaceutical companies, and as a result, few drugs are specifically authorized for them in the UK or worldwide. As a result, most historical data on pharmacokinetics, efficacy and toxicity are of limited application to the single or small-group-housed pet rabbit, and limited high-quality information (i.e. based on peer-reviewed double-blind studies) is available on dosage, safety and efficacy in pet rabbits.

Other sources of information are appropriate: (small animal, exotic) formularies; direct contact with pharmaceutical companies; and discussion with exotic animal practitioners via various fora (see References and further reading). The veterinary surgeon is therefore required to make a case-by-case decision on appropriate therapeutics, ideally using such information where it exists, and where not, using case series or anecdotal data. Extrapolation from other species, including domestic carnivore, equine and human, may be required. However, drug uptake and pharmacokinetics can vary widely among species, and great care is needed with this approach. Carnivores and omnivores have complete emptying from the stomach, ensuring a narrower window of drug uptake. It is possible, in their case, specifically to give oral drugs on an empty or a full stomach, which is not possible in the rabbit. Whilst other hindgut fermenters such as the horse have similar patterns of gastric emptying, rabbits practise caecotrophy, which may recycle drugs. Protein binding is also significantly different between species, which will affect pharmacokinetics.

Accurate bodyweight should always be obtained prior to drug administration because estimates of rabbits' weights are often inaccurate. The therapeutic approach to rabbit diseases is often somewhat different from the more specifically targeted approach often used with other species. Whilst it is important to diagnose rapidly and treat appropriately a rabbit's specific disease problem(s), it is also important, both for welfare reasons and to enhance recovery, to address pain appropriately with suitable analgesia, to maintain nutritional and hydration status and to maintain gastrointestinal motility.

Medicines regulations

It is important to follow local legislation on the selection of therapeutic agents. In the UK, the Prescribing Cascade provides a means of allowing a veterinary surgeon to prescribe unauthorized medicines that would not otherwise be permitted via a pathway of appropriate drug selection (BSAVA, 2012):

1. A veterinary medicine authorized in the UK for use in another animal species or for a different condition in the same species.
2. If there is no such medicine, use either:
   a. A medicine authorized in the UK for human use, or
   b. A veterinary medicine from another Member State or country outside the European Union in accordance with an import certificate from the Veterinary Medicines Directorate (VMD).
3. If there is no such medicine, a medicine prepared extemporaneously by a veterinary surgeon, pharmacist or a person holding an appropriate manufacturer's authorization.

Further explanation is available from the Veterinary Medicines Directorate (www.vmd.defra.gov.uk).

It is important to note that the Cascade does not preclude the use of unauthorized drugs (such as those authorized for other animal species, including human medications), and allows them even where products higher up the Cascade are available, if those are unsuitable. Clinical judgement, guided by appropriate diagnostics where required (e.g. antimicrobial culture and sensitivity testing), is necessary to select a suitable product. For example, lack of efficacy of an authorized product may demonstrate the need for the use of an unauthorized agent.

The SAES (Small Animal Exemption Scheme) covers veterinary medicines marketed in the UK under an exemption from the above. It covers only topical or oral preparations, and does not include antibiotics, anaesthetics, narcotics or psychotropics. It does not include food-producing animals. It is important to realize that a product's inclusion under the SAES does not automatically require it to be used under the Cascade.

Prescriptions for medications may be written in the UK for rabbits as for other species. It is important to include, where the drug is unauthorized, the phrase: 'The medicine is to be used under the prescribing cascade'.

Informed owner consent is essential when using drugs 'off-licence'. *Note that using an authorized product in an unauthorized manner (e.g. a different route, dose or frequency) also requires informed consent.* This should be obtained in writing; however, the fact that written consent is obtained does not automatically demonstrate that INFORMED consent was given by the owner. Model forms are available from the Veterinary Defence Society and useful advice on discussing the issue is available at www.bsava.com. A thorough description and much specific advice about prescribing and labelling drugs for rabbits, particularly 'off-licence' use, may be found at www.vetformulary.com.

Note that the above assumes that rabbits are not potentially destined for the human food chain. Where this may be the case (e.g. meat rabbits, and those bred for showing, but which may end up being eaten at the end of a show career), appropriate withdrawal periods and record-keeping are also necessary.

Routes of drug administration

Choosing the correct route of administration is important to ensure effective uptake and absorption of the drug and to minimize adverse effects and avoid stress.

Systemic routes

Oral
Oral medication is appropriate for many drugs and is the preferred method in most cases for outpatients.

Formulations include powders, solutions, suspensions, tablets and capsules. Human paediatric solutions and suspensions are generally more dilute, and more palatable, than adult versions, and therefore generally more suitable for rabbits. Tablet and capsule preparations are often designed for larger target species, and may require appropriate subdivision, and it is important to divide such formulations accurately. Simply cutting tablets may be straightforward, although this may not be possible with coated tablets, or may affect their absorption characteristics, and becomes highly unreliable for divisions smaller than quarters. Capsules may be opened, the contents divided, and the powder administered directly. If this is likely to affect the uptake of the drug adversely, the contents may be re-encapsulated using plain gelatine capsules, although the grinding action of rabbit cheek teeth makes perforation of the capsule highly likely.

Powder or tablets may be more accurately dosed by weighing out the correct dose. However, unless relatively large amounts of powder are involved, this requires extremely accurate scales. Alternatively, powders or crushed tablets may be suspended in a liquid to allow more accurate titration of medication. The carrier liquid must be inert, palatable, have few or no physiological effects itself, and allow the preparation to dissolve homogeneously into it. Water may be appropriate in some cases, but many preparations do not dissolve in water; methylcellulose or lactulose are more suitable, but excessive quantities may induce diarrhoea.

Compounding drugs in this way creates the potential for errors to occur, and it is vital to recheck calculations and to ensure that owners are fully informed about storage, preparation and dosing requirements such as the importance of thorough mixing before drawing up a liquid. Such methods are unlikely to be scientifically validated pharmacokinetically, and are best used as a last resort. Commercial compounding companies are widely available in the USA, and are starting to compound a limited selection of drugs in other countries (e.g. Doctors Foster and Smith, USA; Nova or Summit in the UK). In-house compounding kits are also available, which may be used to suspend products more reliably for easier dosing.

Direct oral administration is possible in most rabbits.

- Liquid medications are easily delivered, using an appropriately sized syringe. The end of the syringe should be gently introduced into the mouth and passed through the diastema before slowly depressing the plunger. Many rabbits are particularly sensitive about having their lips and noses touched, and approaching from the side of the mouth may be preferred over entering through the philtrum in these cases.
- Whole or fractioned tablets may be placed directly into the mouth, past the first cheek teeth, whereupon they should be ingested by the rabbit. Fingers or pilling instruments designed for cats may be used. A 1 ml syringe with the luer end cut off, and any plastic plunger tips removed, makes a simple pilling device (Figure 21.1).
- Powders, crushed tablets and unpalatable liquids may be mixed into a small carrier volume of semi-liquid recovery diet or other substance. Fruit juice, banana, honey, baby food, yoghurt,

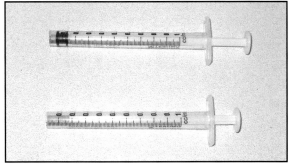

21.1 A simple homemade pill-giving device can be made from a syringe.

jam, nut butters or more palatable medications themselves may be used (e.g. mixing an unpalatable medication such as oral enrofloxacin with oral meloxicam syrup), assuming there are no drug or chemical interactions.

- Use of medicated feed or water is less than ideal because it is difficult to ensure correct dosages and ensure sufficient uptake to sustain effective therapeutic serum concentrations. Where used, Harkness *et al.* (2010) report that adult rabbits daily consume 40–60 g feed/kg bodyweight and 100–120 ml drinking water/kg. In almost every case, direct administration of medication is preferred.

  - Medication may be placed in or on food. This is appropriate for rabbits that reliably eat food items, on which powdered medicine may be sprinkled. Dampened vegetation or forage, dampened or soaked pellets, or small volumes of bread may be used. In most cases, offering a small volume of such food and ensuring it is eaten before offering the rest of the rabbit's food is advised. Medicated pelleted feed is rarely used for pet rabbits, although it is widely used in farmed rabbits and laboratory studies. It may occasionally be used for larger groups of rabbits, where every rabbit requires the product (e.g. in rescue centres), and correct formulation by professional feed mills is advised.

  - In-water administration is rarely appropriate for rabbits. Water intake is highly variable in healthy rabbits, and even more so in ill rabbits, and therefore drug intake is difficult to predict. All group-housed rabbits will be medicated in this case (which may be the intention, but if not, this method is not ideal). Many medications do not dissolve well in water; it may be necessary to restrict the intake of food items of high water content, such as grass, and the palatability of the water may be affected by the medication.

- Gavage via a tube or a blunt needle may also be used, but this is rarely carried out in the conscious pet rabbit. Naso-oesophageal tubes may be placed to assist with oral nutrition and fluid therapy, and if they are present, may be utilized to administer liquid medications.

Transmucosal

Transmucosal administration of some drugs (e.g. buprenorphine) may be a suitable alternative to injection. It is important to ensure that the medication is genuinely placed into contact with the buccal and/ or sublingual mucosa, rather than being swallowed, as oral bioavailability is significantly lower (Nath *et al.*, 1999; Lindhart *et al.*, 2001; Hawkins, 2006).

Transcutaneous

Transcutaneous administration of some drugs may be appropriate. Sustained-release patches containing fentanyl are used for other species and may be used on rabbits to provide long-lasting analgesia. However, fur regrowth can complicate their use after

24 hours (Foley *et al.*, 2001).

Spot-on medications are widely used, particularly for ectoparasite control. In rabbits, there are a variety of authorized (e.g. imidacloprid) and SAES (e.g. ivermectin) products available in the UK. Insect growth hormone regulators such as cyromazine may also be administered this way. Ingestion of the drug directly from the site of application by the treated rabbit, and any in-contact rabbits, should be prevented.

Parenteral

Parenterally administered injections may be given by a variety of routes. The smallest needle through which the preparation can easily pass should be used, to minimize discomfort. With most aqueous solutions, a 25 or 23 G needle is suitable. However, for some injectable antibiotic preparations (penicillins and cephalosporins in particular), wider bore needles such as 21 G will be necessary. Changing the needle for a fresh one after drawing up injectables from multi-dose bottles ensures that the needle used in the rabbit is not blunt, and this causes less trauma and reaction. For a full discussion of intraosseous and intravenous access, see Chapter 7.

Subcutaneous injections: These are easily administered into the large scruff. Most rabbits tolerate subcutaneous injections well, and owners can be instructed in the technique for outpatient care. Uptake is generally slightly slower (Williams and Wyatt, 2007) than by other parenteral routes, but this is not usually a significant issue in outpatients. Some male rabbits have extremely tough skin over the scruff, and other sites may be selected (over the flank or rump).

Intramuscular injections: These are technically more demanding to administer and are not suitable, or necessary, for outpatients. They should be administered into a large muscle group, such as the cranial musculature of the hindlimb, or the lumbar epaxial muscle group. Good restraint is necessary to avoid rabbits jumping and twisting, which may lead to spinal damage. Uptake is slightly faster than via the subcutaneous route, although large volumes or irritant medications can cause muscle damage and pain (Vachan, 1999).

Intraperitoneal injections: These are rarely used in pet rabbits, although they are a rapid, effective method for the delivery of large volumes of fluid. They provide more rapid drug uptake than the subcutaneous and intramuscular routes. However, there is a risk of puncture of the gastrointestinal or urogenital tract (Harcourt-Brown, 2002) with release of contents, and irritant preparations may predispose to intra-abdominal adhesion formation. Intraperitoneal injection is generally carried out in dorsal recumbency, into the caudal left abdominal quadrant. Respiratory embarrassment may be a concern in this position. The site should be aseptically prepared. Aspiration should be performed after penetration, prior to injection of the syringe contents, and if blood, urine or gut content is obtained, the needle should be changed and any contaminated material discarded, before repositioning and reinjection.

Intraosseous route: This is suitable for almost any preparation that may be given intravenously (McClure *et al.*, 1992). Uptake is similar to that using intravenous administration but, in most rabbits, the intravenous route is more suitable. Intraosseous administration may be necessary in very small patients, or those with diminished peripheral circulation, reduced blood pressure, hypothermia or shock, when intravenous access cannot be obtained and where an intraosseous needle has been placed.

Intravenous administration: This provides the most rapid uptake of all routes. In most cases it is relatively straightforward, using the marginal ear vein, or other collateral auricular veins, or the cephalic or lateral saphenous vein. Small patients, or those in shock states, may preclude intravenous access. Use of irritant products (e.g. oil-based diazepam preparations) has been associated with necrosis of the pinna, as has multiple attempts at venepuncture in the vessels of the same ear, and the use of the central auricular artery. Delivery via a preplaced intravenous catheter allows for repeated intravenous access using these relatively fragile vessels, and minimizes the need for repeated subcutaneous or intramuscular injections, and the associated pain and stress, in hospitalized rabbits (Saunders and Whitlock, 2012).

Local routes

Topical medications
Topical agents may be applied to the skin (including the ear canal), or the oral, ophthalmic or other mucosa. They may be absorbed systemically to some degree, and may be ingested and absorbed by the rabbit, or by a companion rabbit during grooming, which may have adverse effects (e.g. the potential for antibiotic-associated enterocolitis), as well as limiting the efficacy of the product.

Topical creams, ointments and sprays may be used as adjunctive or sole treatments for skin disease (Figure 21.2). Particular concerns apply to the use of corticosteroids in topical preparations. While these may be useful in treating inflammatory conditions, systemic uptake may inhibit immune responses, lead to 'flare-ups' of previously subclinical infections (e.g. respiratory pasteurellosis) and may cause transient hepatopathy (Rosenthal, 2004).

Corticosteroids are commonly included in topical ear and skin preparations designed for cats and dogs. Consideration should be given to using a product that does not contain corticosteroids, if they are not specifically required, by following the Cascade.

Shampoos are less commonly used for rabbits than for dogs. Rabbits are not as amenable to being bathed, are more likely to ingest topical treatment during grooming, and do not commonly have the conditions that require shampoos for dogs. Where shampoos are used (e.g. for intractable ectoparasitism or seborrhoeic conditions), it is important to ensure that the water is warm and that the rabbit is dried thoroughly to avoid chilling. The rabbit, and companion rabbits, should be prevented from ingesting any medication during any 'leave in' phase, and should be thoroughly rinsed afterwards.

Aural products may be indicated for treatment of otitis externa. Care should be taken to ensure that the tympanic membrane is intact when using products containing ingredients that can be ototoxic (e.g. aminoglycosides) or irritant to mucous membranes (e.g. chlorhexidine).

Local treatment with protective 'bandage' products may have a role in the treatment of ulcerated areas of oral mucosa such as the lateral aspect of the tongue, or in packing periodontal spaces. Protective 'bandage' products such as Iglu or Orabase may be useful, though temporary, adjunctive treatments to minimize pain during healing.

Some topical ophthalmic drugs are listed in Figure 21.3. Where infection is not confined to the eye (e.g. dacryocystitis), systemic treatment and other treatment methods may also be required.

Nebulization
Nebulization describes the process of creating and delivering a fine mist of liquid (typically saline or water, with or without medication) into the respiratory tract. This mist is generally created by the rapid vibration of a piezoelectric element and does not involve heating the liquid significantly. There is some controversy around how far the fine particles are able to travel down the respiratory tract; this depends on the particle size, turbulence within the respiratory tract, and any electrostatic charge on the particles. Portable nebulizers are readily available (Figure 21.4). They differ in their advertised ability to create sufficiently consistent particles small enough to travel down to the alveoli to treat lower respiratory tract disease (3–5 μm). For upper respiratory tract infections, the particle size is less crucial. See also Chapter 11.

Drug	Dose	Comments	References
Lidocaine, prilocaine	Topical application	Full-thickness local anaesthesia	Harcourt-Brown (2002)
Fusidic acid	Apply q24h for 2–3 days	With or without betamethasone, for topical treatment of skin lesions	Harcourt-Brown (2002)
Silver sulfadiazine	Apply topically q24h	Good Gram-negative activity including *Pseudomonas*	

21.2 Topical agents.

Drug	Dose	Indications/comments	References
Betaxolol	Topical q12h	Glaucoma	Hernandez-Divers (2004)
Chloramphenicol	Topical		Pollock (2006)
Ciclosporin A	Topical q12h	Increases tear production	Pollock (2006)
Ciprofloxacin	Topical q8–12h		Pollock (2006)
Dichlorphenamide	1–2 mg/kg q24h		Richardson (2000)
Dorzolamide	Topical q8–24h		Richardson (2000)
Fusidic acid	Topical q12–24h	Conjunctivitis. Authorized for rabbits (Fucithalmic)	Harcourt-Brown (2002); Flecknell (2005)
Gentamicin	1–2 drops q8h for 5–7 days	Conjunctivitis. Authorized for rabbits (Tiacil)	Harcourt-Brown (2002); Flecknell (2005)

21.3 Ophthalmic agents for topical use.

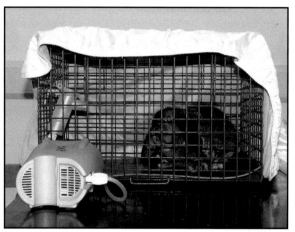

21.4 A portable mains or battery-powered nebulizer can be used to deliver medication.

Water or saline alone can help to moisten and dilute purulent exudate. This assists expulsion of such material from the respiratory tract. The addition of medication to the nebulizing liquid (see Chapter 11) may have additional benefits. Antibiotics are commonly added, for example aminoglycosides, which are often effective against pathogens associated with respiratory tract disease but may cause adverse reactions when given parenterally. Disinfectants, such as quaternary ammonium and biguanide compounds (e.g. F10, Health and Hygiene Pty, SA) may be helpful in treating bacterial, fungal and viral respiratory disease. Mucolytics may aid in loosening of exudates and bronchodilators may assist antibiotic therapy by widening the airway, encouraging expulsion of material, and increasing antibiotic penetration to the alveolus.

Other inhaled therapeutics
Inhalable aerosolized products containing corticosteroids or beta-adrenergic agonists, e.g. fluticasone or salbutamol, administered via an inhaler (e.g. Aero-Kat) may have a role in allergic airway disease (ideally confirmed by bronchoalveolar lavage). These minimize the potential systemic uptake of steroids, although carry a risk of reduction in local immune function, and should only be used after infectious causes have been ruled out or addressed. Dosage is empirical, but feline doses provide a useful starting point, from which the dose and/or frequency may be decreased as necessary.

Local flushing
Flushing infected, impacted or otherwise affected areas such as the nasolacrimal duct is often an effective therapeutic modality (see Chapter 7 for nasolacrimal flushing technique). A single flush of the affected duct(s), with or without topical treatment, may be sufficient in mild cases, e.g. of debris accumulation or foreign body obstruction without significant inflammation. In cases of more significant blockage, and/or associated inflammation of the walls of the duct, repeated gentle flushing over a period of several days, accompanied by appropriate dental treatment, may gradually achieve patency.

Many different flushing agents have been reportedly used. It is therefore suggested that a sterile non-irritant fluid such as normal saline or Hartmann's solution be used, at body temperature, with or without the addition of non-irritant antimicrobials such as topical antibiotic ocular drops (see Figure 21.3).

Local antibiosis in abscess treatment
Local antibiotic treatment of abscess sites, after appropriate debridement, allows high doses of antibiotics to be applied to the residually infected area, while minimizing potential adverse effects seen with systemic administration (e.g. renal damage due to systemic aminoglycosides, or antibiotic-associated enterotoxaemia due to enterally administered clindamycin).

Antibiotics may be soaked into non-absorbable materials (e.g. sterile swabs, bandages) that can be removed a few days later. They can also be mixed into topical debriding wound dressings such as Intrasite gel (Smith and Nephew). Clindamycin, as an intact or perforated capsule or as powder from capsules, has been suggested as a local treatment option (Richardson, 2000), but this carries extremely high risks of oral ingestion and subsequent antibiotic-associated enterotoxaemia if it is accessible to a companion rabbit that licks the wound, or if the abscess cavity communicates with the mouth.

Antibiotic-impregnated polymethylmethacrylate (AIPMMA) beads are produced by mixing an appropriate antibiotic into PMMA (typically used as 'bone cement' to position implants within bones). By itself, PMMA has a slight bacteriostatic effect (Chapman and Hadley, 1976). Antibiotics are added (ideally selected on the basis of bacterial culture and sensitivity from previously obtained samples of abscess capsule). These elute from the beads over a period of weeks to months. Antibiotics are selected as above, and also on their stability during the exothermic cement-hardening process and on the basis of their elution properties (e.g. tetracyclines, chloramphenicol, polymixin, erythromycin and fusidic acid (Wheler *et al.*, 1996) do not elute well). While lincosamides are often extremely effective against bacteria present in abscess cavities, they should be avoided or used with extreme care in abscesses with oral involvement, although as the bead is discrete, rather than a powder, it is less likely to find its way into the gastrointestinal tract. Penicillins and cephalosporins are also highly effective antibiotics to use but, while not as potentially harmful as the lincosamides, should be used with caution. AIPMMA beads may be commercially supplied, or the liquid and powder co-polymers can be obtained and then mixed on site with selected antibiotics (Varga, 2013). If the latter method is selected, a wider variety of antibiotics may be used (the commercial preparations are only available with gentamicin or tobramicin).

Antibiotic-impregnated plaster of Paris (AIPOP) is cheaper than AIPMMA, well tolerated in infected bone cavities and more effectively eliminates dead space. It is absorbed over weeks to months, being replaced by bone (Mackey *et al.*, 1982). POP powder can be heated in a dry oven to 100°C for 4 hours to sterilize it, after which it can be cooled and mixed with antibiotics, thus avoiding the potential damage to the drugs that may occur during the exothermic curing process of PMMA.

Both the above preparations may be made in aseptic conditions, using sterile ingredients, or may be made as a bacteriologically clean process, including, for example, powder from clindamycin capsules, which can then be gamma-irradiated, or sterilized using an electron beam or ethylene oxide gas. Autoclaving is likely to reduce efficacy significantly by denaturing the antibiotics.

Given the refractory nature of abscesses to therapy in many cases, the use of various therapeutics 'off-licence' has been anecdotally suggested, for example, intramammary or ocular antibiotic preparations placed into the abscess cavity. Whilst high local levels of antibiotics may prove effective (see above), they should only be used after, not in place of, thorough debridement and cleaning. For a full discussion of therapeutic options for abscesses see the BSAVA *Manual of Rabbit Surgery, Dentistry and Imaging*.

Local anaesthetics and other agents

These are an extremely useful therapeutic option, used alone or as part of a multimodal analgesic plan. They may be used directly on the mucosa (e.g. the conjunctiva), as local infiltrations into a surgical site, around a peripheral nerve or into the testis prior to removal (McMillan *et al.*, 2012), or epidurally. Other agents such as alpha-2 adrenergic agents and opioids may also be used by the epidural route. See Chapter 10 for further details on local anaesthesia.

Analgesics and anti-inflammatory drugs

In UK surveys postoperative analgesia was administered to 50–70% of dogs and cats, but to only 21% of rabbits and rodents (Hawkins, 2006). Analgesia is particularly important in the rabbit, not only for welfare reasons, but owing to the inhibitory effect of pain on gastrointestinal motility.

Pre-emptive analgesia is more effective in controlling pain (Reichert *et al.*, 2001). However, there are concerns about the use of non-steroidal anti-inflammatory drugs (NSAIDs) in pre-emptive analgesia because of the presence of compromised renal perfusion in the hypovolaemic patient. Note that multimodal analgesia carries the dual advantages of reducing potential toxicity whilst delivering a greater level of analgesia. This allows the use of lower doses of individual drugs, and is of particular benefit in rabbits, where data on safety may be limited (Hawkins, 2006; see also Chapter 10).

Doses of some analgesic and anti-inflammatory agents are given in Figure 21.5.

Drug	Doses	Indications/comments	References
Aspirin	100 mg/kg orally q12–24 h	Analgesic, antipyretic, anti-inflammatory	Richardson (2000)
Buprenorphine	0.01–0.05 mg/kg s.c., i.m., i.v., t.m. q6–12h	Analgesia, sedation. Doses <0.03 mg/kg have very limited analgesic effects but still have some sedative effects	Hawkins (2006)
Butorphanol	0.1–1.0 mg/kg s.c., i.m., i.v. q2–4h	Analgesia, sedation	Hawkins (2006)

21.5 Analgesic and anti-inflammatory drugs. CRI = constant rate infusion; t.d. = transdermally; t.m. = transmucosally. (continues) ▶

Drug	Doses	Indications/comments	References
Carprofen	1–2 mg/kg s.c., orally q12h	Anti-inflammatory, analgesia	Hawkins (2006)
	2–4 mg/kg s.c., orally q24h		Harcourt-Brown (2002); Flecknell (2005)
Fentanyl	0.0074 mg/kg i.v.		Lipman *et al.* (1997)
	30–100 µg/kg/min CRI		Cantwell (2001)
	25 µg per rabbit t.d. for 3 days		Foley *et al.* (2001)
Flunixin	1.1 mg/kg orally, s.c., i.m. q12h	Anti-inflammatory, anti-endotoxic. **Use with caution, especially in hypovolaemic patients, for 3 days maximum**	Harcourt-Brown (2002); Flecknell (2005)
Gabapentin	3–10 mg/kg orally q8–12h	Analgesia, particularly in cases of neurogenic pain	Plumb (2011); Morissey and Carpenter (2012)
Ibuprofen	2–7.5 mg/kg orally q12–24h		Morissey and Carpenter (2012)
Ketoprofen	1–3 mg/kg s.c., orally q12–24 h	Anti-inflammatory, analgesic	Harcourt-Brown (2002)
Meloxicam	0.2–0.6 mg/kg s.c., orally q12–24h	Some rabbits seem to respond better to doses at the lower end of the range given twice daily than to higher doses given once daily	Hawkins (2006); Turner *et al.* (2006)
	≤1.5 mg/kg orally q24h for up to 5 days		Turner *et al.* (2006); Wenger (2012)
Meperidine	5–10 mg/kg s.c., i.m. q2–3h		Morissey and Carpenter (2012)
Methadone	0.7 mg/kg i.v.		Piercy and Schroeder (1980)
	0.3–0.6 mg/kg i.m.	Used by author, based on feline doses	
Morphine	2– 5 mg/kg s.c., i.m. q2–4h		Wixson (1994)
	5–10 mg/kg s.c., i.m. q2–4h		Gillett (1994)
Paracetamol	200–500 mg/kg orally	Analgesia. Short-term use only, hepatic toxicity	Gillett (1994)
Tramadol	4.4–11 mg/kg orally q12h	Analgesia	Souza *et al.* (2008); Egger *et al.* (2009)

21.5 (continued) Analgesic and anti-inflammatory drugs. CRI = constant rate infusion; t.d. = transdermally; t.m. = transmucosally.

Opioids

Opioids are the mainstay of acute pain management, and have a role in the treatment of longer-term pain also. They are categorized as pure agonists, partial agonists, mixed agonists/antagonists, and antagonists, although there is some crossover between categories, depending on the receptor acted upon. Their bioavailability is poor when taken by mouth, owing to the first-pass effect; doses of buprenorphine used orally in rats (Pekow, 1992; Flecknell, 2001) were 8 times higher than the recommended parenteral dose.

Pure agonists

These include morphine, methadone and fentanyl.

- Morphine is not considered to be the first choice of opioid to use in hindgut-fermenting rabbits owing to the risk of reduction in gastrointestinal motility (Hawkins, 2006), although it should be noted that pain also strongly inhibits this motility.

In the UK, fentanyl/fluanisone is authorized for use in rabbits. Methadone is authorized for use in the dog, and according to the Cascade these two agents should be selected in preference to morphine.

- Short-acting agonists, such as fentanyl, without fluanisone, may be used as a bolus or constant rate infusion (CRI) to maintain analgesia following sedation with fentanyl/fluanisone, or other agents such as mixed or partial agonists may be employed. Mixed agonist/antagonists provide continuing analgesia while partially reversing the sedative qualities of the pure agonists. Although pure agonists provide excellent analgesia, they tend to be relatively short acting, requiring frequent administration, which may be stressful to the rabbit.
- Transcutaneous fentanyl patches are often considered for use in rabbits; however, although detectable plasma concentrations are reached there is no good evidence for analgesic efficacy

in rabbits (Weaver *et al.*, 2010). Partial and mixed agonists are more widely used in practice. While not providing the degree of analgesia of the pure agonists, they have a greater duration of action, and fewer side effects (reduced gastrointestinal motility, respiratory depression).

Butorphanol and buprenorphine
These are the most commonly used agents.

- Butorphanol is a mixed agonist/antagonist which has a similar duration of action in rabbits to that in other mammals. A half-life of 3.16 hours with a dose of 0.5 mg/kg s.c. was reported in one study (Portnoy and Hustead, 1992). Butorphanol exerts its agonist effects at kappa receptors and its antagonist effects at mu receptors, making it a good choice of drug for partial reversal of the effects of pure agents. However, its analgesic qualities are questionable, and its ceiling effect limits its usefulness (Lichtenberger and Ko, 2007).
- Buprenorphine has been found to be an effective and safe opioid in many mammalian species, including rabbits (Roughan and Flecknell, 2002). It has a complex profile, exhibiting partial and mixed characteristics at both mu and kappa receptors. Its ceiling effect and slow onset must be taken into consideration, but it provides moderate analgesia for 4–8 hours (Lichtenberger and Ko, 2007).

Non-steroidal anti-inflammatory drugs
NSAIDs are the mainstay of chronic pain and inflammation mitigation in rabbits, as well as having an important role in acute treatment. Their mode of action is the inhibition of cyclooxygenases, therefore reducing prostaglandin synthesis. In hypotensive patients, prostaglandin regulation of renal blood flow may be impaired, leading to acute kidney injury (Harcourt-Brown, 2002). They therefore have more potential adverse effects in the critical patient and those with pre-existing renal disease (Lichtenberger and Ko, 2007) and should ideally only be used after demonstration of normal blood pressure and renal function, and in the absence of gastric bleeding.

The cyclooxygenases COX 1 and COX 2 appear to have less clear-cut roles than previously thought, and therefore specific COX inhibitors may be less effective than expected, and not entirely free of side effects. It should be noted that the most common adverse effects noted in other species involve the gastrointestinal tract. As rabbits do not vomit, and gastrointestinal bleeding is difficult to detect, it is wise to monitor patients closely. The concurrent use of H2 blockers in rabbits is common, and may be beneficial in minimizing such adverse effects.

NSAIDs may be given enterally or parenterally, although oral administration of some products may be complicated by the practicalities of tablet size, especially in smaller rabbits. Commonly used NSAIDs include carprofen, meloxicam and ketoprofen. Ketoprofen is a non-selective COX 1 inhibitor and, as such, is ideally not administered prior to anaesthesia.

Carprofen
Carprofen is a weak COX inhibitor at therapeutic doses, providing anti-inflammatory effects. This may explain its good safety margin, suggesting that other pathways are involved (Hawkins, 2006). This may also suggest its preferential use in cases of gastrointestinal stasis, rather than meloxicam, because prostaglandins are prokinetic in the rabbit caecum/colon.

Meloxicam
Meloxicam is the most widely used NSAID in the rabbit, owing partly to its COX 2-specific action and low incidence of adverse effects, and partly to its liquid formulation and palatability, permitting easy dosing. Doses used in practice are commonly lower than those suggested in the literature, with the consequent risk of providing inadequate analgesia (Carpenter *et al.*, 2009b).

Other NSAIDs
Other NSAIDs such as flunixin, aspirin, ibuprofen, diclofenac and phenylbutazone are generally not used in rabbits, because of the Cascade in the UK, and the presence of suitable alternatives listed above. However, no NSAID is currently authorized for use in the rabbit, and clinical judgement may suggest the use of such drugs in certain situations. For example, flunixin may have a role in the treatment of enterotoxaemia, although its potential nephrotoxicity is a concern (Harcourt-Brown, 2002).

Miscellaneous agents
The analgesic effects of ketamine and alpha-2 adrenergic agents are covered in more detail in Chapter 10.

Tramadol
Tramadol is a synthetic opioid-like drug, which acts on opioid receptors (primarily mu). There is little information on its use in rabbits, and doses have been extrapolated from the literature on human and other veterinary species. It appears to provide good analgesia, and is easily administered long term, providing a useful adjunct or replacement for NSAIDs. Sedation and agitation may be observed, and gastrointestinal disturbance (vomiting, diarrhoea, constipation and inappetence) are noted in other species (Johnston, 2005). However, tramadol given by the oral route at 11 mg/kg in rabbits has been shown not to reach plasma levels equivalent to those required for analgesia in humans, although analgesic effects in the rabbit were not studied (Souza *et al.*, 2008).

Gabapentin
Gabapentin is effective in the control of chronic neurogenic pain in other species, as well as being used for its anticonvulsant activity. Sedation and ataxia may be noted. Starting at the low end of the dose range and slowly increasing is recommended to avoid this. Abrupt discontinuation has led to seizures in humans, and animals should be weaned off slowly (Plumb, 2011).

Paracetamol

Paracetamol (acetaminophen) has a poorly understood mechanism of action, but appears to exert its analgesic and anti-pyretic effects via COX inhibition. It has no anti-inflammatory effects. It may be used in conjunction with other classes of analgesic (Huerkamp, 1995; Hernandez-Divers, 2004). There is potential for renal, hepatic, gastrointestinal and haematological adverse effects in the rabbit (Plumb, 2011).

Corticosteroids

Corticosteroids are occasionally suggested for their anti-inflammatory analgesic qualities. While they are potent anti-inflammatories, and may have a role in neuromuscular and some uncommon skin diseases, allergic and autoimmune disease and neoplasia treatment, as well as the acute treatment of trauma, even small single doses may cause severe pathological changes in rabbits (Rosenthal, 2004). Steroids can stimulate the mobilization of free fatty acids from adipose tissue, contributing to the development of hepatic lipidosis in the anorexic rabbit (particularly if overweight). This makes them a poor choice as appetite stimulants in the inappetent rabbit. Chronic use of steroids impedes wound healing, and chronically diseased rabbits often have low white cell counts and further immune suppression is harmful (Harcourt-Brown, 2002). Immune suppression may lead to (re)activation of subclinical or latent infections such as pasteurellosis (Pollock, 2006).

Antibacterial agents

Antibiotics (Figure 21.6) are widely prescribed therapeutic agents. They may be over-prescribed, in the absence of confirmation or reasonable suspicion of a bacterial pathogen. However, subclinical bacterial disease (particularly respiratory pasteurellosis) is common in the rabbit, and antibiosis may be warranted to prevent recrudescence of infection when managing other conditions.

Drug	Doses	Indications/comments	References
Amikacin	2–3 mg/kg s.c., i.m. q8–12h		Hrapkiewicz *et al.* (1998)
Amoxicillin	7 mg/kg s.c. q24h	**Do not give orally**	Harcourt-Brown (2009)
Azithromycin	15–30 mg/kg orally q24h		Lukehart *et al.* (1990)
Cefalexin	20 mg/kg s.c. q24h		Harcourt-Brown (2009)
	11–22 mg/kg orally q8h	Although there are concerns regarding the use of this drug orally, some authors have done so safely (e.g. Keeble, 2006)	
Chloramphenicol	30–50 mg/kg orally q12h		Keeble (2006)
Ciprofloxacin	5–20 mg/kg orally q12h		Marx and Roston (1996); Hrapkiewicz *et al.* (1998)
Doxycycline	2.5 mg/kg orally q12h		Hrapkiewicz *et al.* (1998)
Enrofloxacin	10–30 mg/kg orally, s.c., i.m. q24h	AUTHORIZED FOR USE IN RABBITS	
	Up to 20 mg/kg orally, s.c., i.m. q24h		Quesenberry (1994); Redrobe (2010)
Florfenicol	25 mg/kg i.m., i.v. q6h	Not for use in food animals	Koc *et al.* (2009)
Gentamicin	1.5–2.5 mg/kg s.c., i.m., i.v. q8h		Hrapkiewicz *et al.* (1998)
Marbofloxacin	2–10 mg/kg orally, i.m., i.v. q24h		Abo-El-Sooud and Goudah (2009); Carpenter *et al.* (2009a); Harcourt-Brown (2009)
Metronidazole	20–40 mg/kg orally q12h	Treatment of choice for enterotoxaemia	Harcourt-Brown (2009)
Oxytetracycline	30 mg/kg s.c. q72h 15 mg/kg s.c. q24h		Harcourt-Brown (2002); Richardson (2000)
Penicillin G	40,000 IU/kg s.c., i.m. q7days for 3 doses	Treponematosis	Harcourt-Brown (2002)
Dihydrostreptomycin/ Penicillin	40 mg/kg penicillin + 50 mg/kg streptomycin s.c. q24h		Harcourt-Brown (2009)

21.6 Antibiotics. (continues) ▶

Drug	Doses	Indications/comments	References
Tilmicosin	10 mg/kg q24h for 3 days or q7days	TEST DOSE of 5 mg/kg is advised first. **DANGER OF DEATH**	Harcourt-Brown (2002)
	12.5 mg/kg orally q24h for 7 days		Gallina *et al.* (2010)
	25 mg/kg once only		McKay *et al.* (1996)
Trimethoprim/ sulfamethoxazole	40 mg/kg orally q12h		Harcourt-Brown (2009)
Tylosin	10 mg/kg orally, s.c., i.m. q12h		Hrapkiewicz *et al.* (1998); Harcourt-Brown (2002)

21.6 (continued) Antibiotics.

Antibacterial selection

Wherever possible, antibiotics should be selected on the basis of (aerobic and anaerobic) culture and sensitivity testing. However, this is often impractical owing to a lack of suitable sample material. There is a risk of antibiotic-associated enterotoxaemia with any antibiotic, although some agents are significantly safer than others, and so the risk-to-benefit ratio should be determined in each case (Harcourt-Brown, 2002). The ability of an antibiotic to penetrate to the area required, and be effective there, depends on local factors such as the presence or absence of pus and the local pH. Bactericidal antibiotics may be preferred, where possible, in the often immunosuppressed rabbit. Some antibiotics may be either bactericidal or bacteriostatic depending on the organism and their concentration at the site of action.

Mitigation of adverse effects

A correct balance of caecal microflora is important for normal digestive function in rabbits. Oral antibiotics may upset this balance, permitting overgrowth of pathogenic species such as *Clostridium spiroforme* and *Escherichia coli*. This can result in enterotoxaemia. This is less likely with parenteral than with oral agents; antibiotics known to cause this problem include penicillins and lincosamides.

Ensuring that rabbits are maintained on suitable high-fibre diets, provision of appropriate supplementary food containing probiotics and electrolytes, and careful monitoring for the development of diarrhoea are all helpful. In cases of antibiotic-associated enterotoxaemia, or to prevent it, metronidazole has been shown to be effective (Carman, 1994). Colestyramine is an ion-exchange resin which has been shown to prevent death in clindamycin-induced enterotoxaemia (Rateau *et al.*, 1986; Lipman *et al.*, 1992).

Pasteurellosis

Pasteurella multocida is a common respiratory pathogen in rabbits. It is considered almost, if not actually, ubiquitous outside of specific pathogen- free collections. It may affect the ear, nasal cavity and lungs, and may be recovered from abscesses and other organs (e.g. uterus, ovaries). Other bacteria (e.g. *Staphylococcus* spp.) may also be recovered from these and other sites, and it is important not to assume that all infections in rabbits are due to *Pasteurella*. Strains resistant to particular antibiotics exist, and bacterial culture and sensitivity testing, performed on abscess capsule, lavage or swabs of affected lesions, is useful. Typically, fluoroquinolones, chloramphenicol, penicillins and aminoglycosides are effective against *P. multocida*. The effect of tetracyclines and potentiated sulphonamides is variable (Harcourt-Brown, 2002; Pollock, 2006). Clinical cure of the animal may not mean that the organism has been completely eliminated, and false negative nasal cultures are common (Redrobe *et al.*, 2010).

Probiotics

Probiotics are products that contain microorganisms that are able to colonize the large intestine. They are usually encapsulated in some way to allow survival, or are otherwise resistant to the low gastric pH. They aim either to compete directly for nutrients with pathogenic bacteria or to act indirectly by supporting the growth of non-pathogenic organisms which do so. They therefore may include bacteria such as *Enterococcus faecium*, or yeasts such as *Saccharomyces cerevisiae*. Other potential benefits include: optimization of caecal pH, by stimulating the growth of lactate-consuming organisms; removing toxins and pathogenic bacteria (e.g. *Salmonella* spp.) directly by adhering to their cell walls; and increasing the number of cellulose-degrading organisms, thus enhancing volatile fatty acid production and improving nutrition. At least some probiotic organisms have been demonstrated to survive rabbit gastrointestinal transit, increase bodyweight, and influence caecal microflora (Benato *et al.*, 2012).

Rabbit-specific products, which avoid ingredients such as montmorillonite clay (used in the symptomatic treatment of diarrhoea in other species), should always be used to avoid possible gastrointestinal tract hypomotility. There are no specific contraindications to their use, and they appear to have no deleterious effects. They may have a role in the prevention and/or treatment of bacterial gastrointestinal diseases, and are often used concurrently with and following antimicrobial treatment, with the aim of reducing the risk of inappropriate bacterial overgrowth in the caecum due to antibiotic use.

Prebiotics such as fructo-oligosaccharides are substrates for non-pathogenic bacterial fermentation, and are often also present alongside probiotics in some preparations. Transfaunation with caecotrophs from healthy rabbits has also been suggested. This requires collection, usually by placing an Elizabethan collar to prevent caecotroph ingestion, and force-feeding of the caecotrophs. Mixing them to a slurry may be less effective than feeding them whole, because it removes their protective mucus coating, but the latter is much less straightforward to perform.

Types of antibacterial

Beta-lactamases

Penicillins: Penicillins are considered the treatment of choice for rabbit syphilis (*Treponema paraluis cuniculi* infection), although tetracyclines are also effective. Penicillins are also used to treat infections involving Gram-positive aerobes and anaerobes, which are commonly found in abscesses (Tyrrell *et al.*, 2002). They are particularly useful in abscess treatment owing to the high prevalence of anaerobes cultured. However, they carry a high risk of inducing caecal dysbiosis when used orally, and should only be used parenterally.

Long-acting formulations may be given every 2–3 days, by owners or in the clinic, to reduce the stress and tissue damage of more frequent injections. Benzyl penicillin, ampicillin and amoxicillin may all be used. The procaine component of procaine penicillin is toxic at high doses or in dependent kits of treated does (Harcourt-Brown, 2002).

Cephalosporins: Cephalosporins are closely related to the penicillins. They appear less toxic, and resistance in *Staphylococcus* spp. is seen less often than with penicillins (Harcourt-Brown, 2009). Long-acting cephalosporins such as cefovectin have much shorter half-lives in the rabbit, however, and therefore do not have suitably long durations of action to be clinically useful. Cefalexin appears to become well distributed in the tissues (including the anterior chamber of the eye), and is well tolerated parenterally.

Carbapenems: The use of carbapenems (e.g. imipenem) has not been documented clinically in the rabbit, but they may have a role in the treatment of resistant *Pseudomonas aeruginosa*.

Lincosamides
Clindamycin can induce fatal dysbiosis in rabbits. However, it is highly effective against anaerobes (Tyrrell *et al.*, 2002), and so may be used with great care in the local treatment of abscesses (see above).

Macrolides
These are a related group to the lincosamides, but they appear to be safer in rabbits. Azithromycin and tylosin, in particular, are effective upper respiratory tract antibiotics, with reasonable safety profiles in this species (Lukehart *et al.*, 1990; Fong, 2000). Erythromycin is often suggested as a prokinetic, but even at the relatively lower doses used in this role, there are more effective products available with a better safety profile.

Tilmicosin is used to treat *Pasteurella* pneumonia in ruminants. It is highly effective, but has caused fatal adverse reactions and therefore cannot be recommended as anything other than a last resort. **It has caused fatalities in humans accidentally injected with the product, and therefore should only be used with great care, with fully informed owner consent, and NEVER dispensed to owners for home use.**

Fluoroquinolones
Enrofloxacin is currently the only systemic antibiotic authorized in the UK for use in the rabbit. It is effective against a wide variety of Gram-negative and some Gram-positive microorganisms. It has good efficacy against *Bordetella* and *Mycoplasma*, as well as *Pasteurella*. It is very safe with regard to digestive problems, even in long-term use. Efficacy is dose related (a concentration-dependent antibiotic effect).

Arthropathies have been reported in some species treated with fluoroquinolones (Sharpnack *et al.*, 1994) and therefore these drugs should be used with care in skeletally immature juvenile rabbits. Antibiotic resistance to fluoroquinolones is increasing, in both domestic animal and human use, and this should be considered when treating rabbits, particularly large groups.

Aminoglycosides
Gentamicin is widely used topically (e.g. Tiacil) and is one of only two topical ocular antibiotics authorized for use in the rabbit in the UK. It is also used locally in the treatment of abscesses. It is nephrotoxic, and therefore not widely used systemically. Amikacin is less nephrotoxic, and therefore might be considered for use against susceptible infections. Aminoglycosides are not absorbed via the enteral route.

Fusidic acid
Fusidic acid is usually used topically on the skin or the eye. It is present in one of only two ocular preparations authorized for use in the rabbit in the UK (Fucithalmic Vet). Unauthorized fusidic acid ointments exist, with or without an accompanying corticosteroid, and may be applied to skin lesions.

Metronidazole
The only commonly available member of the nitroimidazole group, metronidazole is used for the treatment of susceptible anaerobic bacterial infections, and for selected protozoal infections (e.g. *Giardia*) but is not effective against *Encephalitozoon cuniculi*. Used in conjunction with other antibiotics, e.g. enrofloxacin, it provides a wider spectrum of activity.

Potentiated sulphonamides

Sulphonamides are effective against a wide range of bacteria, although they are deactivated by purulent debris. They are also effective against Coccidia and *Toxoplasma*. They are typically potentiated with trimethoprim to reduce the development of resistance. They may precipitate out in acid urine, leading to renal damage. This is not generally a concern in the rabbit, with normal urine pH of 7.5–8.5, but acidic urine may be seen in anorexic or cachexic rabbits, and these drugs should be avoided in such cases.

Tetracyclines

Tetracyclines are broad spectrum, generally bacteriostatic antibiotics, which have been routinely used for many years in rabbits, often via in-water or in-feed medication. There is significant resistance amongst bacteria, especially *Staphylococcus aureus* (Harcourt-Brown, 2002). Use of long-acting parenteral formulations is associated with significant soft tissue damage. Standard preparations may be used at high doses (30 mg/kg) every 72 hours, to good clinical effect (Malley, personal communication).

Chloramphenicol and analogues

Chloramphenicol is not widely available, but related fluorinated analogues such as florfenicol (Park *et al.*, 2007) are available, generally for use in calf pneumonia, and potentially show promise for the treatment of susceptible respiratory tract disease in rabbits.

Antifungals

Topical and systemic antifungal drugs (Figure 21.7) may be used in the treatment of skin conditions such as dermatophytosis, and nasal aspergillosis.

Systemic griseofulvin has been used historically, but the large-sized tablet preparations, teratogenicity, and long treatment courses are not ideal. Azole derivatives may be used topically (miconazole, enilconazole), or systemically (ketoconazole,

itraconazole, voriconazole, pozaconazole). Itraconazole is authorized for use in the cat, and is the first choice under the Cascade in the UK. Unlike the cat, the rabbit does not require a treatment break every 5 days. However, inappetence has been described at the high end of the dose range.

Concurrent topical and systemic treatment may reduce infectivity to the environment and conspecifics, and speed recovery. Treating the environment by removing items that rabbits have rubbed or scratched against helps prevent reinfection. Improving health status generally helps to improve immune status and may often effect spontaneous resolution.

Terbinafine has been used in guinea pigs (Ghannoum *et al.*, 2010) to good effect, and may provide an alternative option in refractory cases.

Antiparasitic agents

The main endoparasites of concern in the rabbit are Coccidia and *Encephalitozoon cuniculi*. Control includes hygiene practices as well as treatment, restricting access to contaminated material (faeces more than 2–3 days old in the case of Coccidia, and urine in the latter). The most widely used treatment option for *E. cuniculi* is fenbendazole (Suter *et al.*, 2001). The main ectoparasites of concern are *Cheyletiella*, *Psoroptes* and *Leporacus*. Doses for some antiparasitic agents are given in Figure 21.8.

Agents acting on specific body systems

The rabbit is extremely susceptible to gastrointestinal disturbance (e.g. enterotoxaemia, stasis, dysbiosis), and treatment of such problems should be a priority (see Chapter 12). Drugs that act on the gastrointestinal system are listed in Figure 21.9.

Figures 21.10–21.13 list drugs used in rabbits that act on the central nervous, urogenital and cardiorespiratory systems, plus miscellaneous agents.

Drug	Doses	Indications/comments	References
Clotrimazole	Topical	Dermatophytosis. Avoid concurrent usage with cisapride	Richardson (2000); Harcourt-Brown (2002)
Enilconazole	Topical, 1:50 dilution	Candidiasis, dermatophytosis	Richardson (2000); Scarff (2000)
Itraconazole	10 mg/kg orally q24h for 15 days	Dermatophytosis	Scarff (2000)
Ketoconazole	10–40 mg/kg orally q24h for 14 days		Harkness and Wagner (1995)
Miconazole	Once daily for 2–4 weeks	Dermatophytosis	Harkness and Wagner (1995)
	1 ml/kg q12h		Dechra product information, 2012
Terbinafine	100 mg/kg q12h		Fiorello and Divers (2012)

21.7 Antifungal agents.

Drug	Doses	Indications/comments	References
Albendazole	15–20 mg/kg orally q24h for 2–4 weeks	*Encephalitozoon cuniculi* **TERATOGENIC**	Richardson (2000); Harcourt-Brown (2002)
Cyromazine	Apply 6% topically every 8–10 weeks		Flecknell (2005)
Fenbendazole	20 mg/kg orally q24h for 9 or 28 days		Suter *et al.* (2001); Keeble (2011)
Imidacloprid	10 mg/kg topically	Fleas	Harcourt-Brown (2002)
Ivermectin	0.4 mg/kg orally, s.c. q10–14 days × 2–3 doses	Ectoparasites	Quesenberry (1994)
Praziquantel	5–10 mg/kg orally, i.m., s.c., topically		Hrapkiewicz *et al.* (1998); Richardson (2000)
Pyrethrin	250 mg/kg t.d.		Xenex: Dechra product information, 2012
Selamectin	6–18 mg/kg topically; repeat after 4 weeks for *Cheyletiella*		Harcourt-Brown (2002)
Sulfamethazine	100 mg/kg orally q24h	Coccidiosis	Hrapkiewicz *et al.* (1998)
Toltrazuril	2.5–5.0 mg/kg orally q24h for 2 days; repeat in 14 days	Coccidiosis	Redrobe *et al.* (2010)
Trimethoprim/ sulfamethoxazole	40 mg/kg orally q12h	Coccidiosis	Harcourt-Brown (2002)

21.8 Antiparasitic agents.

Drug	Doses	Indications/comments	References
Bismuth subsalicylate	0.3–0.6 ml/kg orally q4–6h		Harkness and Wagner (1995); Hrapkiewicz *et al.* (1998)
Butylscopolamine/ Metamizole (Buscopan compositum)	0.1 ml/kg i.v., i.m. q12h	Analgesic, spasmolytic. **Do not use without ruling out intestinal obstruction**	Harcourt-Brown (2002)
Cimetidine	5–10 mg/kg orally q6–12h		Hrapkiewicz *et al.* (1998)
Cisapride	0.5–1.0 mg/kg orally q8–24h	Gastric and intestinal prokinetic. **Do not use without ruling out intestinal obstruction**	Hrapkiewicz *et al.* (1998); Richardson (2000); Harcourt-Brown (2002)
Colestyramine	500 mg/kg orally q12h 2 g per 20 ml drinking water for 14–21 days	Treatment for antibiotic-induced enterocolitis	Richardson (2000); Harcourt-Brown (2002)
Dinoprost	0.2 mg/kg single injection i.m. or s.c.	To assist in emptying impacted caeca, following 3 days' liquid paraffin orally	Harcourt-Brown (2002)
Domperidone	0.5 mg/kg orally q12h	**Do not use without ruling out intestinal obstruction**	Ramsay (2011)
Loperamide	0.04–0.2 mg/kg orally q8–12h		Ramsay (2011)
Metoclopramide	0.2–0.5 mg/kg orally, s.c., i.v. q4–8h	Gastric motility prokinetic. **Do not use without ruling out intestinal obstruction**	Harkness and Wagner (1995); Marx and Roston (1996)
Probiotics	As per package instructions	Many varieties of probiotic are specifically produced for exotic pets, including rabbits	
Ranitidine	2–5 mg/kg orally q8–12h	H2-blocker, prevention and treatment of gastric ulceration. Gastric and intestinal prokinetic. **Do not use without ruling out intestinal obstruction**	Harcourt-Brown (2002). Dose-related prokinetic effect (Kounenis *et al.*, 1992)
Simethicone	100 mg/kg orally q2–8h	For dispersal of gas in gastrointestinal stasis; however, as frothy bloat does not occur in the rabbit, this product may be of limited efficacy	

21.9 Drugs acting on the gastrointestinal system.

Drug	Doses	Indications/comments	References
Atropine	0.05 mg/kg i.m.	Organophosphate toxicity treatment. Approximately 40% of rabbits produce atropinesterase, denaturing atropine	Harcourt-Brown (2002)
Cyclizine	8 mg/rabbit orally q12h	Torticollis	Harcourt-Brown (2002)
Dexamethasone	0.2–0.6 mg/kg s.c., i.v.	Cerebral injury. See text regarding contraindications for corticosteroids	Hrapkiewicz et al. (1998)
Diphenhydramine	2.0 mg/kg orally, s.c. q8–12h	Torticollis	Pollock (2006)
Furosemide	5–10 mg/kg i.m., i.v. q12h	Cerebral oedema	Hrapkiewicz et al. (1998)
Glycopyrollate	0.1 mg/kg s.c., i.m.	Organophosphate toxicity treatment	Harcourt-Brown (2002)
Levetiracetam	20 mg/kg orally q8h		Benedetti et al. (2004)
Meclizine	2–12 mg/kg orally q24h	Torticollis	Harkness and Wagner (1995); Hrapkiewicz et al. (1998)
Naloxone	0.01–1.0 mg/kg i.m., i.v.		Hawk and Leary (1995)
Prednisolone	0.25–0.5 mg/kg orally q12h for 3 days, then q24h for 3 days, then q48h	See text regarding contraindications for corticosteroids	Hrapkiewicz et al. (1998)
Prochlorperazine	0.25 mg/kg orally q8h	Torticollis	Keeble (2011)

21.10 Drugs acting on the central nervous system (see also Chapter 15).

Drug	Doses	Indications/comments	References
Aglepristone	10 mg/kg q24h × 2, on days 6 and 7 after mating	Abortion	Ozalp et al. (2010)
Bendrofluazide	0.6 mg/kg orally q24h	Calcium-sparing diuretic, for use in increasing urine volume and reducing urinary sediment	Malley, personal communication
Bethanecol	2.5–5.0 mg orally q12h	Atonic bladder	Richardson (2000)
Buserelin	0.2 ml/rabbit s.c.	Induces ovulation in breeding does. AUTHORIZED IN UK	Harcourt-Brown (2002); Flecknell (2005)
Chorionic gonadotrophin	20–25 IU i.v.	Induces ovulation in breeding does	Harkness and Wagner (1995)
Diethylstilbestrol	0.5 mg orally 1–2 times weekly	Post-neutering urinary incontinence in does	Richardson (2000)
Furosemide	0.3–2.0 mg/kg i.v., s.c., i.m.		Harcourt-Brown (2002)
	1–4 mg/kg i.m., s.c., orally q4–12h		Marx and Roston (1996)
Oxytocin	0.1–3.0 IU/kg s.c., i.m.	Delayed parturition or agalactia. **Confirm cervix open prior to use**	Harkness and Wagner (1995); Hrapkiewicz et al. (1998)
Phenylpropanolamine	6.25–12.5 mg/rabbit orally q12h	Oestrogen-dependent urinary incontinence	Richardson (2000)
Proligestone	30 mg/kg orally q24h	Pseudopregnancy. Owing to induced ovulation, long-term treatment is necessary	Richardson (2000)

21.11 Drugs acting on the urogenital system.

Drug	Doses	Indications/comments	References
Benazepril	0.25–0.5 mg/kg orally q24h	Vasodilator; less nephrotoxic than enalapril. Beware of hypotensive effects; monitor blood pressure during use	Morissey and Carpenter (2012)
Bromhexine	1 mg/kg orally q12–24h	Upper and lower respiratory hypersecretory and inflammatory disease. Mucolytic	Koyuncu et al. (1989); Ramsay (2011)
Digoxin	0.005–0.01 mg/kg orally q12–24h	Congestive heart failure, atrial fibrillation	Morissey and Carpenter (2012)
Diltiazem	0.5–1.0 mg/kg orally q12–24h	Calcium channel blocker for hypertrophic cardiomyopathy	Morissey and Carpenter (2012)
Enalapril	0.1–0.5 mg/kg orally q24–48h	Vasodilator. Beware of hypotensive effects; monitor blood pressure during use	Jepson (2009)
Fluticasone	50–250 µg q12–72h		Extrapolated from the cat dose, and used empirically by the author
Furosemide	2–5 mg/kg orally s.c., i.m., i.v, q12h prn		Morissey and Carpenter (2012)
Pimobendan	0.1–0.3 mg/kg orally q12–24h	Increases cardiac contractility in dilated cardiomyopathy	Morissey and Carpenter (2012)
Terbutaline	1.25 mg/rabbit orally q8h		Extrapolated from the feline dose; personal anecdotal experience only

21.12 Drugs acting on the cardiorespiratory system.

Drug	Doses	Indications/comments	References
Activated charcoal	1000 mg/kg orally q4–6h	Oral intoxication	Hernandez-Divers (2004)
Aluminium hydroxide	30–60 mg/kg orally q8–12h	Phosphate binder	Hernandez-Divers (2004)
Calcium gluconate	50–100 mg/kg, i.p., i.v. single dose	Hypocalcaemia	Marx and Roston (1996)
Chlorphenamine	0.2–0.4 mg/kg orally q12h		Ramsay (2011)
Chondroitin sulphate	As per feline dose		Uebelhart et al. (1998)
Ciclosporin	5 mg/kg orally q24h	Sebaceous adenitis	Jassies-van der Lee et al. (2009)
Dexamethasone	0.5–2.0 mg/kg i.m., i.v., s.c.	Shock doses for enterotoxaemia	Richardson (2000); Flecknell (2005)
Edetate calcium disodium	27.5 mg/kg s.c. q6h for 5 days, repeat as necessary 1 week later	Heavy metal (lead, zinc) toxicity	Richardson (2000)
Erythropoietin	50–150 IU/kg s.c. q2–3days	Non-regenerative anaemia	Pollock (2006)
Ferrous sulphate	4–6 mg/kg orally q24h		Brown (1997)
Heparin	5 mg/kg i.v.		Hawk and Leary (1995)
Hydroxyzine	2 mg/kg orally q8–12h		Morissey and Carpenter (2012)
Mirtazapine	0.3–0.5 mg/kg orally q24h	Appetite stimulant	Dosage anecdotally reported, extrapolated from the cat (Quimby et al., 2011)
Nandrolone	2 mg/kg s.c., i.m.	Anabolic steroid, appetite stimulant	Harcourt-Brown (2002)
Penicillamine	30 mg/kg orally q12h	Chelating agent for copper and lead toxicity	Harcourt-Brown (2002)
Polysulphated glycosaminoglycan	2.2 mg/kg s.c., i.m. q3days for 21–28 days, then q14days		Hrapkiewicz et al. (1998)
Verapamil	0.2 mg/kg i.p. q8h for 9 doses	Prevention of postoperative adhesions	Hrapkiewicz et al. (1998); Richardson (2000); Harcourt-Brown (2002)
Vitamin K	1–10 mg/kg i.m.		Hrapkiewicz et al. (1998)

21.13 Miscellaneous agents. i.p. = intraperitoneally.

Therapeutic considerations

Dose alteration

Dosing adjustments may be necessary owing to age (incomplete metabolic pathways in younger patients, or reduced efficiency in older rabbits), other disease conditions such as renal or hepatic failure, or the concurrent use of other medications.

Drug interactions

A complete list of drug interactions is outside the scope of this text, and can be found in the relevant drug monographs in the current edition of the *BSAVA Small Animal Formulary*.

Specific therapeutic contraindications in the rabbit

- Fipronil, in both spray and spot-on formulations, has been associated with mortality when used in rabbits, and its use cannot be advised.
- Tilmicosin has been associated with sudden death as a result of cardiovascular failure in a range of species, including rabbits.
- As discussed earlier, enterotoxaemia has been associated with the use of certain antibiotics, especially lincosamides and beta-lactamases, in particular following oral administration.
- Physical agents intended to slow gastrointestinal motility, e.g. to treat hypermotility disorders in other species, including kaolin or montmorillonite clay products, are NOT indicated in the rabbit, because they may precipitate potentially fatal gastric stasis.
- The use of loperamide should be reserved for severe, life-threatening true diarrhoea with associated abdominal pain (Banerjee *et al.*, 1987).

In the event of a suspected adverse reaction (including lack of efficacy), a Suspected Adverse Reaction Form should be completed and submitted to both the drug company and, in the UK, the Veterinary Medicines Directorate (forms available at www.vmd.defra.gov.uk).

References and further reading

Abo-El-Sooud K and Goudah A (2009) Influence of *Pasteurella multocida* infection on the pharmacokinetic behaviour of marbofloxacin after intravenous and intramuscular administration in rabbits. *Journal of Veterinary Pharmacology and Therapeutics* **33**, 63–68

Audeval-Gerard C, Nivet C, el Amrani AI, *et al.* (2000) Pharmacokinetics of ketoprofen in rabbit after a single topical application. *European Journal of Drug Metabolism and Pharmacokinetics* **25**, 227–230

Banerjee AK, Angulo AF, Dhasmana KM and Kong-A-San J (1987) Acute diarrhoeal disease in the rabbit: bacteriological diagnosis and efficacy of oral rehydration in combination with loperamide hydrochloride. *Laboratory Animals* **21**, 314–317

Benato L, Hastie P, Shaw D, Murray J and Meredith A (2012) The semi-quantitative effect of probiotic *Enterococcus faecium* NCIMB 30183 and *Saccaromyces cerevisiae* NCYC Sc47 on the faecal microflora of healthy adult rabbits (*Oryctolagus cuniculus*) using real time PCR. *BSAVA Congress 2012 Scientific Proceedings: Veterinary Programme*, p.460

Benedetti M, Coupez R, Whomsley R, *et al.* (2004) Comparative pharmacokinetics and metabolism of levetiracetam, a new anti-epileptic agent, in mouse, rat, rabbit and dog. *Xenobiotic* **34**, 281–300

Bishop Y (2005) Prescribing for rabbits. In: *The Veterinary Formulary*, pp.62–65. Pharmaceutical Press, London

Bonner J (2008) Coping with the Cascade. *Companion*, pp.7–9

Broome RL, Brooks DL, Babish JG, *et al.* (1991) Pharmacokinetic properties of enrofloxacin in rabbits. *American Journal of Veterinary Research* **52**, 1835–1841

Brown SA (1997) Rabbit urinary tract disease. In: *Proceedings, North American Veterinary Conference*, pp.785–787

BSAVA (2012) *BSAVA Guide to the Use of Veterinary Medicines.* [available at www.bsava.com]

Cabanes A, Arboix M, Garcia-Anton JM and Roig F (1992) Pharmacokinetics of enrofloxacin after intravenous and intramuscular injection in rabbits. *American Journal of Veterinary Research* **53**, 2090–2093

Cantwell CS (2001) Ferret, rabbit and rodent anaesthesia. *Veterinary Clinics of North America: Exotic Animal Practice* **4**, 169–191

Capner CA, Lascelles BD and Waterman-Pearson AE (1999) Current British veterinary attitudes to perioperative analgesia for dogs. *Veterinary Record* **145**, 95–99

Carman RJ (1994) Antibiotic associated diarrhoea of rabbits. *Journal of Small Exotic Animal Medicine* **2**, 69–71

Carpenter JW, Pollack CG, Koch DE, *et al.* (2009a) Single and multiple dose pharmacokinetics of marbofloxacin after oral administration to rabbits. *American Journal of Veterinary Research* **70**, 522–526

Carpenter JW, Pollock CG, Koch DE and Hunter RP (2009b) Single and multiple-dose pharmacokinetics of meloxicam after oral administration to the rabbit (*Oryctolagus cuniculus*). *Journal of Zoo and Wildlife Medicine* **40**(4), 601–606

Chapman MW and Hadley WK (1976) The effect of polymethylmethacrylate and antibiotic combinations on bacterial viability. An in vitro and preliminary in vivo study. *Journal of Bone and Joint Surgery* **58**(1), 76–81

Egger CM, Souza MJ, Greenacre CB, *et al.* (2009) Effect of intravenous administration of tramadol hydrochloride on the minimum alveolar concentration of isoflurane in rabbits. *American Journal of Veterinary Research* **70**, 945–949

Fiorello CV and Divers SJ (2012) *Exotic Animal Formulary, 4th edn*, ed. J Carpenter, pp.517–557. Elsevier, St. Louis

Flecknell PA (1998) Analgesia in small mammals. *Seminars in Avian and Exotic Pet Medicine* **7**, 41–47

Flecknell PA (2001) Analgesia of small mammals. *Veterinary Clinics of North America: Exotic Animal Practice* **4**, 47–56

Flecknell PA (2005) Prescribing for rabbits. In: *The Veterinary Formulary, 6th edn*, ed. Y Bishop, pp.62–65. Pharmaceutical Press, London

Foley PL, Henderson AL, Bissonette EA, Wimer GR and Feldman SH (2001) Evaluation of fentanyl transdermal patches in rabbits: blood concentrations and physiologic response. *Comparative Medicine* **51**(3), 239–244

Fong I (2000) Antibiotic effects in a rabbit model of *Chlamydia pneumoniae*-induced atherosclerosis. *Journal of Infectious Diseases* **181**(Suppl. 3), S514–S518

Gallina G, Lucatello L, Drigoe I, *et al.* (2010) Kinetics and intrapulmonary disposition of tilmicosin after single and repeated oral bolus administrations to rabbits. *Veterinary Research Communications* **34**, s69–s72

Ghannoum MA, Long L, Kim HG, *et al.* (2010) Efficacy of terbinafine compared to lanoconazole and luliconazole in the topical treatment of dermatophytosis in a guinea pig model. *Medical Mycology* **48**(3), 491–497

Gillett CS (1994) Selected drug dosages and clinical reference data. In: *The Biology of the Laboratory Rabbit, 2nd edn*, ed. PJ Manning *et al.*, pp.467–472. Academic Press, London

Harcourt-Brown FM (2002) Therapeutics. In: *Textbook of Rabbit Medicine*, pp.94–120. Butterworth Heineman, Oxford

Harcourt-Brown F (2009) Dental disease in pet rabbits 3. Jaw abscesses. *In Practice* **31**(10), 496–505

Harkness JE, Turner PV, VandeWoude S and Wheler CL (2010) *Harkness and Wagner's Biology of Rabbits and Rodents, 5th edn.* Wiley-Blackwell, Oxford

Harkness JE and Wagner JE (1995) *Biology and Medicine of Rabbits and Rodents, 4th edn.* Blackwell, Oxford

Hawk CT and Leary SL (1995) *Formulary for Laboratory Animals.* Iowa State University Press, Ames

Hawkins, M (2006) The use of analgesics in birds, reptiles and small exotic mammals. *Journal of Exotic Pet Medicine* **15**(3), 177–192

Hernandez-Divers S (2004) Rabbits. In: *Exotic Animal Formulary, 3rd edn*, ed. JW Carpenter, pp.411–444. WB Saunders, Philadelphia

Hrapkiewicz K, Medina L and Holmes DD (1998) *Clinical Medicine of Small Mammals and Primates: An Introduction, 2nd edn.* Manson Publishing/The Veterinary Press, London

Huerkamp M (1995) Anaesthesia and postoperative care of rabbits and pocket pets. In: *Kirk's Current Veterinary Therapy XII SAP*, ed. JD Bonagura, pp.1322–1327. WB Saunders, Philadelphia

Jassies-van der Lee A, van Zeeland Y, Kik M and Shoemaker N (2009) Successful treatment of sebaceous adenitis in a rabbit with ciclosporin and triglycerides. *Veterinary Dermatology* **20**(1), 67–71

Jepson L (2009) *Exotic Animal Medicine: A Quick Reference Guide.* Saunders/Elsevier, Philadelphia

Johnston MS (2005) Clinical approaches to analgesia in ferrets and rabbits. *Seminars in Avian and Exotic Pet Medicine* **14**(4), 229–235

Keeble E (2006) Common neurological and musculosketal problems in rabbits. *In Practice* **28**, 212–218

Keeble E (2011) Encephalitozoonosis in rabbits – what we do and don't know. *In Practice* **33**, 426–435

Koc F, Ozturk M, Kadiogluy Y, *et al.* (2009) Pharmacokinetics of florfenicol after intravenous and intramuscular administration in New Zealand White Rabbits. *Research in Veterinary Science* **87**, 102–105

Kounenis G, Koutsoviti-Papadopoulou M, Elezoglou A and Voutsas A (1992) Comparative study of the H2-receptor antagonists cimetidine, ranitidine, famotidine and nizatidine on the rabbit stomach fundus and sigmoid colon. *Journal of Pharmacobiodynamics* **15**(10), 561–565

Koyuncu M, Yilmaz M, Yalcin S, *et al.* (1989) The existence of sinusitis in rabbits and the use of bromhexine as a mucolytic nose drop in the treatment of sinusitis. *Mikrobiyol Bulletin* **23**(2), 133–44 [in Turkish]

Lascelles BDX, Capner CA and Waterman-Pearson AE (1995) Survey of perioperative analgesic use in small animals. *Veterinary Record* **137**, 676

Lascelles BDX, Capner CA and Waterman-Pearson AE (2000) Current British veterinary attitudes to perioperative analgesia for cats and small mammals. *Veterinary Record* **145**, 601–604

Lichtenberger M and Ko J (2007) Anesthesia and analgesia for small mammals and birds. *Veterinary Clinics of North America: Exotic Animal Practice* **10**, 293–315

Lindhardt K, Bagger M, Andreasen KH and Bechgaard E (2001) Intranasal bioavailability of buprenorphine in rabbit correlated to sheep and man. *International Journal of Pharmaceutics* **217**(1-2), 121–126

Lipman NS, Marini RP and Flecknell PA (1997) Anaesthesia and analgesia in rabbits. In: *Anaesthesia and Analgesia in Laboratory Animals*, ed. DF Kohn, *et al.*, pp.205–237. Academic Press, New York

Lipman NS, Weischedel AK, Connors MJ, *et al.* (1992) Utilisation of cholestyramine resin as a preventative treatment for antibiotic (clindamycin) induced enterotoxaemia in the rabbit. *Laboratory Animals* **26**, 1–8

Lukehart SA, John MJ and Baker-Zander SA (1990) Efficacy of azithromycin for therapy of active syphilis in the rabbit model. *Journal of Antimicrobial Chemotherapy* **25** (Suppl. A), 91–99

Mackey D, Varlet A and Debeaumont D (1982) Antibiotic loaded plaster of Paris pellets: an in vitro study of a possible method of local antibiotic therapy in bone infection. *Clinical Orthopedic and Related Research* **167**, 263–268

Malmberg AB and Yaksh TL (1993) Pharmacology of the spinal action of ketorolac, morphine, ST-91, U50488H, and L-PIA on the formalin test and an isobolographic analysis of the NSAID interaction. *Anesthesiology* **79**, 270–281

Marx KL and Roston MA (1996) *The Exotic Animal Drug Compendium: An International Formulary.* Veterinary Learning Systems, Trenton, NJ

Mauk MD, Olson RD, LaHoste GJ, *et al.* (1981) Tonic immobility produces hyperalgesia and antagonizes morphine analgesia. *Science* **213**, 353–354

McClure SR, Welch RD and Johnson TL (1992) Use of an implant for intraosseous infusion as supportive therapy for a Vietnamese pot-bellied pig with urethral obstruction caused by a polyp. *Journal of the American Veterinary Medicine Association* **201**(10), 1587–1590

McKay SG, Morck DW, Merrill JK, *et al.* (1996) Use of tilmicosin for treatment of pasteurellosis in rabbits. *American Journal of Veterinary Research* **57**, 1180–1184

McMillan MW, Seymoir CJ and Brearley JC (2012) Effect of intratesticular lidocaine on isoflurane requirements in dogs undergoing routine castration. *Journal of Small Animal Practice* **53**(7), 393–397

Morissey JK and Carpenter JW (2012) Appendix: Therapeutics. In: *Ferrets, Rabbits and Rodents, 3rd edn*, ed. KE Quesenberry and JW Carpenter, pp.566–575. Elsevier, St. Louis

Nath RP, Upton RA, Everhart ET, *et al.* (1999) Buprenorphine pharmacokinetics: relative bioavailability of sublingual tablet and liquid formulations. *Journal of Clinical Pharmacology* **39**, 619–623

Ozalp GR, Caliskan C, Seyrek-Intas K and Wehrend A (2010) Effects of the progesterone receptor antagonist aglepristone on implantation administered on days 6 and 7 after mating in rabbits. *Reproduction in Domestic Animals* **45**(3), 505–508

Park BK, Lim JH, Kim MS and Yun HI (2007) Pharmacokinetics of florfenicol and its major metabolite, florfenicol amine, in rabbits. *Journal of Veterinary Pharmacology and Therapeutics* **30**(1), 32–36

Pekow C (1992) Buprenorphine Jell-O recipe for rodent analgesia. *Synapse* **25**, 35–36

Piercy MF and Schroeder LA (1980) A quantitative analgesic assay in the rabbit based on the response to tooth pulp stimulation. *Archives Internationales de Pharmacodynamie* **248**, 294–304

Plumb, DC (2011) *Plumb's Veterinary Drug Handbook, 7th edn.* PharmaVet, Wisconsin

Pollock C (2006) Therapeutics. In: *BSAVA Manual of Rabbit Medicine and Surgery, 2nd edn*, ed. A Meredith and P Flecknell, pp.144–153. BSAVA Publications, Gloucester

Portnoy LG and Hustead DR (1992) Pharmacokinetics of butorphanol tartrate in rabbits. *American Journal of Veterinary Research* **53**, 541–543

Quesenberry KE (1994) Rabbits. In: *Saunders Manual of Small Animal Practice*, ed. HJ Birchard and RG Sherding, pp.1345–1362. WB Saunders Co., Philadelphia

Quimby JM, Gustafson DL, Samber BJ, *et al.* (2011) Studies on the pharmacokinetics and pharmacodynamics of mirtazapine in healthy young cats. *Journal of Veterinary Pharmacology and Therapeutics* **34**(4), 388–396

Ramsey I (2011) *BSAVA Small Animal Formulary, 7th edn.* BSAVA Publications, Gloucester

Rateau JG, Brouillard M, Morgant G and Aymard P (1986) Experimental study in the rabbit of the effect of cholestyramine in the treatment of infectious diarrhoea caused by cholera. *Annals of Gastroenterology and Hepatology* (Paris) **22**, 289–296 [in French]

Redrobe S (2010) Rabbit therapeutics: safe, effective or deadly? *Proceedings of the North American Veterinary Conference*, 2010

Redrobe S, Gakos G, Elliott S, *et al.* (2010) Comparison of toltrazuril and sulphadimethoxine in the treatment of intestinal coccidiosis in pet rabbits. *Veterinary Record* **167**(8), 287–90

Reichert JA, Daughters RS, Rivard R, *et al.* (2001) Peripheral and preemptive opioid antinociception in a mouse visceral pain model. *Pain* **89**, 221–227

Richardson VCG (2000) The skin. In: *Rabbits: Health, Husbandry and Diseases*, pp.29–43. Wiley-Blackwell, Oxford

Rosenthal KL (2004) Therapeutic contraindications in exotic pets. *Seminars in Avian and Exotic Pet Medicine* **13**(1), 44–48

Roughan JV and Flecknell PA (2002) Buprenorphine: a reappraisal of its antinociceptive effects and therapeutic use in alleviating post-operative pain in animals. *Laboratory Animals* **36**, 322–343

Saunders R and Whitlock E (2012) Nursing hospitalized patients. In: *BSAVA Manual of Exotic Pet and Wildlife Nursing*, ed. M Varga, R Lumbis and L Gott, pp.129–166. BSAVA Publications, Gloucester

Scarff DH (2000) Dermatoses. In: *Manual of Rabbit Medicine and Surgery*, ed. PA Flecknell, pp.69–79. BSAVA Publications, Gloucester

Sharpnack DD, Mastin JP, Childress CP and Henningsen GM (1994) Quinolone arthropathy in juvenile New Zealand White rabbits. *Laboratory Animal Science* **44**, 436–442

Souza MJ, Greenacre CB and Cox SK (2008) Pharmacokinetics of orally administered tramadol in domestic rabbit (*Oryctolagus cuniculus*). *American Journal of Veterinary Research* **68**, 979–982

Suter C, Müller-Doblies UU, Hatt JM and Deplazes P (2001) Prevention and treatment of *Encephalitozoon cuniculi* infection in rabbits with fenbendazole. *Veterinary Record* **148**, 478–480

Turner PV, Chen HC and Taylor MW (2006) Pharmacokinetics of meloxicam in rabbits after single and repeat oral dosing. *Comparative Medicine* **56**, 63–67

Tyrrell KL, Citron DM, Jenkins JR and Goldstein EJC (2002) Periodontal bacteria in rabbit mandibular and maxillary abscesses. *Journal of Clinical Microbiology* **40**(3), 1044–1047

Uebelhart D, Thonar EJ, Zhang JW, *et al.* (1998) Protective effects of exogenous chondroitin 4-6-sulphate in the acute degradation of articular cartilage in the rabbit. *Osteoarthritis and Cartilage* **6**(Suppl. A), 6–13

Vachan P (1999) Self-mutilation in rabbits following intramuscular ketamine-xylazine-acepromazine injections. *Journal of the Canadian Veterinary Medical Association* **40**, 581–582

Varga M (2013) *Textbook of Rabbit Medicine, 2nd edn.* Butterworth Heinemann, Oxford

Weaver LA, Blaze CA, Linder DE *et al.* (2010) Model for clinical evaluation of perioperative analgesia in rabbits (*Oryctolagus cuniculus*). *Journal of the American Association of Laboratory Animal Science* **49**(6), 845–851

Wenger S (2012) Anesthesia and analgesia in rabbits and rodents. *Journal of Exotic Pet Medicine* **21**(1), 7–8

Wheler CL, Machin KL and Lew LJ (1996) Use of antibiotic-impregnated polymethylmethacrylate beads in the treatment of chronic osteomyelitis and cellulites in a juvenile bald eagle (*Haliaeetus leucocephalus*). In: *1996 Proceedings of the Annual Conference of the Association of Avian Veterinarians, Tampa, FL*, pp.187–194

Williams AM and Wyatt JD (2007) Comparison of subcutaneous and intramuscular ketamine-medetomidine with and without reversal by atipamezole in Dutch belted rabbits (*Oryctolagus cuniculus*). *Journal of the American Association of Laboratory Animal Science* **46**(6), 16–20

Wixson SK (1994) Anaesthesia and analgesia In: *The Biology of the Laboratory Rabbit, 2nd edn*, ed. PJ Manning *et al.*, pp.87–109. Academic Press, London

Approaches to common conditions

Anna Meredith and Brigitte Lord

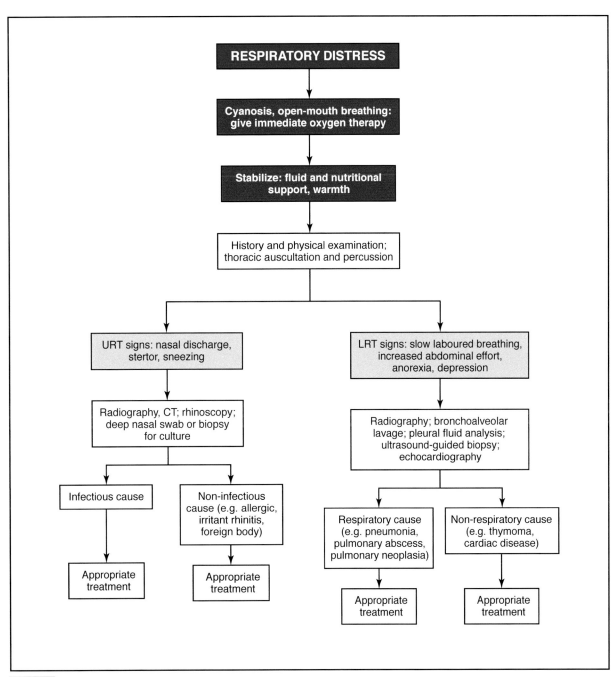

22.1 An approach to the rabbit in respiratory distress.

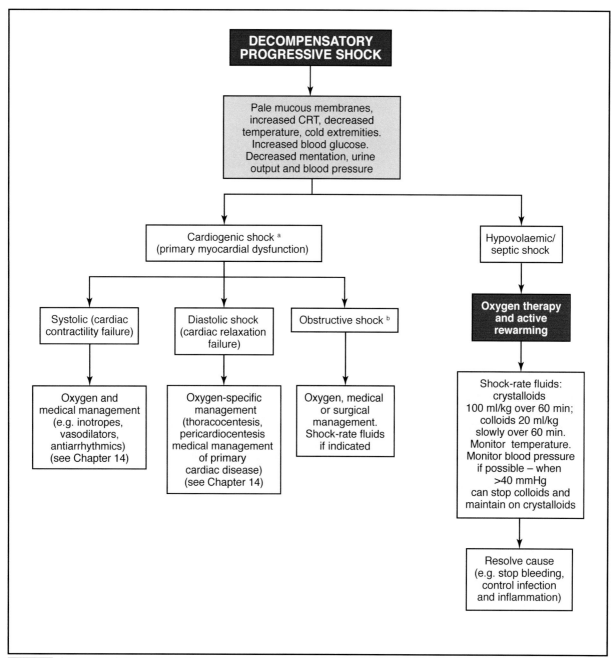

22.2 An approach to shock and/or collapse in the rabbit. Rabbits are usually presented in decompensatory/ progressive shock rather than the initial compensatory stage seen in some other species. [a] It is difficult in rabbits to distinguish cardiogenic from hypovolaemic shock, other than more rapid deterioration; unless a primary myocardial dysfunction is known (e.g. from ECG information) or strongly suspected, assume and treat as hypovolaemic shock. [b] Impedance of the circulation by an intrinsic or extrinsic obstruction, pulmonary embolism, dissecting aneurysm, and pericardial tamponade all result in obstructive shock.

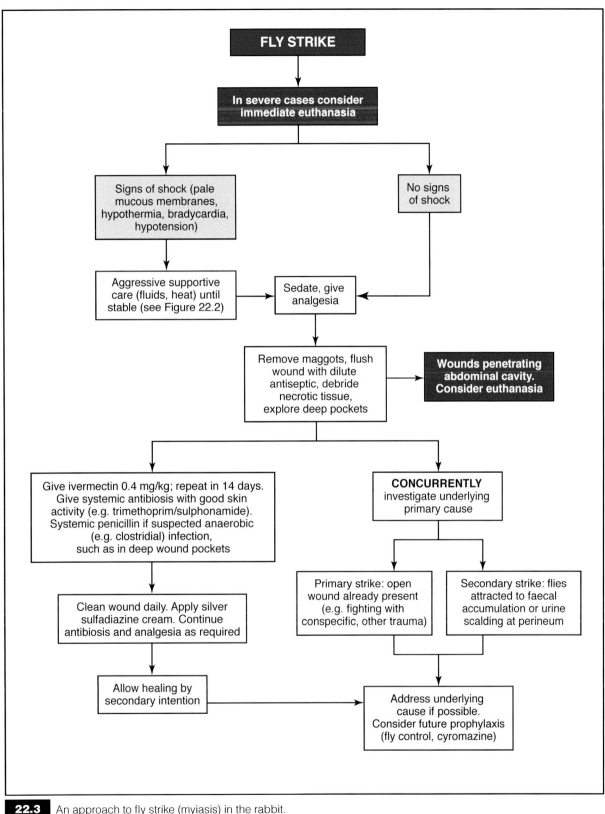

22.3 An approach to fly strike (myiasis) in the rabbit.

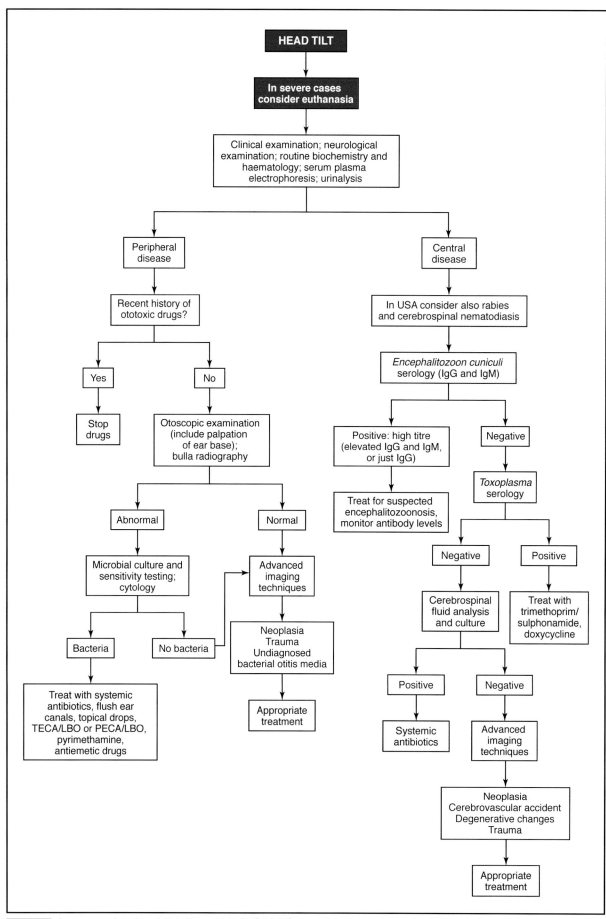

22.4 An approach to head tilt in the rabbit. PECA/LBO = partial ear canal ablation/lateral bulla osteotomy; TECA = total ear canal ablation (see *BSAVA Manual of Rabbit, Surgery, Dentistry and Imaging*)

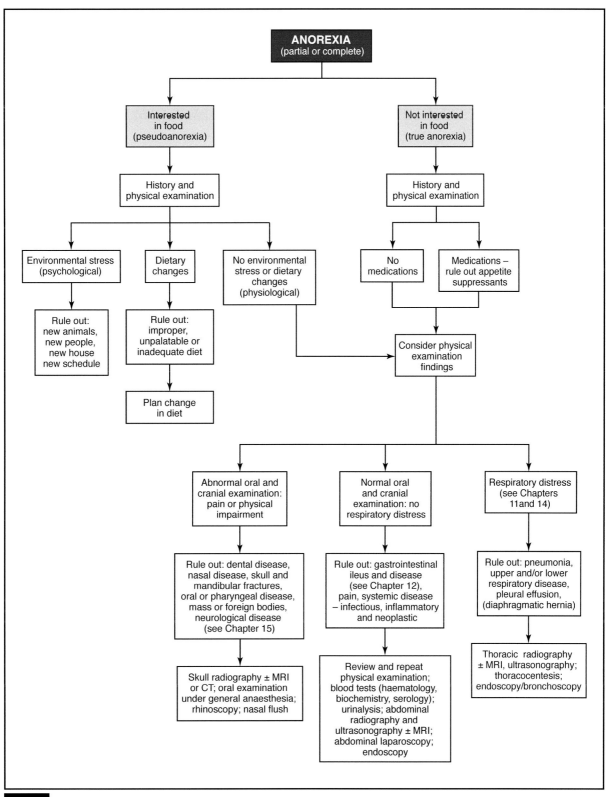

22.5 An approach to evaluating of anorexia in the rabbit. Please see Chapter 12 for further details.

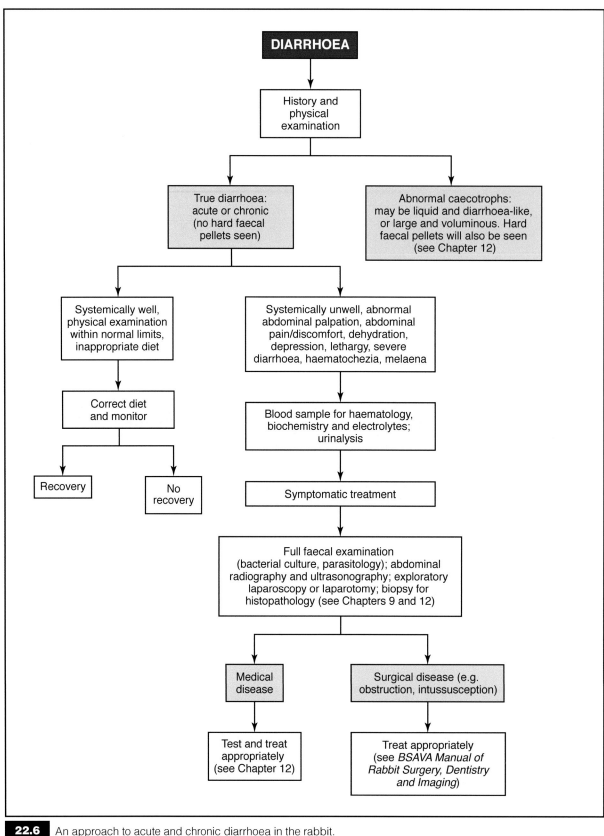

22.6   An approach to acute and chronic diarrhoea in the rabbit.

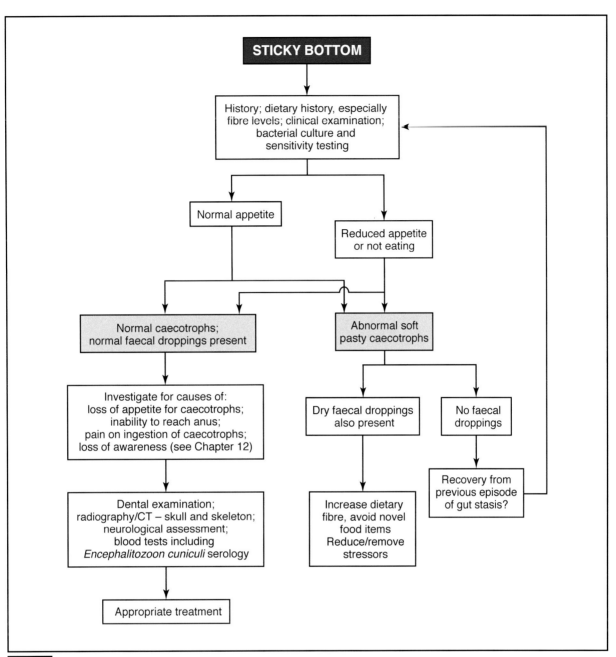

22.7 An approach to the rabbit with a 'sticky bottom'.

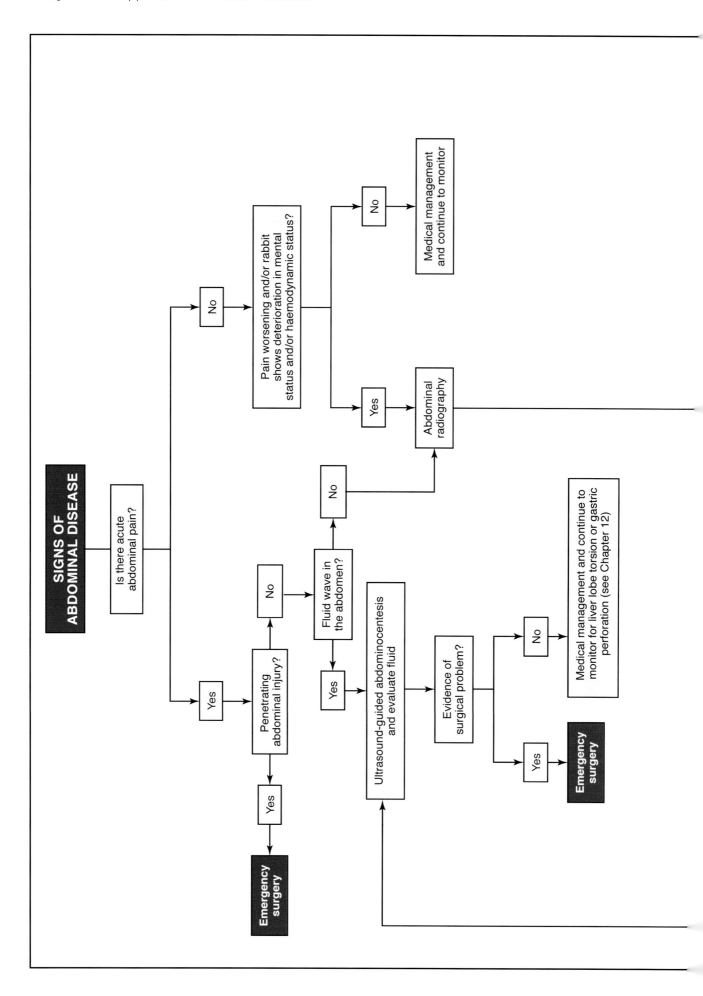

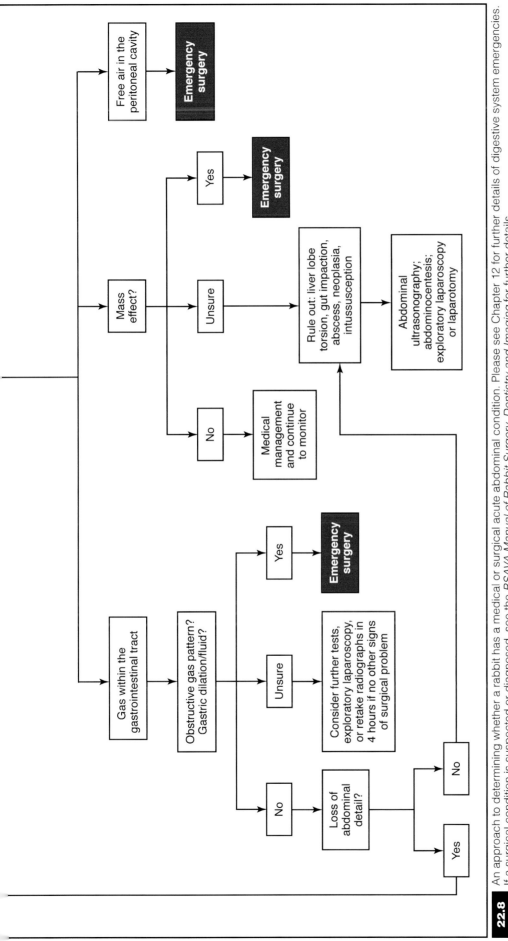

22.8 An approach to determining whether a rabbit has a medical or surgical acute abdominal condition. Please see Chapter 12 for further details of digestive system emergencies. If a surgical condition is suspected or diagnosed, see the *BSAVA Manual of Rabbit Surgery, Dentistry and Imaging* for further details.

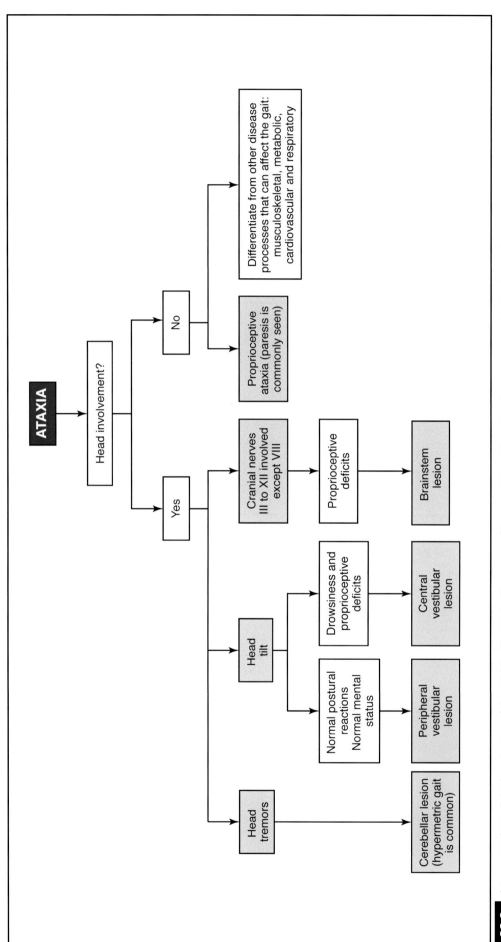

22.9 An approach to clinical evaluation of the rabbit with ataxia. Please see Chapter 15 for differential diagnoses and details of investigation.

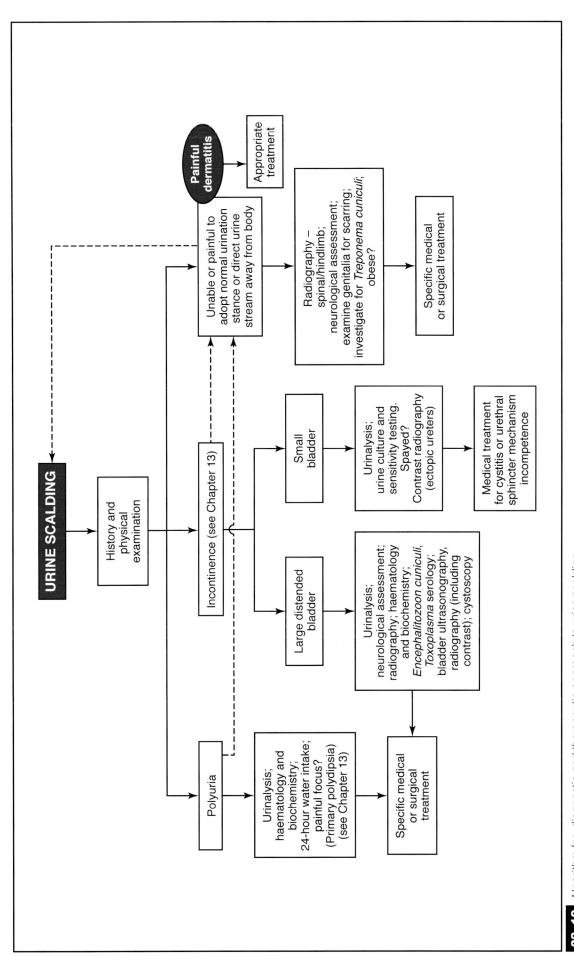

22..10 Algorithm for diagnostic and therapeutic approach to urine scalding.

Appendix 1

Common diseases of rabbits

The reader is advised to refer to the relevant chapters in this Manual for more detail.

Disease/aetiology	Clinical signs	Diagnosis	Treatment/comments
Aberrant conjunctival overgrowth Unique to rabbit. Unknown aetiology	Fold of non-adherent conjunctival tissue arising from limbus and covering variable area of cornea	Clinical signs	Surgical removal results in recurrence. Suturing fold to sclera allows vision
Abscess *Pasteurella multocida*, *Staphylococcus aureus*, *Pseudomonas*, *Proteus*, *Streptococcus*, *Corynebacterium*, *Bacteroides* and other anaerobes. Local entry, e.g. wound or haematogenous spread	Subcutaneous or facial swelling, draining tracts May be dull, anorexic, pyrexic if bacteraemic. Also dyspnoea (pulmonary abscess), neurological signs (cerebral/spinal abscess)	Aspirate, bacterial culture (aerobic and anaerobic), abscess wall is best material for culture; complete blood count (CBC) and biochemistry; radiography, ultrasonography	Surgical removal is treatment of choice. If dental involvement, removal of associated teeth and debridement of bone plus various options, e.g. doxycycline gel, antibiotic-impregnated PMMA beads, sodium hydroxyapatite plus antibiotic, or marsupialization and flushing. If unable to remove surgically, systemic antibiosis: injection of gentamicin into capsule (0.5–1 ml per rabbit empirically)
Accumulation of caecotrophs Excess production {low-fibre, high-protein and high-carbohydrate diet) or reduced ingestion due to overfeeding, altered palatability (e.g. with high-protein diet) or physical problems, such as obesity, spinal pain, dental pain	Caking of caecotrophs around perineum, secondary myiasis (fly strike)	Clinical signs	Address underlying cause. Dietary reform to high-fibre, low- or no-concentrate diet. May take several months on hay alone to resolve
Allergic/irritant rhinitis/bronchitis Environmental allergens or irritants	Sneezing, dyspnoea, nasal discharge	Exclusion of other causes of upper respiratory tract (URT) signs; response to elimination of suspected allergen; response to antihistamines/corticosteroids	Avoidance of allergen. Antihistamines. Corticosteroids (use with extreme care, as highly immunosuppressive; do not use if concurrent *Pasteurella* or other bacterial infection)
Antibiotic toxicity/enterotoxaemia Reported with all antibiotics except fluoroquinolones and potentiated sulphonamides, especially ampicillin, amoxicillin, clindamycin, lincomycin, cephalosporins and erythromycin. Will only occur if clostridia already present in GI tract	Diarrhoea (brown, watery, foetid, bloody), depression, dehydration, hypothermia, abdominal distension, collapse, death	History of antibiotic usage; faecal culture and toxin isloation (rarely performed)	Fluid therapy (intravenous/intraosseous). Colestyramine, ranitidine, metoclopramide, cisapride, metronidazole. High-fibre diet (assisted feeding), probiotics
Bacterial dermatitis (see also pododermatitis) Usually *Staphylococcus aureus* but also other bacteria. Primary bacterial dermatitis rare	Alopecia, erythema, ulceration, pruritus	Bacterial culture	Antibiosis (topical/systemic). Address underlying cause
Bacterial enteritis *Escherichia coli*, *Salmonella*, Tyzzer's disease (*Clostridium piliforme*). High morbidity and mortality in young rabbits	Diarrhoea, depression, weight loss, hypothermia, abdominal distension, collapse, death	Faecal culture; post-mortem examination; histopathology for Tyzzer's disease	Fluid therapy. Appropriate antibiosis, metoclopramide, cisapride, ranitidine. High-fibre diet, probiotics

▶

Disease/aetiology	Clinical signs	Diagnosis	Treatment/comments
'Blue fur' disease Secondary *Pseudomonas aeruginosa* infection of moist skin/fur	Moist dermatitis, blue coloration of fur in moist areas – dewlap, skin folds	Blue coloration pathognomonic; culture of *Pseudomonas aeruginosa*	Clip fur, keep dry. Topical antiseptic. Systemic antibiotics may be required. Address underlying cause
Clostridial overgrowth (see Antibiotic toxicity)			
Coccidiosis *Eimeria* spp., *Eimeria stiedae* (hepatic coccidiosis). Can cause high morbidity and mortality in young rabbits	Diarrhoea, weight loss, anorexia, jaundice, dehydration, ascites, death	Faecal oocysts; post-mortem examination	Sulphonamide drugs, toltrazuril, amprolium, robenidine. Disinfection, good hygiene
Conjunctivitis Bacterial, e.g. *Pasteurella multocida*. Also irritants, e.g. ammonia, dust	Photophobia, blepharospasm, chemosis	Bacterial culture	Topical and subconjunctival antibiosis. Topical corticosteroids if irritant and no corneal ulceration
Cystitis Primary or secondary bacterial infection. Hypercalciuria/urolithiasis may predispose	Urinary incontinence, urine scald, dysuria, haematuria	Urinalysis, culture and cytology; radiography	Antibiosis. Analgesia. Fluid therapy. Reduce calcium content of diet. Potassium citrate
Dacryocystitis Bacterial infection of nasolacrimal duct: *Pasteurella multocida*, *Staphylococcus aureus* and other bacteria	Lacrimation, purulent ocular discharge	Bacterial culture	Flushing of nasolacrimal ducts until clear – may be required over several days. Topical antibiotic instillation. Investigate for underlying incisor and premolar tooth root elongation
Dental disease/malocclusion Primary congenital incisor malocclusion – mandibular prognathism (esp. dwarf breeds); acquired dental disease; cheek teeth malocclusion and overgrowth can lead to secondary incisor malocclusion	Weight loss, ptyalism, dehydration, lack of grooming, lack of caecotrophy, facial/retrobulbar abscesses, ocular discharge, dacryocystitis, incisor wear abnormalities, palpable swellings on ventral border of mandible, ulceration (oral mucosa, tongue, cheek, palate, lip), deep laceration to tongue or cheek, spikes on the edges of cheek teeth occlusal surfaces, pain on palpation of maxillary zygomatic process or mandibular manipulation, food impaction between or around the cheek teeth, missing teeth	Dental examination; skull radiography	Burr sharp edges/spikes, burr crowns to correct form and height. Tooth removal: incisor extraction if primary malocclusion or uncorrectable secondary malocclusion. Antibiosis. Analgesia – may be required long term; oral meloxicam recommended. Euthanasia if severe disease
Dermatophytosis *Trichophyton mentagrophytes* (usually), *Microsporum* (rare)	Alopecia, scaling, crusting, with or without pruritus	Fungal culture	Clip surrounding hair. Topical antifungal agents, e.g. miconazole, clotrimazole, enilconazole for small areas; systemic griseofulvin for widespread lesions; systemic itraconazole
Dysautonomia Cause and incidence unknown. Degeneration of autonomic ganglia leading to GI tract stasis; similar to equine grass sickness	Mucoid diarrhoea, GI tract stasis, caecal impaction, dehydration, anorexia, weight loss, abdominal pain, abdominal distension, death	Histology of mesenteric autonomic ganglia	Fluid therapy. Metoclopramide, cisapride, ranitidine. Analgesia. High-fibre diet. Treatment usually ineffective
Ear mites *Psoroptes cuniculi* (non-burrowing); 3-week life cycle on host	Pruritus, head-shaking, self-trauma, thick crusts in external ear canal, lesions can spread to face and neck	Identification of mite	Ivermectin, moxidectin. Acaricidal ear drops for mild infections. Soften and remove debris – take care not to damage ear canal. Analgesia in severe cases
Encephalitozoonosis *Encephalitozoon cuniculi*, an intracellular microsporidian parasite. Target organs kidney and CNS. Spores shed in urine and ingested or inhaled. Very common, infection often asymptomatic but can cause neurological signs and renal disease. Antibodies not protective	Ataxia, torticollis, posterior paresis/paralysis, 'floppy rabbit syndrome', urinary incontinence, tremors, convulsions, chronic weight loss and polyuria/polydipsia	Clinical signs; serology; post-mortem examination	Fenbendazole. Short-acting steroids if severe neurological signs. Supportive care. Cleaning and disinfection of environment – quaternary ammonium compounds inactivate spores

▶

Disease/aetiology	Clinical signs	Diagnosis	Treatment/comments
Endometrial hyperplasia Common in unmated does. A continuum of aging changes from hyperplasia to adenocarcinoma occurs	Haematuria, bloody vaginal discharge, palpably enlarged uterus	Radiography, ultrasonography; exploratory surgery; histology	Ovariohysterectomy
Endometrial venous aneurysm RARE	Haematuria, blood from vulva	Exclusion of other causes of haematuria; ultrasonography; examination of removed uterus	Blood transfusion if severe haemorrhage. Ovariohysterectomy
Entropion Genetic factors	Keratoconjunctivitis, corneal ulceration	Ocular examination	Corrective surgery
Eosinophilic granuloma Usually secondary to parasitic or other skin disease	Skin ulceration, self-trauma, moist dermatitis	Direct smear; histology of skin biopsy	Address underlying cause. Corticosteroids
Fleas Rabbit flea (*Spillopsylla cuniculi*) important vector for myxomatosis. *Cediopsylla simples* and *Odontopsyllus multispinosus* in USA. Also cat flea (*Ctenocephalides felis*)	Often none, pruritus	Identification of flea or flea faeces	Imidacloprid (authorized in UK), lufenuron, feline/canine pyrethrum products. Avoid fipronil spray – adverse reactions reported. For cat flea, if cat/dog and environment are treated rarely need to treat rabbit
Fur mites *Cheyletiella parasitivorax*: 5-week life cycle on host but can survive off host; ZOONOSIS. *Listrophorus gibbus* not pathogenic or zoonotic; *Demodex cuniculi* rarely reported	Alopecia, scaling, crusting, minimal/no pruritus	Identification of mite	Ivermectin. Treat all in-contacts and environment (can use feline/canine environmental flea products)
Glaucoma/ buphthalmia Inherited in New Zealand White, recessive *bu* gene	Enlarged globe, corneal opacity, non-painful	Clinical signs; tonometry	No treatment
Leptospirosis *Leptospira* spp.: ZOONOSIS. Rabbits can acquire disease via contact with wild rodent hosts	Polyuria, polydipsia, depression, anorexia, renal failure	Serology	Penicillin (not oral) – care, enterotoxaemia. Fluid therapy
Lice *Haemodipsus ventricosis*	Pruritus, anaemia	Identification of louse/ eggs	Feline/canine louse powders or ectoparasite shampoos
Listeriosis RARE *Listeria monocytogenes*: causes a meningoencephalitis	Head tilt/torticollis	Cerebrospinal fluid (CSF) culture; post-mortem examination	Penicillin, tetracycline. (Rarely effective)
Liver lobe torsion	Acute abdominal pain, gut stasis, depression, shock	Anaemia; increased liver enzymes (ALT, ALP, GGT) and CK; ultrasonography, radiography	Stabilize (fluid therapy, analgesia, warmth). Emergency laparotomy, liver lobectomy
Mastitis Bacterial infection of mammary glands in lactation or pseudopregnant does: often *Pasteurella multocida*, *Staphylococcus aureus*, streptococci. Also aseptic cystic mastitis in intact does >3 years	Depression, pyrexia, anorexia, polydipsia, swollen painful abcessated mammary glands, septicaemia, death, non-painful, may exude brown fluid	Clinical signs; bacterial culture; clinical signs; biopsy	Antibiosis. Supportive care. Analgesia. Drainage of abscesses. Surgical excision for severe infections. Wean young. Benign condition. Ovariohysterectomy will resolve
Myiasis (fly strike) Primary or secondary myiasis occurs rapidly in warm weather. Flies usually attracted to accumulated caecotrophs in perineal area, due to dental disease, obesity, spinal disease or any cause of debilitation	Depression, collapse, death	Presence of fly larvae	Fluid therapy and supportive care. Sedate rabbit and remove maggots; clip fur; flush wounds with antiseptic solution. Systemic antibiosis. Ivermectin. Address underlying cause. Fly control for outdoor rabbits. Prevention with cyromazine (Rearguard)

▶

Disease/aetiology	Clinical signs	Diagnosis	Treatment/comments
Myxomatosis Poxvirus spread by the rabbit flea or other biting insects	Facial and genital oedema/swelling, blepharitis, conjunctivitis, ocular and nasal discharge, pyrexia, subcutaneous masses, nasal scabbing only in some cases, depression, death	Clinical signs	Supportive care in mild cases. Euthanasia. Prevention by vaccination
Otitis externa *Psoroptes cuniculi* (see Ear mites)			
Otitis media/interna Usually ascending bacterial infection via eustachian tube from nasopharynx (*Pasteurella multocida* common)	Head tilt/torticollis	Skull radiography, CT; bacterial culture	Antibiosis. Bulla osteotomy
Pasteurellosis *Pasteurella multocida*: common inhabitant of nasal cavity and tympanic bullae; overt disease usually follows injury or stressor, e.g. overcrowding, intercurrent disease. Spread by direct and venereal contact, aerosol (slow), fomites, vertical/perinatal	Nasal discharge, sneezing, conjunctivitis, dacryocystitis, bronchopneumonia, head tilt/torticollis, abscesses, pyometra, mastitis, orchitis, epididymitis, depression, anorexia, pyrexia, death	Bacterial isolation (serology); radiography (turbinate atrophy, pneumonia, pulmonary abscesses)	Antibiosis. Fluid therapy and supportive care. Nebulization with mucolytics (e.g. bromhexine, *N*-acetylcysteine, hyaluronidase) to break up nasal secretions. See treatment for abscesses, pyometra, mastitis, metritis, orchitis, epididymitis
Pinworm *Passalurus ambiguus*: usually non-pathogenic even in large numbers	Usually none. Can be seen within gut during abdominal surgery	Identification of adult worm/ova in faeces or cellophane tape test for ova from perineum	Fenbendazole 10–20 mg/kg orally, repeated offer 14 days
Pododermatitis Bacterial infection (often *Staphylococcus aureus*, streptococci) secondary to poor husbandry (wet soiled bedding), obesity, inactivity, genetic factors (Rex rabbits lack guard hairs on plantar surface)	Alopecia, erythema, skin thickening, lameness, ulceration, abscessation, osteomyelitis	Clinical signs; bacterial culture	Antibiosis – topical and systemic. Analgesia/NSAIDs. Bandaging. Surgical debridement if severe. Improve husbandry. Weight reduction
Pregnancy toxaemia/hepatic lipidosis Affects pregnant, postpartum and pseudopregnant does or obese rabbits if for any reason anorexia occurs	Depression, incoordination, collapse, dyspnoea, convulsions, coma, death	Clinical signs: ketonuria, proteinuria, aciduria	Intravenous lactated Ringer's solution and 5% glucose. Corticosteroids. Assisted feeding
Rabbit haemorrhagic disease Calicivirus: spread by direct or indirect contact (fomites)	Usually sudden death, pyrexia, depression, haemorrhagic discharge from nose and mouth	Post-mortem examination	No treatment. Prevention by vaccination
Rabbit syphilis/venereal spirochaetosis *Treponema paraluis cuniculi*: direct contact/venereal spread; kits can be infected at birth. Symptomless carrier state	Ulcerative crusting lesions around genitalia and on face and legs from autoinocculation; secondary bacterial infection and eosinophilic granuloma formation can occur	Detection of organism in direct smear (dark field background) or biopsy sample (silver stain)	Penicillin (not oral) – care, enterotoxaemia
Splay leg Inherited disease, several genes involved. 1 to 4 legs affected. Subluxation of hip in some cases	One or more legs held adducted	Clinical signs; radiography	No treatment
Spondylosis/ spondylitis Ankylosis/osteomyelitis of a vertebral joint. Degenerative change, infection, usually by haematogenous spread, e.g. *Pasteurella*	Reluctance to move, paresis, lack of caecotrophy	Radiography, CT	NSAIDs. Antibiosis
Toxoplasmosis RARE *Toxoplasma gondii*	Ataxia, tremors, paresis/paralysis	Serology	Trimethoprim/sulphonamide. Avoid clindamycin (enterotoxaemia). Prevent contact with cat faeces

▶

Disease/aetiology	Clinical signs	Diagnosis	Treatment/comments
Tyzzer's disease *Clostridium piliforme*: can cause high morbidity and mortality in young rabbits	Watery diarrhoea, depression, death, chronic weight loss (older rabbits)	Post-mortem examination	Poor response to antibiosis: treatment only palliative once clinical signs observed – try supportive care and tetracyclines. Prevention by good husbandry. 0.3% sodium hypochlorite kills spores
Urolithiasis/hypercalciuria Associated with obesity, inactivity, low water intake, neurological bladder disease and high calcium intake	Haematuria, dysuria, abdominal pain	Radiography, ultrasonography; cystoscopy; urinalysis	Bladder lavage. Cystotomy and urolith removal. Antibiosis. Lower dietary calcium content. Not possible to acidify urine. Oral potassium citrate may be beneficial. Weight loss and increased exercise
Uterine adenocarcinoma Extremely common in older unmated does. Progressive uterine changes from hyperplasia to adenocarcinoma. Rapidly metastasizes locally and to lungs	Haematuria, vulval discharge, weight loss	Abdominal palpation; radiography; exploratory surgery	Ovariohysterectomy. Always radiograph thorax for pulmonary metastases
Viral enteritis Rotavirus. Coronavirus (RARE)	Diarrhoea, depression, anorexia, death. High morbidity/mortality in young rabbits	Viral isolation	No treatment

Differential diagnoses based on clinical signs

The differentials listed are not comprehensive. The reader is advised to refer to the relevant chapters in this Manual for more detail.

Clinical sign	Differential diagnoses	Further investigations
Abdominal distension	Ileus and gaseous distension of bowel Gastric dilation (fluid/gas) Ascites (see below) Abdominal mass (see below) Pregnancy Obesity	Radiography, contrast studies; ultrasonography; peritoneal tap; exploratory surgery
Abdominal mass	Dehydrated stomach contents (gastric stasis) Foreign body (esp. at sacculus rotundus) Impaction (usually caecal – right hemiabdomen) Neoplasia Uterine hyperplasia Pyometra Metritis Hydrometra Abdominal fat Fetus/es	Radiography, contrast studies; ultrasonography; exploratory surgery
Alopecia	*Cheyletiella*, *Listrophorus* (RARE) Barbering Normal moult Dermatophytosis	Cellophane tape test; skin scrape; microscopic examination of hair; fungal culture
Anaemia	Renal disease Any chronic disease Uterine hyperplasia/adenocarcinoma Uterine venous aneurysm Lead toxicity	Complete blood count (CBC) and blood biochemistry; serum lead levels; radiography; ultrasonography; exploratory surgery
Anorexia	Dental disease Any systemic disease, especially gastrointestinal Pain Any stressor	CBC and blood biochemistry; dental examination; radiography – skull and body; ultrasonography; CT
Ascites	Abdominal neoplasia Hepatic coccidiosis Liver disease Cardiac disease Pleural effusion disease (coronavirus – RARE)	CBC and blood biochemistry; peritoneal tap; radiography; ultrasonography; liver biopsy; faecal analysis (coccidia); virology
Dermatitis	Ectoparasites Bacterial dermatitis (usually *Staphylococcus aureus*, and secondary. Also 'blue fur' disease – *Pseudomonas aeruginosa*) Eosinophilic granuloma Dermatophytosis Self-trauma Venereal spirochaetosis (*Treponema paraluis cuniculi*) Urine scald Viral infection (pox, herpes, myxomatosis – nose) Injection site reaction Sebaceous adenitis	Cellophane tape test; skin scrape; bacterial culture; fungal culture; skin biopsy; investigate urinary tract disease (see below)

▶

Clinical sign	Differential diagnoses	Further investigations
Diarrhoea	Bacterial enteritis (*Escherichia coli*, *Salmonella*, Tyzzer's disease) Viral enteritis (rotavirus – young rabbits, coronavirus – RARE) Coccidiosis (young rabbits) Clostridial enterotoxaemia – antibiotic toxicity, stress Low-fibre, high-carbohydrate diet Gastric stasis/ileus Dysautonomia	Dietary history; faecal analysis – culture, parasitology; radiography/contrast studies; post-mortem examination
Dyspnoea/collapse	Any respiratory disease (see below) Cardiac disease Intrathoracic mass (e.g. thymoma, lymphoma) Pregnancy toxaemia/hepatic lipidosis Severe pain	Radiography; echocardiography; electrocardiography; urinalysis (ketones); CBC and blood biochemistry
Facial swelling	Myxomatosis Facial/dental abscess Cellulitis Neoplasia	Vaccination/contact history; skull radiography; dental examination; CT
Haematuria	False haematuria – red/brown porphyrin pigments in urine Cystitis Urolithiasis/hypercalciuria Uterine hyperplasia Uterine adenocarcinoma Uterine venous aneurysm Bladder polyps Renal infarcts Disseminated intravascular coagulation (DIC)	Urinalysis – dipstick, culture, cytology; CBC and biochemistry; radiography/contrast studies; ultrasonography
Lower respiratory signs	Bacterial pneumonia (esp. pasteurellosis) Pulmonary abscess Pleural effusion disease (coronavirus – RARE) Pulmonary neoplasia (esp. metastases from uterine adenocarcinoma) Thymoma Cardiac disease	Radiography; pleural fluid analysis; bronchoalveolar lavage; ultrasound-guided biopsy; echocardiography
Neurological signs	Encephalitozoonosis Otitis media/interna Heat stroke Trauma Toxoplasmosis Listeriosis Epilepsy (RARE) Pregnancy toxaemia Splay leg Hypovitaminosis A, E (RARE)	Radiography (skull, spine); CBC and blood biochemistry; serology (*Encephalitozoon cuniculi*, *Toxoplasma*); CT; CSF analysis
Paresis/paralysis	Spinal trauma (fracture/luxation) Spondylosis/spondylitis Spinal abscess Intervertebral disc disease Encephalitozoonosis Toxoplasmosis	Spinal radiography; serology; CT
Subcutaneous mass	Abscess Lipoma Other neoplasia Myxomatosis – typical or atypical (vaccinated rabbit) Injection reaction Coenurus/cysticercus cyst	Fine-needle aspirate; biopsy; vaccination/contact history
Testicular swelling	Orchitis Epididymitis Myxomatosis Venereal spirochaetosis Testicular neoplasia	Fine-needle aspirate; bacterial culture; histology

▶

Clinical sign	Differential diagnoses	Further investigations
Torticollis	Encephalitozoonosis Otitis media/interna Meningitis Listeriosis Toxoplasmosis Cerebral abscess Hypovitaminosis A (RARE)	Aural examination; skull radiography; CT; MRI; bacterial culture; serology (*Encephalitozoon cuniculi*, *Toxoplasma*); CBC and blood biochemistry
Upper respiratory signs	Pasteurellosis Other bacterial upper respiratory tract disease, e.g. *Staphylococcus aureus* *Bordetella bronchiseptica* High environmental ammonia levels Myxomatosis Allergic/irritant rhinitis	Bacterial culture; skull radiography; CT; environmental history
Urinary incontinence/ urine scald	Cystitis Urolithiasis/hypercalciuria Posterior paralysis/paresis (see above) Encephalitozoonosis Obesity Renal failure Hormone-responsive incontinence (spayed does) Ectopic ureter (RARE)	Urinalysis; radiography; CT; serology (*Encephalitozoon cuniculi*, *Leptospira*); CBC and blood biochemistry; response to stilbestrol
Vaginal discharge	Pyometra Metritis Uterine hyperplasia/adenocarcinoma Dystocia	Culture and cytology of discharge; radiography; ultrasonography; exploratory surgery
Weight loss	Dental disease Any infectious or metabolic disease Neoplasia Bullying	Dental examination; radiography; ultrasonography; CT; CBC and biochemistry; appropriate serology; faecal sample

Appendix 3

Dorsal immobility response in rabbits

Sally Everitt

Rabbits, along with many other prey species, may display fight, flight or freeze behaviour when they perceive a threat. It is thought that the freeze response is intended to deceive a predator into thinking that the animal is already dead and is believed to be an adaptive response to limit injury and allow the possibility of escape. This response has been described as a 'death feint', 'playing dead' or 'playing possum'.

A similar response may also be produced in the restraint of rabbits, most often by holding a rabbit in dorsal recumbency, with the head slightly below the body and stroking the abdomen until the rabbit is completely relaxed. In this condition the rabbit becomes immobile and does not appear to respond to mild noxious stimuli.

There has been some research into the physiological changes that take place in this condition; most studies are small and have produced varied and even contradictory results. Although animals in this state may at the time show bradycardia, reduced blood pressure and apparent lack of response to noxious stimuli, they may also show tachycardia and raised cortisol following the procedure, indicating that this is not a stress-free state.

This state has been variously described as 'hypnosis', 'trance', 'thanatosis' (playing dead) and 'tonic immobility', although all of these terms have problems in that they may suggest similarities with other physical or psychological states which cannot be substantiated. It may therefore be better to adopt a neutral descriptive term, e.g. dorsal immobility response.

There does seem to be variation between rabbits in the ease with which the dorsal immobility response can be induced and there may also be differences dependent on the experience of the handler and circumstances in which the animal is being handled. While the rabbit may remain in this state for some time it should also be remembered that they can come out of this state and 'take flight' very suddenly.

Veterinary surgeons sometimes use the dorsal immobility response to enable the rabbit to be examined or for minor, non-invasive procedures to be carried out. A document produced by the RSPCA and UFAW (*Refining rabbit care – A resource for those working with rabbits in research*; available at www.rspca.org) has advised that it is not acceptable to rely on the immobility response alone to 'facilitate any type of procedure that would normally require sedation, anaesthesia or analgesia'.

Whether it is appropriate to rely on the dorsal immobility response for radiography will depend on a number of factors, including the experience of the handler in using this technique, the positioning required, and the ability to ensure that the rabbit will not be injured if it regains mobility.

Index

Index

Index